Chronic Kidney Disease: Latest Findings

Chronic Kidney Disease: Latest Findings

Editor: Dakota Beckett

FOSTER ACADEMICS
www.fosteracademics.com

www.fosteracademics.com

FOSTER ACADEMICS

Cataloging-in-Publication Data

Chronic kidney disease : latest findings / edited by Dakota Beckett.
p. cm.
Includes bibliographical references and index.
ISBN 978-1-63242-706-9
1. Kidneys--Diseases. 2. Chronic diseases. 3. Nephrology. I. Beckett, Dakota.
RC902 .C47 2019
616.61--dc23

Foster Academics,
118-35 Queens Blvd., Suite 400,
Forest Hills, NY 11375, USA

ISBN 978-1-63242-706-9 (Hardback)

Printed and bound in China.

Contents

Preface

This book was inspired by the evolution of our times; to answer the curiosity of inquisitive minds. Many developments have occurred across the globe in the recent past which has transformed the progress in the field.

The form of kidney disease which results in the gradual loss of kidney function over a period of time is known as chronic kidney disease. It is commonly caused by high blood pressure, glomerulonephritis, diabetes and polycystic kidney disease. Fatigue, loss of appetite, swelling of the legs, etc. are some of the symptoms of this disease. Chronic kidney disease can result in an increased risk of cardiovascular disease. Renal replacement and hemodialysis are the most common treatment methods for this disease. Different approaches and evaluations and advanced studies on chronic kidney disease have been included in this book. Clinicians, nephrologists and students in the field of nephrology will find this book full of crucial and unexplored information.

This book was developed from a mere concept to drafts to chapters and finally compiled together as a complete text to benefit the readers across all nations. To ensure the quality of the content we instilled two significant steps in our procedure. The first was to appoint an editorial team that would verify the data and statistics provided in the book and also select the most appropriate and valuable contributions from the plentiful contributions we received from authors worldwide. The next step was to appoint an expert of the topic as the Editor-in-Chief, who would head the project and finally make the necessary amendments and modifications to make the text reader-friendly. I was then commissioned to examine all the material to present the topics in the most comprehensible and productive format.

I would like to take this opportunity to thank all the contributing authors who were supportive enough to contribute their time and knowledge to this project. I also wish to convey my regards to my family who have been extremely supportive during the entire project.

Editor

Early Nephrology Referral Reduces the Economic Costs among Patients Who Start Renal Replacement Therapy: A Prospective Cohort Study in Korea

Jeonghwan Lee[1,2], Jung Pyo Lee[2,3], Ji In Park[2,4], Jin Ho Hwang[2,5], Hye Min Jang[2,6], Ji-Young Choi[2,7], Yong-Lim Kim[2,7], Chul Woo Yang[2,8], Shin-Wook Kang[2,9], Nam-Ho Kim[2,10], Yon Su Kim[2,4], Chun Soo Lim[2,3,4]*, CRC for ESRD investigators[2]

1 Department of Internal Medicine, Hallym University Hangang Sacred Heart Hospital, Seoul, Korea, **2** Clinical Research Center for End Stage Renal Disease (CRC for ESRD), Daegu, Korea, **3** Department of Internal Medicine, Seoul National University Boramae Medical Center, Seoul, Korea, **4** Department of Internal Medicine, Seoul National University College of Medicine, Seoul, Korea, **5** Department of Internal Medicine, Chung-Ang University Hospital, Seoul, Korea, **6** Department of Statistics, Kyungpook National University, Daegu, Korea, **7** Department of Internal Medicine, Kyungpook National University School of Medicine, Daegu, Korea, **8** Department of Internal Medicine, The Catholic University of Korea College of Medicine, Seoul, Korea, **9** Department of Internal Medicine, Yonsei University College of Medicine, Seoul, Korea, **10** Department of Internal Medicine, Chonnam National University Medical School, Gwangju, Korea

Abstract

Background: The nature of cost-saving effects of early referral to a nephrologist in patients with chronic kidney disease (CKD) is not fully evaluated. We evaluated the health care costs before and after dialysis according to the referral time.

Methods: A total of 879 patients who were newly diagnosed as having end-stage renal disease from August 2008 to June 2011 were prospectively enrolled. The early referral (ER) group was defined as patients who were referred to a nephrologist more than a year before dialysis and had visited a nephrology clinic 2 or more times. Patients whose referral time was less than a year were considered the late referral (LR) group. Information about medical costs was acquired from the claim data of the Korea Health Insurance Review and Assessment Service.

Results: The total medical costs during the first 12 months after the initiation of dialysis were not different between the 526 ER patients and the 353 LR patients. However, the costs of the ER patients during the first month were significantly lower than those of the LR patients (ER vs. LR: 3029±2219 vs. 3438±2821 US dollars [USD], P = 0.025). The total 12-month health care costs before the initiation of dialysis were significantly lower in the ER group (ER vs. LR: 6206±5873 vs. 8610±7820 USD, P<0.001). In the multivariate analysis, ER significantly lowered the health care costs during the 12 months before (2534.0±436.2 USD, P<0.001) and the first month (428.5±172.3 USD, P = 0.013) after the initiation of dialysis.

Conclusions: The ER of patients with CKD to a nephrologist is associated with decreased medical costs during the pretreatment period of renal replacement therapy and the early period of dialysis initiation.

Editor: Leighton R. James, University of Florida, United States of America

Funding: This study was supported by a grant of the Korea Healthcare technology R&D Project, Ministry of Health and Welfare, Republic of Korea. (HI10C2020). The funders had no role in study design, data collection and analysis, decision to publish, or preparation of the manuscript.

Competing Interests: The authors have declared that no competing interests exist.

* Email: cslimjy@snu.ac.kr

Introduction

Chronic kidney disease (CKD) is a major public health problem that is continually growing worldwide. The overall prevalence of CKD around the world is 10–16% [1–3]. In the United States, the prevalence estimate for CKD rose from 12.3% to 14.0% over the past 20 years [4]. Kidney function progressively declines in a proportion of CKD patients without adequate therapy, eventually progressing to devastating end-stage renal disease (ESRD) [5]. In accordance with the increasing prevalence of CKD, the prevalence of ESRD has also increased. The total treated ESRD population in the United States rose from 450,000 in 2004 to 593,086 in 2010 [4]. In Korea, the overall number of ESRD patients was 56,396, and the prevalence was 738.3 per million population, at the end of 2009 [6]. The prevalence increased by approximately 12% during the period 2000–2009.

Along with the increase in ESRD prevalence, the economic costs resulting from the care of these patients have increased. In the United States, the annual medical cost of dialysis patients borne by the Centers for Medicare and Medicaid in 2008 was 26.8 billion USD, which was 5.9% of the total costs of the entire population, and the annual increase rate reached 13.2% [7]. Among patients starting dialysis, the proportion of elderly patients and those with diabetes have increased compared with the past [8], and thus the economic burden of patients on dialysis is serious.

Therefore, proper management or intervention of CKD patients is required to improve clinical outcomes and reduce medical costs.

The late referral (LR) of patients to a nephrologist in the course of CKD progression has increased the morbidity and mortality [9–19]. The timely referral of CKD patients to a nephrologist is associated with a higher quality of care before the start of renal replacement therapy [20–26] and with improved outcomes after the initiation of dialysis [27–31]. The increased morbidity of patients referred late to a nephrologist is likely to result in a greater usage of health care resources. Our previous investigation revealed that timely referral (1 year before dialysis) to a nephrologist integrated with education about dialysis was associated with reduced usage of temporary vascular catheters and improved survival [32]. Although early referral (ER) has been suggested to produce cost savings in addition to the health benefits for the patient, there are few reports that have directly analyzed the effects of referral time on medical costs before and after the start of dialysis. To evaluate the economic benefits of ER to a nephrologist, we investigated the difference in the economic burden according to the referral time using national health insurance claim data in a prospective cohort ESRD patients.

Methods

Cohort Description

This study was nested within an ongoing cohort study (Clinical Research Center for End Stage Renal Disease, CRC for ESRD) of patients with ESRD in South Korea. The CRC for ESRD is a nationwide multi-center web-based comprehensive prospective cohort of CKD patients on dialysis whose aim is to analyze the treatment effects on survival or quality of life and cost-effectiveness by dialysis modality [32,33]. All enrolled patients are adults aged 20 years old or older and who started dialysis for ESRD without a schedule for kidney transplantation within 3 months. The patients began to be registered in July 2008, and 31 hospitals in Korea are currently participating in the CRC for ESRD cohort study. Until September 2012, a total of 1620 CKD patients who had newly started dialysis and 2917 patients who had already been on dialysis had been enrolled. All patients provided their written consent to participate voluntarily in this study. The study was approved by the institutional review board at each center [The Catholic University of Korea, Bucheon St. Mary's Hospital; The Catholic University of Korea, Incheon St. Mary's Hospital; The Catholic University of Korea, Seoul St. Mary's Hospital; The Catholic University of Korea, St. Mary's Hospital; The Catholic University of Korea, St. Vincent's Hospital; The Catholic University of Korea, Uijeongbu St. Mary's Hospital; Cheju Halla General Hospital; Chonbuk National University Hospital; Chonnam National University Hospital; Chung-Ang University Medical Center; Chungbuk National University Hospital; Chungnam National University Hospital; Dong-A University Medical Center; Ehwa Womens University Medical Center; Fatima Hospital, Daegu; Gachon University Gil Medical Center; Inje University Pusan Paik Hospital; Kyungpook National University Hospital; Kwandong University College of Medicine, Myongji Hospital; National Health Insurance Corporation Ilsan Hospital; National Medical Center; Pusan National University Hospital; Samsung Medical Center, Seoul; Seoul National University, Boramae Medical Center; Seoul National University Hospital; Seoul National University, Bundang Hospital; Yeungnam University Medical Center; Yonsei University, Severance Hospital; Yonsei University, Gangnam Severance Hospital; Ulsan University Hospital; Wonju Christian Hospital (in alphabetical order)]. All clinical investigators followed the Ethics for Medical Research and conducted this study in accordance with the guidelines of the 2008 Declaration of Helsinki.

Study Participants

We selected and studied 1011 adult patients who were newly diagnosed as having ESRD and started dialysis between August 2008 and June 2011 from the new patient registry in the CRC for ESRD cohort. Of the 132 patients who were excluded, the data regarding visits to a nephrologist were missing for 61 patients, and data regarding the type of initial dialysis were unknown for 33 patients. In addition, 38 patients were excluded due to the lack of cost data because of an unmatched identifier. The early referral group (ER) was defined as patients who were referred to a nephrologist more than 1 year before dialysis initiation and who had visited a nephrology clinic 2 or more times; the remaining patients whose referral time was less than a year were considered the late referral group (LR) [32].

Clinical Data Acquisition

Information about the participants was primarily collected from the data server of the CRC for ESRD for analysis. All traceable identifiers were removed prior to the analysis to ensure patient confidentiality. The clinical and laboratory data had been stored in the form of web-based medical questionnaires. The questionnaire items were filled in by data coordinators, who were trained in each center to collect patient data by a combination of chart reviews and direct interviews using a standardized form. The questionnaires included data on demographics, previous medical history, laboratory results, dialysis modality and prescription, type of permanent access used for the first dialysis, and medications. The estimated glomerular filtration rate (eGFR) was calculated by CKD-EPI equations [34]. The modified Charlson co-morbidity index (CCI) and Davies co-morbidity index (DCI) at the initiation of dialysis were recorded for each patient. The modified CCI and DCI values were calculated using the method described in a previous study [35–37]. The patients were asked to respond to the questionnaire when they first visited a nephrologist before starting dialysis.

Health Care Costs

Information about the medical costs during the 1 year periods just before and after the initiation of dialysis was acquired from the claim data of the Korea Health Insurance Review and Assessment Service (HIRA). In Korea, government-initiated public health insurance is mandatory, and private health insurance without national health insurance is not allowed for direct medical costs. All populations are obligatorily registered in the national health insurance service, and almost all legitimate medical costs are controlled and reimbursed via the Korea HIRA. We calculated the medical costs by an official request for the claim data of medical costs from the Korea HIRA and data integration by the coded identifiers of patients in the CRC for ESRD. To determine the economic cost of an illness, three types of costs should be considered: direct costs, indirect costs (productivity loss), and intangible costs. In this study, we evaluated direct medical expenditures, including physician visit costs, admission costs, surgery costs, physical therapy costs, and total medicine costs. The following costs were excluded: traffic costs, which are considered a direct non-medical cost; traditional Chinese herbal medicine costs; indirect costs; and intangible costs, which cannot be directly collected through the claim data of the Korea HIRA. All of the costs were calculated in the currency unit of the Korean Won (KRW) (US$1 = 1,100 KRW in 2013).

Statistical Analysis

In the descriptive analysis of the demographic and clinical characteristics and laboratory results, continuous variables were expressed as the mean and standard deviation, and categorical variables were described numerically with a percentage. Comparisons between the groups based on referral time were performed using a t-test for continuous variables and Chi-square or Fisher's exact tests for categorical variables when appropriate. We presented the mean with the standard error of the mean for the entire cost. The associations between medical costs and independent parameters were assessed using univariate and multivariate linear regression methods. Variables in the univariate models were selected *a priori* and by clinical significance, and included the type of referral, age, sex, type of dialysis modality, body mass index, causes of underlying kidney disease, hemoglobin level, and serum albumin level. Multivariate model included variables that were proved to be associated (P value <0.10) with the total medical costs. SAS/STAT 9.2 (SAS Institute Inc., Cary, NC, USA) was used in the analysis of the medical costs, and IBM SPSS ver. 20.0 was used to compare the demographic and clinical parameters. A P value <0.05 was considered statistically significant.

Results

Patients Characteristics by Referral Pattern

The patients' clinical and laboratory characteristics are summarized in Table 1. The mean age was 55.8±14.1 years old, and 59.5% of patients were male. Of the 879 patients enrolled in the cost analysis, 526 patients were in the ER group, and 353 were in the LR group. The time from referral to dialysis was significantly longer in the ER group than in the LR group (63.9±62.1 months vs. 2.7±3.4 months, P<0.001). In the LR group, the proportion of patients who visited a nephrologist less than 2 times before dialysis initiation reached up to 34.8%. The most common cause of renal disease was diabetic nephropathy in both groups.

At the time of the referral to a nephrologist, ages were younger, the blood pressure (BP) and serum creatinine level were lower, and the hemoglobin level and eGFR were higher in the ER group than in the LR group. At the time of dialysis initiation, most findings, including the age, sex, co-morbidity index, serum creatinine, eGFR, hemoglobin levels, calcium and phosphate levels, urate levels, and total cholesterol levels were similar in both groups. However, diastolic BP (77.5±13.4 vs. 79.5±14.8 mmHg, P = 0.041) and LDL cholesterol levels (89.9±39.0 vs. 98.7±58.6 mmHg, P = 0.018) were lower in the ER group.

Medical Costs

The monthly medical costs before and after the initiation of dialysis are summarized in table 2 and figure 1. The total medical costs during the first 12 months after the initiation of dialysis were not different between the two groups (ER vs. LR: 18947±11864 vs. 19104±11501 USD, P = 0.845). However, the costs of the ER patients during the first month were significantly lower than those of the LR patients (ER vs. LR: 3029±2219 vs. 3438±2821 USD, P = 0.025). The total 12-month health care costs before the initiation of dialysis were significantly lower in the ER group (ER vs. LR: 6206±5873 vs. 8610±7820 USD, P<0.001).

We evaluated the impact of various clinical and laboratory parameters on medical costs by univariate and multivariate analyses. Table 3 summarizes the results of the costs during the first month after dialysis initiation. The referral type (ER) reduced the costs (409.1±174.3 USD, P = 0.019) and the dialysis modality (hemodialysis) increased the medical costs (823.8±184.3 USD, P< 0.001) during the first month in the univariate analysis. The patients' age, gender, body mass index, causes of renal disease, hemoglobin level, and serum albumin level were not associated with the medical costs. In the multivariate analysis, ER significantly reduced the medical costs (428.5±172.3 USD, P = 0.013) during the first month after dialysis initiation.

The univariate and multivariate analyses on the costs during the 1 year before dialysis also showed a significant association of the referral time with the medical costs (Table 4). In the univariate analysis, ER (2404.1±447.4 USD, P<0.001) and the cause of renal disease reduced the costs, and age (30.1±15.7 USD, P = 0.055) and hemoglobin level (89.9±47.3 USD, P = 0.057) showed an association with increased medical costs. In the multivariate analysis, ER was also proved to be significantly associated with reduced medical costs (2534.0±436.2 USD, P< 0.001).

Medications and Vascular Access

Frequency of medication use, including antihypertensive drug, antiplatelet agents, anticoagulants, vitamin D, and phosphate binders, were not different between the two groups. Erythropoiesis-stimulating agents use was more (68.0 vs. 59.3%, P = 0.007) in the ER group. In the ER group, frequency of native arteriovenous fistula was higher (30.7% vs. 20.1%, P = 0.003) and temporary tunneled-catheter use was lower (40.2% vs. 49.0%, P = 0.031).

Discussion

We evaluated the benefit of ER to a nephrologist with respect to economic costs in a prospective cohort of patients who started dialysis for ESRD. We found that ER to a nephrologist significantly reduced medical costs during the periods of 1 year before and 1 month after the initiation of renal replacement therapy using national health insurance claim data. Patients with advanced CKD are frequently complicated with anemia, electrolyte imbalances, hypertension, mineral bone disorders, and other risk factors of cardiovascular diseases. Therefore, correcting and reversing the causes of renal impairment and managing the comorbidities in CKD are important to improve clinical outcomes and patient survival. Education of CKD patients about dialysis can reduce the incidence of emergent hemodialysis via a central venous catheter [38,39]. Recently, we reported that the timely referral of patients with CKD to a nephrologist is associated with the reduced usage of a central venous catheter for hemodialysis, improved patient survival, and decreased cardiovascular mortality [32]. The participants of this study are slightly different from our previous investigation in that the duration of patients' enrollment of this study was shorter by about 4 months and the definition of the ER group was defined as patients who had been referred 1 year before dialysis and who had visited nephrology clinic at least two times irrespective to the status of education about dialysis. In this study, we also proved that early referral to a nephrologist could reduce the usage of temporary vascular catheter for hemodialysis, and improve patients' blood pressure and lipid level control. The economic benefits of ER to a nephrologist were expected due to reduced morbidities and improved patient survival. To date, there have been several reports that ER to a nephrologist is cost-effective. However, those studies were retrospective analyses or included indirect estimations of medical costs [21,25,40,41]. In this study, we directly proved the cost-saving effect of ER by the integration of the clinical data of patients who started dialysis for ESRD from a prospective cohort and the claim data of a national health insurance organization.

Despite the various benefits of early nephrology referral, there are still many patients who are referred to a nephrology clinic too

Table 1. Patient characteristics by referral pattern at the time of referral and dialysis initiation.

	Total ESRD			
	Total	Early referral	Late referral	P Value
	(*N*=879)	(*N*=526)	(*N*=353)	
Age at the time of referral (year)	52.5±15.1	50.6±15.1	55.4±14.6	<0.001
Findings at the time of referral to nephrologist				
Underlying kidney disease (%)				0.003
Diabetes mellitus	48.7	49.6	47.4	
Hypertension	17.4	15.4	20.5	
Glomerulonephritis	16.4	18.7	12.9	
Polycystic kidney disease	2.5	3.5	1.1	
Others	10.5	9.3	12.1	
Unknown	4.5	3.5	5.9	
Systolic BP (mmHg)	146.3±26.8	142.9±25.1	150.2±28.1	0.001
Diastolic BP (mmHg)	84.4±16.6	83.4±16.0	85.4±17.1	0.132
Serum creatinine (mg/dL)	4.94±4.50	2.82±2.70	7.41±4.90	<0.001
eGFR (mL/min/1.73 m^2)	23.9±23.3	34.3±25.2	11.8±12.7	<0.001
Hemoglobin (g/dL)	10.1±5.3	11.3±6.8	8.8±1.8	<0.001
Number of visits to a nephrologist from referral to dialysis (%)				<0.001
None	7.1	0	17.7	
1 time	6.9	0	17.1	
2 times or more	86.0	100	65.2	
Time from referral to dialysis (month)	39.2±56.6	63.9±62.1	2.7±3.4	<0.001
Age at the time of dialysis (year)	55.8±14.1	55.9±13.8	55.6±14.6	0.761
Gender (male, %)	59.5	59.2	60.1	0.774
Findings at the time of dialysis				
Modified Charlson co-morbidity index	5.1±2.6	5.2±2.6	5.0±2.5	0.337
Davies co-morbidity index2	1.0±0.9	1.0±0.9	1.0±1.0	0.836
Systolic BP (mmHg)	139.7±22.2	138.9±22.2	140.8±22.1	0.222
Diastolic BP (mmHg)	78.3±14.0	77.5±13.4	79.5±14.8	0.041
BMI (kg/m^2)	23.1±3.5	23.1±3.3	23.1±3.7	0.882
Serum creatinine (mg/dL)	8.48±4.41	8.48±4.17	8.48±4.73	0.996
eGFR (mL/min/1.73 m^2)	7.6±7.4	7.3±6.6	7.9±8.4	0.214
Hemoglobin (g/dL)	8.8±1.7	8.9±1.7	8.8±1.6	0.287
Uric acid (mg/dL)	8.1±2.6	8.0±2.6	8.1±2.5	0.593
Calcium (mg/dL)	7.8±1.0	7.8±1.0	7.7±1.1	0.368
Phosphate (mg/dL)	5.4±1.8	5.4±1.8	5.5±1.9	0.672
Total cholesterol (mg/dL)	161.3±53.6	158.6±49.9	165.5±58.6	0.063
LDL cholesterol (mg/dL)	93.5±48.1	89.9±39.0	98.7±58.6	0.018

Values for continuous variables are expressed as the means ± standard deviation; values for categorical variables are expressed as proportions.
BMI, body mass index; BP, blood pressure; eGFR, estimated glomerular filtration rate; HDL, high-density lipoprotein; LDL, low-density lipoprotein

late for impending renal replacement therapy. The problems related to LR are common in many countries, and the proportion of patients who are referred when facing the impending dialysis is up to 31–38% [9,42,43]. The LR of CKD patients to a nephrologist can increase the medical costs due to increased mortality and comorbidities. The increased incidence of emergent hemodialysis and the frequent use of a temporary central venous catheter for hemodialysis contribute to the increased medical costs associated with LR [23,44]. Moreover, the increased duration of admission for the first dialysis is an important factor for the increased economic burden [16]. Although we could not compare the duration of admission between the two groups, more patients in the ER group started hemodialysis with their own native arteriovenous fistula without insertion of temporary central venous catheter. Reduced catheter usage contributed to the cost-saving effects in the ER group. The increased medical costs in the LR group may have resulted from the increased number or severity of the comorbidities associated with rapidly aggravating renal dysfunction. However, in this study, the cost-saving effects of ER were independent of comorbid conditions because we could not find a difference in the severity of illness between the ER and LR groups. Cost-saving effects of ER did not persist more than 1 months after dialysis start. It can be possible that main factors influencing on the decreased medical costs of ER work on during the predialysis period or early period of dialysis initiation. Detrimental effects of LR have been reported to be influential on 3 months short-term mortality, but not on long-term mortality [45]. After dialysis start, all patients are treated by nephrologists, patterns of clinical practice affecting on medical costs necessarily come to be similar between the ER and LR groups. Interestingly, medical costs in the ER groups were remarkably decreased before dialysis start. Advanced CKD patients are complicated with various medical problems, including hypertension, dyslipidemia, diabetes, and mineral bone disease. If patients were not referred to a nephrologist at the right time, inappropriate or overlapped laboratory tests would increase the medical costs in the LR group. In addition, detailed and appropriate medical therapy in the ER group would decrease the morbidities and medical costs before dialysis initiation. In this study, although more patients in the ER group were prescribed erythropoiesis-stimulating agents and the usage of antihypertensive drugs was not different between the two groups, blood pressure and lipid level were better controlled and medical costs were decreased through cost-effective care in the ER group.

There are several causes of the LR of patients with CKD to a nephrologist despite the clinical benefits of ER. With respect to clinicians or medical facilities, the lack of communication between doctors or hospitals, the absence of definite guidelines for the referral time to a nephrologist, and ambivalent opinions about dialysis in the elderly or high risk patients are factors that affecting LR [46]. With respect to patients, the refusal of dialysis, a lack of knowledge about CKD and dialysis, and economic poverty might function as factors that affect LR. Economic difficulties have been reported several times as the main cause of LR [29,47]. When patients with CKD are referred late due to economic difficulties, adequate treatment and preparation for dialysis are inevitably delayed. Increased metabolic complications related to ESRD eventually raise the medical costs related to dialysis and hospital admission, which in turn deteriorate the patients' economic status. The timely referral of patients with CKD, especially those with a poor socioeconomic status, to a nephrologist is necessary to prevent delayed dialysis due to a lack of knowledge and negative thinking about renal replacement therapy and to reduce the unnecessary medical expenses related to delayed referral.

Despite the unique findings and advantages, this study has several limitations. At first, there can be concerns about the lead time bias that patients in the ER group had better renal function, lower blood pressure, less severe anemia, and lower LDL cholesterol levels at the time of referral, and these reduced comorbidities could influence to the reduced medical costs in the ER group. These facts that patients in the ER group showed better clinical conditions are not surprising because they were referred about 5 years earlier than those in the LR group. At least, almost all parameters including age and co-morbidity index at the time of dialysis were similar between the ER and LR groups, and it is hard to say that patients in the ER group had better renal function or lesser comorbidities at the same time 6 or 12 months before dialysis initiation. If we could adjust parameters at the 12 months before dialysis instead of parameters at the time of dialysis initiation, multivariate regression model would be more accurately fitted to predict medical costs during the 12 months before dialysis initiation. However, due to the limited data collection in this cohort study, we could not gather clinical parameters or laboratory data at the 12 months before dialysis initiation, but only get data at the time of referral and at the time of dialysis initiation. Secondly, we only analyzed and compared the medical costs during the 12 months before and after dialysis initiation, not the whole or average medical costs from referral to dialysis initiation. Considering the 5 year mean duration from referral to dialysis in the ER group, if we could have compared the total 5 year medical costs or yearly medical costs during the 5 years between the two groups, the cost-saving effects of ER would be proved apparently without bias. The reasons why we focused on the medical costs during the 12 months before dialysis initiation were that we had divided the ER and LR groups by the referral time of 12 months and aimed to compare the medical costs around the time just before and after dialysis initiation. Actually, during the 12 months before dialysis initiation, monthly medical costs and the difference of medical costs between the ER and LR groups increased steadily. A considerable part of cost-saving effects of ER derived from the reduced medical costs during the several months of impending dialysis. It is still important that patients in the LR group spend much more medical costs probably due to the increased length of hospital stay and increased use of temporary vascular catheters immediately before dialysis initiation. Lastly, we could not investigate the relationship between medical costs and other clinical and laboratory parameters including eGFR, co-morbidity index, blood pressure, and cholesterol levels in univariate analysis. However, it might not lessen the strength of our results because these parameters were similar between the two groups.

The care of patients with CKD requires not only evaluation and treatment of decreased renal function but also a multidisciplinary

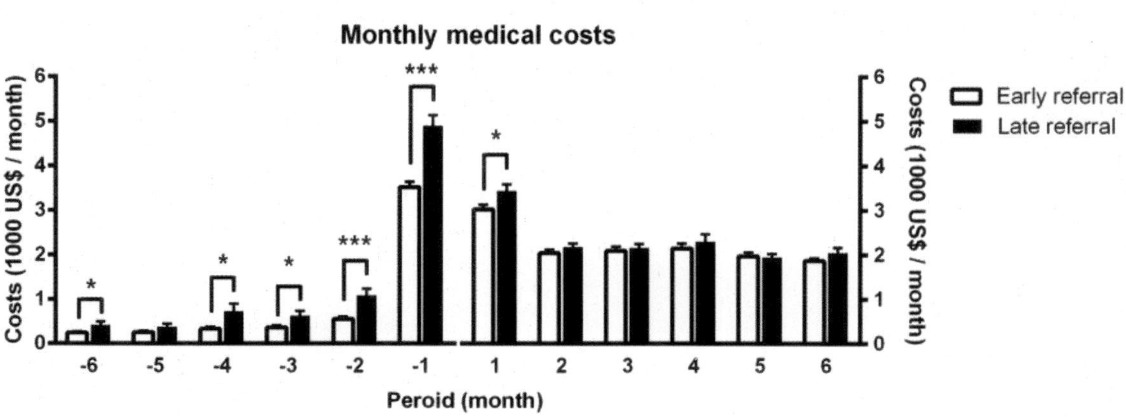

Figure 1. Monthly medical costs before and after the initiation of dialysis. The monthly medical costs are represented, comparing 'early referral' and 'late referral' according to the time period. The values (unit: US dollars) are expressed as the mean ± SEM. *P<0.05, ***P<0.001.

Table 2. Medical costs during the first year before and after dialysis therapy.

	Periods	Costs (USD)		
		Early referral	Late referral	P Value
After dialysis initiation (month)	0~1	3029±2219	3438±2821	0.025
	1~2	2044±1679	2181±1515	0.223
	2~3	2091±2087	2162±1669	0.597
	3~4	2148±2317	2301±3079	0.456
	4~5	1975±1623	1953±1258	0.844
	5~6	1871±1148	2046±2086	0.215
	0~12	18947±11864	19104±11501	0.845
Before dialysis initiation (month)	−1~0	3529±2696	4896±4629	<0.001
	−2~−1	555±1297	1092±2624	<0.001
	−3~−2	367±922	635±1779	0.015
	−4~−3	333±1003	725±3092	0.032
	−5~−4	259±705	382±1180	0.108
	−6~−5	247±520	417±1352	0.042
	−6~0	4926±3811	7162±6762	<0.001
	−12~0	6206±5873	8610±7820	<0.001

Costs are expressed as the mean ± standard deviation values.

approach, including proper blood pressure control, appropriate selection of medications and their dosages, the avoidance of nephrotoxic drugs, education about diet, preparation for renal placement therapy, psychological consultations, and economic evaluations. Timely referral is essential to improve patient outcomes and survival, but a considerable proportion of patients are referred late to dialysis for various reasons, including a lack of knowledge, negative preconceptions about dialysis, and economic difficulties. In this study, we demonstrated that the ER of CKD patients could reduce economic costs during the period before and after the initiation of renal replacement therapy. Considering the benefits of ER to a nephrologist in both economic and clinical terms, clinicians should focus on the timely referral of patients with CKD.

Acknowledgments

A proportion of this work was selected for oral presentation and presented at Kidney Week 2013, American Society of Nephrology Annual Meeting, on November 9 at the Georgia World Congress Center in Atlanta, GA. We express our gratitude to all participants and investigators of the cohort study (Clinical Research Center for End Stage Renal Disease, CRC for ESRD) in South Korea. Jeonghwan Lee (Hallym University Hangang Sacred Heart Hospital, Seoul, Korea), Jung Pyo Lee, Chun Soo Lim (Seoul National University Boramae Medical Center, Seoul, Korea), Ji In Park, Yon Su Kim (Seoul National University College of Medicine, Seoul, Korea), Jin Ho Hwang (Chung-Ang University Hospital, Seoul, Korea), Hye Min Jang, Ji-Young Choi, Yong-Lim Kim (Kyungpook National University, Daegu, Korea), Chul Woo Yang (The Catholic University of Korea College of Medicine, Seoul, Korea), Shin-Wook Kang (Yonsei University College of Medicine, Seoul, Korea), Nam-Ho Kim (Chonnam

Table 3. Multivariate analysis for the medical costs during the first month after dialysis initiation.

	Univariate model		Multivariate model	
Variables	Parameter estimates	P Value	Parameter estimates	P Value
Type of referral (early referral)	−409.1±174.3	0.019	−428.5±172.3	0.013
Age (years)	−1.2±6.1	0.846		
Gender (female)	53.9±175.3	0.759		
Type of dialysis (hemodialysis))	823.8±184.3	<0.001	845.7±184.8	<0.001
BMI	−26.7±22.0	0.226		
Causes of renal disease				
Diabetes mellitus	−197.2±236.0	0.404		
Glomerulonephritis	−571.9±295.5	0.053		
Hypertension	−285.0±302.6	0.347		
Hemoglobin (g/dL)	−14.0±22.4	0.532		
Serum albumin (g/dL)	−4.1±6.1	0.503		

Parameter estimates (unit: USD) are expressed with β ± standard error values.

Table 4. Multivariate analysis for medical costs during the 1 year before dialysis initiation.

	Univariate model		Multivariate model	
Variables	Parameter estimates	P Value	Parameter estimates	P Value
Type of referral (early referral)	−2404.1±447.4	<0.001	−2534.0±436.2	<0.001
Age (years)	30.1±15.7	0.055	27.9±15.7	0.076
Gender (female)	−431.4±449.8	0.338		
Type of dialysis (hemodialysis)	389.2±478.5	0.416		
BMI	8.1±55.3	0.883		
Causes of renal disease				
Diabetes mellitus	−637.6±571.5	0.265	−860.2±596.7	0.150
Glomerulonephritis	−2520.9±720.0	<0.001	−2247.6±749.5	0.003
Hypertension	−1507.3±717.3	0.036	−1814.4±737.1	0.014
Hemoglobin (g/dL)	89.9±47.3	0.057	81.4±46.3	0.080
Serum albumin (g/dL)	7.2±8.8	0.412		

Parameter estimates (unit: USD) are expressed with β ± standard error values.

National University Medical School, Gwangju, Korea) are participating CRC for ESRD, and Chun Soo Lim (email: cslimjy@snu.ac.kr) is the lead author of this article.

Author Contributions

Conceived and designed the experiments: JL JPL YSK CSL. Performed the experiments: JPL JIP JHH JYC YLK CWY SWK NHK YSK. Analyzed the data: JL JPL HMJ JYC CSL. Contributed reagents/materials/analysis tools: YLK CSL. Wrote the paper: JL JPL CSL.

References

1. Levey AS, Coresh J (2012) Chronic kidney disease. Lancet 379: 165–180.
2. James MT, Hemmelgarn BR, Tonelli M (2010) Early recognition and prevention of chronic kidney disease. Lancet 375: 1296–1309.
3. Kim S, Lim CS, Han DC, Kim GS, Chin HJ, et al. (2009) The prevalence of chronic kidney disease (CKD) and the associated factors to CKD in urban Korea: a population-based cross-sectional epidemiologic study. J Korean Med Sci 24 Suppl: S11–21.
4. Collins AJ, Foley RN, Herzog C, Chavers B, Gilbertson D, et al. (2013) US Renal Data System 2012 Annual Data Report. Am J Kidney Dis 61: A7, e1–476.
5. Keith DS, Nichols GA, Gullion CM, Brown JB, Smith DH (2004) Longitudinal follow-up and outcomes among a population with chronic kidney disease in a large managed care organization. Arch Intern Med 164: 659–663.
6. Jin DC (2011) Current status of dialysis therapy in Korea. Korean J Intern Med 26: 123–131.
7. Collins AJ, Foley RN, Herzog C, Chavers B, Gilbertson D, et al. (2009) United States Renal Data System 2008 Annual Data Report. Am J Kidney Dis 53: S1–374.
8. Seok SJ, Kim JH, Gil HW, Yang JO, Lee EY, et al. (2010) Comparison of patients starting hemodialysis with those underwent hemodialysis 15 years ago at the same dialysis center in Korea. Korean J Intern Med 25: 188–194.
9. Hommel K, Madsen M, Kamper AL (2012) The importance of early referral for the treatment of chronic kidney disease: a Danish nationwide cohort study. BMC Nephrol 13: 108.
10. Chan MR, Dall AT, Fletcher KE, Lu N, Trivedi H (2007) Outcomes in patients with chronic kidney disease referred late to nephrologists: a meta-analysis. Am J Med 120: 1063–1070.
11. Innes A, Rowe PA, Burden RP, Morgan AG (1992) Early deaths on renal replacement therapy: the need for early nephrological referral. Nephrol Dial Transplant 7: 467–471.
12. Arora P, Obrador GT, Ruthazer R, Kausz AT, Meyer KB, et al. (1999) Prevalence, predictors, and consequences of late nephrology referral at a tertiary care center. J Am Soc Nephrol 10: 1281–1286.
13. Jungers P, Zingraff J, Page B, Albouze G, Hannedouche T, et al. (1993) Detrimental effects of late referral in patients with chronic renal failure: a case-control study. Kidney Int Suppl 41: S170–173.
14. Metcalfe W, Khan IH, Prescott GJ, Simpson K, MacLeod AM (2000) Can we improve early mortality in patients receiving renal replacement therapy? Kidney Int 57: 2539–2545.
15. Ifudu O, Dawood M, Homel P, Friedman EA (1996) Excess morbidity in patients starting uremia therapy without prior care by a nephrologist. Am J Kidney Dis 28: 841–845.
16. Jungers P, Zingraff J, Albouze G, Chauveau P, Page B, et al. (1993) Late referral to maintenance dialysis: detrimental consequences. Nephrol Dial Transplant 8: 1089–1093.
17. Stack AG (2003) Impact of timing of nephrology referral and pre-ESRD care on mortality risk among new ESRD patients in the United States. Am J Kidney Dis 41: 310–318.
18. Roderick P, Jones C, Drey N, Blakeley S, Webster P, et al. (2002) Late referral for end-stage renal disease: a region-wide survey in the south west of England. Nephrol Dial Transplant 17: 1252–1259.
19. Kazmi WH, Obrador GT, Khan SS, Pereira BJ, Kausz AT (2004) Late nephrology referral and mortality among patients with end-stage renal disease: a propensity score analysis. Nephrol Dial Transplant 19: 1808–1814.
20. Yokoyama Y, Yamazaki S, Hasegawa T, Wakita T, Hayashino Y, et al. (2009) Impact of early referral to nephrologist on mental health among hemodialysis patients: a Dialysis Outcomes and Practice Patterns Study (DOPPS). Nephron Clin Pract 113: c191–197.
21. Levin A, Lewis M, Mortiboy P, Faber S, Hare I, et al. (1997) Multidisciplinary predialysis programs: quantification and limitations of their impact on patient outcomes in two Canadian settings. Am J Kidney Dis 29: 533–540.
22. Winkelmayer WC, Glynn RJ, Levin R, Owen W Jr, Avorn J (2001) Late referral and modality choice in end-stage renal disease. Kidney Int 60: 1547–1554.
23. Astor BC, Eustace JA, Powe NR, Klag MJ, Sadler JH, et al. (2001) Timing of nephrologist referral and arteriovenous access use: the CHOICE Study. Am J Kidney Dis 38: 494–501.
24. Avorn J, Winkelmayer WC, Bohn RL, Levin R, Glynn RJ, et al. (2002) Delayed nephrologist referral and inadequate vascular access in patients with advanced chronic kidney failure. J Clin Epidemiol 55: 711–716.
25. Schmidt RJ, Domico JR, Sorkin MI, Hobbs G (1998) Early referral and its impact on emergent first dialyses, health care costs, and outcome. Am J Kidney Dis 32: 278–283.
26. Stehman-Breen CO, Sherrard DJ, Gillen D, Caps M (2000) Determinants of type and timing of initial permanent hemodialysis vascular access. Kidney Int 57: 639–645.
27. Smart NA, Titus TT (2011) Outcomes of early versus late nephrology referral in chronic kidney disease: a systematic review. Am J Med 124: 1073–1080.
28. Chen SC, Hwang SJ, Tsai JC, Liu WC, Hwang SC, et al. (2010) Early nephrology referral is associated with prolonged survival in hemodialysis patients even after exclusion of lead-time bias. Am J Med Sci 339: 123–126.
29. Kinchen KS, Sadler J, Fink N, Brookmeyer R, Klag MJ, et al. (2002) The timing of specialist evaluation in chronic kidney disease and mortality. Ann Intern Med 137: 479–486.
30. Avorn J, Bohn RL, Levy E, Levin R, Owen WF Jr, et al. (2002) Nephrologist care and mortality in patients with chronic renal insufficiency. Arch Intern Med 162: 2002–2006.

31. Winkelmayer WC, Glynn RJ, Levin R, Mittleman MA, Pliskin JS, et al. (2002) Late nephrologist referral and access to renal transplantation. Transplantation 73: 1918–1923.
32. Kim do H, Kim M, Kim H, Kim YL, Kang SW, et al. (2013) Early referral to a nephrologist improved patient survival: prospective cohort study for end-stage renal disease in Korea. PLoS One 8: e55323.
33. Choi JY, Jang HM, Park J, Kim YS, Kang SW, et al. (2013) Survival advantage of peritoneal dialysis relative to hemodialysis in the early period of incident dialysis patients: a nationwide prospective propensity-matched study in Korea. PLoS One 8: e84257.
34. Levey AS, Stevens LA, Schmid CH, Zhang YL, Castro AF 3rd, et al. (2009) A new equation to estimate glomerular filtration rate. Ann Intern Med 150: 604–612.
35. Charlson ME, Pompei P, Ales KL, MacKenzie CR (1987) A new method of classifying prognostic comorbidity in longitudinal studies: development and validation. J Chronic Dis 40: 373–383.
36. Davies SJ, Russell L, Bryan J, Phillips L, Russell GI (1995) Comorbidity, urea kinetics, and appetite in continuous ambulatory peritoneal dialysis patients: their interrelationship and prediction of survival. Am J Kidney Dis 26: 353–361.
37. Chae JW, Song CS, Kim H, Lee KB, Seo BS, et al. (2011) Prediction of mortality in patients undergoing maintenance hemodialysis by Charlson Comorbidity Index using ICD-10 database. Nephron Clin Pract 117: c379–384.
38. Caskey FJ, Wordsworth S, Ben T, de Charro FT, Delcroix C, et al. (2003) Early referral and planned initiation of dialysis: what impact on quality of life? Nephrol Dial Transplant 18: 1330–1338.
39. Jones C, Roderick P, Harris S, Rogerson M (2006) Decline in kidney function before and after nephrology referral and the effect on survival in moderate to advanced chronic kidney disease. Nephrol Dial Transplant 21: 2133–2143.
40. Ledoux F, Rasamimanantsoa D, Moulin B, Hannedouche T (2001) From the first symptoms to terminal renal failure: need for a nephrologic follow-up. Rev Med Interne 22: 245–254.
41. Smith DH, Gullion CM, Nichols G, Keith DS, Brown JB (2004) Cost of medical care for chronic kidney disease and comorbidity among enrollees in a large HMO population. J Am Soc Nephrol 15: 1300–1306.
42. Roderick P, Jones C, Tomson C, Mason J (2002) Late referral for dialysis: improving the management of chronic renal disease. QJM 95: 363–370.
43. Roubicek C, Brunet P, Huiart L, Thirion X, Leonetti F, et al. (2000) Timing of nephrology referral: influence on mortality and morbidity. Am J Kidney Dis 36: 35–41.
44. Eadington DW (1996) Delayed referral for dialysis. Nephrol Dial Transplant 11: 2124–2126.
45. Kessler M, Frimat L, Panescu V, Briancon S (2003) Impact of nephrology referral on early and midterm outcomes in ESRD: EPidemiologie de l'Insuffisance REnale chronique terminale en Lorraine (EPIREL): results of a 2-year, prospective, community-based study. Am J Kidney Dis 42: 474–485.
46. Ismail N, Neyra R, Hakim R (1998) The medical and economical advantages of early referral of chronic renal failure patients to renal specialists. Nephrol Dial Transplant 13: 246–250.
47. Obialo CI, Ofili EO, Quarshie A, Martin PC (2005) Ultralate referral and presentation for renal replacement therapy: socioeconomic implications. Am J Kidney Dis 46: 881–886.

2

Fluctuation between Fasting and 2-H Postload Glucose State Is Associated with Chronic Kidney Disease in Previously Diagnosed Type 2 Diabetes Patients with HbA1c ≥ 7%

Chuan Wang[1]⁹, Jun Song[1]⁹, Zeqiang Ma[2], Weifang Yang[3], Chengqiao Li[4], Xiuping Zhang[5], Xinguo Hou[1], Yu Sun[1], Peng Lin[1], Kai Liang[1], Lei Gong[1], Meijian Wang[1], Fuqiang Liu[1], Wenjuan Li[1], Fei Yan[1], Junpeng Yang[1], Lingshu Wang[1], Meng Tian[1], Jidong Liu[1], Ruxing Zhao[1], Li Chen[1]*

1 Department of Endocrinology, Qilu Hospital of Shandong University, Jinan, Shandong, China, **2** China National Heavy Duty Truck Group Corporation Hospital, Jinan, Shandong, China, **3** Lukang Hospital of Jining, Jining, Shandong, China, **4** Department of Endocrinology, Second People's Hospital of Jining, Jining, Shandong, China, **5** Shantui Community Health Center, Jining, Shandong, China

Abstract

Objective: To investigate how the glucose variability between fasting and a 2-h postload glucose state (2-h postload plasma glucose [2hPG]-fasting plasma glucose [FPG]) is associated with chronic kidney disease (CKD) in middle-aged and elderly Chinese patients previously diagnosed with type 2 diabetes.

Design and Methods: This cross-sectional study included 1054 previously diagnosed type 2 diabetes patients who were 40 years of age and older. First, the subjects were divided into two groups based on a glycated hemoglobin (HbA1c) value of 7%. Each group was divided into two subgroups, with or without CKD. The Chronic Kidney Disease Epidemiology Collaboration (CKD-EPI) equation was used to estimate the glomerular filtration rate (GFR). CKD was defined as eGFR< 60 mL/min/1.73 m^2. Multiple linear regression analysis was used to estimate the association between the 2hPG-FPG and eGFR. The 2hPG-FPG value was divided into four groups increasing in increments of 36 mg/dl (2.0 mmol/L): 0–72, 72–108, 108–144 and ≥144 mg/dl, based on the quartiles of patients with HbA1c levels ≥7%; then, binary logistic regression analysis was used to investigate the association between 2hPG-FPG and the risk of CKD.

Results: In the patients with HbA1c levels ≥7%, the 2hPG-FPG was significantly associated with decreased eGFR and an increased risk of CKD independent of age, gender, body mass index (BMI), systolic blood pressure (BP), diastolic BP, smoking, and drinking, as well as fasting insulin, cholesterol, triglyceride, and HbA1c levels. The patients with 2hPG-FPG values ≥144 mg/dl showed an increased odds ratio (OR) of 2.640 (P=0.033). Additionally, HbA1c was associated with an increased risk of CKD in patients with HbA1c values ≥7%.

Conclusions: The short-term glucose variability expressed by 2hPG-FPG is closely associated with decreased eGFR and an increased risk of CKD in patients with poor glycemic control (HbA1c≥7%).

Editor: Mohammad E. Khamseh, Institute of Endocrinology and Metabolism, Iran, Islamic Republic of

Funding: This study was supported by grants from the Chinese Society of Endocrinology, the National Natural Science Foundation of China (No. 81100617), the Medical and Health Science and Technology Development Projects of Shandong Province (2011HD005), the National Science and Technology Support Plan (2009BAI80B04), the Natural Science Foundation of Shandong Province (ZR2012HM014), the International Science and Technology Projects of Shandong Province (2012GGE27126), the Business Plan of Jinan Students Studying Abroad (20110407), and the special scientific research fund of clinical medicine of Chinese Medical Association (12030420342). The funders had no role in study design, data collection and analysis, decision to publish, or preparation of the manuscript.

Competing Interests: The authors have declared that no competing interests exist.

* Email: wangchuansdu.edu@163.com

⁹ These authors contributed equally to this work.

Introduction

Chronic kidney disease (CKD), which is characterized by albuminuria or reduced kidney function, is a rapidly increasing global public health problem [1,2] that significantly increases the risk of cardiovascular events and mortality [3,4]. Effective treatment for end-stage renal disease (ESRD) is limited to renal replacement therapy, and treatment is predominantly aimed at preventing or slowing disease progression by controlling the risk factors, such as diabetes, hypertension, and dyslipidemia [2,5,6].

Among the risk factors, diabetes is the most frequent cause of CKD [5,7]. Hyperglycemia is closely related to the development of CKD and could be prevented by strict control of blood glucose levels [8]. A growing body of research suggests that glucose variability might accelerate the renal complications of diabetes independently of hyperglycemia; however, the results are inconsistent. One study of type 1 diabetes patients revealed that short-term glucose variability did not predict the development of nephropathy [9]. Two studies indicated that long-term glucose variability could affect CKD in patients with type 2 diabetes [10,11]. Because of the conflicting results and limited data on the influence of short-term glucose variability on renal function in type 2 diabetes, it is necessary to further clarify this issue.

Monitoring glucose variability is complicated, which greatly limits its application in clinical practice and large epidemiological studies. The most common short-term glucose variability occurs after a meal. It should be determined whether the difference between the fasting and postprandial glucose levels relates to CKD. The calories in a diet differs among subjects because of dietary variations. Thus, the standardization of postprandial glucose levels is greatly limited. The 75-g oral glucose tolerance test (OGTT) is the gold standard test for diagnosing diabetes, and the variability between the fasting plasma glucose (FPG) and the 2-h postload plasma glucose (2hPG) reflects, to some extent, short-term glucose variability. Therefore, a 75-g OGTT was performed for all participants to investigate whether the glucose variability between the FPG and 2hPG states (2hPG-FPG) is associated with CKD.

Materials and Methods

Ethics Statement

This work is part of the baseline survey in the REACTION study of the association of diabetes and cancer, which included 259,657 adults (40 years of age and older) in 25 communities across mainland China from 2011 to 2012 [12]. The study was approved by the Ruijin Hospital Ethics Committee of the Shanghai Jiao Tong University School of Medicine. Written informed consent was obtained from the study participants.

Study population

This study randomly recruited 10,028 subjects (40 years of age and older) in Shandong province from January to April 2012. Based on previous medical history, which was obtained using a standard questionnaire, we selected 1181 patients who were previously diagnosed with type 2 diabetes. The following exclusion criteria were applied: (1) lower 2hPG than FPG; (2) missing data for calculating the eGFR; (3) previously diagnosed kidney disease, including autoimmune or drug-induced kidney disease, nephritis, renal fibrosis or renal failure; (4) previously diagnosed hepatic disease, including fatty liver, liver cirrhosis and autoimmune hepatitis; and (5) any malignant disease. A total of 1054 subjects (604 women) were eligible for the analysis.

Data collection

A standard questionnaire was used by trained investigators to collect data regarding the demographic characteristics, lifestyle and previous medical histories of the subjects. Body mass index (BMI) was calculated as weight (kg) divided by height squared (m^2). Blood pressure (BP) was measured 3 consecutive times (OMRON Model HEM-752 FUZZY, Omron Company, Dalian, China) on the left arm after the subjects had remained seated for at least 5 min; the average reading was used for the analysis. After at least 10 h of overnight fasting, venous blood samples were collected between 07:00 and 09:00 to measure the FPG, fasting insulin, cholesterol, triglycerides and creatinine levels. The 2hPG was measured after the subjects had completed a 75-g OGTT. HbA1c was measured by high-performance liquid chromatography (VARIANT II and D-10 Systems, BIO-RAD, USA). The homeostasis model assessment of insulin resistance (HOMA-IR) index was calculated as follows: fasting insulin concentration (mIU/L)×FPG concentration (mmol/L)/22.5 [13]. The eGFR was calculated from the creatinine levels using the CKD-EPI formula [14] as shown in Table 1.

Definition

According to the Kidney Disease Outcomes Quality Initiative provided by the US National Kidney Foundation, CKD was defined as eGFR<60 mL/min/1.73 m^2 [15].

Diabetic patients who were previously diagnosed based on the 1999 World Health Organization (WHO) criteria (FPG≥126 mg/dl [7.0 mmol/L] and/or 2hPG≥200 mg/dl [11.1 mmol/L]) [16] were identified after reviewing their medical histories.

To explore the association between 2hPG-FPG and CKD in diabetic patients with glycemic control variations, we divided the subjects into the following two groups, according to the target HbA1c value (7.0%) [17]: patients with good glycemic control (HbA1c<7%) and patients with poor glycemic control (HbA1c≥7%).

Statistical analysis

The continuous variables with normal distribution are expressed as the mean ± standard deviation (SD), and the variables with non-normal distribution are presented as the median (interquartile range). The categorical variables are presented as numbers (%). Between-group differences were detected using Student's *t*-test (the continuous variables in normal distribution), Mann-Whitney U-test (the skewed continuous variables), or chi-squared test (categorical variables). Multiple linear regression analysis was used to estimate the association between 2hPG-FPG and eGFR. The following three models were constructed: Model 1 = not adjusted; Model 2 = adjusted for age, gender, BMI, systolic BP and diastolic BP; Model 3 = Model 2 plus Log (fasting insulin), cholesterol, Log (triglyceride), drinking, smoking and HbA1c. The assumption of a linear relationship between the dependent and independent variables was assessed using a histogram of the residuals, with a scatter plot of the standardized residuals to the standardized predicted values in different models. The 25th, 50th, and 75th percentiles for 2hPG-FPG in the subjects with HbA1c≥7% were 75.6 mg/dl (4.2 mmol/L), 108 mg/dl (6.0 mmol/L) and 144 mg/dl (8.0 mmol/L), respectively. The 2hPG-FPG quartiles in the subjects with HbA1c levels <7% were 50.4 mg/dl (2.8 mmol/L), 84.6 mg/dl (4.7 mmol/L) and 108 mg/dl (6.0 mmol/L). Based on the multiple linear regression analysis, we focused on the subjects with HbA1c levels ≥7% in the following analysis. To facilitate use in clinical practice, the 2hPG-FPG values were divided into four groups increasing in increments of 36 mg/dl (2.0 mmol/L): 0–72, 72–108, 108–144 and ≥144 mg/dl. The association of 2hPG-FPG (the 2hPG-FPG groups were introduced as ordinal dummy variables) with the risk of CKD was estimated using binary logistic regression analysis, and $P<0.05$ was considered to be statistically significant. The data were analyzed using the SPSS 16.0 software (SPSS, Inc., Chicago, IL, USA).

Table 1. eGFR calculated from the creatinine levels using the CKD-EPI formula.

Sex	Cr (mg/dl)	eGFR (mL/min/1.73 m^2)
Females	≤0.7	$144\times(Cr/0.7)^{-0.329}\times(0.993)^{age}$
	>0.7	$144\times(Cr/0.7)^{-1.209}\times(0.993)^{age}$
Males	≤0.9	$141\times(Cr/0.9)^{-0.411}\times(0.993)^{age}$
	>0.9	$141\times(Cr/0.9)^{-1.209}\times(0.993)^{age}$

eGFR, estimated glomerular filtration rate; Cr: creatinine.

Results

Characteristics of study participants

We included 1054 subjects (604 women) who were previously diagnosed with diabetes. The subjects were divided into two groups based on their HbA1c values, using 7% as the cut-off value. Each group was divided into two subgroups, with or without CKD. As shown in Table 2, compared with the non-CKD patients, the CKD patients were more likely to be older, male and smokers in both groups. The CKD patients had higher levels of FPG, 2hPG, 2hPG-FPG and HbA1c in the group with HbA1c values ≥7%.

Multiple linear regression analysis

As shown in Table 3, three models were constructed to analyze the association between 2hPG-FPG and eGFR (HOMA-IR and 2hPG-FPG are involved in the calculation of FPG, and we added fasting insulin instead of HOMA-IR to model 3). A linear relationship between the dependent and independent variables in each model was confirmed. A significantly negative association between 2hPG-FPG and eGFR was observed, independent of age, gender, BMI, systolic BP, diastolic BP, smoking, and drinking, as well as fasting insulin, cholesterol, triglyceride, and HbA1c levels only in previously diagnosed diabetes patients with HbA1c values ≥7%. In addition, a close relationship between HbA1c and decreased eGFR levels was observed in both groups.

Binary logistic regression analysis

The subjects were divided into four groups based on their 2hPG-FPG values, in increasing increments of 36 mg/dl (2.0 mmol/L), as follows: 0–72, 72–108, 108–144 and ≥ 144 mg/dl. As shown in Table 4, we analyzed the association between the increased 2hPG-FPG levels and the risk of CKD in three models. As expected, 2hPG-FPG could significantly increase the risk of CKD in patients with HbA1c values ≥7%; but not in subjects with HbA1c<7%. In model 1, the patients with 2hPG-FPG values ranging from 108–144 and ≥144 mg/dl had a significantly increased risk of CKD (odds ratio [OR] = 2.339 and 3.298, respectively). After adjusting for age, gender, BMI, systolic

Table 2. Characteristics of the study participants by HbA1c and CKD.

	HbA1c (%) <7 (n = 276)		HbA1c (%) ≥7 (n = 778)	
Characteristics	**CKD (n = 25)**	**non-CKD (n = 251)**	**CKD (n = 86)**	**non-CKD (n = 692)**
Female (%)	3 (12.0%)	144 (57.4%)**	21 (24.4%)	436 (63.0%)**
Age (years)	70.80±7.48	62.84±9.74**	69.35±8.86	62.62±8.25**
BMI (kg/m^2)	26.73±3.74	26.80±3.66	26.71±3.23	27.24±3.62
Systolic BP (mmHg)	149.50±22.23	145.45±21.67	149.93±21.12	145.71±21.87
Diastolic BP (mmHg)	76.09±9.61	79.51±10.34	79.89±11.44	80.04±11.74
FPG (mg/dl)	146.61±27.11	137.35±20.13	194.89±64.46	174.13±47.36*
2hPG (mg/dl)	219.67±49.98	218.42±44.30	327.37±84.81	283.66±73.01**
2hPG-FPG (mg/dl)	73.06±44.56	81.08±43.36	132.48±52.02	109.52±49.53**
HbA1c (%)	6.50 (6.10–6.80)	6.50 (6.20–6.80)	8.40 (7.68–9.93)	8.20 (7.50–9.30)*
Fasting insulin (mIU/L)	9.00 (7.05–14.80)	8.90 (6.10–11.90)	9.10 (5.90–1.38)	9.40 (6.48–13.73)
HOMA-IR index	3.33 (2.46–4.67)	2.96 (1.98–4.03)	3.98 (2.70–6.43)	3.77 (2.65–5.90)
Cholesterol (mg/dl)	223.36±44.14	202.36±38.02*	210.41±45.51	215.46±40.08
Triglyceride (mg/dl)	136.44 (91.70–167.90)	129.36 (93.92–183.40)	157.27 (108.98–206.44)	139.10 (100.12–207.32)
Smoking (%)	4 (16.0%)	22 (8.8%)	17 (19.8%)	74 (10.7%)*
Drinking (%)	2 (8.0%)	24 (9.6%)	6 (7.0%)	42 (6.1%)
Creatinine (mg/dl)	1.08 (1.00–1.19)	0.74 (0.68–0.83)**	1.08 (0.99–1.25)	0.75 (0.69–0.82)**
eGFR (mL/min/1.73 m^2)	52.62 (16.92–58.05)	84.35 (74.45–92.45)**	53.49 (43.57–56.60)	85.26 (75.62–93.09)**

The data are expressed as the means ± SD or numbers (%). CKD, chronic kidney disease; BMI, body mass index; BP, blood pressure; FPG, fasting plasma glucose; 2hPG, 2-h postload plasma glucose; HOMA-IR, homeostasis model assessment of insulin resistance; eGFR, estimated glomerular filtration rate. *$P<0.05$ vs the CKD group; **$P<0.01$ vs the CKD group.

Table 3. Multiple linear regression analysis of the relationship between 2hPG-FPG and eGFR.

		HbA1c (%) <7		HbA1c (%) ≥7	
Models	**Independent variable**	**β Coefficient (95% CI)**	***P*-value**	**β Coefficient (95% CI)**	***P*-value**
Model 1	2hPG-FPG, per mg/dl	−0.018 (−0.062 to 0.026)	0.417	−0.042 (−0.064 to −0.020)	**<0.001**
Model 2	2hPG-FPG, per mg/dl	0.013 (−0.018 to 0.043)	0.417	−0.035 (−0.053 to −0.017)	**<0.001**
Model 3	2hPG-FPG, per mg/dl	0.011 (−0.020 to 0.041)	0.492	−0.023 (−0.041 to −0.004)	**0.018**
	Log (HbA_{1c}), per unit	−46.082 (−90.153 to −2.012)	**0.040**	−23.194 (-35.654 to −10.733)	**<0.001**

Model 1: not adjusted; Model 2: adjusted for age, gender, BMI, systolic BP and diastolic BP; Model 3: Model 2 plus Log (fasting insulin), cholesterol, Log (triglyceride), drinking and smoking.

BP and diastolic BP, these two groups also presented increased ORs (2.397 and 3.662, respectively). With further adjusting for fasting insulin, cholesterol, triglycerides, smoking, drinking and HbA1c, the patients with a 2hPG-FPG value ≥144 mg/dl showed an increased risk of CKD (OR = 2.640, $P = 0.033$) Additionally, HbA1c was associated with an increased risk of CKD in patients with HbA1c levels ≥7%.

Discussion

There has been no consensus to define glucose variability, although the concept is intuitively comprehensible. The most common understanding of glucose variability refers to the within-day glucose variability, which is evaluated using the blood glucose values obtained by self-monitoring or continuous glucose monitoring (CGM) [18]. The other predominant concepts are between-day fasting glycemia variability, postprandial glycemic peaks, variability of HbA1c over time, and hypoglycemic episodes [18]. Numerous indices are calculated to estimate glucose variability [18]. Regardless of which index is used, continuous glucose monitoring within one day or longer is required, which complicates and greatly limits its application in clinical practice and large epidemiological studies. Because the most common glucose variability occurs after a meal and the definition of glucose variability is uncertain, the difference between fasting and postprandial glucose levels might reflect the state of glucose variability (to some extent). Moreover, to standardize the calories intake in the meal, 75 g OGTT was done for all subjects and 2hPG was used to express postprandial glucose. Therefore, in this study, glucose variability is expressed by the 2hPG-FPG.

Although the effect of glucose variability on the development of complications of diabetes has been postulated and discussed in recent years [19,20,21,22], the study results are controversial. Kilpatrick et al. analyzed Diabetes Control and Complications Trial (DCCT) patients with type 1 diabetes and observed that the within-day glucose variability (calculated using the SD and mean amplitude of glycemic excursions) in the DCCT did not predict the development of retinopathy or nephropathy [9]. Two recent studies revealed that HbA1c variability (expressed by the SD of

Table 4. Binary logistic regression analysis of the relationship between 2hPG-FPG and CKD.

		HbA1c (%) <7		HbA1c (%) ≥7	
Models	**Independent variable**	**Odds ratio (95% CI)**	***P*-value**	**Odds ratio (95% CI)**	***P*-value**
Model 1	2hPG-FPG, mg/dl				
	Group 1 (0–72)	1 (reference)		1 (reference)	
	Group 2 (72–108)	1.292 (0.509–3.279)	0.589	1.385 (0.611–3.138)	0.435
	Group 3 (108–144)	0.762 (0.232–2.508)	0.655	2.339 (1.094–4.999)	**0.028**
	Group 4 (≥144)	0.472 (0.058–3.852)	0.483	3.298 (1.577–6.895)	**0.002**
Model 2	2hPG-FPG, mg/dl				
	Group 1 (0–72)	1 (reference)		1 (reference)	
	Group 2 (72–108)	0.862 (0.266–2.788)	0.804	1.448 (0.589–3.558)	0.420
	Group 3 (108–144)	0.364 (0.088–1.511)	0.164	2.397 (1.038–5.534)	**0.041**
	Group 4 (≥144)	0.200 (0.017–2.325)	0.198	3.662 (1.575–8.514)	**0.003**
Model 3	2hPG-FPG, mg/dl				
	Group 1 (0–72)	1 (reference)		1 (reference)	
	Group 2 (72–108)	0.812 (0.233–2.832)	0.743	1.220 (0.477–3.120)	0.678
	Group 3 (108–144)	0.330 (0.068–1.606)	0.170	2.076 (0.874–4.929)	0.098
	Group 4 (≥144)	0.240 (0.020–2.878)	0.260	2.640 (1.083–6.436)	**0.033**
	HbA_{1c}, per % unit	0.717 (0.232–2.222)	0.565	1.295 (1.096–1.529)	**0.002**

Model 1: not adjusted; Model 2: adjusted for age, gender, BMI, systolic BP and diastolic BP; Model 3: Model 2 plus Log (fasting insulin), cholesterol, Log (triglyceride), drinking and smoking.

HbA1c) independently affected the development of CKD in type 2 diabetes patients [10,11]. The conflicting results might be attributed to the different study populations and various indices used to express glucose variability in the various studies. The latter two studies [10,11] observed the effect of long-term glycemic variability (the SD of HbA1c) on renal complications. Whether short-term glucose variability affects change in renal function in type 2 diabetes remains to be explored. To verify this hypothesis, we investigated the association between short-term glucose variability (expressed by 2hPG-FPG) and the risk of CKD in type 2 diabetes. To analyze this association, we divided the subjects into two groups based on their glycemic control, with 7% HbA1c as the cut-off value. In diabetes patients with good glycemic control (HbA1c<7%), 2hPG-FPG and HbA1c levels were not associated with the risk of CKD, indicating that, with good glycemic control, short-term glucose variability would not significantly affect the development of CKD. The small sample of CKD in the group with HbA1c<7% might influence the accuracy of the results. Additional studies with a larger sample size of CKD patients should be performed to verify this observation. In the subjects with poor glycemic control (HbA1c≥7%), both 2hPG-FPG and HbA1c levels were significantly associated with decreased eGFR and an increased risk of CKD, which suggested that, with poor glycemic control, both the average blood glucose and the short-term glucose variability contributed to the development of CKD. The underlying mechanism for this phenomenon might be found in diabetic rodent studies. One study found that blood glucose fluctuation could accelerate the trend of kidney fibrosis through the ERK/MAPK and TGF-β/Smad signaling pathways in diabetic mice by increasing collagen production and inhibiting collagen degradation [23]. Another study observed that diabetic rodents with higher blood glucose fluctuation always showed a more serious degree of glomerular sclerosis compared with that shown in rodents with sustained high blood glucose levels [24].

In addition to hyperglycemia, the traditional risk factors of CKD include sex, age, obesity, hypertension, smoking, drinking, dyslipidemia and insulin resistance [2,6]. We adjusted for age, gender, BMI, systolic BP, diastolic BP, smoking, and drinking, as well as fasting insulin, cholesterol, triglycerides, and HbA1c levels, to ensure that our results were more reliable. Because HOMA-IR and 2hPG-FPG included FBG in the calculation, we added fasting insulin instead of HOMA-IR to model 3. After adjusting for the above risk factors, 2hPG-FPG was significantly associated with decreased eGFR and an increased risk of CKD in patients with HbA1c levels ≥7%; there was not a significant association regarding patients with HbA1c levels <7%.

Our study has some limitations. First, a cross-sectional study could not infer causality between 2hPG-FPG and CKD. Second, the fluctuation between a fasting and postprandial glucose state (2hPG-FPG) could not precisely reflect the glucose fluctuation. As a simple indicator of glucose fluctuation, 2hPG-FPG might be easily applicable to clinical practice. Third, our study included only middle-aged and elderly Chinese subjects; therefore, these results might not be applicable to subjects of different ages or ethnicities. Fourth, the sample size of CKD patients in the group with HbA1c levels <7% was limited, which would lead to an erroneous estimation of the effect of 2hPG-FPG on the risk of CKD. Fifth, the duration of diabetes was unknown; a longer disease duration could increase the risk of CKD. Additionally, other risk factors for CKD, such as uric acid, were not included in this study, which might affect the results. Finally, without measuring protein in the urine, the GFR based on creatinine and estimated by the CKD-EPI equation might not accurately reflect the kidney function, which might influence the accurate estimation of CKD. The gold standard method for measuring the GFR (isotope clearance measurement) is expensive and time-consuming, and the use of creatinine-based equations to estimate the GFR is reasonable for large epidemiological studies. The CKD-EPI equation is more accurate and precise than the MDRD study equation and the Cockcroft-Gault equation, particularly for the subjects with eGFR levels <60 mL/min/1.73 m^2 [25]. The CKD-EPI equation might be an optimum estimation of the GFR.

We found that 2hPG-FPG was closely associated with decreased eGFR and an increased risk of CKD in previously diagnosed type 2 diabetes patients with HbA1c levels ≥7%; it was not associated in patients with HbA1c levels <7%. In patients with poor glycemic control, the average blood glucose (expressed by HbA1c) and the short-term glucose variability (expressed by 2hPG-FPG) could increase the risk of CKD. With blood glucose control within the target HbA1c value (7.0%), the short-term glucose variability might not continue to affect the change in renal function, which indicates the fundamental role of good control of the average blood glucose in CKD prevention. Additional longitudinal studies are needed to verify these study results and to explore the degree to which the 2hPG-FPG value should be controlled in clinical practice to benefit CKD patients.

Author Contributions

Conceived and designed the experiments: CW JS. Performed the experiments: CW JS ZM WY CL XZ XH YS PL KL LG MW FL WL FY JY LW MT JL RZ LC. Analyzed the data: CW JS. Contributed reagents/materials/analysis tools: CW JS. Contributed to the writing of the manuscript: CW JS LC.

References

1. Tomonaga Y, Risch L, Szucs TD, Ambuehl PM (2013) The prevalence of chronic kidney disease in a primary care setting: a Swiss cross-sectional study. PLoS One 8: e67848.
2. Zhang L, Wang F, Wang L, Wang W, Liu B, et al. (2012) Prevalence of chronic kidney disease in China: a cross-sectional survey. Lancet 379: 815–822.
3. Chen YC, Su YC, Lee CC, Huang YS, Hwang SJ (2012) Chronic kidney disease itself is a causal risk factor for stroke beyond traditional cardiovascular risk factors: a nationwide cohort study in Taiwan. PLoS One 7: e36332.
4. Hallan SI, Matsushita K, Sang Y, Mahmoodi BK, Black C, et al. (2012) Age and association of kidney measures with mortality and end-stage renal disease. JAMA 308: 2349–2360.
5. Pyram R, Kansara A, Banerji MA, Loney-Hutchinson L (2012) Chronic kidney disease and diabetes. Maturitas 71: 94–103.
6. Chen W, Wang H, Dong X, Liu Q, Mao H, et al. (2009) Prevalence and risk factors associated with chronic kidney disease in an adult population from southern China. Nephrol Dial Transplant 24: 1205–1212.
7. Collins AJ, Foley RN, Herzog C, Chavers B, Gilbertson D, et al. (2011) US Renal Data System 2010 Annual Data Report. Am J Kidney Dis 57: A8, e1–526.
8. The Diabetes Control and Complications Trial Research Group (1993) The effect of intensive treatment of diabetes on the development and progression of long-term complications in insulin-dependent diabetes mellitus. The Diabetes Control and Complications Trial Research Group. N Engl J Med 329: 977–986.
9. Kilpatrick ES, Rigby AS, Atkin SL (2006) The effect of glucose variability on the risk of microvascular complications in type 1 diabetes. Diabetes Care 29: 1486–1490.
10. Penno G, Solini A, Bonora E, Fondelli C, Orsi E, et al. (2013) HbA1c variability as an independent correlate of nephropathy, but not retinopathy, in patients with type 2 diabetes: the Renal Insufficiency And Cardiovascular Events (RIACE) Italian multicenter study. Diabetes Care 36: 2301–2310.
11. Luk AO, Ma RC, Lau ES, Yang X, Lau WW, et al. (2013) Risk association of HbA1c variability with chronic kidney disease and cardiovascular disease in type 2 diabetes: prospective analysis of the Hong Kong Diabetes Registry. Diabetes Metab Res Rev 29: 384–390.
12. Ning G (2012) Risk Evaluation of cAncers in Chinese diabeTic Individuals: a lONgitudinal (REACTION) study. J Diabetes 4: 172–173.
13. Matthews DR, Hosker JP, Rudenski AS, Naylor BA, Treacher DF, et al. (1985) Homeostasis model assessment: insulin resistance and beta-cell function from

fasting plasma glucose and insulin concentrations in man. Diabetologia 28: 412–419.
14. Levey AS, Stevens LA, Schmid CH, Zhang YL, Castro AF 3rd, et al. (2009) A new equation to estimate glomerular filtration rate. Ann Intern Med 150: 604–612.
15. National Kidney Foundation (2002) K/DOQI clinical practice guidelines for chronic kidney disease: evaluation, classification, and stratification. Am J Kidney Dis 39: S1–266.
16. Alberti KG, Zimmet PZ (1998) Definition, diagnosis and classification of diabetes mellitus and its complications. Part 1: diagnosis and classification of diabetes mellitus provisional report of a WHO consultation. Diabet Med 15: 539–553.
17. American Diabetes Association (2009) Standards of medical care in diabetes–2009. Diabetes Care 32 Suppl 1: S13–61.
18. Frontoni S, Di Bartolo P, Avogaro A, Bosi E, Paolisso G, et al. (2013) Glucose variability: An emerging target for the treatment of diabetes mellitus. Diabetes Res Clin Pract 102: 86–95.
19. Brownlee M, Hirsch IB (2006) Glycemic variability: a hemoglobin A1c-independent risk factor for diabetic complications. JAMA 295: 1707–1708.
20. Cameron FJ, Baghurst PA, Rodbard D (2010) Assessing glycemic variation: why, when and how? Pediatr Endocrinol Rev 7 Suppl 3: 432–444.
21. Siegelaar SE, Holleman F, Hoekstra JB, DeVries JH (2010) Glucose variability; does it matter? Endocr Rev 31: 171–182.
22. Weber C, Schnell O (2009) The assessment of glycemic variability and its impact on diabetes-related complications: an overview. Diabetes Technol Ther 11: 623–633.
23. Cheng X, Gao W, Dang Y, Liu X, Li Y, et al. (2013) Both ERK/MAPK and TGF-Beta/Smad signaling pathways play a role in the kidney fibrosis of diabetic mice accelerated by blood glucose fluctuation. J Diabetes Res 2013: 463740.
24. Wang H, Wang A, Lei M, Liao J, Hu W (2013) [Effect of blood glucose fluctuation and the sustained high blood glucose on renal pathological change and collagen IV expression in diabetic rats]. Zhong Nan Da Xue Xue Bao Yi Xue Ban 38: 818–823.
25. Jessani S, Levey AS, Bux R, Inker LA, Islam M, et al. (2014) Estimation of GFR in South Asians: a study from the general population in Pakistan. Am J Kidney Dis 63: 49–58.

Axl Tyrosine Kinase Protects against Tubulo-Interstitial Apoptosis and Progression of Renal Failure in a Murine Model of Chronic Kidney Disease and Hyperphosphataemia

Gareth D. Hyde[1,2], Rebecca F. Taylor[1,2], Nick Ashton[3], Samantha J. Borland[1], Hon Sing Geoffrey Wu[3], Andrew P. Gilmore[2,3], Ann E. Canfield[1,2]*

1 Institute of Cardiovascular Sciences, Faculty of Medical and Human Sciences, University of Manchester, Manchester, United Kingdom, **2** Wellcome Trust Centre for Cell-Matrix Research, University of Manchester, Manchester, United Kingdom, **3** Faculty of Life Sciences, University of Manchester, Manchester, United Kingdom

Abstract

Chronic kidney disease (CKD) is defined as the progressive loss of renal function often involving glomerular, tubulo-interstitial and vascular pathology. CKD is associated with vascular calcification; the extent of which predicts morbidity and mortality. However, the molecular regulation of these events and the progression of chronic kidney disease are not fully elucidated. To investigate the function of Axl receptor tyrosine kinase in CKD we performed a sub-total nephrectomy and fed high phosphate (1%) diet to Axl+/+ and Axl−/− mice. Plasma Gas6 (Axl' ligand), renal Axl expression and downstream Akt signalling were all significantly up-regulated in Axl+/+ mice following renal mass reduction and high phosphate diet, compared to age-matched controls. Axl−/− mice had significantly enhanced uraemia, reduced bodyweight and significantly reduced survival following sub-total nephrectomy and high phosphate diet compared to Axl+/+ mice; only 45% of Axl−/− mice survived to 14 weeks post-surgery compared to 87% of Axl+/+ mice. Histological analysis of kidney remnants revealed no effect of loss of Axl on glomerular hypertrophy, calcification or renal sclerosis but identified significantly increased tubulo-interstitial apoptosis in Axl−/− mice. Vascular calcification was not induced in Axl+/+ or Axl−/− mice in the time frame we were able to examine. In conclusion, we identify the up-regulation of Gas6/Axl signalling as a protective mechanism which reduces tubulo-interstitial apoptosis and slows progression to end-stage renal failure in the murine nephrectomy and high phosphate diet model of CKD.

Editor: David Long, UCL Institute of Child Health, United Kingdom

Funding: This work was supported by the British Heart Foundation [PG/08/075/25545] and the Wellcome Trust [097820/Z/11/Z]. The Wellcome Trust Centre for Cell-Matrix Research, University of Manchester, is supported by core funding from the Wellcome Trust [088785/Z/09/Z]. The Bioimaging Facility microscopes used were purchased with grants from BBSRC, Wellcome Trust and the University of Manchester Strategic Fund. The funders had no role in study design, data collection and analysis, decision to publish, or preparation of the manuscript.

* Email: ann.canfield@manchester.ac.uk

Introduction

Chronic kidney disease (CKD) is a major healthcare burden and significant cause of death worldwide. Although CKD can be initiated by several different insults, it is believed to converge on common progressive pathways leading to loss of renal function and end-stage renal failure [1]. Cardiovascular disease accounts for a significant proportion of mortality within CKD patients. Indeed, vascular calcification (VC) is detected in over 80% of end-stage renal disease patients and its extent associates with increased morbidity and mortality [2,3,4].

Axl is a member of the TAM (Tyro3, Axl and Mertk) family of receptor tyrosine kinases which are all activated by the ligand Gas6. Binding of Gas6 to Axl leads to receptor dimerisation, autophosphorylation and activation of downstream signalling pathways including PI3-Kinase/Akt and Erk1/2 resulting in pro-survival and proliferative responses, respectively [5,6].

We have shown previously that Axl is down-regulated during phosphate-driven calcification of vascular smooth muscle cells (VSMC) and pericytes [7,8]. Activation of Axl/PI3-kinase signalling reduces VSMC apoptosis and *in vitro* mineralisation, suggesting that Axl is protective against vascular calcification [7,8,9,10]. Conversely, previous studies using Gas6−/− mice have shown a pathological role for Gas6 in nephrotoxic nephritis and streptozotocin-induced diabetic nephropathy [11,12]. Loss of Gas6 protected against mesangial cell proliferation and glomerular hypertrophy and improved proteinuria and survival [11,12]. These data suggest that inhibitors of the Gas6/Axl pathway may be of therapeutic benefit in these renal pathologies. However, the function of Axl in CKD and associated VC has not been investigated and whether Axl has a protective or pathological role in this setting is unknown.

Therefore, the purpose of this study was to investigate the function of Axl in CKD using a well-established murine sub-total nephrectomy and high phosphate diet model [13,14,15,16,17,18].

We demonstrate that renal Axl and circulating Gas6 are up-regulated in Axl+/+ mice following sub-total nephrectomy and high phosphate diet. Furthermore, we show that in the absence of Axl, mice undergo rapid deterioration following sub-total nephrectomy and we uncover a novel role of Axl in protecting against tubulo-interstitial apoptosis and progression of renal failure.

Methods and Materials

Animal breeding and surgery

All experiments involving animals were carried out in accordance with the UK Animals (Scientific Procedures) Act 1986 (project licence number PPL 40/3518) and received local approval from the University of Manchester Ethical Review Process. All surgery was performed under isoflurane anaesthesia (4% in oxygen at 2 L/min) and with buprenorphine analgesia (0.003 mg). All efforts were made to minimize suffering.

Axl−/− mice were provided by Dr Angelillo-Scherrer (University of Lausanne, Switzerland) with permission of Prof Lemke (Salk Institute, USA) [19]. The mice had a C57/SV129 mixed background. Mice were genotyped with the following primers: Axl forward 5-TCTGGCTGGGAAAGTCAGAT-3, Axl reverse 5-CAGCCGAGGTATAGGCTGTC-3; Neo forward 5-ATGACTGGGCACAAACAGACA-3, Neo reverse 5-AATATCACGGGTAGCCAACG-3. PCR conditions were: 94°C for 10 minutes followed by 35 cycles of 94°C, 1 minute; 65°C, 1 minute; 72°C, 2 minutes and a final 10 minute incubation at 72°C. The absence of Axl in these mice was confirmed by western blotting of kidney lysates (results not shown). Initially an Axl+/− breeding pair was set up from which an Axl+/+ breeding trio (1 male, 2 females) and an Axl−/− breeding trio was derived. These 2 breeding trios produced the 23 Axl+/+ (9 males, 14 females) and 24 Axl−/− mice (10 males, 14 females) that underwent surgery in this study. Additional Axl+/+ and Axl−/− mice were bred for use as controls (no surgery, normal phosphate diet).

Sub-total nephrectomy was performed in a two-stage procedure. Mice underwent an approximate 2/3rd resection of the left kidney at 11 weeks of age. This was performed by surgically removing the poles of the left kidney and applying tissue glue (Histoacryl, Braun) to curtail bleeding. One week later a complete right side nephrectomy was performed. Percentage renal mass removed was calculated by weighing the material removed in the initial partial nephrectomy, combining this with the weight of the right kidney when removed and assuming that total kidney mass was double that of the right kidney upon removal. On average 72.1% (n = 22, Std. Dev. 3.57) of renal mass was removed from Axl+/+ and 70.8% (n = 23, Std. Dev. 4.46) from Axl−/− animals, with no statistically significant difference between the groups.

Animals were placed on a 1% phosphate diet (rodent maintenance diet 1, containing 1% phosphate, Special Diet Services, UK) 1 week after the second surgery. Following surgery animals were checked daily and weighed twice per week. Animals were killed by cervical dislocation at the end of the experiment or when the predetermined humane end-point had been reached. Decisions to humanly cull animals post-surgery were based on the presence of 2 or more of the following criteria: blood present in the urine and/or faeces, weight loss of 15% or more compared to pre-surgery or 10% in the previous 72 hours, BUN greater than 100 mg/dL, piloerection and lack of response to external stimuli.

Plasma analysis

Blood was collected by tail vein sampling during the study and by cardiac puncture at the end of the study. Blood Urea Nitrogen (BUN) levels were determined using the BUN enzymatic end point test kit (Stanbio labs, Texas, USA). Creatinine levels were determined using the mammalian serum and plasma creatinine detection kit (Arbor assays, Ann Arbor, USA). Plasma Gas6 concentrations were determined using the mouse Gas6 ELISA kit (Adipo Bioscience, Santa Clara, USA). Plasma phosphate and total calcium concentrations were determined using a Roche P8000 analyser.

Western Blotting

Kidneys were snap frozen in liquid nitrogen, ground into a powder using a Mikro-dismembrator S (Braun Biotech International), and solubilised in lysis buffer (20 mM Tris-HCl pH 7.6, 150 mM sodium chloride, 1 mM EDTA, 1% (v/v) Igepal, 50 mM sodium fluoride, 1 mM sodium orthovanadate, 1 mM sodium pyrophosphate, and 1x protease inhibitor cocktail set 1 (Calbiochem)). Protein was quantified using the Pierce BCA protein assay kit (Thermo Scientific, UK). Samples (50 µg) were run on 10% SDS-PAGE gels and blotted with anti: Axl (1:1000) (Santa Cruz, SC-1096, raised against a peptide mapping to the C-terminus of human Axl), phosphoAkt (1:1000) (Cell Signalling, 9271), Akt (1:1000) (Cell Signalling, 9272) or α-tubulin (1:1000) (Abcam, ab4074). Membranes were incubated for 1 hour with either HRP-conjugated secondary antibodies (1:2000) (Dako), washed, incubated with SuperSignal Chemiluminescent substrate (Pierce) and exposed to Hyperfilm (GE Healthcare) or with AlexaFluor 680-conjugated secondary antibodies (1:5000) (Life Technologies, A21109) and visualized using an Odyssey Imaging system (LI-COR Biosciences, UK).

Histology

Kidney remnants and thoracic aortas were washed in PBS. The adventitia was removed from aorta and tissues were fixed overnight in 4% (v/v) formaldehyde in PBS at 4°C. Samples

Table 1. Kidney mass pre- and post-surgery.

	Kidney mass at baseline	Percentage of kidney mass removed	Kidney remnant mass 14 weeks post-surgery
Axl+/+ females	1.47 (13, 0.18)	70.7 (13, 3.15)	0.66 (13, 0.13)
Axl−/− females	1.57 (14, 0.23)	69.9 (14, 2.55)	0.77 (8, 0.12)
Axl+/+ males	1.72 (9, 0.15)	74.0 (9, 4.40)	0.71 (7, 0.26)
Axl −/− males	1.70 (9, 0.16)	72.2 (9, 3.97)	0.70 (3, 0.09)

Kidney mass at baseline and the kidney remnant mass are expressed as a percentage of the animal's weight at these time points. When calculating kidney mass at baseline and the percentage kidney mass removed, total kidney mass was assumed to be twice that of the right kidney upon removal. The n number and standard deviation are in brackets. There is no statistically significant difference between genotypes.

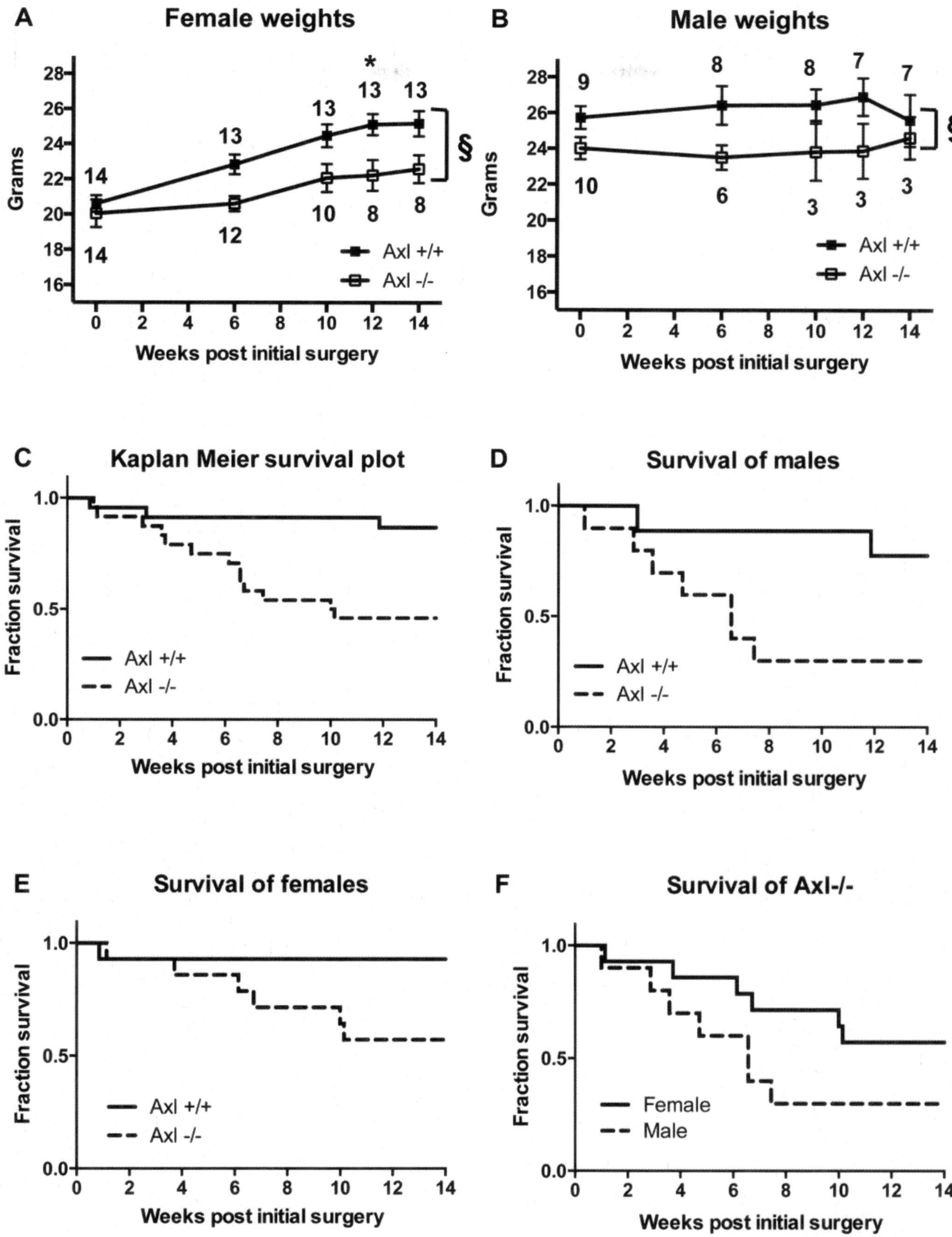
A
Female weights
Grams
Weeks post initial surgery
Axl +/+
Axl -/-
§
*
B
Male weights
Grams
Weeks post initial surgery
Axl +/+
Axl -/-
§
C
Kaplan Meier survival plot
Fraction survival
Weeks post initial surgery
Axl +/+
Axl -/-
D
Survival of males
Fraction survival
Weeks post initial surgery
Axl +/+
Axl -/-
E
Survival of females
Fraction survival
Weeks post initial surgery
Axl +/+
Axl -/-
F
Survival of Axl-/-
Fraction survival
Weeks post initial surgery
Female
Male

Figure 1. Axl−/− mice have significantly reduced body weight and survival following sub-total nephrectomy and high phosphate diet. Weight in grams of (A) females and (B) males expressed as means +/− standard error of the mean (SEM). Statistical test is a 2-way ANOVA with a Sidak compensation for multiple comparison, § = $p \leq 0.005$ for difference between genotypes and * = $p \leq 0.05$ for individual time points, n number (surviving animals) in brackets. (C–F) Kaplan-Meier survival plots of Axl+/+ and Axl−/− mice following nephrectomy and high phosphate diet. (C) All mice, (D) males, (E) females, (F) Axl−/− mice alone.

were dehydrated and paraffin wax embedded using a microm STP 120 processor and a Microm EC 350-1/2 embedder. Seven-micron sections were cut using a Microm HM 355S and dried overnight at 37°C. All analyses were performed in a blinded manner.

Sections were stained with haematoxylin and eosin using a varistain 24-2 (Thermo-Shandon) or with picrosirius red, digitised with a 3D Histech Pannoramic 250 slide scanner and analysed using Pannoramic Viewer image analysis software. To determine the mean maximal glomeruli diameter, at least 15 glomeruli per animal were measured.

TUNEL staining was performed using the DeadEnd Fluorometric TUNEL kit (Promega, UK). TUNEL positive cells were quantified by a blinded individual (6 images per animal, 3 of the inner cortex and 3 of the outer cortex). TUNEL positive cells were expressed per unit area.

Kidney calcification was analysed by von Kossa staining. Slides were digitised with a 3D Histech Pannoramic 250 slide scanner. Calcification was quantified using HistoQuant analysis software and expressed as percentage of total surface area. VC was analysed by both von Kossa and alizarin red staining. At least 3 sections per animal were analysed. The extent of calcification for each animal was graded: 0 = no calcification in any sections, 1 = 1 or 2 deposits in a single section, 2 = 1 or 2 deposits in multiple sections, 3 = multiple deposits in multiple sections, 4 = heavily calcified in multiple sections.

Statistical Analysis

Statistical analysis was performed using GraphPad Prism. Where repeated measures of the 2 genotypes were made over time a two-way ANOVA was used to analyse the difference between genotypes followed by post hoc analysis of individual time points with Sidak compensation for multiple comparisons. Where 3 or more groups were analysed one-way ANOVA with Sidak compensation was used for parametric data and Kruskal-Wallis with Dunn' compensation for non-parametric data. Where only two groups were being compared a Student's *t*-test was used for parametric data and a Mann-Whitney test for non-parametric data. Differences in survival were determined using a Gehan-Breslow-Wilcoxon test.

Results

Loss of Axl results in significantly reduced survival following sub-total nephrectomy and high phosphate diet

Equal amounts of renal mass were removed from both genotypes. No difference in kidney mass was observed between the genotypes either at the start of the study, upon right side nephrectomy or at the end of the study (Table 1). However, following sub-total nephrectomy and high phosphate diet Axl+/+ and Axl−/− mice exhibited marked differences in body mass (Figure 1A&B). Female Axl−/− mice did not gain weight at the same rate as Axl+/+ females, resulting in significantly lower body weights (Figure 1A). Male Axl−/− mice lost weight initially again resulting in significantly lower body weights compared to Axl+/+ controls (Figure 1B).

Axl−/− mice also had significantly reduced survival following nephrectomy and high phosphate diet (Figure 1C). Only 45% (11/24) of Axl−/− mice survived to 14 weeks post-surgery compared with 87% (20/23) of Axl+/+ mice ($p = 0.0053$, hazard ratio 5.22, 95% CI 1.62–11.65). This effect was most marked in males (Figure 1D&F); only 30% of male Axl−/− mice survived to 14 weeks post-surgery, compared to 78% male Axl+/+ mice ($p = 0.0370$, hazard ratio 4.52, 95% CI 1.14–15.91). These mice exhibited rapid weight loss and severe uraemia (see below) and were culled before the end of the experiment having reached the predetermined humane end-point. In contrast, 57% of female Axl−/− mice survived to 14 weeks post-surgery compared to 93% of female Axl+/+ mice ($p = 0.0529$, hazard ratio 6.72, 95% CI 1.07–20.90) (Figure 1E&F).

Axl−/− mice have elevated uraemia post sub-total nephrectomy and high phosphate diet

As uraemia is a surrogate marker of renal function and drives VC, blood urea nitrogen (BUN) levels were monitored. In addition, plasma creatinine levels were measured at the end of the study. By 6 weeks post-surgery, BUN levels were significantly increased in Axl+/+ and Axl −/− mice (Figure 2A), confirming induction of a uraemic state. At 6 weeks, BUN levels were also significantly higher in Axl−/− compared to Axl+/+ mice (Figure 2A). Beyond 6 weeks post-surgery the BUN levels of the Axl−/− mice appeared to improve; falling below those of the Axl+/+ mice (Figure 2B). Plasma creatinine analysis 14 weeks post-surgery supported these findings (Axl+/+0.18 mg/dL, Std Dev 0.27, n = 11; Axl−/− 0.04 mg/dL, Std Dev 0.07, n = 8). The reduction in the average BUN level in the Axl−/− group is due to two reasons. Firstly, the loss of the more severely affected Axl−/− mice and their absence from later data points contributes to the reduced average BUN level in this population. By 6 weeks post-surgery, 25% of Axl−/− mice had been culled as their condition had reached the humane end-point defined in our license. Analysis confirmed severe uraemia in these mice with an average BUN concentration of 105.3±29.5 mg/dL (Figure 2C). Between 6 and 10 weeks more Axl−/− mice were lost (average BUN concentration of 85.33±8.1 mg/dL; Figure 2C). Secondly, there was an improvement in the remaining sub-population of Axl−/− mice that survived until the end of the study (Figure 2C).

Female and male Axl−/− mice showed the same trend in BUN levels (Figure 2D, E&G). However, female Axl−/− mice tolerated sub-total nephrectomy and high phosphate diet better than the Axl−/− males, and greater numbers survived to the end of the study, as shown in the Kaplan-Meier plot (Figure 1F). BUN levels were significantly higher in male Axl+/+ mice than female Axl+/+ mice 12 and 14 weeks post-nephrectomy (Figure 2F), suggesting that males progress to renal failure more quickly than females.

Renal Axl expression is up-regulated following sub-total nephrectomy and high phosphate diet and protects against tubulo-interstitial apoptosis

To determine what happens to the expression of Axl and Gas6 following sub-total nephrectomy and high phosphate diet, we analysed kidney protein extracts and plasma Gas6 concentrations.

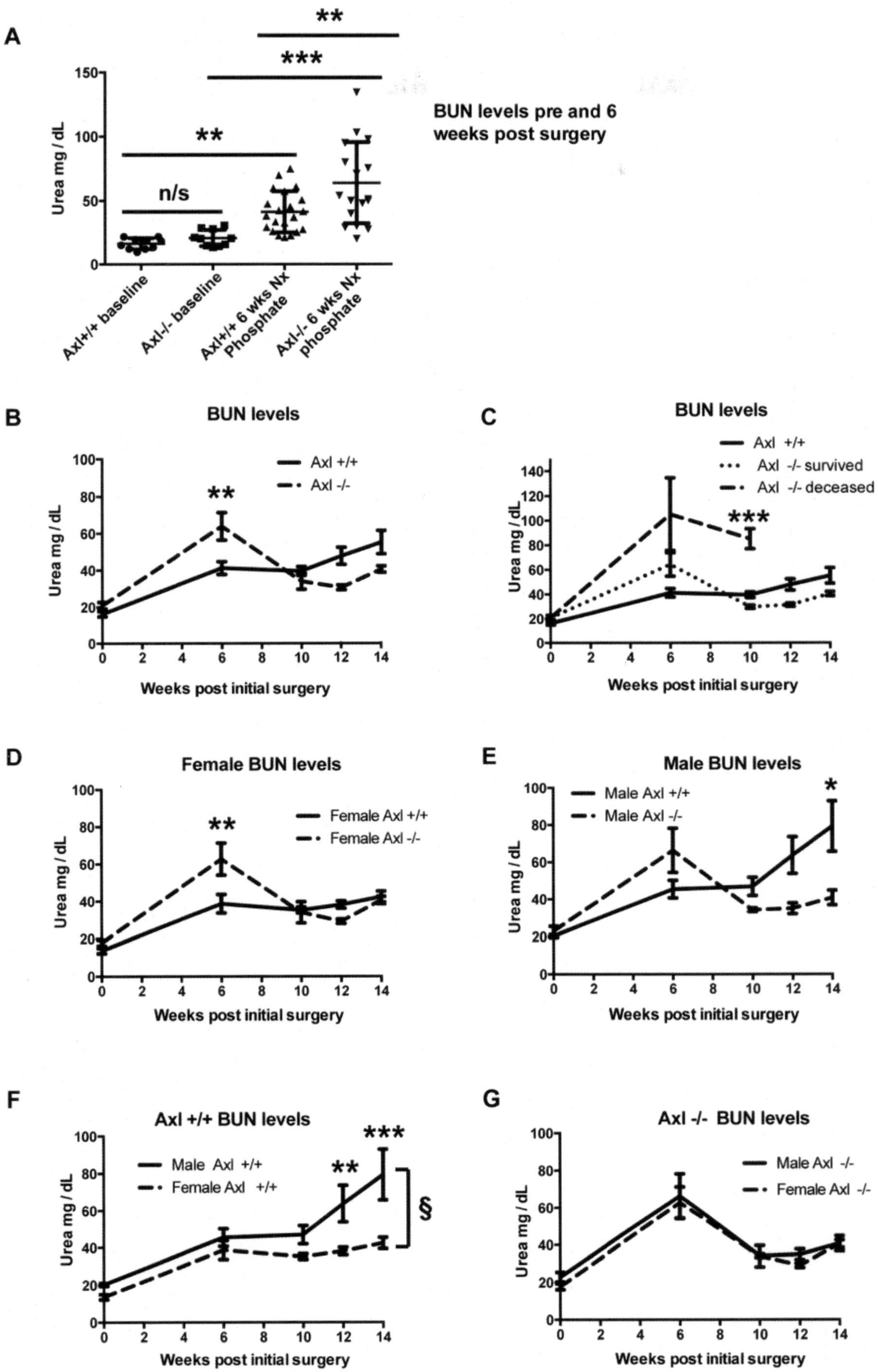
A
BUN levels pre and 6 weeks post surgery
Urea mg / dL
n/s
**
***
**
Axl+/+ baseline
Axl-/- baseline
Axl+/+ 6 wks Nx Phosphate
Axl-/- 6 wks Nx phosphate
B
BUN levels
Axl +/+
Axl -/-
Weeks post initial surgery
C
BUN levels
Axl +/+
Axl -/- survived
Axl -/- deceased
D
Female BUN levels
Female Axl +/+
Female Axl -/-
E
Male BUN levels
Male Axl +/+
Male Axl -/-
F
Axl +/+ BUN levels
Male Axl +/+
Female Axl +/+
§
G
Axl -/- BUN levels
Male Axl -/-
Female Axl -/-

Figure 2. Axl−/− mice develop elevated uraemia following sub-total nephrectomy and high phosphate diet. (A) Blood Urea Nitrogen (BUN) levels expressed as individual data points with means +/− standard deviation (Std Dev). Statistical test is a 1-way ANOVA with Sidak compensation for multiple comparisons. (B–G) BUN levels of Axl+/+ and Axl−/− mice expressed as means +/− SEM; (B) all mice, (C) Axl−/− sub-populations (survived/deceased), (D) females analysed by genotype, (E) males analysed by genotype, (F) Axl+/+ mice analysed by gender, (G) Axl−/− mice analysed by gender. Statistical test is a 2-way ANOVA with Sidak compensation for multiple comparisons. § = $p \leq 0.05$ for difference between genotypes, * = $p \leq 0.05$, ** = $p \leq 0.01$, *** = $p \leq 0.005$.

Renal Axl expression was down-regulated with age in Axl+/+ mice which had not undergone surgery (11 week vs 25 week mice) (Figure 3A). However, the expression of Axl and its downstream signalling partner (Akt and pAkt) were significantly increased (6–9 fold; $p<0.05$) following sub-total nephrectomy and high phosphate diet compared to age-matched controls (Figure 3A). As both Akt and pAkt were upregulated the pAkt/Akt ratio did not change. Plasma Gas6 concentration also tended to decrease with age in control non-nephrectomised mice (11 vs 25 weeks); albeit not significantly. Gas6 concentrations in WT mice were significantly up-regulated following sub-total nephrectomy and high phosphate diet (Figure 3B). Furthermore circulating Gas6 concentrations were significantly reduced in Axl−/− mice, both at baseline and post-nephrectomy compared to Axl+/+ mice (Figure 3B), suggesting that Axl positively regulates the production of its ligand. Gas6 concentration did not differ between female and male Axl+/+ mice and the downward trend in Gas6 levels in Axl−/− mice was observed in both genders (Figure 3C).

To further investigate the effect of loss of Axl, sub-total nephrectomy and high phosphate diet on kidney ultrastructure, histological analyses were performed. These showed that loss of Axl had no overt effect on kidney ultrastructure at baseline (Figure S1). Sub-total nephrectomy and high phosphate diet were associated with hypercellularity, tubular dilation and the recruitment of cells tentatively identified as inflammatory cells on the basis of their characteristic staining (Figure S1). However, when sections were graded for these characteristics by a blinded individual, no significant difference between genotypes was detected (data not shown).

Gas6/Axl signalling has been implicated in mesangial proliferation, glomerular hypertrophy and sclerosis [11,12,20,21,22]. We show that sub-total nephrectomy and high phosphate diet induced glomerular hypertrophy; however no significant difference between Axl+/+ and Axl−/− mice was seen (Figure S2). Sub-total nephrectomy also increased renal collagen content, but loss of Axl did not appear to modulate this effect (Figure S3).

As signalling downstream of Axl commonly results in anti-apoptotic effects [5] we hypothesised that increased cell death may be occurring in the Axl−/− kidneys, contributing to the observed phenotype. We show that the number of TUNEL positive cells was significantly increased in Axl−/− kidneys compared to Axl+/+ kidneys post-nephrectomy and high phosphate diet (Figure 4A&B). No difference in TUNEL positive cells was detected within the glomeruli; however a significant increase was detected in the tubulo–interstitial regions of Axl−/− kidneys compared to Axl+/+ controls (Figure 4B).

Sub-total nephrectomy and phosphate feeding did not induce significant vascular calcification, but increased renal calcification

Hyperphosphataemia and hypercalcaemia mediate CKD-associated VC [23]; therefore, we measured plasma phosphate and calcium concentrations at baseline and the end of the study (Table 2). Axl+/+ female mice had significantly elevated plasma phosphate and calcium concentrations 14 weeks post-surgery, as previously observed [13,17]. Axl+/+ male mice also tended to have higher plasma phosphate and calcium concentrations, although this did not reach statistical significance. Neither female nor male Axl−/− mice exhibited hyperphosphataemia or hypercalcaemia at the end of the study.

We have shown that Axl expression is down-regulated during VSMC and pericyte mineralisation *in vitro* and activation of Axl reduces phosphate-driven mineralisation [7,8]. Therefore, to determine whether loss of Axl affects calcification we performed von Kossa staining on kidney remnants and both von Kossa and alizarin red staining on aortic sections. The majority of kidney remnants analysed (10/13 WT and 9/15 Axl nulls) exhibited calcification post-nephrectomy and high phosphate diet. There was a downward trend in the number of animals with renal calcification and in the amount of calcification in the Axl−/− group; however histomorphometric analysis revealed no statistically significant difference between the two genotypes (Figure 5). Calcification was only detected in a minority of aorta analysed (3/10 Axl+/+ and 3/8 Axl−/− aortas); the calcium deposits were small and no significant difference was detected between the groups (results not shown). TUNEL staining did not reveal any significant induction of apoptosis in the aortas of either Axl+/+ or Axl−/− mice.

Discussion

In this study we investigated the role of Axl tyrosine kinase in the murine sub-total nephrectomy and high phosphate diet model of CKD and VC. We demonstrate for the first time that plasma Gas6, renal Axl and downstream Akt signalling are up-regulated following sub-total nephrectomy and high phosphate diet, and that loss of Axl results in significantly elevated tubulo-interstitial apoptosis, uraemia and mortality.

Based on these results we hypothesise that the loss of Axl-dependent cell survival signalling in the tubulo-interstitium is likely to be the primary cause of accelerated renal disease and reduced survival in these animals. This is supported, first, by the fact that Axl mediates cell survival signalling in many cell types [5]. Second, tubular interstitial injury is a common mediator of CKD progression [1,24] and finally, that we did not detect any glomerular or sclerotic defects that have previously been shown to be modified by Gas6/Axl signalling in other models of kidney disease [11,12].

Within the kidney, Axl and Gas6 are expressed by VSMCs, glomerular mesangial cells and tubular cells in both mice and humans [22,25,26]. There is low expression in the basal state, but Axl and Gas6 are up-regulated in several murine models of renal disease including: Thy1.1 antibody induced glomerulonephritis, [21] nephrotoxic nephritis [12], streptozotocin-induced diabetic nephropathy [11] and a podocyte ablation model of glomerular albuminuria [26]. Furthermore, Axl and Gas6 are elevated in patients with inflammatory kidney disease [25] and IgA nephropathy [27]. Plasma Gas6 levels are also increased in patients with CKD [28]. In the disease context, Gas6/Axl signalling has been implicated mainly in cell proliferation and glomerular hypertrophy. Loss of Gas6 protected against glomerular proliferation, sclerosis and proteinuria in the nephrotoxic nephritis model [12] and reduced mesangial hypertrophy in streptozotocin-induced

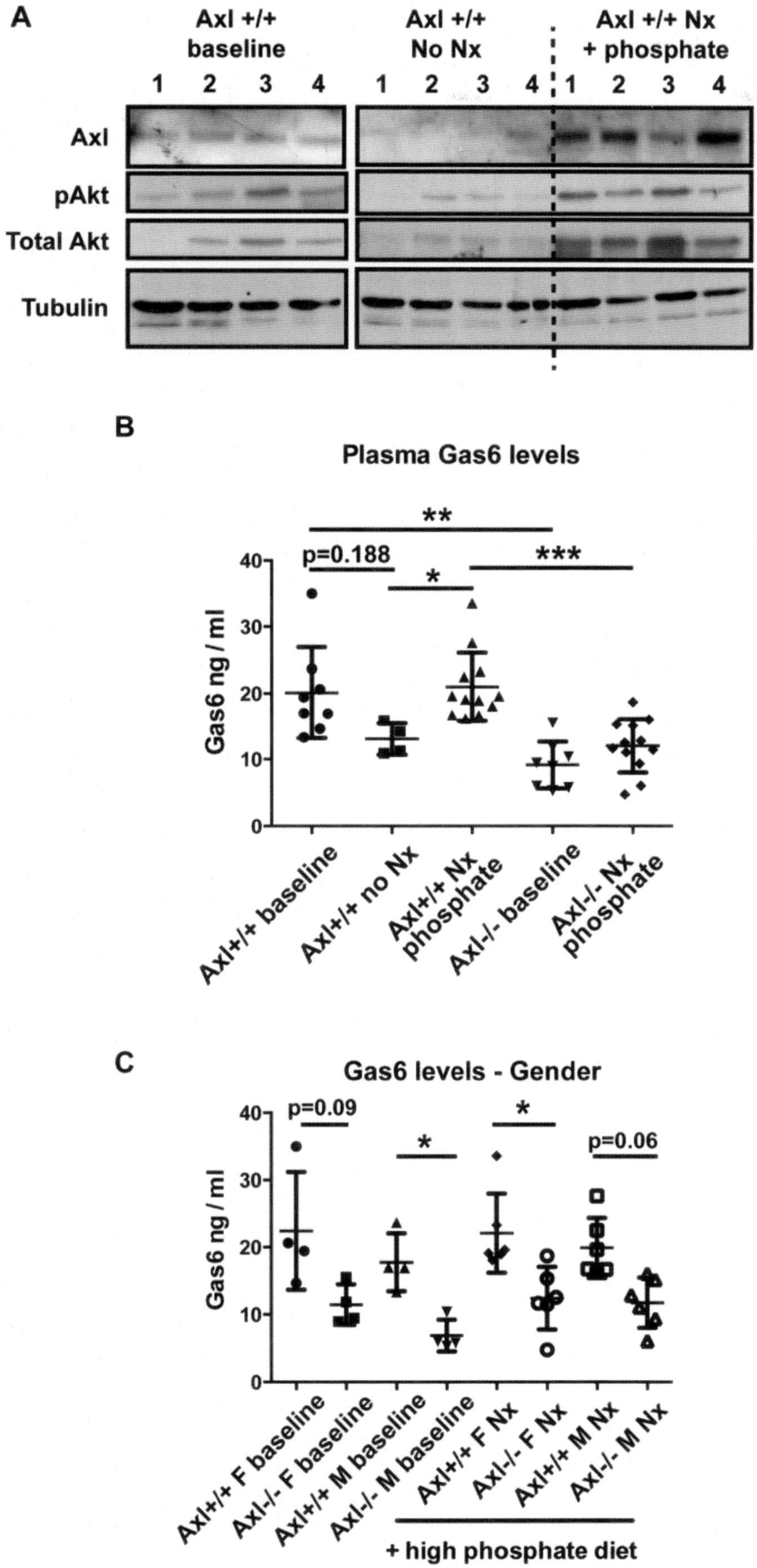
A
Axl +/+
baseline
Axl +/+
No Nx
Axl +/+ Nx
+ phosphate
1 2 3 4 1 2 3 4 1 2 3 4
Axl
pAkt
Total Akt
Tubulin
B
Plasma Gas6 levels
**
p=0.188
***
*
Gas6 ng / ml
0
10
20
30
40
Axl+/+ baseline
Axl+/+ no Nx
Axl+/+ Nx phosphate
Axl-/- baseline
Axl-/- Nx phosphate
C
Gas6 levels - Gender
p=0.09
*
*
p=0.06
Gas6 ng / ml
0
10
20
30
40
Axl+/+ F baseline
Axl-/- F baseline
Axl+/+ M baseline
Axl-/- M baseline
Axl+/+ F Nx
Axl-/- F Nx
Axl+/+ M Nx
Axl-/- M Nx
+ high phosphate diet

Figure 3. Axl and its ligand Gas6 are up-regulated following sub-total nephrectomy and high phosphate diet. (A) Western blots of kidney lysates for Axl, pAkt, total Akt and α-tubulin; 4 individual animals per group. The groups are Axl+/+ animals at baseline (11 weeks of age), 25 week old Axl+/+ animals with no nephrectomy (age-matched controls; no Nx), and 25 week old Axl+/+ animals that had a sub-total nephrectomy (Nx) at 11 weeks (Nx + phosphate). (B, C) Plasma Gas6 levels determined by ELISA; (B) Gas6 levels by genotype, (C) Gas6 levels by gender. A minimum of 4 animals were analysed per group. Results expressed as individual data points with means +/− Std Dev. Statistical test is a Kruskal-Wallis test with Dunn's compensation for multiple comparisons, * = p≤0.05, ** = p≤0.01, *** = p≤0.005.

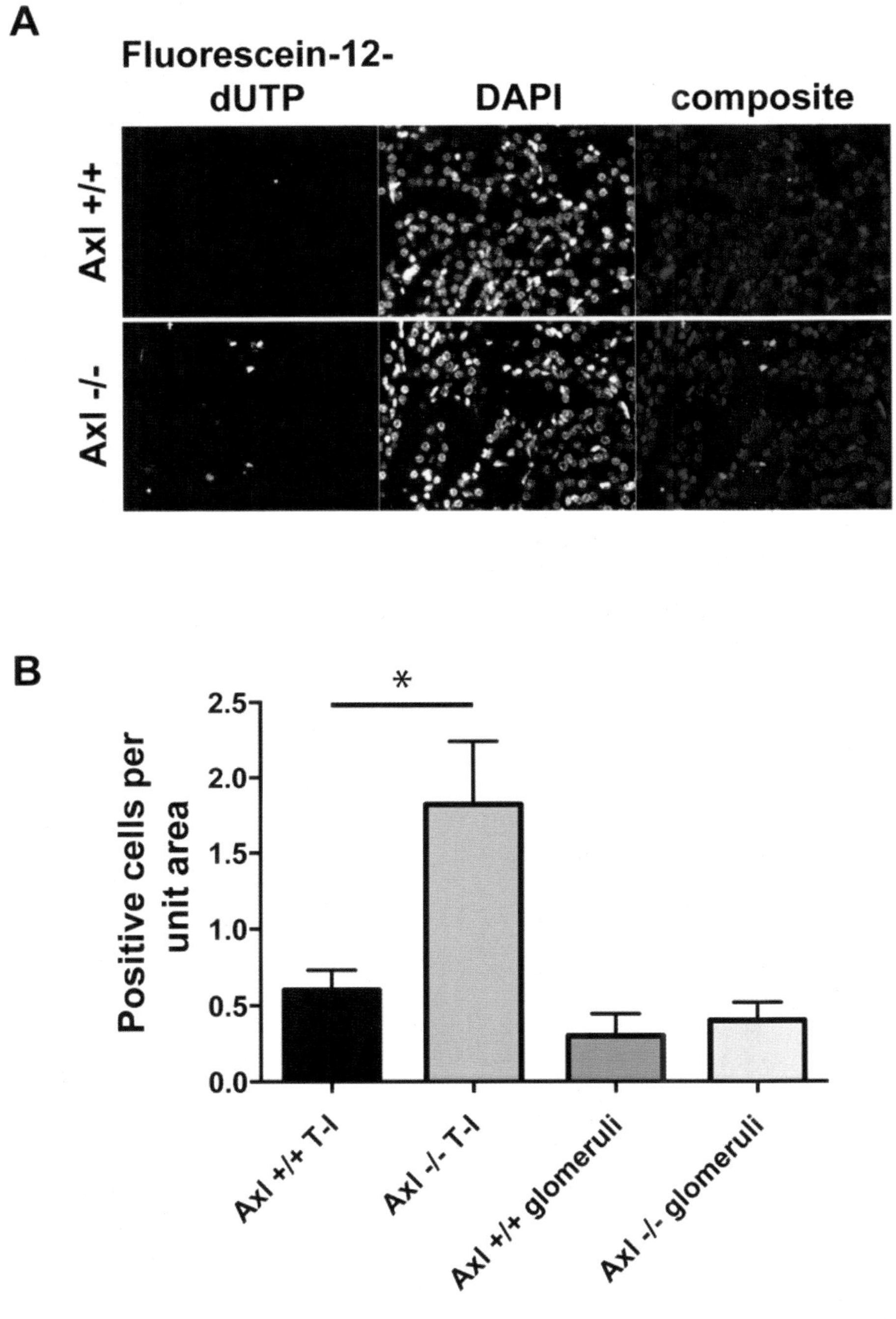

Figure 4.: Loss of Axl results in elevated renal tubulo-interstitial apoptosis. (A) Representative TUNEL- and DAPI-stained kidney sections post-sub-total nephrectomy and high phosphate diet. Tubulo-interstitial areas of the kidney are shown, bar = 50 microns. (B) Quantification of TUNEL staining expressed as mean +/− SEM, n = 10 per group. Statistical test is Student's *t*-test; ns = not significant, * = p≤0.05.

Table 2. Plasma phosphate and calcium concentrations.

	Baseline, no Nx (11 weeks of age)	14 weeks post Nx + elevated Phosphate (25 weeks of age)
Phosphate (mM)		
Female Axl+/+	1.51+/−0.11 (5)	1.78+/−0.21 (13) *
Male Axl+/+	2.02+/−0.38 (5)	2.66+/−1.24 (7)
Female Axl−/−	1.65+/−0.37 (4)	1.69+/−0.31 (8)
Male Axl−/−	1.98+/−0.38 (8)	1.74+/−0.23 (3)
Calcium (mM)		
Female Axl+/+	2.02+/−0.13 (5)	2.42+/−0.29 (13) *
Male Axl+/+	2.19+/−0.37 (5)	2.51+/−0.41 (7)
Female Axl−/−	2.12+/−0.14 (4)	2.3+/−0.22 (8)
Male Axl−/−	2.34+/−0.16 (8)	2.13+/−0.06 (3)

Plasma phosphate and calcium levels in mM +/− Std Dev, n number in brackets. Statistical test is Student's *t*-test, * = $p \leq 0.05$. Nx = nephrectomy.

diabetic nephropathy [11]. Conversely, increased Gas6/Axl signalling was associated with a protective tubular proliferative response in a podocyte ablation model of glomerular albuminuria [26].

Our data together with those of other groups, suggest that Gas6/Axl signalling potentiates toxin-induced glomerular inflammatory disease but has a protective function within the tubulo-interstitium, as identified here and in the podocyte-ablation model [26]. Renal Axl expression having a protective function in kidney pathology is also consistent with a recent report examining the role of haematopoietic and non-haematopoietic Axl in DOCA salt-induced hypertension and kidney dysfunction [29]. This study demonstrated that while haematopoietic Axl had a pathological role in the model, non-haematopoietic Axl protected against renal reactive oxygen species production [29].

Gas6 can also signal via Mertk and Tyro3 which are also expressed in the kidney [30,31]. Gas6 signalling via Mertk has been shown to be protective in the nephrotoxic nephritis model [32]. As we observed a significant reduction in plasma Gas6 concentrations in Axl−/− mice compared to Axl+/+ mice, we cannot rule out the contribution of reduced Gas6 signalling via Tyro3/Mertk to the phenotype we have characterised. It is also possible that loss of Axl modulates the expression of Tyro3/Mertk. The reduced Gas6 concentration in the Axl−/− mouse is seen in the basal state as well as the disease model. As a result, this finding has implications for all studies performed with the Axl−/− mouse when the phenotype has been attributed exclusively to reduced signalling via Axl.

Gender differences in the progression of CKD in patients [33,34,35] and in the rat nephrectomy model [36] have been documented previously. Here we also demonstrated clear differences between male and female nephrectomised mice. In Axl+/+ animals, sub-total nephrectomy resulted in an initial increase in uraemia which then stabilised for several weeks prior to a deterioration of only the male mice within the time frame of this study. In Axl−/− mice, both genders showed significantly elevated levels of uraemia compared to Axl+/+ mice 6 weeks post-initial surgery. However, male mice were generally unable to recover from this state, and progressed more rapidly to renal failure. Several mechanisms have been suggested to contribute to the more rapid progression of CKD in males. These include sex-dependent differences in kidney structure, glomerular hemodynamics and sex hormones. It has been proposed that estrogens have anti-apoptotic and anti-fibrotic effects on the kidney, whereas androgens promote renal apoptosis and fibrosis and thereby progression of renal disease [37,38].

One of the objectives of this study was to investigate the role of Axl in VC associated with CKD. Surprisingly, Axl−/− mice did not demonstrate hyperphosphataemia or hypercalcaemia at the end of the study. In the absence of a full endocrine profile and a detailed assessment of renal calcium and phosphate handling, it is difficult to say why this was the case. There may have been differences in intestinal uptake; similarly renal losses of phosphate and calcium may have been greater in the Axl−/− mice. In any case, significant VC was not induced in either Axl+/+ or Axl−/− animals in the time-frame we were able to examine. We had intended to feed the high phosphate diet for a longer period in order to induce calcification; however the profound effect of the loss of Axl on renal function led to the cessation of the study after 12 weeks of phosphate feeding. The genetic background of our mice (C57/SV129 mix) may also have contributed to their reduced susceptibility to VC. Mice on this genetic background have been used for similar *in vivo* studies previously [14], although the majority of published articles use female DBA/2J mice that are particularly susceptible to calcification [13,15,17]. Therefore, Axl's role in VC *in vivo* remains unresolved.

Although significant vascular calcification was not induced in the model, renal calcification was induced. The calcium deposition appeared to be consistent and to occur at the cortico-medullary boundary. The conditions within the tubules of the nephrectomised mice on a high phosphate diet (e.g. low tubular fluid flow rate, high phosphate concentration) are likely to favour crystal formation, so we speculate that the calcium deposits that we observed are precursors of renal stones. However without further detailed analysis of the calcium deposits seen in the remnant kidneys, this notion remains speculation.

Axl inhibitors have received much attention in recent years, particularly in the field of oncology [39,40]. While previous studies using Gas6−/− mice suggest that such inhibitors may be of therapeutic use in some renal pathology this article and previous work on Axl in VC [7,8,9,10] indicate that such inhibitors should be studied in humans with caution, particularly in patients with renal disease.

In conclusion we have identified for the first time the up-regulation of Axl as a protective mechanism in a murine model of CKD and demonstrate that it functions to reduce tubulo-interstitial apoptosis and slow the progression of renal failure.

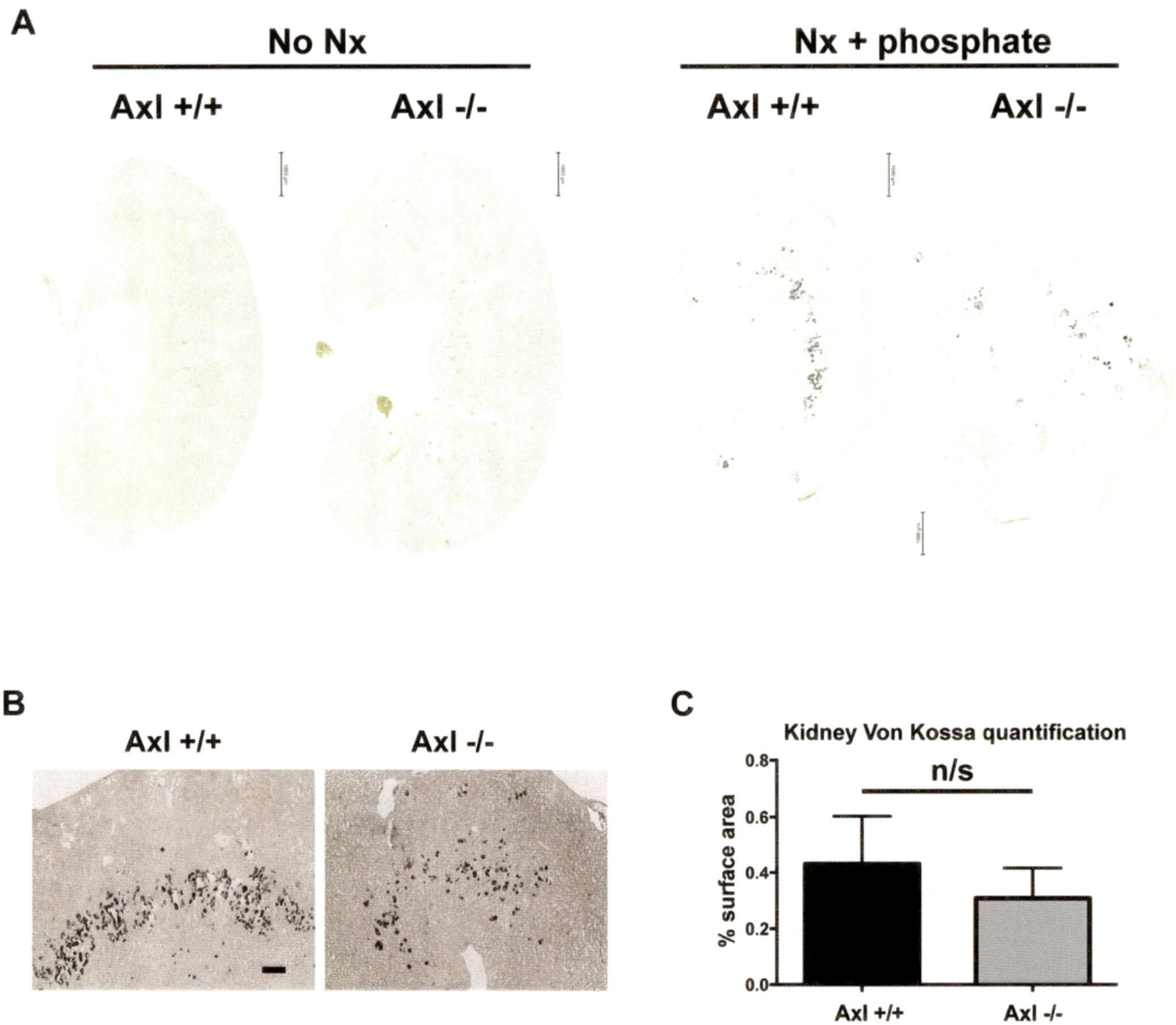

Figure 5. Loss of Axl did not affect the extent of renal calcification following sub-total nephrectomy and high phosphate diet. Histological analysis of kidney calcification (A) Representative scans of von Kossa stained sections from Axl+/+ and Axl−/− kidneys with and without nephrectomy and high phosphate diet. Bar = 1000 microns. (B) Magnified images of kidney calcification 14 weeks post-initial surgery. Bar = 200 microns. (C) Quantification of von Kossa staining, Axl+/+ n = 13, Axl−/− n = 15. Statistical test is Student's *t*-test. ns = not significant. Nx = nephrectomy.

Supporting Information

Figure S1 Histological analysis of Axl+/+ and Axl−/− kidneys pre- and post- sub-total nephrectomy and high phosphate diet. H&E stained sections of Axl+/+ and Axl−/− kidneys pre and post-nephrectomy (Nx) and high phosphate diet (14 weeks post initial surgery). Bar = 50 microns,

Figure S2 Loss of Axl does not modulate glomerular hypertrophy post sub-total nephrectomy and high phosphate diet. Representative H&E stained glomerular sections. Bar = 20 microns. Arrow indicates how maximal diameter of glomeruli was measured. (B) Quantification of mean maximal glomerular diameter. Axl+/+ n = 4, Axl −/− n = 3, Axl+/+ Nx n = 13, Axl −/− n = 15. Results expressed as means +/− SEM. Statistical test is a Kruskal-Wallis test with Dunn' compensation for multiple comparisons, * = $p \leq 0.05$.

Figure S3 Loss of Axl does not modulate renal collagen content post sub-total nephrectomy and high phosphate diet. (A) Representative images of picrosirius red stained kidney sections. Bar = 100 microns. (B) Frequency of positive picrosirius red staining in Axl+/+ and Axl−/− kidney post sub-total nephrectomy.

Acknowledgments

We are grateful to Mary Birch for performing the phosphate and calcium assays, Sally Price for pathological analysis of the kidney sections, Peter

March and Roger Meadows for their help with the bioimaging, and Rachel Lennon for critically reading the manuscript.

Author Contributions

Conceived and designed the experiments: GDH RFT NA SJB HSGW APG AEC. Performed the experiments: GDH RFT SJB HSGW. Analyzed the data: GDH RFT NA SJB HSGW APG AEC. Wrote the paper: GDH RFT NA SJB HSGW APG AEC.

References

1. Hodgkins KS, Schnaper HW (2012) Tubulointerstitial injury and the progression of chronic kidney disease. Pediatric nephrology 27: 901–909.
2. Blacher J, Guerin AP, Pannier B, Marchais SJ, London GM (2001) Arterial calcifications, arterial stiffness, and cardiovascular risk in end-stage renal disease. Hypertension 38: 938–942.
3. London GM, Guerin AP, Marchais SJ, Metivier F, Pannier B, et al. (2003) Arterial media calcification in end-stage renal disease: impact on all-cause and cardiovascular mortality. Nephrology, dialysis, transplantation: official publication of the European Dialysis and Transplant Association - European Renal Association 18: 1731–1740.
4. Okuno S, Ishimura E, Kitatani K, Fujino Y, Kohno K, et al. (2007) Presence of abdominal aortic calcification is significantly associated with all-cause and cardiovascular mortality in maintenance hemodialysis patients. American journal of kidney diseases: the official journal of the National Kidney Foundation 49: 417–425.
5. Hafizi S, Dahlback B (2006) Signalling and functional diversity within the Axl subfamily of receptor tyrosine kinases. Cytokine & growth factor reviews 17: 295–304.
6. Korshunov VA (2012) Axl-dependent signalling: a clinical update. Clinical science 122: 361–368.
7. Collett G, Wood A, Alexander MY, Varnum BC, Boot-Handford RP, et al. (2003) Receptor tyrosine kinase Axl modulates the osteogenic differentiation of pericytes. Circulation research 92: 1123–1129.
8. Collett GD, Sage AP, Kirton JP, Alexander MY, Gilmore AP, et al. (2007) Axl/phosphatidylinositol 3-kinase signaling inhibits mineral deposition by vascular smooth muscle cells. Circulation research 100: 502–509.
9. Son BK, Kozaki K, Iijima K, Eto M, Kojima T, et al. (2006) Statins protect human aortic smooth muscle cells from inorganic phosphate-induced calcification by restoring Gas6-Axl survival pathway. Circulation research 98: 1024–1031.
10. Son BK, Kozaki K, Iijima K, Eto M, Nakano T, et al. (2007) Gas6/Axl-PI3K/Akt pathway plays a central role in the effect of statins on inorganic phosphate-induced calcification of vascular smooth muscle cells. European journal of pharmacology 556: 1–8.
11. Nagai K, Arai H, Yanagita M, Matsubara T, Kanamori H, et al. (2003) Growth arrest-specific gene 6 is involved in glomerular hypertrophy in the early stage of diabetic nephropathy. The Journal of biological chemistry 278: 18229–18234.
12. Yanagita M, Ishimoto Y, Arai H, Nagai K, Ito T, et al. (2002) Essential role of Gas6 for glomerular injury in nephrotoxic nephritis. The Journal of clinical investigation 110: 239–246.
13. El-Abbadi MM, Pai AS, Leaf EM, Yang HY, Bartley BA, et al. (2009) Phosphate feeding induces arterial medial calcification in uremic mice: role of serum phosphorus, fibroblast growth factor-23, and osteopontin. Kidney international 75: 1297–1307.
14. Hu MC, Shi M, Zhang J, Quinones H, Griffith C, et al. (2011) Klotho deficiency causes vascular calcification in chronic kidney disease. Journal of the American Society of Nephrology: JASN 22: 124–136.
15. Lau WL, Leaf EM, Hu MC, Takeno MM, Kuro-o M, et al. (2012) Vitamin D receptor agonists increase klotho and osteopontin while decreasing aortic calcification in mice with chronic kidney disease fed a high phosphate diet. Kidney international 82: 1261–1270.
16. Li KL, Chen J, Li ZH, Zhao L, He YN (2012) p53 negatively regulates the osteogenic differentiation of vascular smooth muscle cells in mice with chronic kidney disease. Cardiovascular journal of Africa 23: e1–9.
17. Pai A, Leaf EM, El-Abbadi M, Giachelli CM (2011) Elastin degradation and vascular smooth muscle cell phenotype change precede cell loss and arterial medial calcification in a uremic mouse model of chronic kidney disease. The American journal of pathology 178: 764–773.
18. Westenfeld R, Schafer C, Smeets R, Brandenburg VM, Floege J, et al. (2007) Fetuin-A (AHSG) prevents extraosseous calcification induced by uraemia and phosphate challenge in mice. Nephrology, dialysis, transplantation: official publication of the European Dialysis and Transplant Association - European Renal Association 22: 1537–1546.
19. Lu Q, Gore M, Zhang Q, Camenisch T, Boast S, et al. (1999) Tyro-3 family receptors are essential regulators of mammalian spermatogenesis. Nature 398: 723–728.
20. Nagai K, Matsubara T, Mima A, Sumi E, Kanamori H, et al. (2005) Gas6 induces Akt/mTOR-mediated mesangial hypertrophy in diabetic nephropathy. Kidney international 68: 552–561.
21. Yanagita M, Arai H, Ishii K, Nakano T, Ohashi K, et al. (2001) Gas6 regulates mesangial cell proliferation through Axl in experimental glomerulonephritis. The American journal of pathology 158: 1423–1432.
22. Yanagita M, Ishii K, Ozaki H, Arai H, Nakano T, et al. (1999) Mechanism of inhibitory effect of warfarin on mesangial cell proliferation. Journal of the American Society of Nephrology; JASN 10: 2503–2509.
23. Shanahan CM, Crouthamel MH, Kapustin A, Giachelli CM (2011) Arterial calcification in chronic kidney disease: key roles for calcium and phosphate. Circulation research 109: 697–711.
24. Nath KA (1992) Tubulointerstitial changes as a major determinant in the progression of renal damage. American journal of kidney diseases: the official journal of the National Kidney Foundation 20: 1–17.
25. Fiebeler A, Park JK, Muller DN, Lindschau C, Mengel M, et al. (2004) Growth arrest specific protein 6/Axl signaling in human inflammatory renal diseases. American journal of kidney diseases: the official journal of the National Kidney Foundation 43: 286–295.
26. Guo JK, Marlier A, Shi H, Shan A, Ardito TA, et al. (2012) Increased tubular proliferation as an adaptive response to glomerular albuminuria. Journal of the American Society of Nephrology: JASN 23: 429–437.
27. Nagai K, Miyoshi M, Kake T, Fukushima N, Matsuura M, et al. (2013) Dual involvement of growth arrest-specific gene 6 in the early phase of human IgA nephropathy. PloS one 8: e66759.
28. Lee IJ, Hilliard B, Swami A, Madara JC, Rao S, et al. (2012) Growth arrest-specific gene 6 (Gas6) levels are elevated in patients with chronic renal failure. Nephrology, dialysis, transplantation: official publication of the European Dialysis and Transplant Association - European Renal Association 27: 4166–4172.
29. Batchu SN, Hughson A, Gerloff J, Fowell DJ, Korshunov VA (2013) Role of axl in early kidney inflammation and progression of salt-dependent hypertension. Hypertension 62: 302–309.
30. Yin JL, Hambly BD, Bao SS, Painter D, Bishop GA, et al. (2003) Expression of growth arrest-specific gene 6 and its receptors in dysfunctional human renal allografts. Transplant international: official journal of the European Society for Organ Transplantation 16: 681–688.
31. Yin JL, Pilmore HL, Yan YQ, McCaughan GW, Bishop GA, et al. (2002) Expression of growth arrest-specific gene 6 and its receptors in a rat model of chronic renal transplant rejection. Transplantation 73: 657–660.
32. Shao WH, Zhen Y, Rosenbaum J, Eisenberg RA, McGaha TL, et al. (2010) A protective role of Mer receptor tyrosine kinase in nephrotoxic serum-induced nephritis. Clinical immunology 136: 236–244.
33. Eriksen BO, Ingebretsen OC (2006) The progression of chronic kidney disease: a 10-year population-based study of the effects of gender and age. Kidney international 69: 375–382.
34. Halbesma N, Brantsma AH, Bakker SJ, Jansen DF, Stolk RP, et al. (2008) Gender differences in predictors of the decline of renal function in the general population. Kidney international 74: 505–512.
35. Neugarten J, Acharya A, Silbiger SR (2000) Effect of gender on the progression of nondiabetic renal disease: a meta-analysis. Journal of the American Society of Nephrology: JASN 11: 319–329.
36. Lemos CC, Mandarim-de-Lacerda CA, Dorigo D, Coimbra TM, Bregman R (2005) Chronic renal failure in male and female rats. Journal of nephrology 18: 368–373.
37. Carrero JJ (2010) Gender differences in chronic kidney disease: underpinnings and therapeutic implications. Kidney & blood pressure research 33: 383–392.
38. Silbiger S, Neugarten J (2008) Gender and human chronic renal disease. Gender medicine 5 Suppl A: S3–S10.
39. Linger RM, Keating AK, Earp HS, Graham DK (2010) Taking aim at Mer and Axl receptor tyrosine kinases as novel therapeutic targets in solid tumors. Expert opinion on therapeutic targets 14: 1073–1090.
40. Verma A, Warner SL, Vankayalapati H, Bearss DJ, Sharma S (2011) Targeting Axl and Mer kinases in cancer. Molecular cancer therapeutics 10: 1763–1773.

4

The Need for Improved Identification and Accurate Classification of Stages 3–5 Chronic Kidney Disease in Primary Care: Retrospective Cohort Study

Poorva Jain[1]*, Melanie Calvert[1], Paul Cockwell[2,3], Richard J. McManus[4]

1 Primary Care Clinical Sciences, NIHR School of Primary Care Research, University of Birmingham, Birmingham, United Kingdom, 2 Department of Renal Medicine, Queen Elizabeth Hospital Birmingham, University Hospital Birmingham, Birmingham, United Kingdom, 3 Division of Immunity and Infection, Medical School, University of Birmingham, Birmingham, United Kingdom, 4 Department of Primary Care Health Sciences, NIHR School of Primary Care Research, University of Oxford, Oxford, United Kingdom

Abstract

Background: Around ten percent of the population have been reported as having Chronic Kidney Disease (CKD), which is associated with increased cardiovascular mortality. Few previous studies have ascertained the chronicity of CKD. In the UK, a payment for performance (P4P) initiative incentivizes CKD (stages 3–5) recognition and management in primary care, but the impact of this has not been assessed.

Methods and Findings: Using data from 426 primary care practices (population 2,707,130), the age standardised prevalence of stages 3–5 CKD was identified using two consecutive estimated Glomerular Filtration Rates (eGFRs) seven days apart. Additionally the accuracy of practice CKD registers and the relationship between accurate identification of CKD and the achievement of P4P indicators was determined. Between 2005 and 2009, the prevalence of stages 3–5 CKD increased from 0.3% to 3.9%. In 2009, 30,440 patients (1.1% unadjusted) fulfilled biochemical criteria for CKD but were not on a practice CKD register (uncoded CKD) and 60,705 patients (2.2% unadjusted) were included on a practice CKD register but did not fulfil biochemical criteria (miscoded CKD). For patients with confirmed CKD, inclusion in a practice register was associated with increasing age, male sex, diabetes, hypertension, cardiovascular disease and increasing CKD stage ($p<0.0001$). Uncoded CKD patients compared to miscoded patients were less likely to achieve performance indicators for blood pressure (OR 0.84, 95% CI 0.82–0.86 $p<0.001$) or recorded albumin-creatinine ratio (OR 0.73, 0.70–0.76, $p<0.001$).

Conclusions: The prevalence of stages 3–5 CKD, using two laboratory reported eGFRs, was lower than estimates from previous studies. Clinically significant discrepancies were identified between biochemically defined CKD and appearance on practice registers, with misclassification associated with sub-optimal care for some people with CKD.

Editor: Darwin Ang, University of South Florida, United States of America

Funding: RJM and PJ were funded as part of an NIHR Career Development Fellowship awarded to RJM. The funders had no role in study design, data collection and analysis, decision to publish, or preparation of the manuscript. The views expressed in this paper are those of the authors and not necessarily those of the NHS, the NIHR or the Department of Health.

Competing Interests: The authors have declared that no competing interests exist.

* Email: p.jain@bham.ac.uk

Introduction

Chronic Kidney Disease (CKD) is defined by a reduced glomerular filtration rate (GFR) and/or evidence of kidney damage and in clinical practice a reduced eGFR is usually estimated using the Modification of Diet in Renal Disease (MDRD) four-variable equation [1]. Patients with an eGFR below 60 mls/min/1.73 m^2 (stages 3–5 CKD) are at increased risk of cardiovascular disease (CVD), in comparison to the general population [2–4]. Between 2009–2010, CKD accounted for 1.3% of the UK health care budget directly and indirectly up to 25% of the healthcare budget in the United States in patients aged over 65 [5,6]. In the past decade there have been sustained efforts to improve the identification, management and monitoring of CKD [7]. In the UK this has included the incorporation of stages 3–5 CKD into the Quality and Outcomes Framework (QOF), a primary care based pay for performance system (P4P) [8,9]. Incentivised payments within the CKD domain depend on blood pressure control and appropriate prescribing [10].

Previous estimates of the prevalence of stages 3–5 CKD have varied widely (depending on the methodology) from 4.3% (all clinically coded patients in QOF) to 8.5% in UK primary care databases [11]. Potential sources of bias include ascertainment problems (reliance on coding, limited coverage of population), intra patient variation in renal function (single eGFR likely to overestimate prevalence) and intra-laboratory variation (use of raw creatinines to calculate eGFR does not take into account calibration issues between labs) [12]. Accurate identification and subsequent clinical coding of CKD is important, as previous work suggests that inclusion on a chronic disease register affects quality of care [13].

This study aimed to determine the prevalence of stages 3–5 CKD based on objective evidence from at least two laboratory reported eGFRs and to assess the accuracy of QOF CKD (stages 3–5) registers on this basis. The quality of care for patients with stages 3–5 CKD was compared between those who were included on a CKD register and those who had laboratory evidence of stages 3–5 CKD but were not included on a register.

Materials and Methods

Data source

A retrospective cohort study was undertaken using anonymised records from The Health Improvement Network (THIN) database. In brief this is a large UK primary care database that contains data from patients registered in 426 primary care centres using VISION clinical software; in 2009 2.7 million patients were included [14]. The THIN database has previously been validated for use in pharmaco-epidemiological research [14,15]. Permission to obtain and analyse this data has to be sought from the THIN Scientific Review Committee and was granted for our study in May 2010 (reference number 10-006).

Data were extracted from the THIN database concerning renal function, age (on 1st April of the year of the prevalence estimate), registration status, gender, Read codes indicating co-morbidity (cardiovascular disease, diabetes, hypertension, chronic kidney disease, and hypercholesterolemia) and cardiovascular risk factors (smoking status, blood pressure, ACR and total cholesterol). Read codes are a system of hierarchal clinical codes that specify types of diseases, symptoms, diagnoses or other medical information from consultations or letters. Co-morbidities were defined using previously described code groupings and the authors' clinical expertise [16,17].

Prevalence: study population

Adults with stages 3–5 CKD, permanently registered on the THIN database for a minimum of six months, were identified if the last two laboratory eGFRs in each UK financial year (April – March) between 2005 and 2009, taken at least seven days apart, were both <60 ml/min/1.73 m^2 (Figure 1). This definition was used as a pragmatic operationalization of UK pay for performance (QOF) guidance which states that stages 3–5 CKD is defined as an eGFR <60 mls/min/1.73 m^2 "...confirmed with at least two separate readings over a three month period". Note this is different to the KDIGO/KDOQI definition of CKD [7,18]. Ethnicity data were not available for the large majority of patients who were therefore assumed to be not of black ethnicity [19].

Patients identified as having CKD in a given year could be reclassified in following years if their eGFRs changed. Where two laboratory eGFRs were in different CKD stages, the lowest corresponding CKD stage was used; i.e. the more conservative estimate. Patients with a laboratory biochemical definition of stages 3 -5 CKD were defined as having confirmed CKD (Figure 1) for use in the subsequent QOF CKD disease register analysis. In common with previous work, people without a kidney function measurement were assumed not to have CKD [20].

QOF outcomes: population

This analysis considered QOF performance between April 2008 and March 2009 and included risk factor data from January 2008. Stages 3–5 CKD was defined on the basis of laboratory eGFRs, to avoid issues with laboratory to laboratory variation and assuming that practices had not calculated eGFR themselves. Appearance on practice CKD registers was defined by a relevant clinical (Read) code specified by the UK pay for performance, QOF business rules which include only patients with stages 3–5 CKD [16]. On this basis, patients were categorised as having either 'confirmed CKD' or 'labelled CKD' dependent on biochemical evidence and/or Read coding. These were further divided into subgroups of 'appropriately coded' CKD patients, 'uncoded CKD patients' or 'miscoded CKD patients' as defined below.

- **Confirmed CKD:** sustained biochemical evidence of stages 3–5 CKD, i.e. a laboratory eGFR under 60 mls/min/1.73 m^2 on the last two consecutive eGFRs before 1st April 2009 that were at least seven days apart.
- **Labelled CKD:** patients recorded as having stages 3–5 CKD by a Read code according to the UK pay for performance (QOF) Business Rules [10,21].
- **Appropriately coded:** patients with both a Read Code for CKD and biochemical evidence of an eGFR under 60 mls/min/1.73 m^3 on the last two consecutive eGFRs before 1st April 2009 that were at least seven days apart.
- **Uncoded CKD:** patients with biochemical evidence of stages 3–5 CKD but no CKD Read code entered into their records.
- **Miscoded CKD:** patients with a Read code for stages 3–5 CKD but no biochemical evidence of stages 3–5 CKD (using above definition).

Statistical analyses

The prevalence of CKD was ascertained and tabulated by stage and year for the years 2005–2009. Prevalence estimates were age standardised using the relevant Office of National Statistics yearly estimates of age and gender distribution for the United Kingdom and 95% confidence intervals were calculated [22]. The management of each subgroup according to the CKD indicators of the QOF for the period of 1st January 2008 and 1st of April 2009 was evaluated [16].

Factors associated with the likelihood of being excluded from the practice CKD register were analysed in two subgroups:

- uncoded compared to appropriately coded
- uncoded compared to miscoded

These subgroups were examined in two multivariable models using backward stepwise selection ($\alpha = 0.05$ as criteria for model inclusion). Multivariable models allow a series of factors to be assessed simultaneously to take into account possible confounding. Non-linear functional forms were considered for continuous candidate variables. More complex functional forms were included in the final model only when they provided a statistically significantly improved model fit assessed using Akaike's Information Criterion [23]. The final model included the selected variables in a mixed linear model with logit link and with general practice as a random effect to account for clustering [24,25].

The following pre-specified explanatory variables were included in the backwards selection process: age, gender, Townsend quintiles, coronary heart disease, stroke, peripheral vascular disease, cardiovascular disease (coronary heart disease, stroke, peripheral vascular disease combined), hypertension, diabetes mellitus, smoking status and hypercholesterolaemia.

Achievement for each quality indicator was compared between miscoded and uncoded CKD patients using Pearson Chi-Square tests. Blood pressure and cholesterol comparisons were carried out using t-tests or Mann Whitney tests depending on the distribution of the variable.

All statistical analyses were performed in SAS v9.2 (Cary, USA).

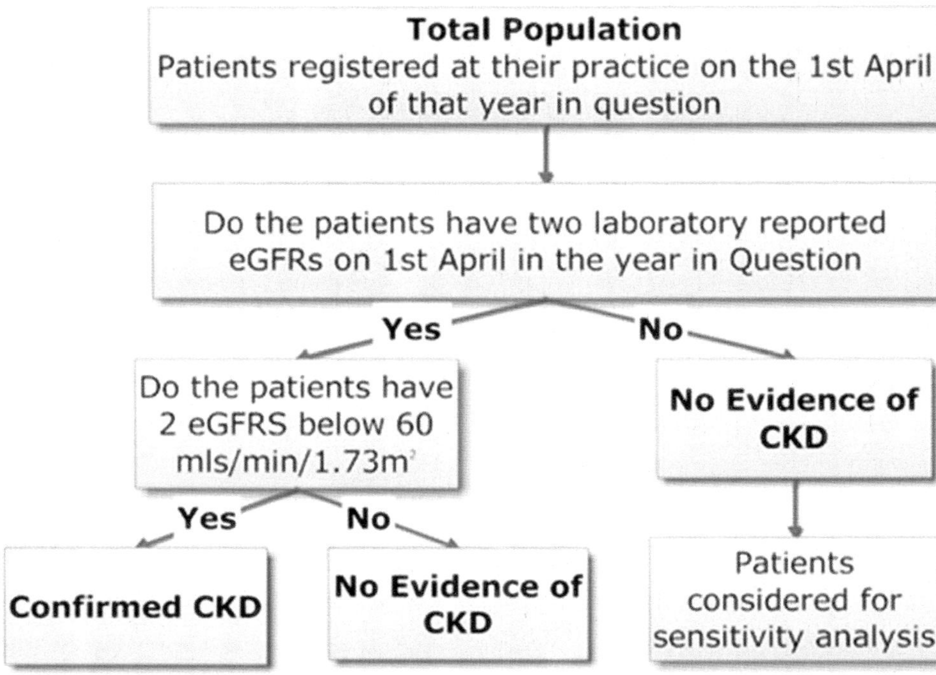

Figure 1. The definition of Stages 3–5 CKD in the prevalence cohort.

Sensitivity Analysis

A separate sensitivity analysis ascertained the prevalence of stage 3–5 CKD from the last two consecutive creatinines, taken at least 7 days apart, utilising the four variable MDRD equation to calculate the eGFR, when laboratory eGFRs were not available [26]. This analysis was undertaken as it was anticipated that prior to 2007 many patients would not have reported laboratory eGFR. The standardised Isotope Dilution Mass Spectrometry (IDMS) method for creatinine measurement was in use in less than 50% of UK laboratories during the study timeframe hence it was assumed that this method had not been used [12].

Results

Results were adjusted for age and gender where possible but are presented as crude proportions where this is not stated.

Prevalence of Chronic Kidney Disease

Between 2005 and 2009, the number of patients with two lab eGFRs, at least seven days apart, in the given year increased from 53 176(2%) to 614 590 (23%). The median time apart from each laboratory report in our study was 171 days (Interquartile range 56–351 days) and by 2009 this was 280 days (125–425 days). The age and gender adjusted prevalence of stages 3–5 CKD increased from 0.28% (95% CI 0.28 to 0.29) to 3.93% (3.91 to 3.95) between 2005 and 2009 (Figure 2). The majority of patients had stage 3a CKD with an adjusted prevalence in 2009 of 2.86% (2.84 to 2.87), followed by stage 3b CKD (0.86%, 0.86 to 0.87), stage 4 CKD (0.18%, 0.176 to 0.184) and stage 5 CKD (0.03, CI 0.28 to 0.03).

Practice Registers of CKD

In 2009, 108 911/2 701 730 (4.03% 95% CI 4.01–4.05) of the adult population had biochemically confirmed chronic kidney disease (see methods for definitions) and 139 176 (5.15%, 95% CI 5.13–5.18) appeared on practice registers (labelled CKD) [Table 1]. Of those with biochemically confirmed CKD, 78 471/108 911 (72.1%, 95% CI 71.8–72.3) were labelled with a Read code for stages 3–5 CKD. A further 60 705/139 176 (43.6%, 95% CI 43.3–43.9) of labelled CKD patients had a Read code but no biochemical evidence of stages 3–5 CKD (i.e. were miscoded) and 30 440/108 911 (27.9%, 95% CI 27.7–28.2%) fulfilled biochemical criteria for stages 3–5 CKD but were not on a practice CKD register (uncoded CKD). The demographic and clinical features are shown in Table 1.

Multivariable analysis

In the multivariable analyses, uncoded CKD patients in comparison with appropriately coded patients were more likely to be younger (for an increase in one year of age OR 0.991, 95% CI 0.989–0.993), female (OR 1.20, 95% CI 1.16–1.25), have no comorbidity and have a lower CKD stage [Table 2].

In the second model uncoded patients were more likely to be older (for every year increase, OR 1.027, 95% CI 1.026–1.208), have hypertension (OR 1.11, 95% CI 1.02–1.15), cardiovascular disease (OR 1.21, 95% CI 1.13–1.30), and to smoke (OR 1.21, 95% CI 1.16–1.30) compared to miscoded patients. They were less likely to have diabetes (OR 0.84, 95% CI 0.77–0.89), coronary heart disease (OR 0.80, 95% CI 0.74–0.86), and have hypercholesterolaemia (OR 0.90, 95% CI 0.84–0.97) [Table 2].

Pay for Performance

The management of CKD patients according to QOF P4P indicators is shown in Table 3. There was significant underachievement in QOF outcomes in the uncoded CKD group compared to both the miscoded CKD group and the appropriately coded CKD group: uncoded CKD patients were less likely to have a blood pressure measurement (90% versus 91% in miscoded group, $p<0.0001$, 90% vs. 97% in appropriately coded group, $p<0.0001$), a blood pressure on target (47% vs. 51%, $p<0.0001$, 47% vs. 55%, $p<0.0001$). or have an albumin-creatinine ratio recorded

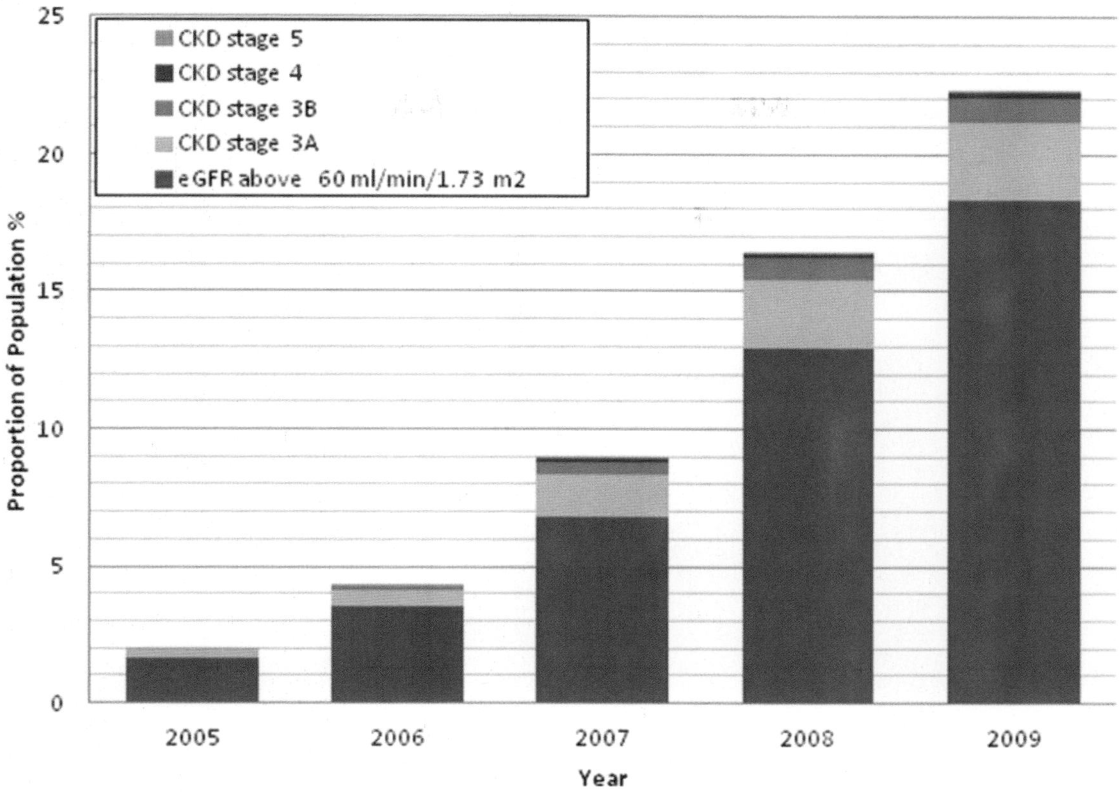

Figure 2. Age standardised prevalence (%) of stages 3–5 CKD from 2005–2009. CKD stage was defined by the last two consecutive laboratory eGFRS at least seven days apart in the year in question. Note figures are approximated to the nearest decimal place and therefore may be slightly different from the total figure.

(12% vs. 16%, p<0.0001, 12% vs. 20%, p<0.0001). Mean systolic blood pressure, in mmHg, was significantly higher in patients with uncoded CKD [136.2 (95% CI 136.0 to 136.4)/75.8 (75.7 to 75.9) compared to miscoded CKD 134.5 (134.3 to 134.6)/76.3 (75.0 to 75.1)]. Cholesterol was measured in 92% of individuals regardless of group. There was no difference in serum cholesterol level between miscoded and uncoded CKD (median cholesterol 4.7 vs. 4.7 mmol/l, p = 0.9455). All patients with proteinuria as defined by an ACR ≥30 mg/mmol and with a Read code for hypertension (n = 1018) were on angiotensin blockade regardless of CKD coding [Table 3].

Sensitivity Analysis including calculated eGFR from serum creatinine. Inclusion of patients with stages 3–5 CKD calculated from two consecutive serum creatinine results seven days apart gave an adult adjusted prevalence of 4.05% (95% CI 4.03 to 4.10%) in 2005 and 4.66% (95% CI 4.64 to 4.69%) in 2009, peaking at 5.00% (95% CI 4.97 to 5.02%) in 2007. [Figure 3].

Discussion

This large primary care based database study has found evidence that the current management of stages 3–5 CKD in UK primary care is systemically suboptimal. Major misclassification of individuals with stages 3–5 CKD was found including both inappropriate labelling as stages 3–5 CKD of those without evidence of stages 3–5 CKD and no labelling of stages 3–5 CKD of others with clear evidence of a reduced eGFR. The finding of an age adjusted prevalence of stages 3–5 CKD in the UK by laboratory reported estimated GFR of 4% in 2008–9, using a definition requiring a confirmed reduction in eGFR to <60 ml/min/1.73 m^2, was lower than most previous UK primary care estimates of between 4.1 and 8.5% which included patients classified on the basis of a single available eGFR [10,11,20,27].

In patients with stages 3–5 CKD, exclusion from the practice CKD register ('uncoded' CKD), was associated with decreasing age, female gender, less co-morbidity (with the exception of hypercholesterolaemia) and lower CKD stage. When comparing uncoded patients with miscoded patients, uncoded patients were less likely to have cardiovascular disease and diabetes but more likely to have hypertension, be older and smoke.

The widespread misclassification shown by this study is important: individuals without an appropriate Read code, despite increased co-morbidity, were less likely to have received adequate care as defined by UK pay for performance targets. Comparison of outcomes for two cardiovascular risk factors (blood pressure and cholesterol) provides some evidence that clinical coding mediates performance for QOF P4P indicators. Uncoded stages 3–5 CKD patients had worse blood pressure control (included in QOF) but similar cholesterol levels (not in QOF) in comparison to miscoded stages 3–5 CKD patients. This also suggests an inappropriate targeting of resources away from individuals in need which could be reversed by better identification of stages 3–5 CKD without increasing workload.

In the sensitivity analysis where patients with either two lab eGFRs or two calculated eGFRs were included the prevalence in 2009 varied from 4% to 4.7%. This suggests a further potential cause of misclassification where laboratory reported eGFR is not available.

Table 1. Demographics of CKD patients between 1st January 2008 to 1st April 2009 (The proportions in brackets are not adjusted and crude percentages).

	Total Population	Patients with biochemical evidence of CKD[a]	Practice CKD Register (with or without biochemical evidence)[b]	Patients on CKD register with biochemical evidence[c]	Practice CKD Register but no biochemical evidence of Stages 3–5 CKD[d]	Patients with biochemical evidence of CKD not on Practice Register[e]
True CKD status	Baseline Population	Confirmed CKD	Labelled CKD	Appropriately coded CKD	Miscoded CKD	Uncoded CKD
Number (crude %)	2 707 130 (100)	108 911 (4.0%)	139 176 (5.1%)	78 471 (2.9%))	60 705 (2.2%)	30 440 (1.1%)
Age in years (median (IQR))	47(19–114)	79(19–106)	76 (19–106)	78 (19–106)	71(19–105)	76(19–105)
Female Gender	1378 422(51%)	67 352 (62%)	82 949 (60%)	47 666(60%)	35 283 (58%)	19 686 (65%)
Ethnic Group[f]						
Black	11 329(0.40%)	528 (0.48%)	592(0.43%)	324(0.41%)	268(0.44%)	204(0.67%)
White	355 121(13%)	25 381 (23%)	29 820(21.4%)	18 764(23%)	11 056(18%)	6617(21%)
South Asian	20 032(0.70%)	594 (0.54%)	1051(0.76%)	468(0.59%)	583(0.96%)	126(0.41%)
Diabetes Mellitus[gf]	174 622(6%)	26 985 (25%)	33 083(23%)	20 970(26%)	12 113(20%)	6015(19%)
Hypertension	413 235(16%)	63 917(59%)	73 037(52%)	48 587(62%)	24 450(40%)	15 330 (50%)
CHD[gf]	158 701(6%)	31 234(29%)	35 471(25%)	24 254(30.8%)	11 217(18%)	6980(23%)
PVD[gf]	35 033(1%)	8330(8%)	9011(6%)	6656(8.5%)	2355(4%)	1674(5.5%)
Stroke[gf]	67 075(3%)	14 339((13%)	15 370(11%)	11 020(13.9%)	4350(7%)	3319(11%)
Ever Smoked	446 034(17%)	20 805(19%)	24 301(17%)	15 296(19%)	9005(15%)	5509(18%)

[a]Patients with two consecutive eGFRS under 60 at least seven days apart.
[b]Patients with a QOF business Rule Read code for Chronic Kidney Disease.
[c]Patients with 2 consecutive eGFRS <60 at least 7 days apart and a QOF business rule Read code.
[d]Patients with a QOF business Rule Read code for CKD but no sustained eGFRs below 60.
[e]Patients with 2 consecutive eGFRS <60 at least 7 days apart but no QOF Read code for CKD.
[f]Where reported as not all patients have Ethnic group reported.
[g]Diabetes Mellitus – Type 1&2, CHD = Coronary Heart Disease, PVD = peripheral vascular disease.

Table 2. Multivariate Logistic Regression Model for significant predictors for inclusion on CKD QOF register.

Risk Factor	Odds Ratio of Uncoded CKD compared to appropriately Coded CKD	Odds Ratio of Uncoded CKD compared to miscoded CKD
	Odds Ratio (95% CI)	**Odds Ratio (95% CI)**
Age[i]	0.991(0.990–0.993)	1.027(1.026–1.028)*
Female sex[ii]	1.20(1.16–1.24)	1.23(1.17–1.26)*
CKD stage		NA
3a[iii]	1*	
3b	0.37(0.35–0.38)	
4	0.24(0.22–0.27)	
5	0.24(0.19–0.31)	
Coronary Heart Disease[iv]	0.81(0.76–0.86)*	0.80(0.74–0.86)*
Hypertension[iv]	0.61(0.59–0.63)*	1.11(1.02–1.15)*
Diabetes Mellitus	0.72(0.69–0.75)*	0.84(0.77–0.89)*
Cardiovascular Disease(composite of Coronary Heart Disease, Peripheral Vascular Disease and Stroke)	0.83(0.78–0.88)*	1.21(1.13–1.30)*
Peripheral Vascular Disease[iv]	0.88(0.82–0.95)*	NS
Hypercholesterolaemia[iv]	0.80(0.76–0.84)*	0.90(0.84–0.97)*
Smoking[iv]	NS	1.21(1.16–1.30)*

*$p < 0.0001$.
[i]For an increase in years from the mean age.
[ii]In comparison with male gender.
[iii]Indicates the reference indicator.
[iv]The presence of the disease in comparison to those without it. The disease was ascertained by having a Read code for the disease.

Table 3. CKD Management according to QOF standards between 1st January 2008 to 1st April 2009[+].

	Patients with biochemical evidence of CKD[a]	Practice CKD Register(with or without biochemical evidence)[b]	Patients on CKD register with biochemical evidence[c]	Practice CKD Register but no biochemical evidence of Stages 3-5 CKD[d]	Patients with biochemical evidence of CKD not on Practice Register[e]
True CKD status	Confirmed CKD	Labelled CKD	Appropriately coded CKD	Miscoded CKD	Uncoded CKD
Total Number	108 911	139 176	78 471	60 705	30 440
Proportion with Blood pressure in last 15 months*	104 213(96%)	132 343(95%)	76 602(97%)	55 741(91%)	27 611(90%)
Patients whose last BP is less than 140/85 in last 15 months*	57 169(52%)	73 852(53%)	42 986(55%)	30 866(51%)	14 183(47%)
Patients with CKD who have an ACR*	19 483(18%)	25 445(18%)	15 806(20%)	9639(16%)	3677(12%)
Patients with CKD who have Proteinuria *	1358(1.2%)	1474(0.9%)	1153(1.4%)	320(0.5%)	205(0.7%)
Patients with Hypertension and proteinuria (ACR>30) on angiotensin blockade*	1018(100%)	1073(100%)	883(100%)	190(100%)	135(100%)

[a]Patients with two consecutive eGFRS under 60 at least seven days apart.
[b]Patients with a QOF business Rule Read code for CKD.
[c]Patients with two consecutive eGFRS under 60 at least seven days apart and a QOF business rule Read code.
[d]Patients with a QOF business Rule Read code for CKD but no sustained eGFRs below 60.
[e]Patients with two consecutive eGFRS under 60 at least seven days apart but no QOF business Rule Read code for CKD.
Proportions quoted are of the total in that group.
*When comparing groups d and e/c and e, $p<0.0001$.
[+]QOF pay for performance business rules look back 15 months hence time period.

Strengths and Limitations

This is the largest UK cohort study to date to examine stages 3–5 CKD prevalence and comprised approximately 4% of the total UK population. Accounting for the chronicity of stages 3–5 CKD by using two laboratory results rather than a single point estimate has allowed the true burden of stages 3–5 CKD to be more clearly estimated. Although the study aimed to capture stages 3–5 CKD patients diagnosed according to the QOF guidelines, by 2009 the majority of patients diagnosed with stages 3–5 CKD would meet the KDIGO/KDOQI guidelines with lab eGFRs over 90 days apart. It is however possible that some patients who met the QOF guidelines for CKD in fact had acute kidney injury hence did not have CKD on two samples more than three months apart and these would have been incorrectly categorised as miscoded by our study. The methodology differs from other studies by reporting stages 3–5 CKD stages using laboratory reported eGFR, thereby reducing the variation of calculated eGFR due to different creatinine assays [1].

In this study we have performed a multivariable model with a random effects term for primary care practice location, to determine which factors are independently associated with exclusion from the practice register. This model is the most favourable as it takes into account clustering at the practice level.

A limitation of the use of routine data is that 77% of the population did not have two consecutive lab eGFRs reported in the study period. This is likely to result in over-representation of patients with increased co-morbidity (who will have more kidney function tests) and therefore have a higher risk of stages 3–5 CKD. Conversely, it is likely that some individuals with stages 3–5 CKD will not have undergone testing during the time period of the study; however most of the risk factors for CKD (e.g. hypertension, diabetes) are also conditions where routine blood testing is common therefore the majority with stage 3–5 CKD should have been captured.

Ethnicity was not satisfactorily reported in the THIN database and therefore eGFR could not be adjusted for those of black ethnicity. Whilst this could theoretically lead to over-reporting of stages 3–5 CKD prevalence, individuals of black ethnicity only comprise 3.3% of the United Kingdom population so the effect of this limitation should be small [28]. When undertaking the sensitivity analysis there were limitations in calculating the eGFR. The method of creatinine analysis used in the laboratories contributing data to this cohort was not known and therefore analysis did not incorporate the IDMS method as this was not in widespread use during the time period of this study. Prevalence using both serum creatinine and laboratory eGFR appeared to rise and fall over time; this may have been due to changes in the number of laboratories analysing creatinine with the IDMS method.

Laboratory eGFRs and creatinines that were utilised for stages 3–5 CKD prevalence estimates in this study were derived directly from data that were downloaded into the primary care record. Whilst this is complete for patients who had their laboratory tests done from primary care, some patients who were under follow-up in secondary care CKD clinics may not have had their results available. This may have impacted on the prevalence estimates of patients with stage 4 CKD and stage 5 CKD, many of whom are under secondary care follow-up, explaining rates (0.21%) below those reported in other studies.

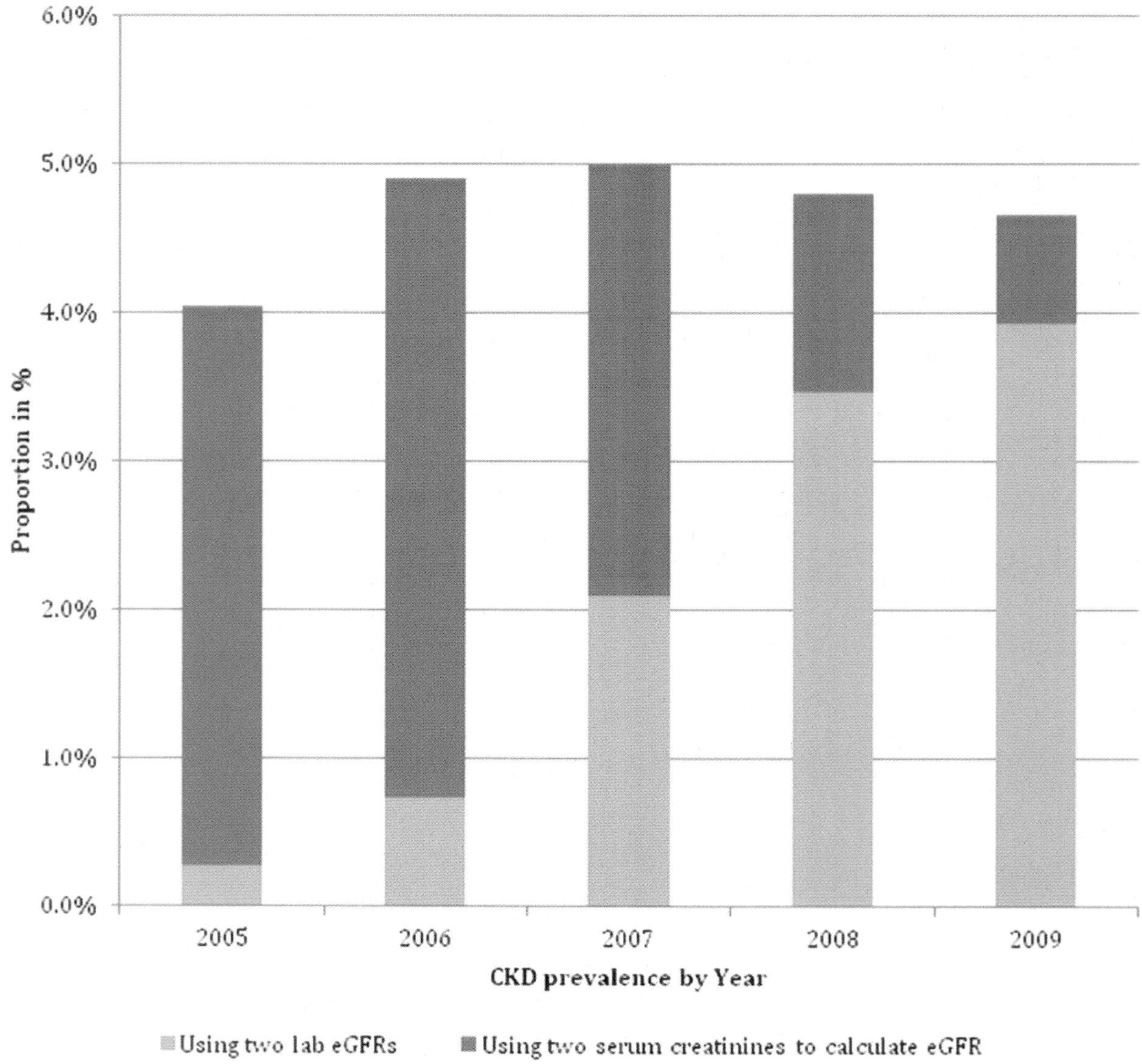

Figure 3. Prevalence of CKD by year combining CKD stage derived from laboratory eGFRs and eGFR calculated from serum creatinine.

Finally, it is plausible that GPs may calculate the eGFR themselves and place patients on the CKD practice register. However the GP would have to do this manually as the Vision electronic patient record does not automatically perform this function hence this seems unlikely to have happened on a large scale. Furthermore, this does not explain the issue of uncoded patients and the sensitivity analyses showed that relatively few (0.7%) patients would have been reclassified as stages 3–5 CKD had physicians calculated eGFR themselves. This would therefore not explain the observed miscoding.

Comparison to the literature

The prevalence estimates for stages 3–5 CKD in this study, with 3.1% of men and 4.8% women affected, were lower than other UK based studies (Appendix A). However the current results were based on two contemporary laboratory reported eGFRs whereas most other UK studies have used a single renal function test to calculate eGFR and therefore have the potential for bias [20,29–31]. Two previous studies need special mention: the QICKD study which included two eGFRs where available and the Health Survey of England which used a single measurement but screened its population [11,21].

QICKD estimated the "headline" prevalence of stages 3–5 CKD to be 6.8% in a large primary care population but 25% of those labelled as stages 3–5 CKD only had a single eGFR and the study combined laboratory and externally calculated eGFRs. If those with only one eGFR were excluded the prevalence dropped to approximately 5% or under 3% if only laboratory eGFRs were included.

The Health Survey of England Screening study (HSE), using a single eGFR result, reported the prevalence of stages 3–5 CKD as 5% in Men and 7% in women and found the overall prevalence to be 6% [21]. This was a higher proportion than other larger international screening studies which found prevalences of 3.8% (United States) and 4.7% (Norway) also on the basis of a single eGFR [32,33]. All three of these screening studies are therefore likely to have overestimated the prevalence of stages 3–5 CKD which arguably requires two laboratory eGFRs and a minimum time period between these, as in the KDOQI definition (3 months) or the current study (at least 7 days) [7].

A relationship between increased co-morbidity and appropriate labelling is potentially important, particularly as early CKD may not be associated with higher mortality in otherwise well older people, unlike younger individuals [34–36]. The multivariate model in this paper builds on a previous analysis that looked at primary care practitioners in other UK cities. This study showed increasing co-morbidity, age and deprivation at practice level were associated with QOF CKD recording. The current work expands this to individual patients with stage 3–5 CKD: age, male gender, increasing CKD stage, cardiovascular disease and peripheral vascular disease are all associated with appropriate coding [37].

Clinical Implications

These results suggest that the mechanism for recording stages 3–5 CKD prevalence in primary care needs re-evaluation: relying on manual coding of CKD appears to have resulted in significant misclassification with under treatment of those uncoded and potentially inappropriate intervention in those miscoded. This is consistent with results from a study in Type II diabetes which showed higher $HbA1_c$ and worse cholesterol control in patients with diabetes not on the QOF diabetes register [17]. Furthermore, almost twice as many were miscoded as uncoded meaning that improving the accuracy of CKD classification might also reduce workload. One solution for this would be automatic coding on the basis of eGFR results to highlight those at higher risk and similar reclassification of those apparently mislabelled.

These findings may also have implications for estimates of CKD resource use. A recent paper modelled the costs of CKD suggesting these comprised 1.3% of the NHS budget [5]. However this may be an over estimation as some of the costs are based systematically miscoded individuals as seen here [5].

Conclusions

In summary this paper has shown that robust estimation of the prevalence of stage 3–5 CKD results in generally lower prevalence than previously reported but more importantly uncovers significant misclassification and subsequent sub optimal management of chronic kidney disease. Definitive estimates of prevalence await ongoing screening studies. In the meantime, Primary Care physicians should consider the use of automatic methods to reclassify their CKD population as this may lead to both improved outcomes for patients and reduced workload for primary care practitioners.

Author Contributions

Conceived and designed the experiments: PJ MC PC RJM. Performed the experiments: PJ MC PC RJM. Analyzed the data: PJ MC PC RJM. Contributed reagents/materials/analysis tools: PJ MC PC RJM. Wrote the paper: PJ MC PC RJM.

References

1. Levey AS, Coresh J, Greene T, Stevens LA, Zhang YL, et al (2006) Using standardized serum creatinine values in the modification of diet in renal disease study equation for estimating glomerular filtration rate. Annals of Internal Medicine 145: 247–254.
2. Anavekar NS, McMurray JJV, Velazquez EJ, Solomon SD, Kober L, et al (2004) Relation between Renal Dysfunction and Cardiovascular Outcomes after Myocardial Infarction. N Engl J Med 351: 1285–1295. doi: 10.1056/NEJMoa041365.
3. Go AS, Chertow GM, Fan D, McCulloch CE, Hsu CY (2004) Chronic kidney disease and the risks of death, cardiovascular events, and hospitalization. N Engl J Med 351: 1296–1305. 10.1056/NEJMoa041031 [doi];351/13/1296 [pii].
4. Tonelli M, Muntner P, Lloyd A, Manns BJ, James MT, et al (2011) Using Proteinuria and Estimated Glomerular Filtration Rate to Classify Risk in Patients With Chronic Kidney DiseaseA Cohort Study. Annals of Internal Medicine 154: 12–21. doi: 10.1059/0003-4819-154-1-201101040-00003.
5. Kerr M, Bray B, Medcalf J, O'Donoghue DJ, Matthews B (2012) Estimating the financial cost of chronic kidney disease to the NHS in England. Nephrol Dial Transplant 27 Suppl 3: iii73–iii80. gfs269 [pii];10.1093/ndt/gfs269 [doi].
6. Collins AJ, Chen SC, Gilbertson DT, Foley RN (2009) CKD surveillance using administrative data: impact on the health care system. American Journal of Kidney Diseases 53: S27–S36. S0272-6386(08)01724-1 [pii];10.1053/j.ajkd.2008.07.055 [doi].
7. Levey AS, Coresh J, Balk E, Kausz AT, Levin A, et al (2003) National Kidney Foundation practice guidelines for chronic kidney disease: evaluation, classification, and stratification. Ann Intern Med 139: 137–147. 200307150-00013 [pii].
8. Department of Health. (2005) The National Service Framework for renal services. Pt. 2, Chronic Kidney Disease, Acute Renal Failure and End of Life Care. London: Department of Health.
9. Joint Specialty Committee on Renal Medicine of the Royal College of Physicians of London and the Renal Association (2006) identification, management and referral of adults with chronic kidney disease. guidelines for general physicians and general practitioners. JAMA.
10. NHS Information Centre (2010) Quality and Outcomes Framework Achievement Data 2009/10. Kidney Int.
11. de Lusignan S, Tomson C, Harris K, Van VJ, Gallagher H (2011) Creatinine fluctuation has a greater effect than the formula to estimate glomerular filtration rate on the prevalence of chronic kidney disease. Nephron Clinical Practice 117: c213–c224. 000320341 [pii];10.1159/000320341 [doi].
12. Mackenzie F. (2011) Notes from Birmingham Quality, UK NEQAS, February 2010.
13. Calvert M, Shankar A, McManus RJ, Lester H, Freemantle N (2009) Effect of the quality and outcomes framework on diabetes care in the United Kingdom: retrospective cohort study. BMJ 338.
14. Arellano FM, Yood MU, Wentworth CE, Oliveria SA, Rivero E, et al (2006) Use of cyclo-oxygenase 2 inhibitors (COX-2) and prescription non-steroidal anti-inflammatory drugs (NSAIDS) in UK and USA populations. Implications for COX-2 cardiovascular profile. Pharmacoepidemiol Drug Saf 15: 861–872.
15. Hippisley-Cox J, Coupland C, Vinogradova Y, Robson J, Brindle P (2008) Performance of the QRISK cardiovascular risk prediction algorithm in an independent UK sample of patients from general practice: a validation study. Heart 94: 34–39.
16. NHS Primary Care Commissioning (2009) QOF Implementation: Business Rules. BMJ.
17. Calvert MJ, Shankar A, McManus RJ, Ryan R, Freemantle N (2009) Evaluation of the management of heart failure in primary care. Family Practice 26: 145.
18. 2013) Chapter 1: Definition and classification of CKD. Kidney Int Suppl 3: 19–62.
19. Office for National Statistics (2004) Census 2001: National report for England and Wales.
20. Stevens PE, O'Donoghue DJ, de Lusignan S, Van VJ, Klebe B, et al (2007) Chronic kidney disease management in the United Kingdom: NEOERICA project results. Kidney Int 72: 92–99. 5002273 [pii];10.1038/sj.ki.5002273 [doi].
21. Aresu M, Chaudhury M, Diment E, Fuller E, Gordon-Dseagu V, et al (2010) Health Survey of England 2009.
22. Office for National Statistics (2012) All releases of Population Estimates for UK, England and Wales, Scotland and Northern Ireland.
23. Akaike H (1981) Likelihood of a model and information criteria. Journal of Econometrics 16: 3–14.
24. Blundell R, Windmeijer F (1997) Cluster effects and simultaneity in multilevel models. Health Econ 6: 439–443. 10.1002/(SICI)1099-1050(199707)6:4<439::AID-HEC276>3.0.CO;2-B [pii].
25. Gardiner JC, Luo Z, Roman LA (2009) Fixed effects, random effects and GEE: what are the differences? Stat Med 28: 221–239. 10.1002/sim.3478 [doi].
26. Levey AS, Bosch JP, Lewis JB, Greene T, Rogers N, et al (1999) A more accurate method to estimate glomerular filtration rate from serum creatinine: a new prediction equation. Modification of Diet in Renal Disease Study Group. Annals of Internal Medicine 130: 461–470. 199903160-00002 [pii].
27. O'Callaghan CA, Shine B, Lasserson DS (2011) Chronic kidney disease: a large-scale population-based study of the effects of introducing the CKD-EPI formula for eGFR reporting. BMJ Open 1: e000308. bmjopen-2011-000308 [pii];10.1136/bmjopen-2011-000308 [doi].
28. Office for National Statistics (2012) All releases of Population Estimates for UK, England and Wales, Scotland and Northern Ireland.
29. Gifford FJ, Methven S, Boag DE, Spalding EM, MacGregor MS (2011) Chronic kidney disease prevalence and secular trends in a UK population: the impact of MDRD and CKD-EPI formulae. QJM 104: 1045–1053.

30. Glynn LG, Anderson J, Reddan D, Murphy AW (2009) Chronic kidney disease in general practice: prevalence, diagnosis, and standards of care. Ir Med J 102: 285–288.
31. Carter JL, Stevens PE, Irving JE, Lamb EJ (2011) Estimating glomerular filtration rate: comparison of the CKD-EPI and MDRD equations in a large UK cohort with particular emphasis on the effect of age. QJM 104: 839–847.
32. Hallan SI, Coresh J, Astor BC, Asberg A, Powe NR, et al (2006) International comparison of the relationship of chronic kidney disease prevalence and ESRD risk. J Am Soc Nephrol 17: 2275–2284. ASN.2005121273 [pii] 10.1681/ASN.2005121273.
33. Coresh J, Byrd-Holt D, Astor BC, Briggs JP, Eggers PW, et al (2005) Chronic kidney disease awareness, prevalence, and trends among U.S. adults, 1999 to 2000. J Am Soc Nephrol 16: 180–188. 10.1681/ASN.2004070539.
34. O'Hare AM, Bertenthal D, Covinsky KE, Landefeld CS, Sen S, et al (2006) Mortality risk stratification in chronic kidney disease: one size for all ages? J Am Soc Nephrol 17: 846–853. ASN.2005090986 [pii] 10.1681/ASN.2005090986.
35. Haynes RB, Sackett DL, Taylor DW, Gibson ES, Johnson AL (1978) Increased absenteeism from work after detection and labeling of hypertensive patients. N Engl J Med 299: 741–744. 10.1056/NEJM197810052991403 [doi].
36. Johnston ME, Gibson ES, Terry CW, Haynes RB, Taylor DW, et al (1984) Effects of labelling on income, work and social function among hypertensive employees. J Chronic Dis 37: 417–423.
37. Walker N, Bankart J, Brunskill N, Baker R (2011) Which factors are associated with higher rates of chronic kidney disease recording in primary care? A cross-sectional survey of GP practices. Br J Gen Pract 61: 203–205. 10.3399/bjgp11X561212 [doi].

5

Impact of Chronic Kidney Disease on Use of Evidence-Based Therapy in Stable Coronary Artery Disease: A Prospective Analysis of 22,272 Patients

Paul R. Kalra[1,2]*, Xavier García-Moll[3], José Zamorano[4], Philip A. Kalra[5], Kim M. Fox[2,6], Ian Ford[7], Roberto Ferrari[8], Jean-Claude Tardif[9], Michal Tendera[10], Nicola Greenlaw[7] and Ph. Gabriel Steg for the CLARIFY Investigators[6,11,12,13]¶

1 Portsmouth Hospitals NHS Trust, Portsmouth, United Kingdom, **2** NHLI Imperial College, ICMS, London, United Kingdom, **3** Unitat Hospitalització, Servei de Cardiologia, Hospital de la Santa Creu i Sant Pau, Barcelona, Spain, **4** University Hospital Ramón y Cajal, Madrid, Spain, **5** Salford Royal NHS Foundation Trust, Salford, United Kingdom, **6** Royal Brompton Hospital, London, United Kingdom, **7** University of Glasgow, Glasgow, United Kingdom, **8** Department of Cardiology, Azienda Ospedaliero-Universitaria di Ferrara, Ospedale di Cona, Cona, Italy, **9** Montreal Heart Institute, Université de Montreal, Montreal, Canada, **10** Medical University of Silesia, Katowice, Poland, **11** Université Paris-Diderot, Sorbonne-Paris Cité, Paris, France, **12** INSERM U-1148, Paris, France, **13** Département Hospitalo-Universitaire FIRE, Hôpital Bichat, Assistance Publique – Hôpitaux de Paris, Paris, France

Abstract

Purpose: To assess the frequency of chronic kidney disease (CKD), define the associated demographics, and evaluate its association with use of evidence-based drug therapy in a contemporary global study of patients with stable coronary artery disease.

Methods: 22,272 patients from the ProspeCtive observational LongitudinAl RegIstry oF patients with stable coronary arterY disease (CLARIFY) were included. Baseline estimated glomerular filtration rate (eGFR) was calculated (CKD-Epidemiology Collaboration formula) and patients categorised according to CKD stage: >89, 60–89, 45–59 and <45 mL/min/1.73 m^2.

Results: Mean (SD) age was 63.9±10.4 years, 77.3% were male, 61.8% had a history of myocardial infarction, 71.9% hypertension, 30.4% diabetes and 75.4% dyslipidaemia. Chronic kidney disease (eGFR<60 mL/min/1.73 m^2) was seen in 22.1% of the cohort (6.9% with eGFR<45 mL/min/1.73 m^2); lower eGFR was associated with increasing age, female sex, cardiovascular risk factors, overt vascular disease, other comorbidities and higher systolic but lower diastolic blood pressure. High use of secondary prevention was seen across all CKD stages (overall 93.4% lipid-lowering drugs, 95.3% antiplatelets, 75.9% beta-blockers). The proportion of patients taking statins was lower in patients with CKD. Antiplatelet use was significantly lower in patients with CKD whereas oral anticoagulant use was higher. Angiotensin-converting enzyme inhibitor use was lower (52.0% overall) and inversely related to declining eGFR, whereas angiotensin-receptor blockers were more frequently prescribed in patients with reduced eGFR.

Conclusions: Chronic kidney disease is common in patients with stable coronary artery disease and is associated with comorbidities. Whilst use of individual evidence-based medications for secondary prevention was high across all CKD categories, there remains an opportunity to improve the proportion who take all three classes of preventive therapies. Angiotensin-converting enzyme inhibitors were used less frequently in lower eGRF categories. Surprisingly the reverse was seen for angiotensin-receptor blockers. Further evaluation is required to fully understand these associations. The CLARIFY (ProspeCtive observational LongitudinAl RegIstry oF patients with stable coronary arterY disease) Registry is registered in the ISRCTN registry of clinical trials with the number ISRCTN43070564. http://www.controlled-trials.com/ISRCTN43070564.

Editor: Jaap A. Joles, University Medical Center Utrecht, Netherlands

Funding: The study was designed and conducted by the investigators and funded via research grants from Servier, France, including a grant to the academic statistical centre. The sponsor had no role in study design, data collection and analysis, decision to publish, or preparation of the manuscript, but did assist with the set up and management of the study in each country. Sophie Rushton-Smith provided editorial assistance, limited to editing, checking content and language, formatting, and referencing, and was compensated by the sponsor. The CLARIFY registry enforces a no ghost-writing policy. This manuscript was written by the authors, who take full responsibility for its content.

Competing Interests: PRK reports research grants from Servier; consultancy fees/honoraria from A Menarini and Servier. Support for travel to meetings from Servier. XG-M reports advisory and conference fees from Servier. JZ reports speaker fees from Servier. IF reports research grants, honoraria for committee membership, and support for conference attendance from Servier. RF reports Speaker's bureau for Servier, Novartis, Merck Serono; research grants from Servier, Boehringer Ingelheim; and advisory board for Servier, Boehringer Ingelheim and Novartis. J-CT reports that his institution received grants and consulting fees from Servier; he also received a consulting fee or honorarium from Servier; support for travel to meetings for the study or other purposes from Servier; and payment for lectures from Servier. MT reports fees, honoraria, and research grants from Amgen, Bayer, and Servier. PGS reports that his institution received grants and consulting fees from Servier; he also received a consulting fee or honorarium from Servier; support for travel to meetings for the study or other purposes from consulting fees from Servier; he also received a consulting fee or honorarium from Servier; support for travel to meetings for the study or other purposes from Servier; and payment for lectures from Servier.

* Email: paulkalra@doctors.org.uk

¶Membership of the CLARIFY Investigators is included in Table S1.

Introduction

Chronic kidney disease (CKD) is a powerful independent predictor of adverse prognosis following myocardial infarction (MI) [1,2] or coronary revascularization [3,4]. A recent study has shown that post MI the presence of CKD (defined as estimated glomerular filtration rate, eGFR, <60 mL/min/1.73 m^2) was a stronger predictor of all-cause mortality than either a history of MI or diabetes [2]. Compared with a reference population without a history of MI, CKD or diabetes, the presence of CKD was associated with a 3.6-fold unadjusted relative rate of all-cause mortality; the respective rates for patients with history of MI or diabetes were 2.7 and 1.9.

A number of plausible reasons might explain this link. CKD may merely represent a bystander marker of advancing age and comorbidities. Alternatively pathophysiological derangements in patients with CKD such as activation of the renin-angiotensin-aldosterone systems, inflammatory immune activation or disordered calcium-phosphate metabolism might contribute to cardiovascular disease progression or expression [5,6]. Underutilization of evidence-based treatments in patients with CKD and coronary artery disease (CAD) may also play a role. Historical data have suggested that despite major advances in secondary prevention following MI, patients with CKD are less commonly prescribed prognostically beneficial drugs. For example, data from 14,527 patients with acute MI complicated by heart failure (Valsartan in Acute Myocardial Infarction Trial) showed that declining eGFR was associated with increased risk of death and non-fatal cardiovascular outcomes [1]. Whilst patients with eGFR <45 mL/min/1.73 m^2 were at highest risk of events, the use of aspirin, beta-blockers, statins or coronary revascularization was lowest in this group. A retrospective cohort study of Medicare patients with acute MI showed that those with CKD stage 4 (eGFR 15–29 mL/min/1.73 m^2) were infrequently prescribed aspirin with beta-blockers (27.1%) and fewer than one in 10 were prescribed the combination of aspirin, beta-blockers and angiotensin-converting enzyme (ACE) inhibitors [7]. Similar data were found in a single-centre prospective study for patients discharged after acute MI [8].

Patients with CKD and CAD are at higher absolute risk of adverse events and many are therefore likely to derive marked benefit from secondary prevention. Identifying and subsequently rectifying deficiencies of care in such patients has the potential to impact positively on outcomes. The aims of the current study were to assess the frequency of CKD, define the associated demographics, and evaluate the impact of CKD on medical therapy in a large contemporary global study of patients with stable CAD: the ProspeCtive observational LongitudinAl RegIstry oF patients with stable coronary arterY disease (CLARIFY) [9]. We hypothesized that patients with advanced CKD would receive suboptimal secondary prevention compared to patients with preserved renal function. This unique, contemporary cohort study has enabled us to evaluate these objectives in detail.

Methods

Ethics Statement

The study was conducted in accordance with the principles in the Declaration of Helsinki and local ethical approval was obtained as necessary in all countries prior to recruitment. All patients gave written informed consent.

Study Design

CLARIFY is an ongoing international, prospective, observational, longitudinal cohort study in outpatients with stable CAD. The study rationale and methods have been published elsewhere (further information can be found online at www.clarify-registry.com) [9,10]. Briefly, the registry was designed to collect data on the current status of outpatients with stable CAD, including their demographic characteristics, clinical profiles, therapeutic strategies, and outcomes. More than 33,000 patients were enrolled in 45 countries in Africa, Asia, Australia, Europe, the Middle East, and North, Central and South America. A detailed list of countries, sites, and investigators has already been published [10]. Patients are followed up for 5 years with data collected prospectively at annual visits, and interim phone calls every 6 months. Patients are treated according to usual clinical practice at each institution, with no specific tests or therapies defined in the study protocol. The current study relates to data collected at baseline assessment.

Study Design and Patients

The 2,884 participating physicians were selected on the basis of their geographic distribution; each was requested to recruit 10–15 consecutive stable outpatients with CAD to meet a predefined country target of 25 patients per million inhabitants (range 12.5–50) and obtain an epidemiologically representative population in each country. Eligible patients had stable CAD proven by a history of at least one of the following: documented MI (>3 months before enrolment); angiographic demonstration of coronary stenosis >50%; chest pain with evidence of myocardial ischaemia (stress electrocardiogram, stress echocardiograph or myocardial perfusion imaging); or coronary artery bypass graft (CABG) or percutaneous coronary intervention (PCI) performed >3 months before enrolment. These criteria were not mutually exclusive. Exclusion criteria included hospital admission for cardiovascular reasons (including revascularization) in the past 3 months, planned revascularization, or conditions hampering participation for the 5-year follow-up, such as limited cooperation, inability to provide informed consent, serious non-cardiovascular disease or conditions interfering with life expectancy (e.g. cancer, drug abuse) or severe other cardiovascular disease (e.g. advanced heart failure, severe valve disease, history of valve repair/replacement). CKD *per se* was not an exclusion criterion. To ensure that the study population was representative of stable CAD outpatients, recruitment of sites and subjects was based on predefined selection of physicians (cardiologists, as well as office-based primary care physicians and physicians based in hospitals with outpatient clinics) by national coordinators, using the best available epidemiological data in each country reflecting the burden of CAD; this was done in an attempt to provide a distribution of physicians across regions and locations (i.e. urban, suburban, or rural areas) mimicking the epidemiological patterns in each country. In each practice, patient enrolment was restricted over a brief period to achieve near consecutive patient enrolment in order to avoid selection bias. The first patient was included on 26 November 2009 and recruitment was completed on 30 June 2010.

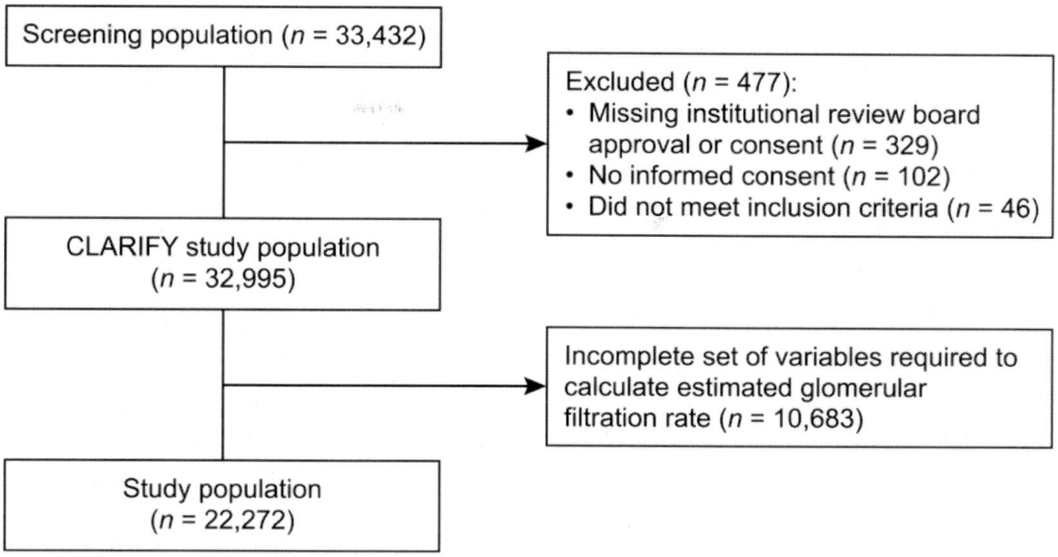

Figure 1. Patient flow chart.

Data Collection

The investigators completed standardized electronic case report forms (eCRFs) at baseline. All forms were sent electronically to the data management centre where checks for completeness, internal consistency and accuracy were run. A number of measures were implemented to ensure data quality, including onsite monitoring visits of all data in randomly selected centres (1% per annum). Data quality control happened at face-to-face quality control visits involving review of source documents supporting the adequacy and accuracy of data collected on the case report forms. At baseline data were collected on demographics, medical history, risk factors and lifestyle, physical condition and vital signs, current symptoms and treatments. Available results of laboratory tests, invasive and non-invasive tests were collected, but no test was mandated by the study and there was no standardized measurement of the left ventricular ejection fraction.

Patient confidentiality was ensured by utilizing patient identification code numbers to correspond to the computer files. The study is registered (ISRCTN43070564).

Statistical Analysis

All CLARIFY data are collected and analysed at an independent academic statistics centre at the Robertson Centre for Biostatistics, University of Glasgow, United Kingdom, which is responsible for the management of the database, all analyses (using the SAS statistical program, version 9.2 or higher), and storing the data according to regulations. Baseline characteristics for the whole population, according to renal function, are presented using descriptive statistics with mean (standard deviation [SD]) or median (quartile 1, quartile 3 [Q1, Q3]) for continuous variables, depending on the distribution of the data, and as counts (percentages) for categorical data.

We analysed the CLARIFY population at baseline grouped by eGFR according to the CKD-Epidemiology Collaboration (CKD-EPI) formula [11] (Table S2). Patients were categorized according to CKD stage [12]: stage 1, >89 mL/min/1.73 m^2; stage 2, 60–89 mL/min/1.73 m^2; stage 3a, 45–59 mL/min/1.73 m^2; and stage 3b–5: <45 mL/min/1.73 m^2. CKD-EPI was selected since data suggest that it may be more accurate than other creatinine-based formulae when applied to a population of patients in which a large proportion have eGFR>60 mL/min/1.73 m^2 [11]. Patients with CKD stages 3b, 4 and 5 (eGFR<45 mL/min/1.73 m^2) were grouped since it was anticipated that there would be small numbers with stages 4 or 5 in particular. The prevalence of renal dysfunction and the differential characteristics of these patients are described. Management of these patients is also depicted.

In order to explore medication use further, an analysis of how many patients received all cardiovascular preventive measures was performed. Data for each renal function group were analysed according to the number (%) of patients who received 'all secondary preventive measures', defined as taking at least one medication from all three of the following drug categories: (i) antiplatelet, (ii) statin, and (iii) ACE inhibitor or angiotensin receptor blocker (ARB).

Comparisons between the renal function groups were made using either one-way analysis of variance or the Kruskal–Wallis test for continuous data, depending on the distribution of the data, or the chi-square test for categorical data.

Univariate and multivariable logistic regression analyses were also performed to ascertain the relationship between renal dysfunction and management. Analyses were performed to examine the effect of renal dysfunction on the use of ACE inhibitors and then separately the use of ARBs. The multivariable analyses were adjusted for other clinical and demographic variables known to have a relationship with the use of these therapies, and included the following: age, body mass index (BMI), systolic blood pressure, diastolic blood pressure, gender, heart rate, smoking status, history of heart failure, angina, diabetes mellitus and hypertension.

Results

Of the 33,432 patients screened, 329 patients were missing institutional review board approval or consent, 102 did not provide consent and 46 did not meet the inclusion criteria, leaving 32,955 patients for analysis. Of these, 22,272 patients had all of the baseline variables available to permit eGFR calculation and thereby formed the final study group (Figure 1). The mean age was 63.9±10.4 years, 77.3% were male, 61.8% had a history of MI, 71.9% had treated hypertension, 30.4% were diabetic, 75.4%

Table 1. Demographic data: characteristics of the study population classified according to eGFR group calculated using the CKD-EPI.

Variable	Total (n=22,272)	eGFR (mL/min/1.73 m^2)				p-value[a]
		<45 (n=1,528)	45–59 (n=3,389)	60–89 (n=11,826)	≥90 (n=5,529)	
Age, mean (SD), years	63.9±10.4	71.4±9.5	69.8±8.8	64.7±9.5	56.5±8.8	<0.0001
Men, n (%)	17,221 (77.3)	968 (63.4)	2,283 (67.4)	9,331 (78.9)	4,639 (83.9)	<0.0001
BMI, median (Q1, Q3), kg/m^2	27.5 (24.9, 30.5)	27.5 (24.7, 30.8)	27.5 (24.9, 30.7)	27.4 (25.0, 30.4)	27.5 (24.9, 30.8)	0.25
Time since 1st CAD diagnosis, median (Q1, Q3), years	4 (2, 9)	6 (2, 12)	6 (2, 11)	5 (2, 10)	3 (1, 7)	<0.0001
Myocardial infarction, n (%)	13,759 (61.8)	956 (62.6)	2,015 (59.5)	7,255 (61.4)	3,533 (63.9)	0.0002
PCI, n (%)	12,606 (56.6)	755 (49.4)	1,729 (51.0)	6,643 (56.2)	3,479 (62.9)	<0.0001
CABG, n (%)	5,386 (24.2)	462 (30.3)	977 (28.8)	2,901 (24.5)	1,046 (18.9)	<0.0001
Internal cardiac defibrillator, n (%)	284 (1.3)	54 (3.5)	56 (1.7)	132 (1.1)	42 (0.8)	<0.0001
Pacemaker, n (%)	489 (2.2)	88 (5.8)	117 (3.5)	237 (2.0)	47 (0.9)	<0.0001
Stroke, n (%)	951 (4.3)	137 (9.0)	205 (6.0)	484 (4.1)	125 (2.3)	<0.0001
Transient ischaemic attack, n (%)	694 (3.1)	92 (6.0)	178 (5.3)	311 (2.6)	113 (2.0)	<0.0001
Peripheral artery disease, n (%)	2,122 (9.5)	240 (15.7)	420 (12.4)	1,075 (9.1)	387 (7.0)	<0.0001
Hospitalization for CHF, n (%)	1,120 (5.0)	202 (13.2)	237 (7.0)	504 (4.3)	177 (3.2)	<0.0001
Treated hypertension, n (%)	16,000 (71.9)	1,297 (84.9)	2,660 (78.5)	8,423 (71.2)	3,620 (65.5)	<0.0001
Diabetes, n (%)	6,763 (30.4)	688 (45.0)	1,159 (34.2)	3,276 (27.7)	1,640 (29.7)	<0.0001
Dyslipidaemia, n (%)	16,794 (75.4)	1,189 (77.8)	2,542 (75.0)	8,969 (75.9)	4,094 (74.1)	0.009
Atrial fibrillation/flutter, n (%)	1,615 (7.3)	211 (13.8)	384 (11.3)	839 (7.1)	181 (3.3)	<0.0001
Asthma/COPD, n (%)	1,750 (7.9)	156 (10.2)	300 (8.9)	964 (8.2)	330 (6.0)	<0.0001
Smoking status, n (%)						
Current	2,828 (12.7)	99 (6.5)	254 (7.5)	1,436 (12.2)	1,039 (18.8)	
Former	10,302 (46.3)	669 (43.8)	1,479 (43.6)	5,619 (47.5)	2,535 (45.9)	
Never	9,137 (41.0)	760 (49.7)	1,656 (48.9)	4,768 (40.3)	1,953 (35.3)	
Angina and CCS class, n (%)						<0.0001
No Angina	1,6921 (76.0)	1,142 (74.7)	2,512 (74.1)	8,961 (75.8)	4,306 (77.9)	
CCS class I	1,527 (6.9)	98 (6.4)	222 (6.6)	832 (7.0)	375 (6.8)	
CCS class II	2,802 (12.6)	193 (12.6)	498 (14.7)	1,486 (12.6)	625 (11.3)	
CCS class III	953 (4.3)	90 (5.9)	151 (4.5)	506 (4.3)	206 (3.7)	
CCS class IV	61 (0.3)	5 (0.3)	6 (0.2)	35 (0.3)	15 (0.3)	

Abbreviations: CABG, coronary artery bypass graft; CAD, coronary artery disease; CCS, Canadian Cardiovascular Society; CHF, chronic heart failure; CKD-EPI, Chronic Kidney Disease–Epidemiology Collaboration; COPD, chronic obstructive pulmonary disease; eGFR, estimated glomerular filtration rate; NYHA, New York Heart Association; PCI, percutaneous coronary intervention; SD, standard deviation.
[a]p-value tests for differences across eGFR groups.

were dyslipidaemic and 5.0% had a prior hospitalization for chronic heart failure (Table 1). The majority of patients were white (74.3%). Just over half of the study population had received PCI (56.6%) and 24.2% CABG; most (76.0%) were free of symptomatic angina.

Table 1 also shows the demographics of patients by eGFR status. Chronic kidney disease (eGFR<60 mL/min/1.73^2) was seen in 22.1%. Patients with lower eGFR were older, with a higher prevalence of women, comorbidities, cardiovascular risk factors and overt vascular disease. Patients with CKD were more likely to have undergone CABG but less likely to have had PCI compared to those with preserved renal function. The prevalence of atrial fibrillation/flutter (AF) and chronic heart failure increased in stepwise fashion whereas the proportion of active smokers decreased in patients with lower eGFR.

Clinical findings and investigations according to eGFR category are shown in Table 2. Patients with lower eGFR exhibited higher systolic blood pressures whilst the converse was seen for diastolic pressure. There were no clinically meaningful differences in heart rate or lipid profile. Haemoglobin concentration was progressively lower according to worse CKD class.

Drug therapy is detailed in Table 3. High use of secondary prevention was seen across all CKD stages (overall 93.4% for lipid-lowering drugs, 95.3% antiplatelets, 75.9% beta-blockers). When considering the whole study population, statins were being taken by 84.3% of patients; a small but significant stepwise reduction in use was seen in patients with lower eGFR. Antiplatelet use was progressively reduced in patients with lower eGFR; the converse was seen for oral anticoagulant use. When considering patients with a history of AF, the proportion receiving oral anticoagulation significantly increased in a step-wise fashion as CKD class

Table 2. Clinical finding and investigations of the study population classified according to eGFR group calculated using the CKD-EPI.

Variable	Total available	Total (n=22,560)	eGFR (mL/min/1.73 m^2)				p-value[a]
			<45 (n=1,528)	45–59 (n=3,389)	60–89 (n=11,826)	≥90 (n=5,529)	
Heart rate palpation, mean (SD), beats per min	22,269	68.5±10.7	69.4±11.4	68.6±11.1	68.0±10.6	69.1±10.5	<0.0001
Systolic BP, mean (SD), mm Hg	22,268	131.1±16.9	132.8±18.4	132.6±17.5	131.2±16.7	129.5±16.4	<0.0001
Diastolic BP, mean (SD), mm Hg	22,268	77.3±10.1	75.5±11.0	76.7±10.4	77.3±10.0	78.1±9.8	<0.0001
Left bundle branch block, n (%)	16,719	814 (4.9)	107 (9.6)	169 (6.9)	399 (4.5)	139 (3.3)	<0.0001
LVEF, mean (SD), %	15,998	55.6±11.2	52.0±12.9	54.8±11.8	56.1±10.9	56.0±10.5	<0.0001
Fasting blood glucose, median (Q1, Q3), mmol/L	19,811	5.7 (5.1, 6.7)	5.9 (5.1, 7.3)	5.8 (5.2, 6.7)	5.6 (5.1, 6.5)	5.7 (5.1, 6.7)	<0.0001
HbA_{1C}, mean (SD), %	6,747	6.8 (1.9)	7.1 (1.6)	6.9 (2.4)	6.7 (1.6)	6.9 (2.0)	<0.0001
Total cholesterol, median (Q1, Q3), mmol/L	21,185	4.3 (3.6, 5.0)	4.2 (3.5, 4.9)	4.3 (3.6, 5.1)	4.3 (3.6, 5.0)	4.2 (3.6, 5.0)	0.002
High-density lipoprotein	18,839	1.1 (1.0, 1.4)	1.1 (0.9, 1.3)	1.1 (1.0, 1.4)	1.1 (1.0, 1.4)	1.1 (0.9, 1.3)	<0.0001
Low-density lipoprotein	17,812	2.3 (1.9, 2.9)	2.3 (1.8, 2.9)	2.3 (1.8, 2.9)	2.4 (1.9, 2.9)	2.4 (1.8, 3.0)	0.0012
Fasting triglycerides, median (Q1, Q3), mmol/L	19,586	1.4 (1.0, 2.0)	1.5 (1.1, 2.1)	1.4 (1.1, 2.0)	1.4 (1.0, 1.9)	1.4 (1.0, 2.0)	<0.0001
Haemoglobin, median (Q1, Q3), mmol/L	18,714	8.7 (8.1, 9.3)	8.0 (7.2, 8.7)	8.5 (7.8, 9.1)	8.8 (8.2, 9.4)	8.9 (8.3, 9.4)	<0.0001

Abbreviations: BP, blood pressure; CKD-EPI, Chronic Kidney Disease–Epidemiology Collaboration; eGFR, estimated glomerular filtration rate; LVEF, left ventricular ejection fraction; SD, standard deviation.
[a]p-value tests for differences across eGFR groups.

Table 3. Drug treatment for all patients with available data according to eGFR group calculated using the CKD-EPI.

Variable	Total (*n* = 22,272)	eGFR (mL/min/1.73 m²)				*p*-value[a]
		<45 (*n* = 1,570)	45–59 (*n* = 3,443)	60–89 (*n* = 11,958)	≥90 (*n* = 5,589)	
Antiplatelet, *n* (%)	21,228 (95.3)	1,385 (90.6)	3,152 (93.0)	11,288 (95.5)	5,403 (97.7)	<0.0001
Aspirin, *n* (%)	19,876 (89.3)	1,238 (81.1)	2,900 (85.6)	10,578 (89.5)	5,160 (93.4)	<0.0001
Thienopyridine, *n* (%)	5,707 (25.7)	404 (26.5)	797 (23.6)	2,872 (24.3)	1,634 (29.6)	<0.0001
Other antiplatelet, *n* (%)	2,067 (9.3)	153 (10.0)	299 (8.8)	1,050 (8.9)	565 (10.2)	0.02
Oral anticoagulant, *n* (%)	1,734 (7.8)	205 (13.5)	353 (10.4)	890 (7.5)	286 (5.2)	<0.0001
Oral anticoagulants in AF[b], *n* (%)	753 (43.9)	110 (51.2)	192 (46.5)	374 (42.4)	77 (37.7)	0.02
Neither antiplatelet nor oral anticoagulant, *n* (%)	399 (1.8)	35 (2.3)	81 (2.4)	216 (1.8)	67 (1.2)	0.0002
Beta-blocker, *n* (%)	16,906 (75.9)	1,160 (75.9)	2548 (75.2)	8,861 (74.9)	4,337 (78.5)	<0.0001
Ivabradine, *n* (%)	2,177 (9.8)	150 (9.8)	362 (10.7)	1,162 (9.8)	503 (9.1)	0.11
Calcium antagonist, *n* (%)	6,069 (27.3)	513 (33.6)	1,076 (31.7)	3,204 (27.1)	1,276 (23.1)	<0.0001
Verapamil or diltiazem, *n* (%)	1,287 (5.8)	86 (5.6)	196 (5.8)	720 (6.1)	285 (5.2)	0.11
Dihydropyridine, *n* (%)	4,827 (21.7)	431 (28.2)	884 (26.1)	2,509 (21.2)	1,003 (18.1)	<0.0001
ACE inhibitor, *n* (%)	11,586 (52.0)	676 (44.2)	1,715 (50.6)	6,190 (52.3)	3,005 (54.4)	<0.0001
ARB, *n* (%)	5,951 (26.7)	570 (37.3)	1,086 (32.1)	3,086 (26.1)	1,209 (21.9)	<0.0001
Neither ACE nor ARB, *n* (%)	5,169 (23.2)	342 (22.4)	674 (19.9)	2,763 (23.4)	1,390 (25.1)	<0.0001
Lipid lowering, *n* (%)	20,791 (93.4)	1,412 (92.4)	3,110 (91.8)	11,054 (93.5)	5,215 (94.3)	<0.0001
Statin, *n* (%)	18,776 (84.3)	1,251 (81.9)	2,783 (82.1)	10,033 (84.8)	4,709 (85.2)	<0.0001
Diuretic, *n* (%)	6,614 (29.7)	836 (54.7)	1,399 (41.3)	3233 (27.3)	1,146 (20.7)	<0.0001
Other antihypertensive drug, *n* (%)	1,660 (7.5)	245 (16.0)	303 (8.9)	790 (6.7)	322 (5.8)	<0.0001
Digoxin and derivatives, *n* (%)	599 (2.7)	94 (6.2)	141 (4.2)	279 (2.4)	85 (1.5)	<0.0001
Amiodarone/dronedarone, *n* (%)	632 (2.8)	90 (5.9)	179 (5.3)	289 (2.4)	74 (1.3)	<0.0001
NSAID, *n* (%)	1,186 (5.3)	94 (6.2)	217 (6.4)	659 (5.6)	216 (3.9)	<0.0001
Insulin, *n* (%)	1,533 (6.9)	245 (16.0)	283 (8.4)	656 (5.5)	349 (6.3)	<0.0001
Oral antidiabetic agent, *n* (%)	4,833 (21.7)	425 (27.8)	813 (24.0)	2,364 (20.0)	1,231 (22.3)	<0.0001
All secondary preventive measures, n (%)	13,936 (62.6)	893 (58.4)	2,110 (62.3)	7,465 (63.1)	3,468 (62.7)	0.0049

Abbreviations: ACE, angiotensin converting enzyme; AF, atrial fibrillation; ARB, angiotensin receptor blocker; CKD-EPI, Chronic Kidney Disease–Epidemiology Collaboration; eGFR, estimated glomerular filtration rate; NSAID, non-steroidal anti-inflammatory drug.
[a]*p*-value tests for differences across eGFR groups.
[b]For patients with history of (or currently in) AF.

deteriorated. The use of calcium channel antagonists, ARBs, diuretics, digoxin, amiodarone and insulin was increased in those patients with lower eGFR. ACE inhibitor use was lower and inversely related to lower eGFR. A similar pattern of use was seen for patients (n = 13,759) with a history of MI (data not shown).

In the overall study population, 62.6% received all three secondary prevention treatments (antiplatelet plus statin plus ACE or ARB), with a significant reduction seen with lower eGFR (Table 3).

We explored the relationship between renal function and the use of ACE/ARB further (Figures 2 and 3). Univariate analysis demonstrated that renal function (eGFR) was a significant and independent predictor for both ACE inhibitor and ARB use when considered as a continuous (data not shown) or categorical variable; lower eGFR values had reduced odds of ACE inhibitor use, whereas the converse was seen for ARB use. These associations were consistent following adjustment for a number of variables (age, body mass index, systolic blood pressure, diastolic blood pressure, gender, heart rate, smoking status, history of heart failure, angina, diabetes and hypertension). The odds of taking ACE inhibitors in the severely impaired renal function group were 0.75 (95% confidence interval [CI] 0.67, 0.84) compared to those with eGFR 60–89 mL/min/1.73 m², whilst the odds of taking ARBs for the same group were 1.33 (95% CI 1.18, 1.49) compared to those with renal function 60–89 mL/min/1.73 m². Patients with eGFR>90 mL/min/1.73 m² had very similar results to those in the 60–89 mL/min/1.73 m² group.

Discussion

Published data on the prevalence of CKD in patients with stable CAD are scarce. The CLARIFY study population represents a unique, contemporary, global cohort of patients with stable CAD. In our study, where 22,272 patients were included, CKD (defined as eGFR <60 mL/min/1.73 m²) is seen in just under one-quarter of patients with CAD and is associated with increasing age, female sex, cardiovascular risk factors, overt vascular disease, other comorbidities, and higher systolic but lower diastolic blood pressure. Severe CKD (eGFR<45 mL/min/1.73 m²), which has previously been shown to be associated with poor prognosis, is as common as AF (6.9% and 7.3%, respectively).

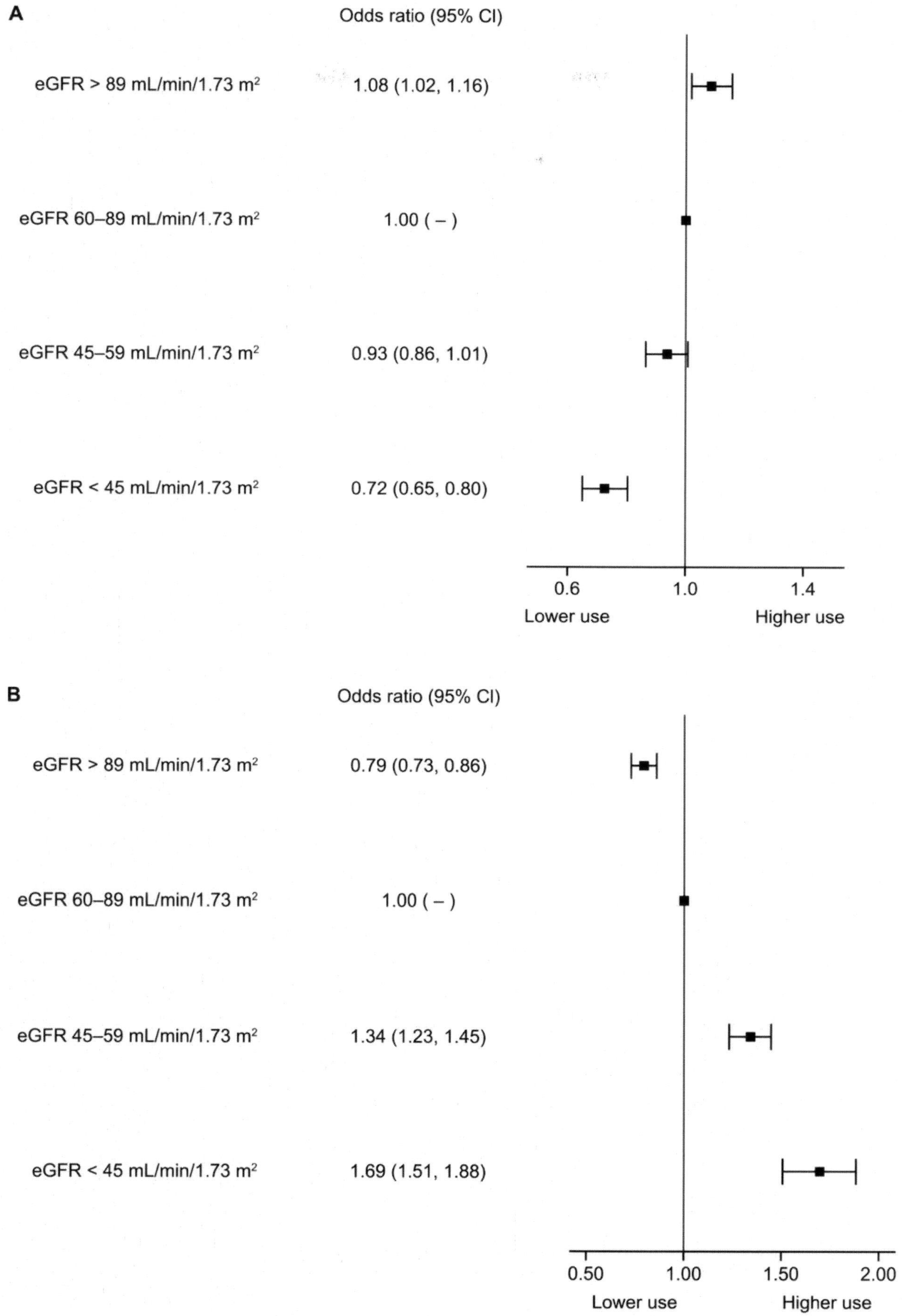
A
Odds ratio (95% CI)
eGFR > 89 mL/min/1.73 m²
1.08 (1.02, 1.16)
eGFR 60–89 mL/min/1.73 m²
1.00 (–)
eGFR 45–59 mL/min/1.73 m²
0.93 (0.86, 1.01)
eGFR < 45 mL/min/1.73 m²
0.72 (0.65, 0.80)
0.6
1.0
1.4
Lower use
Higher use
B
Odds ratio (95% CI)
eGFR > 89 mL/min/1.73 m²
0.79 (0.73, 0.86)
eGFR 60–89 mL/min/1.73 m²
1.00 (–)
eGFR 45–59 mL/min/1.73 m²
1.34 (1.23, 1.45)
eGFR < 45 mL/min/1.73 m²
1.69 (1.51, 1.88)
0.50
1.00
1.50
2.00
Lower use
Higher use

Figure 2. Univariate relationship between chronic kidney disease class and use of (A) angiotensin-converting enzyme inhibitors and (B) angiotensin receptor blocker.

Compared with recent published data, the prevalence of CKD in patients with CAD is greater than that seen in the general population. For example, contemporary data from a representative sample of the Canadian general population demonstrated a prevalence of CKD (any stage) of 12.5% [13]. The estimated prevalence of patients with CKD stages 3–5 (eGFR<59 mL/min/1.73 m^2) was 3.1%, increasing to 18.6% when considering only subjects >65 years of age. The latter figure is perhaps more relevant, since the mean age of subjects in our study was 64 years. A recent study of consecutive patients receiving primary PCI for myocardial infarction in the UK demonstrated a mean age of approximately 64 years, with 17.6% exhibiting CKD stages 3–5 [14]. In the Canadian study [13], the prevalence of comorbidities such as hypertension and diabetes mellitus was greater in those with CKD, but no real difference in lipid profile (excepting triglycerides) was seen. A similar finding in relation to lipid profile was seen in our population, where no meaningful clinical difference in lipids levels was seen across the CKD stages. The United States National Health and Nutrition Examination Survey dataset show a total crude CKD prevalence estimate for adults aged ≥20 years to be 16.8%, of which 5.4% were in CKD stage 3 and 0.4% in stages 4 or 5 [15]. The prevalence of renal disease was significantly associated with age. The finding that almost one-quarter of subjects in the current study had CKD is likely to be explained in part by age but also by the high presence of comorbidities in patients with CAD, when compared with the general unselected population. For example, when considering all subjects, 30.4% had a history of diabetes mellitus, 71.9% treated hypertension, 75.4% dyslipidaemia and 61.8% prior myocardial infarction. Patients with severe CKD demonstrated a significantly higher prevalence of diabetes mellitus (45.0%) and hypertension (84.9%). Female sex was associated with lower eGFR; this relationship is likely to be influenced by increasing age and is in keeping with previous studies of patients with CAD [1].

It is not possible from the current study to determine if the presence of comorbid conditions led to the development of concomitant CAD and CKD (i.e. shared aetiological risk) or whether when present they contribute to accelerated decline in renal function. Alternatively renal impairment *per se* may contribute to adverse risk factor profile, such as hypertension. For example, the finding that wider pulse pressure, a marker of increased vascular stiffness [16], was more apparent in subjects with CKD could lead to the conclusion that it may underlie (at least in part) the renal dysfunction; yet it is equally plausible that it might be secondary to it (or perhaps both). It is hoped that the prospective nature of the CLARIFY study, with annual data collection, may help to tease out some of these complex relationships in more detail.

Secondary prevention was generally very good across all categories of renal function with no meaningful differences in use of beta-blockers. This is a major difference when the current data are compared with historical datasets, most of which were obtained in an acute or subacute care setting [8,17–19]. These findings were consistent across subgroups of patients, such as those with a history of MI or CABG. A small but significant stepwise reduction in statin use was seen in patients with lower eGFR. Antiplatelet therapy use declined with lower eGFR; this may be explained by the concomitant increase in use of anticoagulant therapy and higher prevalence of AF with impaired renal function.

To try to identify any gap in implementation of secondary prevention in clinical practice, we assessed the number of patients within each renal function group who were taking evidence-based therapy in the form of an antiplatelet, a statin, and an ACE inhibitor or ARB. Just under two-thirds (62.6%) of the patients were found to be on this combination of drugs and a significant reduction was seen in patients with CKD (e.g. 58.4% in patients with CKD stage 3b–5). It is possible that the appropriate utilization of anticoagulant therapy for patients with AF may have influenced use of antiplatelet therapy.

Just over three-quarters (76.8%) of the overall patient group received either an ACE inhibitor or ARB (or both), and this order of magnitude was even seen when considering patients with severe CKD (stages 3b–5, 77.6%). However, ACE inhibitors were not used in a similar proportion across the eGFR groups; a step-wise reduction in use was seen in patients with lower eGFR. The opposite was seen for ARBs. These findings were independent of a number of clinical variables that might impact on use of these drugs, including history of hypertension, diabetes and age. A similar trend of higher use of ARBs following PCI for ST-elevation MI was seen in patients with severe CKD in a recently published UK study [14]. Guidelines relating to the management of patients with CKD do not differentiate between the use of ACE inhibitors or ARBs [20]. Further evaluation is required to fully understand these associations.

When considering patients with a history of AF, the proportion receiving oral anticoagulation significantly increased in step-wise fashion as CKD class deteriorated (37.8% amongst patients with CKD stage 1 to 51.2% in stages 3b–5). Renal impairment has recently been shown to be associated with higher risk of stroke and peripheral embolism in patients with AF [21].

Significant differences in the rates of use of other drug classes were seen across CKD stages. For example, dihydropyridine calcium channel blockers, diuretics, other antihypertensive drugs, digoxin and amiodarone were more frequently prescribed in patients with lower eGFR, most likely reflecting the associated high prevalence of comorbidities, including hypertension and AF.

This study has a number of limitations. For example, there are no data available with respect to albuminuria, and data on left ventricular function (e.g. from echocardiogram) were not systematically required for the study. The current study population comprises 68% of the total CLARIFY population, due to insufficient baseline data being available in the remainder. In some countries ethnicity data were not collected due to legal or ethical reasons (hence eGFR could not be calculated) and not all subjects had recent local laboratory data available (not mandated for the study). Whilst CKD *per se* was not an exclusion criterion, it is plausible that subjects with more severely impaired renal function may have been excluded on the basis of this being considered as hampering the collection of 5-year follow-up data. Renal function has been analysed according to eGFR, which is derived from a single serum creatinine assessment. This might lead to an overestimate of the prevalence of CKD stages 3–5. Whilst most western laboratories use a creatinine method that has calibration traceable to an isotope dilution mass spectrometry reference measurement procedure, given the international scope of this collaborative study it was difficult to establish the creatinine validation technique for all laboratories. It is plausible that this may have led to some error in attribution of diagnosis of CKD, but which was unavoidable. We chose to use CKD-EPI, as it performs

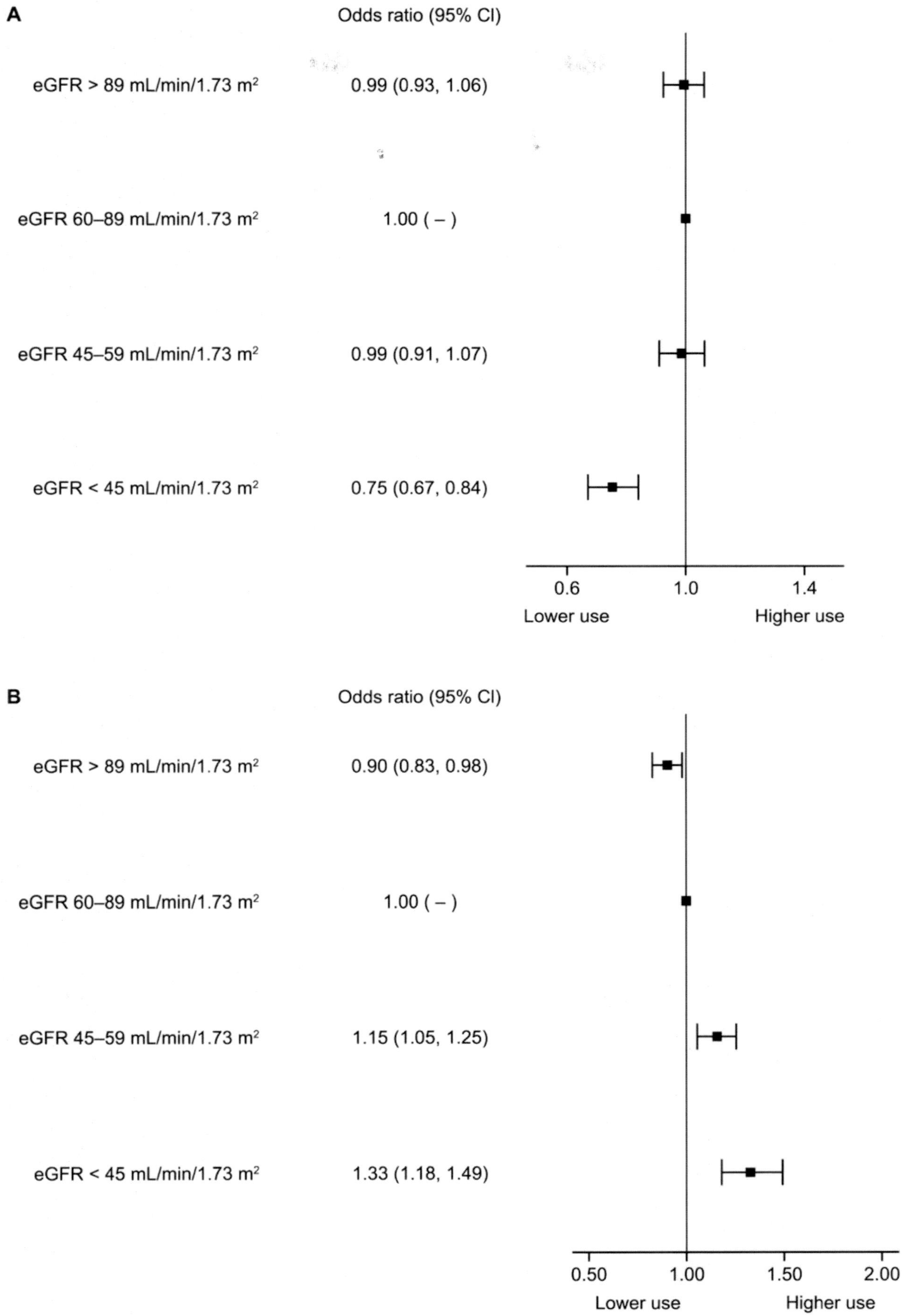
A
Odds ratio (95% CI)
eGFR > 89 mL/min/1.73 m2
0.99 (0.93, 1.06)
eGFR 60–89 mL/min/1.73 m2
1.00 (–)
eGFR 45–59 mL/min/1.73 m2
0.99 (0.91, 1.07)
eGFR < 45 mL/min/1.73 m2
0.75 (0.67, 0.84)
0.6
1.0
1.4
Lower use
Higher use
B
Odds ratio (95% CI)
eGFR > 89 mL/min/1.73 m2
0.90 (0.83, 0.98)
eGFR 60–89 mL/min/1.73 m2
1.00 (–)
eGFR 45–59 mL/min/1.73 m2
1.15 (1.05, 1.25)
eGFR < 45 mL/min/1.73 m2
1.33 (1.18, 1.49)
0.50
1.00
1.50
2.00
Lower use
Higher use

Figure 3. The association of use of (A) angiotensin-converting enzyme inhibitors and (B) angiotensin receptor blocker with chronic kidney disease following adjustment for age, body mass index, systolic blood pressure, diastolic blood pressure, gender, heart rate, smoking status, history of heart failure, angina, diabetes and hypertension.

better at higher GFRs, and data suggest that it may provide enhanced cardiovascular risk prediction compared with the Modification of Diet in Renal Disease (MDRD) method [21]. It is acknowledged that in clinical practice, decision-making regarding medical treatment by the responsible clinician is most likely to be influenced by serum creatinine and/or eGFR (e.g. in several countries MDRD-derived eGFR is routinely reported by laboratories). We believe that these potential limitations are overcome by the large size of the described cohort and the fact that the key findings are consistent irrespective of the method used to analyse renal function (in general qualitatively similar results with the MDRD formula [data not shown]). The data presented relate to 'current treatments' (i.e. those being taken when the patients were assessed at baseline). Owing to the nature of an observation study, it is not possible to ascertain whether patients were actually taking their prescribed medications.

In summary, baseline data from the CLARIFY study show that CKD is common in patients with stable CAD and is associated with age and comorbidities. Secondary prevention on the whole appears to be good, with high use of antiplatelet agents, statins, and beta-blockers. Around three-quarters of patients were prescribed either an ACE inhibitor or ARB, irrespective of renal function. In patients with severe CKD, there is lower use of ACE inhibitors, whereas ARBs are increasingly used. Yet the study shows opportunities for improvement in terms of increasing the proportion of patients taking all three evidence-based therapies for cardiovascular prevention. Many questions regarding the relationship between CKD and CVD remain unanswered. We believe that prospective data from the CLARIFY study will, in due course, help shed further light on this by permitting evaluation of the association of renal function on cardiovascular outcomes and mortality. The study will also assess the prognostic importance of and predictors for change in renal function over time.

Acknowledgments

Editorial support was provided by Sophie Rushton-Smith, PhD (MedLink Healthcare Communications) and was funded by Servier.

Author Contributions

Conceived and designed the experiments: PRK XG-M JZ PAK KMF IF RF J-CT MT PGS. Performed the experiments: PRK XG-M JZ PAK KMF IF RF J-CT MT NG PGS. Analyzed the data: NG IF. Wrote the paper: PRK XG-M PAK KMF IF MT NG PGS.

References

1. Anavekar NS, McMurray JJ, Velazquez EJ, Solomon SD, Kober L, et al. (2004) Relation between renal dysfunction and cardiovascular outcomes after myocardial infarction. N Engl J Med 351: 1285–1295.
2. Tonelli M, Muntner P, Lloyd A, Manns BJ, Klarenbach S, et al. (2012) Risk of coronary events in people with chronic kidney disease compared with those with diabetes: a population-level cohort study. Lancet 380: 807–814.
3. Latif F, Kleiman NS, Cohen DJ, Pencina MJ, Yen CH, et al. (2009) In-hospital and 1-year outcomes among percutaneous coronary intervention patients with chronic kidney disease in the era of drug-eluting stents: a report from the EVENT (Evaluation of Drug Eluting Stents and Ischemic Events) registry. JACC Cardiovasc Interv 2: 37–45.
4. Roghi A, Savonitto S, Cavallini C, Arraiz G, Angoli L, et al. (2008) Impact of acute renal failure following percutaneous coronary intervention on long-term mortality. J Cardiovasc Med (Hagerstown) 9: 375–381.
5. Sarnak MJ, Levey AS, Schoolwerth AC, Coresh J, Culleton B, et al. (2003) Kidney disease as a risk factor for development of cardiovascular disease: a statement from the American Heart Association Councils on Kidney in Cardiovascular Disease, High Blood Pressure Research, Clinical Cardiology, and Epidemiology and Prevention. Circulation 108: 2154–2169.
6. Tripepi G, Mallamaci F, Zoccali C (2005) Inflammation markers, adhesion molecules, and all-cause and cardiovascular mortality in patients with ESRD: searching for the best risk marker by multivariate modeling. J Am Soc Nephrol 16 Suppl 1: S83–88.
7. Krause MW, Massing M, Kshirsagar A, Rosamond W, Simpson RJ Jr (2004) Combination therapy improves survival after acute myocardial infarction in the elderly with chronic kidney disease. Ren Fail 26: 715–725.
8. Wright RS, Reeder GS, Herzog CA, Albright RC, Williams BA, et al. (2002) Acute myocardial infarction and renal dysfunction: a high-risk combination. Ann Intern Med 137: 563–570.
9. Steg PG (2009) Heart rate management in coronary artery disease: the CLARIFY registry. Eur Heart J 11(suppl D): D13–D18.
10. Steg PG, Ferrari R, Ford I, Greenlaw N, Tardif JC, et al. (2012) Heart rate and use of beta-blockers in stable outpatients with coronary artery disease. PLoS One 7: e36284.
11. Levey AS, Stevens LA, Schmid CH, Zhang YL, Castro AF 3rd, et al. (2009) A new equation to estimate glomerular filtration rate. Ann Intern Med 150: 604–612.
12. National Kidney F (2002) K/DOQI clinical practice guidelines for chronic kidney disease: evaluation, classification, and stratification. Am J Kidney Dis 39: S1–266.
13. Arora P, Vasa P, Brenner D, Iglar K, McFarlane P, et al. (2013) Prevalence estimates of chronic kidney disease in Canada: results of a nationally representative survey. CMAJ 185: E417–423.
14. Zachariah D, Brown R, Kanagala P, Bashir A, Mohan M, et al. (2014) The impact of age and chronic kidney disease on secondary prevention post-primary percutaneous coronary intervention. QJM 107: 185–192.
15. Centers for Disease Control and Prevention National Health and Nutrition Examination Survey. http://www.cdc.gov/nchs/nhanes.htm. Access date: 2014 March 7.
16. Eddington H, Sinha S, Li E, Hegarty J, Ting J, et al. (2009) Factors associated with vascular stiffness: cross-sectional analysis from the Chronic Renal Insufficiency Standards Implementation Study. Nephron Clin Pract 112: c190–198.
17. Choi JS, Kim CS, Bae EH, Ma SK, Jeong MH, et al. (2012) Suboptimal medical care of patients with ST-elevation myocardial infarction and renal insufficiency: results from the Korea Acute Myocardial Infarction Registry. BMC Nephrol 13: 110.
18. Fox CS, Muntner P, Chen AY, Alexander KP, Roe MT, et al. (2010) Use of evidence-based therapies in short-term outcomes of ST-segment elevation myocardial infarction and non-ST-segment elevation myocardial infarction in patients with chronic kidney disease: a report from the National Cardiovascular Data Acute Coronary Treatment and Intervention Outcomes Network registry. Circulation 121: 357–365.
19. Hanna EB, Chen AY, Roe MT, Saucedo JF (2012) Characteristics and in-hospital outcomes of patients presenting with non-ST-segment elevation myocardial infarction found to have significant coronary artery disease on coronary angiography and managed medically: stratification according to renal function. Am Heart J 164: 52–57 e51.
20. Piccini JP, Stevens SR, Chang Y, Singer DE, Lokhnygina Y, et al. (2013) Renal dysfunction as a predictor of stroke and systemic embolism in patients with nonvalvular atrial fibrillation: validation of the R(2)CHADS(2) index in the ROCKET AF (Rivaroxaban Once-daily, oral, direct factor Xa inhibition Compared with vitamin K antagonism for prevention of stroke and Embolism Trial in Atrial Fibrillation) and ATRIA (AnTicoagulation and Risk factors In Atrial fibrillation) study cohorts. Circulation 127: 224–232.
21. KDIGO (2012) CKD evaluation and management. KDIGO 2012 Clinical Practice Guideline for the Evaluation and Management of Chronic Kidney Disease. http://kdigo.org/home/guidelines/ckd-evaluation-management/. Access date: 2014 March 7.

6

Smoking Is a Risk Factor for the Progression of Idiopathic Membranous Nephropathy

Makoto Yamaguchi[1], Masahiko Ando[2], Ryohei Yamamoto[3], Shinichi Akiyama[1], Sawako Kato[1], Takayuki Katsuno[1], Tomoki Kosugi[1], Waichi Sato[1], Naotake Tsuboi[1], Yoshinari Yasuda[1], Masashi Mizuno[1], Yasuhiko Ito[1], Seiichi Matsuo[1], Shoichi Maruyama[1]*

1 Department of Nephrology, Nagoya University Graduate School of Medicine, Nagoya, Japan, **2** Center for Advanced Medicine and Clinical Research, Nagoya University Hospital, Nagoya, Japan, **3** Department of Geriatric Medicine and Nephrology, Osaka University Graduate School of Medicine, Suita, Japan

Abstract

Background: Multiple studies have shown cigarette smoking to be a risk factor for chronic kidney disease. However, it is unknown whether smoking similarly increases the risk for progression of membranous nephropathy.

Methods: This study used the Nagoya Nephrotic Syndrome Cohort Study (N-NSCS), including 171 patients with idiopathic membranous nephropathy (IMN) from 10 nephrology centers in Japan. The dose-response relationships between cigarette smoking and the outcomes were assessed by using multivariate Cox proportional hazards models adjusted for clinically relevant factors. The primary outcome was a 30% decline in the estimated glomerular filtration rate (eGFR). The secondary outcome was first complete remission (CR) of proteinuria.

Results: During the observation period (median, 37 months; interquartile range, 16–71 months), 37 (21.6%) patients developed a 30% decline in eGFR and 2 (1.2%) progressed to ESRD. CR occurred in 103 (60.2%) patients. Multivariate Cox proportional hazards models revealed current smoking (adjusted hazard ratio [HR], 7.81 [95% confidence interval (CI), 3.17–19.7]), female sex (adjusted HR, 3.58 [95% CI, 1.87–8.00]), older age (adjusted HR, 1.71 [95% CI, 1.13–2.62] per 10 years), the number of cigarettes smoked daily (adjusted HR, 1.61 [95% CI, 1.23–2.09] per 10 cigarettes daily), and cumulative smoking of ≥40 pack-years (adjusted HR, 5.56 [95% CI, 2.17–14.6]) to be associated with a 30% decline in eGFR. However, smoking was not associated with CR.

Conclusion: Smoking is a significant and dose-dependent risk factor for IMN progression. All patients with IMN who smoke should be encouraged to quit.

Editor: Chris Bullen, The University of Auckland, New Zealand

Funding: This study was supported by a Grant-in-Aid for Progressive Renal Diseases Research, Research on Rare and Intractable Disease, from the Ministry of Health, Labour, and Welfare of Japan. The funders had no role in study design, data collection and analysis, decision to publish, or preparation of the manuscript.

Competing Interests: The authors have declared that no competing interests exist.

* Email: marus@med.nagoya-u.ac.jp

Introduction

Membranous nephropathy (MN) is a very common cause of nephrotic syndrome in adults [1,2]. Spontaneous remission occurs in 30–50% of patients, whereas another 30–50% experience progressive renal failure [3,4]. Previously identified clinical predictors of poor renal survival include older age, male sex, elevated serum creatinine level at the time of diagnosis, and the severity of proteinuria at the time of disease onset and during follow-up [5–9]. However, most of these cannot be modified, and the long-term outcome is not unfavorable regardless: the 10-year renal survival ranges from 60 to 80% [10,11]. The optimal management strategy for MN remains unclear.

It has recently become apparent that cigarette smoking, in addition to promoting cardiovascular disease (CVD), is an important independent renal risk factor [12–21]. However, these studies included patients with heterogeneous causes of CKD, such as diabetes, nephrosclerosis, and other diseases. Therefore, it was uncertain whether all kidney diseases were equally exacerbated by cigarette smoking. Elisabeth et al. reported in a nationwide population-based case-control study that the relationship between cigarette smoking and kidney impairment varied with the underlying kidney disease [22].

Yamamoto et al. reported in a large-scale retrospective cohort study that cigarette smoking was a key, dose-dependent prognostic factor in patients with IgA nephropathy [23]. The link between smoking and nephrotic syndrome has been investigated in only one case-control study of 80 patients with MN [24]. Although that study showed no relationship between smoking and MN, it was limited by the omission of two potentially significant independent variables, baseline proteinuria and kidney function at the time of study entry.

This study aimed to determine whether a history of smoking is an independent risk factor for the progression of MN and whether such risk is dose-dependent. This multicenter observational cohort study was organized as part of the Nagoya Nephrotic Syndrome Cohort Study (N-NSCS) based at 10 major nephrology centers in Nagoya, Japan.

Subjects and Methods

Study Population and Data Source

This cohort study included patients aged >18 years who had been diagnosed with membranous nephropathy (MN) on the basis of kidney biopsy between January 2003 and December 2012 at Nagoya University, Chubu Rosai Hospital, Japanese Red Cross Nagoya Daiichi Hospital, Tsushima City Hospital, Kasugai Municipal Hospital, Nagoya Kyoritsu Hospital, Anjo Kosei Hospital, Ichinomiya Municipal Hospital, Handa City Hospital, or Tosei General Hospital. Of the 272 such patients, we excluded patients with conditions generally considered to cause secondary MN, such as exposure to drugs associated with MN, diabetes mellitus, systemic lupus erythematosus, malignancy, or any other systemic disease known to be associated with secondary MN [25].

After exclusion of an additional 7 (3.9%) patients with missing data related to smoking status, 171 (62.9%) patients with idiopathic membranous nephropathy (IMN) were enrolled and followed up until September 2013. Clinically relevant factors at the baseline of those excluded (n = 7) and enrolled (n = 171) were not significantly different.

Our study was conducted by using linkable anonymous data set. No informed consent was obtained. The study protocol and consent procedure were approved by the ethics committees of Nagoya University, Chubu Rosai Hospital, Japanese Red Cross Nagoya Daiichi Hospital, Tsushima City Hospital, Kasugai Municipal Hospital, Nagoya Kyoritsu Hospital, Anjo Kosei Hospital, Ichinomiya Municipal Hospital, Handa City Hospital, and Tosei General Hospital Approval number:2012–0268.

Data Collection

Data pertaining to the patients' clinical characteristics at baseline were collected retrospectively from their medical records. The time of kidney biopsy was used as the baseline if the patient had not received immunosuppressive therapy or had received immunosuppressive therapy only after kidney biopsy. In patients who had received immunosuppressive therapy before kidney biopsy, the time of the initiation of immunosuppressive treatment was used as the baseline. The clinical characteristics included age, sex, body mass index, systolic and diastolic blood pressure, serum total cholesterol level, serum creatinine level, glomerular filtration rate (GFR; estimated using the equation recently generated by the Japanese Society of Nephrology: eGFR [mL/min/1.73 m^2] = $194 \times Scr^{-1.094} \times Age^{-0.287} \times 0.739$ [if female] [26]), serum albumin level, 24-hour urinary protein excretion or urinary protein-to-creatinine ratio, smoking status, use of any antihypertensive drugs, and initial use of corticosteroids and/or other immunosuppressive agents. Urinary protein excretion and eGFR data were collected from the medical record at each checkup in 1 to 3 month intervals.

We obtained detailed information about each patient's smoking status at the time of kidney biopsy, including the amount smoked (cigarettes/day), starting and stopping dates, and changes in use over time, from the medical records. The relationships between smoking and outcome measures were then studied for the following variables: (1) smoking status (all patients): never smoked, ex-smoker, or current smoker; (2) number of cigarettes smoked daily (current and ex-smokers); and (3) cumulative quantity smoked (current and ex-smokers): 0, 1–20, 21–39, or ≥40 pack-years (PY; 1 PY = 1 pack of 20 cigarettes/day ×1 year). Because we were most interested in whether a history of smoking was a risk factor for the progression of IMN, current smokers and ex-smokers were combined into a single group (current/ex-smokers).

The antihypertensive drugs used in this cohort were angiotensin-converting enzyme (ACE) inhibitors or angiotensin II receptor blockers (ARB), calcium channel blockers, β-blockers, and thiazides. The drugs used for therapeutic intervention, including the prescription of ACE inhibitors/ARB and corticosteroids or other immunosuppressive agents within 6 months of kidney biopsy, were also examined.

Nephrotic syndrome was defined as urinary protein excretion of ≥3.5 g/day (or a urinary protein/creatinine ratio of ≥3.5) and a serum albumin level of <3.0 mg/dL.

Complete remission (CR) of proteinuria was defined as urinary protein excretion of <0.3 g/day, a urinary protein/creatinine ratio of <0.3, and/or a negative/trace result for urinary protein on a dipstick test.

Partial remission (PR) of proteinuria was defined as urinary protein excretion of <3.5 g/day and a urinary protein/creatinine ratio of <3.5.

Relapse was defined as urinary protein excretion of ≥1.0 g/day, a urinary protein/creatinine ratio of ≥1.0, or a urinary protein dipstick result of ≥2+ on at least 2 occasions after achievement of CR.

The rate of decline in eGFR per year (mL/min per 1.73 m^2/year) was determined by plotting the eGFR against the observation time.

The anonymous data set is available in the Table S4.

Outcomes

The primary outcome was a 30% decline in eGFR before end-stage renal disease (ESRD). The secondary outcome was first CR.

The serum creatinine level was measured as required for each patient. Patients were followed up until September 2013 and censored at the time of death (if before ESRD or CR) or as of the last serum creatinine measurement before September 2013.

Statistical Analysis

Differences in clinical characteristics between those who had never smoked and current-/ex-smokers were compared by using the Wilcoxon rank-sum test or Fisher's exact test. To identify predictors independently associated with each outcome, potential covariates were examined by using the log-rank test and/or univariate and multivariate Cox proportional hazards models. The proportional hazards assumption for covariates was tested by using scaled Schoenfeld residuals. For continuous variables, the Wilcoxon rank-sum test was performed to assess the significance of inter-group differences. Categorical variables were expressed as percentages and compared by using Fisher's exact test. The rate of survival without a 30% decline in eGFR and the cumulative probability of achieving a first CR were calculated by using the Kaplan-Meier method and the log-rank test. The trend in each outcome with respect to the cumulative quantity smoked was examined statistically by scoring never smoking as 0 and current-/ex-smokers with 1–20, 21–39, and ≥40 pack-years' exposure as 1, 2, and 3, respectively; the resulting scores were then included in the regression model. The level of statistical significance was set at $P<0.05$. All statistical analyses were performed by using JMP version 10.0.0 (SAS Institute, Cary, NC, USA; www.jmp.com) and STATA version 13.0 (STATA Corp, www.stata.com).

Results

Study participants and clinical characteristics

The present study included 171 patients with IMN, of whom 108 (63.2%) had never smoked, 28 (16.4%) were ex-smokers, and 35 (20.5%) were current smokers. The clinical characteristics of the two groups (those who had never smoked and current/ex-smokers) are summarized in Table 1.

The two groups differed significantly in age, proportion of males, body mass index, urinary protein excretion, and rate of therapeutic intervention with an ACE inhibitor or ARB within 6 months of kidney biopsy. At baseline, 114 patients (66.7%) had nephrotic syndrome as previously defined. The median follow-up period of those who had never-smoked, ex-smokers, and current-smokers was 36 (15–71), 33 (16–63), and 46 (18–87) months, respectively ($P = 0.288$).

We obtained the number of cigarettes smoked daily for 62 (98.4%) of the current/ex-smokers (1–10 cigarettes for 10 [16.1%], 11–20 cigarettes for 32 [51.6%], 21–30 cigarettes for 9 [14.5%], and 31–50 cigarettes for 11 [17.7%] patients) and the cumulative smoking dose for 60 (95.2%) of the current-/ex-smokers (≤20 pack-years for 11 [18.3%], 21–39 pack-years for 15 [25.0%], and ≥40 pack-years for 34 [56.7%] patients).

Table 1. Clinical Characteristics of the 171 Patients with IMN.

	Never smoked	Smokers (Current/Ex-)	*P* value
Number	108	63 (35/28)	
Baseline characteristics			
Age (years)	66 (59–73)	63 (53–68)	0.012
Male [n (%)]	63 (58.3)	55 (87.3)	<0.001
Body mass index (kg/m^2)	22.9 (21.1–24.7)	23.5 (22.3–26.2)	0.046
Systolic blood pressure (mmHg)	130 (120–145)	132 (121–143)	0.873
Diastolic blood pressure (mmHg)	76 (70–84)	79 (72–86)	0.156
Serum creatinine (mg/dL)	0.78 (0.66–1.00)	0.80 (0.71–1.00)	0.171
eGFR (mL/min/1.73 m^2)	76 (58–92)	76 (63–86)	0.639
Serum albumin (g/dL)	2.6 (2.1–3.2)	2.4 (2.0–3.2)	0.518
Urinary protein (g/day)	3.9 (2.4–6.1)	4.8 (3.2–8.4)	0.025
Urinary protein >3.5 (g/day) [n (%)]	68 (63.0)	46 (73.0)	0.239
Total cholesterol (mg/dL)	283 (238–375)	295 (247–368)	0.617
Use of antihypertensive drugs [n (%)]	33 (30.6)	25 (39.7)	0.244
Smoking status			
Number of cigarettes smoked daily	NA	20 (20–30)	
Pack-years	NA	40 (24–49)	
Therapeutic interventions within 6 months after kidney biopsy			
ACE inhibitor or ARB therapy [n (%)]	65 (60.2)	48 (76.2)	0.044
Immunosuppressive treatment			0.413
No immunosuppressive agent	58 (53.7)	28 (44.4)	
Prednisolone [n (%)]	19 (17.6)	11 (17.5)	
Prednisolone + cyclosporine [n (%)]	31 (28.7)	24 (38.1)	
Outcomes			
30% reduction in eGFR [n (%)]	16 (14.8)	21 (33.3)	0.007
50% reduction in eGFR [n (%)]	6 (5.6)	11 (17.5)	0.017
Decline in eGFR (mL/min per 1.73 m^2 per year)	2.42 (−1.44 to 6.91)	4.01 (0.51–8.78)	0.046
ESRD [n (%)]	1 (0.9)	1 (1.6)	1.000
Death [n (%)]	8 (7.4)	3 (4.8)	0.748
Remission			
Complete remission [n (%)]	63 (58.3)	40 (63.5)	0.522
Partial remission [n (%)]	96 (88.9)	54 (85.7)	0.631
Relapse [n (%)]	14 (16.1)	12 (26.7)	0.170
Observation period (months)	36 (15–71)	39 (18–74)	0.375

Median (interquartile range), Conversion factors for units: SCr in mg/dL to μmol/L, ×88.4; eGFR (mL/min/1.73 m^2) = $194 \times Scr^{-1.094} \times Age^{-0.287} \times 0.739$ (if female), total cholesterol in mg/dL to mmol/L, ×0.02586.

Abbreviations: IMN, idiopathic membranous nephropathy; eGFR, estimated glomerular filtration rate; ACE inhibitor/ARB, angiotensin-converting enzyme inhibitor/angiotensin receptor blocker; SCr, serum creatinine; ESRD, end-stage renal disease; NA, not applicable.

Treatment during the observation period

An ACE inhibitor or ARB was newly prescribed within 6 months of kidney biopsy in 113 (66.1%) patients and was used by 156 (91.2%) by the end of follow-up. The enrolled patients were divided according to the treatment within 6 months of kidney biopsy into three groups: (1) the prednisolone group, comprising 30 patients (17.5%) who received prednisolone alone; (2) the cyclosporine group, comprising 55 patients (32.1%) who received prednisolone and cyclosporine; and (3) the supportive therapy group, comprising 86 patients (50.3%) who received neither prednisolone nor other immunosuppressive drugs. One patient in the cyclosporine group (0.6%) also received mizoribine. Most of the patients in the prednisolone group were prescribed prednisolone starting at 0.8–1.0 mg/kg/day orally and tapered according to the response to therapy, whereas most in the cyclosporine group started with cyclosporine at 1 to 2 mg/kg and prednisolone at 0.4–0.6 mg/kg. The cyclosporine dosage was adjusted to achieve the target whole-blood trough level, and the prednisolone dose was tapered according to the response to therapy. The time from renal biopsy to the initiation of immunosuppressive therapy was 0.7 months (interquartile range, 0.3–3.3 months). The duration of prednisolone use was 11 months (interquartile range, 8–25 months) in the prednisolone group and 14 months (interquartile range, 9–17 months) in the cyclosporine group.

Outcome data

The median observation time for the entire cohort was 37 months (interquartile range, 15–72 months). In total, 37 (21.6%) patients developed a 30% decline in eGFR before ESRD, 17 (9.9%) developed a 50% decline in eGFR before ESRD, and 2 (1.2%) progressed to ESRD.

The rates of avoiding a 30% decline in eGFR for 1, 5, and 10 years were 0.82 (95% confidence interval [CI], 0.71–0.90), 0.61 (95% CI, 0.46–0.74), and 0.56 (95% CI, 0.40–0.71), respectively, in current-/ex-smokers and 0.93 (95% CI, 0.86–0.97), 0.80 (95% CI, 0.69–0.88), and 0.74 (95% CI, 0.57–0.86) in those who had never smoked; therefore, current/ex-smokers were at higher risk for developing a 30% decline in eGFR ($P = 0.012$; Fig. 1).

The eGFR decreased significantly faster in current/ex-smokers than in those who had never smoked (4.01 mL/min per 1.73 m^2 per year [interquartile range, 0.51–8.78 mL/min per 1.73 m^2 per year] versus 2.42 mL/min per 1.73 m^2 per year [interquartile range, −1.44 to 6.91 mL/min per 1.73 m^2 per year]).

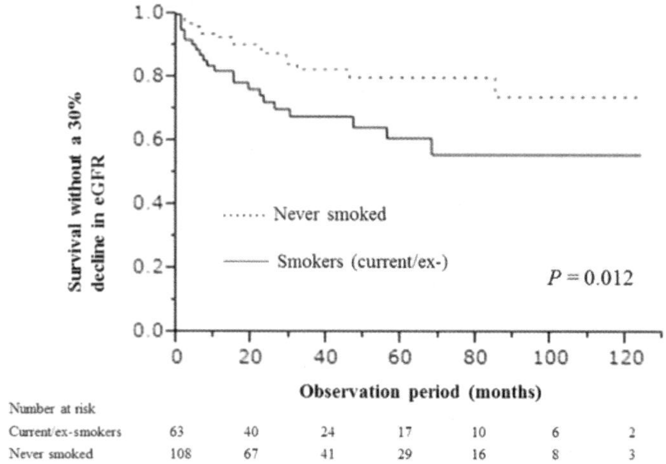

Figure 1. Time to 30% decline in eGFR in current/ex-smokers and those who never smoked.

The eGFR did not improve by the last follow-up visit in any of the 37 patients who experienced a 30% decline in eGFR.

Meanwhile, 103 (60.2%) patients achieved CR of proteinuria after a median follow-up of 14 months (interquartile range, 6–25 months). The cumulative probabilities of achieving CR within 1, 5, and 10 years were 0.31 (95% CI, 0.20–0.44), 0.77 (95% CI, 0.62–0.87), and 0.81 (95% CI, 0.65–0.90) in current-/ex-smokers and 0.43 (95% CI, 0.33–0.54), 0.80 (95% CI, 0.67–0.88), and 0.81 (95% CI, 0.65–0.92) in those who had never smoked. Therefore, smoking was not associated with the achievement of CR ($P = 0.570$).

Among the patients who achieved a first remission, 26 (25.2%) relapsed at least once.

No patient progressed to ESRD before developing a 30% decline in eGFR.

Eleven (6.4%) patients died during follow-up, one due to infection, and one each to acute subdural hematoma, traffic accident, sudden death, and intestinal bleeding. Malignancy occurred in 5 (2.9%) patients; the diagnoses were esophageal cancer, stomach cancer, colon cancer, prostate cancer, and malignant lymphoma in one patient each.

Predictors of a 30% decline in eGFR

Univariate Cox proportional hazards models revealed that older age, female sex, initial use of cyclosporine combination therapy, and current smoking were significantly associated with the primary outcome (Table 2). Adjustment for clinically relevant factors revealed current smoking (adjusted hazard ratio [HR], 7.81 [95% CI, 3.17–19.7], $P < 0.001$), female sex (adjusted HR, 3.58 [95% CI, 1.87–8.00], $P = 0.002$), older age (adjusted HR, 1.71 [95% CI, 1.13–2.62], per 10 years, $P = 0.010$), and use of cyclosporine in combination with prednisolone (adjusted HR, 2.67 [95% CI, 1.08–6.59], $P = 0.034$) to be significant predictors of the primary outcome.

No interactive effect on the primary outcome was detected between use of cyclosporine and smoking (adjusted HR, 1.16 [95% CI, 0.61–2.24], $P = 0.644$).

To confirm the robustness of our results, we similarly assessed predictors of a 50% decline in eGFR and found that current smoking (adjusted HR, 9.85 [95% CI, 2.68–41.0], $P < 0.001$) and female sex (adjusted HR, 4.20 [95% CI, 1.19–15.3], $P = 0.027$) were also significant predictors of this outcome (Table S1).

Table 2. Predictors of a 30% decline in eGFR.

	Univariate model		Multivariate model	
	HR (95% CI)	*P* value	HR (95% CI)	*P* value
Age (per 10 years)	1.47 (1.07–2.07)	0.018	1.71 (1.13–2.62)	0.010
Male (versus female)	0.43 (0.22–0.83)	0.012	0.28 (0.13–0.63)	0.002
Systolic blood pressure (per 10 mmHg)	1.06 (0.90–1.23)	0.455	1.07 (0.86–1.32)	0.546
Diastolic blood pressure (per 10 mmHg)	1.20 (0.94–1.53)	0.142	1.08 (0.77–1.52)	0.660
Serum albumin (per 1.0 g/dL)	0.80 (0.51–1.24)	0.317	1.32 (0.73–2.36)	0.359
Serum creatinine (per 1.0 mg/dL)	0.67 (0.18–1.98)	0.501	0.90 (0.19–3.13)	0.885
Urinary protein excretion (per 1.0 g/day)	1.03 (0.94–1.12)	0.519	1.02 (0.91–1.13)	0.673
Therapeutic interventions within 6 months after kidney biopsy				
ACE inhibitor or ARB therapy	0.72 (0.26–2.99)	0.598	0.90 (0.29–3.96)	0.874
Immunosuppressive treatment				
No immunosuppressive agent	Reference		Reference	
Prednisolone	0.84 (0.24–2.33)	0.758	1.30 (0.33–4.21)	0.687
Prednisolone + cyclosporine	2.18 (1.09–4.42)	0.027	2.67 (1.08–6.59)	0.034
Smokers (Current/Ex-)	2.24 (1.17–4.35)	0.015	4.00 (1.87–8.79)	<0.001
Ex-smokers	1.68 (0.64–3.93)	0.273	2.23 (0.79–5.79)	0.127
Current smokers	2.68 (1.29–5.52)	0.009	7.81 (3.17–19.7)	<0.001

HR, hazard ratio; CI, confidence interval.
Data are the HR, 95% CI, and *P* value from Cox proportional hazard regression analyses.
"Never smoked" was used as the reference category.
Adjusted for baseline characteristics (age, sex, systolic/diastolic pressure, serum creatinine level, urinary protein, use of ACE inhibitor or ARB within 6 months after kidney biopsy, and immunosuppressive therapy within 6 months after kidney biopsy).
Abbreviations: IMN, idiopathic membranous nephropathy; ACE, angiotensin-converting enzyme; ARB, angiotensin receptor blocker.

Dose-dependent association between smoking and a 30% decline in eGFR

Table 3 shows that the total smoking dose had a strong independent effect on the risk of renal progression. Both univariate and multivariate Cox proportional hazards models showed a significant association between the number of cigarettes per day and the primary outcome (adjusted HR, 1.61 [95% CI, 1.23–2.09], $P<0.001$, multivariate model 1). Cumulative smoking of ≥ 40 pack-years was also significantly associated with the primary outcome (adjusted HR, 5.56 [95% CI, 2.17–14.6], $P<0.001$, multivariate model 2). These results suggested that the risk of renal progression increased almost linearly with the number of cigarettes smoked.

Predictors of first complete remission

Univariate Cox proportional hazards models revealed a lower serum creatinine level, initial use of prednisolone monotherapy, and initial use of cyclosporine in combination with prednisolone to be significantly associated with first CR of proteinuria (Table S2). After adjustment for clinically relevant factors, the initial use of prednisolone monotherapy (adjusted HR, 2.15 [95% CI, 1.17–3.84], $P=0.015$) and cyclosporine in combination with prednisolone (adjusted HR, 2.90 [95% CI, 1.68–5.00], $P<0.001$) remained significant predictors of first CR of proteinuria. Neither a history of smoking (Table S2) nor the total smoking dose (Table S3) was associated with CR.

Discussion

We found that smoking increased the risk of renal dysfunction in Japanese patients with IMN in a dose-dependent manner, although former smoking did not appear to be a risk factor. These results highlight the clinical importance of smoking cessation in the treatment of patients with IMN.

Several cohort studies in the general population have suggested a dose-dependent association between smoking and CKD. The Cardiovascular Health Study identified smoking as a risk factor related to CKD progression in 4142 U.S. participants aged >65 years but did not include proteinuria as an independent variable [12]. The NHANRS II study followed 9082 middle-aged (49.3±13.3 years) U.S. participants for 13.2 years and showed a higher adjusted risk of end-stage kidney disease among those smoking >20 cigarettes per day. Baggio et al. studied 2981 elderly subjects from Italy and found smoking ≥21 cigarettes per day to be a very strong risk factor for pathological loss of kidney function [17]. Furthermore, the HUNT II study of 65,589 Norwegian participants revealed that the risk increased significantly as the cumulative amount of smoking (pack-years) increased; however, the risk significantly decreased as the years elapsed since smoking cessation increased among male ex-smokers aged <70 years [27]. Yamagata reported in a 10-year follow-up study of 123,764 Japanese participants aged ≥40 years who received community-based annual examinations that current smoking increased the risk of developing proteinuria, but that study did not evaluate the dose-dependency of the relationship between smoking and CKD [21]. These reports collectively identify smoking as a risk factor for the progression of CKD in the general population. Our present results were consistent with this literature, particularly the HUNT II study, in which current/ex-smokers reporting larger cumulative numbers of cigarettes smoked were at significantly higher risk of renal progression than were those who had never smoked.

Table 3. Influence of smoking dose on the risk of a 30% decline in eGFR.

	Univariate model		Multivariate model	
	HR (95% CI)	***P* value**	**HR (95% CI)**	***P* value**
Model 1				
No. of cigarettes (/10/d)	1.32 (1.05–1.63)	0.021	1.61 (1.23–2.09)	<0.001
Model 2				
1–20 pack-years	1.07 (0.17–3.75)	0.933	1.36 (0.20–5.94)	0.715
21–39 pack-years	1.64 (0.47–4.49)	0.399	3.51 (0.87–12.5)	0.076
≥40 pack-years	2.61 (1.21–5.48)	0.016	5.56 (2.17–14.6)	<0.001
Test for trend		0.015		<0.001

HR, hazard ratio; CI, confidence interval.
Data are the HR, 95% CI, and *P* value from Cox proportional hazard regression analyses.
"Never smoked" was used as the reference category. Models 1 and 2 are based on data from 168 patients because the number of cigarettes was missing for 1 current and 2 ex-smokers. Adjusted for baseline characteristics (age, sex, systolic/diastolic pressure, serum creatinine level, urinary protein, use of angiotensin-converting enzyme inhibitor or angiotensin receptor blocker within 6 months after kidney biopsy, and immunosuppressive therapy within 6 months after kidney biopsy).

Only a few studies of primary kidney disease have found a dose-dependent association between cigarette smoking and progression of primary glomerulonephritis. Yamamoto et al. identified cigarette smoking as a key dose-dependent prognostic factor for IgA nephropathy in a multivariate model. There has been only one case-control study addressing the relationship between smoking and nephrotic syndrome, which revealed no relationship between smoking and kidney progression in patients with MN [24]. However, that study failed to include baseline proteinuria and kidney function at study entry as independent variables. In contrast, we included those variables and identified smoking as an important dose-dependent prognostic factor in patients with IMN after adjustment for relevant confounders.

The present study identified immunosuppressive therapy as both a risk factor for renal progression (although urinary protein excretion was greater in such patients than in those who initially received supportive therapy) and the most significant independent predictor of achievement of CR. These results may, however, reflect indication bias, for which the present retrospective cohort study did not control. Furthermore, we should consider that unmeasured factors associated with treatment may not be included in the model.

Combination therapy with cyclosporine and prednisolone was frequently used for treatment of IMN in our cohort. Cattran et al. demonstrated that cyclosporine significantly decreased the rate of renal progression and reduced proteinuria in patients with IMN at high risk for progression and persistent nephrotic-range proteinuria [28,29]. Alexopoulos et al. also found that cyclosporine with or without corticosteroids effectively induced remission in the majority of nephrotic patients with IMN and well-preserved renal function [30]. Based on these findings, we often use cyclosporine in combination with corticosteroids for first-line treatment of patients with IMN. Although the 2012 Kidney Disease Improving Global Outcomes (KDIGO) clinical practice guideline for IMN recommends a cytotoxic agent (cyclophosphamide) for patients at high risk of progression [31], no patient in our study was treated with cyclophosphamide. This should be considered when interpreting our results.

Interestingly, our study identified female sex as an independent risk factor after adjustment for relevant clinical factors. Previous studies had shown male sex to be associated with a higher risk of developing ESRD [5–9]. In contrast, female sex has generally been associated with a relatively benign course [32]. However, these studies did not include smoking status as an independent variable, which may have caused overestimation of the relationship between male sex and risk of renal progression. Furthermore, Mina Yu reported in a cross-sectional study that menopause was an independent risk factor for CKD because of the accompanying loss of possibly cardioprotective estradiol production [33]. Previous studies of membranous nephropathy have generally enrolled younger patients than our study, suggesting that our study may have included a relatively large number of postmenopausal patients. Therefore, membranous nephropathy may lead to more rapid decline in GFR in postmenopausal women, who are already in an unfavorable hormonal state (i.e., estrogen deficient) with respect to the kidney. The generalizability of our results should be confirmed in another cohort study.

Although the exact mechanisms of the nephrotoxic effects of smoking are poorly understood, we can present some potential explanations of the relationship between smoking and CKD onset and progression. First, nephrotic syndrome increases oxidative stress by impairing antioxidant pathways [34]. The addition of smoking-induced oxidative stress to nephrotic syndrome-associated oxidative stress may accelerate renal progression [35–38]. Second, ex vivo studies have suggested that nicotine could promote mesangial cell proliferation and increase production of critical molecules involved in extracellular matrix production [39,40]. Third, smoking (or nicotine) could increase the plasma endothelin level [41], which has been shown to correlate with effective renal plasma flow in smokers [42]. Furthermore, Alves et al. reported that smoking aggravates the cyclosporine-induced impairment of GFR and that smoking in combination with cyclosporine induced periglomerular structural lesions and oxidative stress in a rat model of cyclosporine nephrotoxicity [43]. However, our results showed no interactive effect on renal function between use of cyclosporine and smoking. The external validity of the result should be confirmed in another study.

It is also possible that smoking might relate to medication adherence in some other way. A cross-sectional study showed that current smokers were less compliant with medication use than nonsmokers [44]. Therefore, we should consider the possibility of medication adherence in smokers. Moreover, we are aware that MN can itself have extra-renal associations and these should be considered for their possible relationship with smoking.

Our study has some limitations that must be discussed. First, underreporting of smoking and changes in smoking habits during the follow-up period can cause misclassification and tend to overestimate the effect of smoking on renal progression. Second, we did not address the relationship between smoking cessation and renal progression because our sample size was insufficient to evaluate it. Third, the patients in this study may not be representative of patients with IMN in other countries: different consequences of smoking have been reported in different populations [45]. We therefore advise caution when interpreting and generalizing our results.

Allowing for these methodological issues, our study has several advantages: it is one of the largest multicenter adult MN cohorts in Japan ever reported and is also, to the best of our knowledge, the first description of a relationship between smoking and renal dysfunction in patients with IMN.

In conclusion, our retrospective cohort study in patients with IMN showed cigarette smoking to be a key, dose-dependent predictor of IMN progression. All patients with IMN who smoke should be encouraged to quit.

Acknowledgments

We are grateful for the time and efforts of the nephrologists who supported the present study: Dr. Shizunori Ichida, Dr. Hideaki Shimizu, Dr. Junichiro Yamamoto, Dr. Tomohiko Naruse, Dr. Hirofumi Tamai, Dr. Kei Kurata, Dr. Hirotake Kasuga, Dr. Arimasa Shirasaki, and Dr. Makoto Mizutani.

Author Contributions

Conceived and designed the experiments: MY MA SK S. Maruyama. Performed the experiments: MY MA RY SA SK T. Katsuno T. Kosugi WS NT YY MM YI S. Matsuo S. Maruyama. Analyzed the data: MY MA RY. Contributed reagents/materials/analysis tools: MY MA RY SK S. Maruyama. Contributed to the writing of the manuscript: MY MA S. Maruyama. Critically revised manuscript: MY MA S. Maruyama.

References

1. Fervenza FC, Sethi S, Specks U (2008) Idiopathic membranous nephropathy: diagnosis and treatment. Clin J Am Soc Nephrol 3: 905–919.
2. Cattran DC (2001) Idiopathic membranous nephropathy. Kidney Int 59: 1983–1994.
3. van den Brand JAJG, Hofstra JM, Wetzels JFM (2011) Low-molecular-weight proteins as prognostic markers in idiopathic membranous nephropathy. Clin J Am Soc Nephrol 6: 2846–2853.
4. du Buf-Vereijken PW, Branten AJ, Wetzels JF (2005) Idiopathic membranous nephropathy: outline and rationale of a treatment strategy. Am J Kidney Dis 46: 1012–1029.
5. Shiiki H, Saito T, Nishitani Y, Mitarai T, Research Group on Progressive Renal Diseases in Japan, et al. (2004) Prognosis and risk factors for idiopathic membranous nephropathy with nephrotic syndrome in Japan. Kidney Int 65: 1400–1407.
6. Marx BE, Marx M (1999) Prediction in idiopathic membranous nephropathy. Kidney Int 56: 666–673.
7. Troyanov S, Wall CA, Miller JA, Scholey JW, Cattran DC (2004) Idiopathic membranous nephropathy: definition and relevance of a partial remission. Kidney Int 66: 1199–1205.
8. Cattran DC, Pei Y, Greenwood CM, Ponticelli C, Passerini P, et al. (1997) Validation of a predictive model of idiopathic membranous nephropathy: its clinical and research implications. Kidney Int 51: 901–907.
9. Pei Y, Cattran D, Greenwood C (1992) Predicting chronic renal insufficiency in idiopathic membranous glomerulonephritis. Kidney Int 42: 960–966.
10. Noel LH, Zanetti M, Droz D, Barbanel C (1979) Long-term prognosis of idiopathic membranous glomerulonephritis. Study of 116 untreated patients. Am J Med 66: 82–90.
11. Zucchelli P, Ponticelli C, Cagnoli L, Passerini P (1987) Long-term outcome of idiopathic membranous nephropathy with nephrotic syndrome. Nephrol Dial Transplant 2: 73–78.
12. Bleyer AJ, Shemanski LR, Burke GL, Hansen KJ, Appel RG (2000) Tobacco, hypertension, and vascular disease: risk factors for renal functional decline in an older population. Kidney Int 57(5): 2072–2079.
13. Tozawa M, Iseki K, Iseki C, Oshiro S, Ikemiya Y, et al. (2002) Influence of smoking and obesity on the development of proteinuria. Kidney Int 62: 956–962.
14. Haroun MK, Jaar BG, Hoffman SC, Comstock GW, Klag MJ, et al. (2003) Risk factors for chronic kidney disease: a prospective study of 23,534 men and women in Washington County, Maryland. J Am Soc Nephrol 14(11): 2934–2941.
15. Stengel B, Tarver-Carr ME, Powe NR, Eberhardt MS, Brancati FL (2003) Lifestyle factors, obesity and the risk of chronic kidney disease. Epidemiology 14(4): 479–487.
16. Fox CS, Larson MG, Leip EP, Culleton B, Wilson PW, et al. (2004) Predictors of new-onset kidney disease in a community-based population. JAMA 29(7): 844–850.
17. Baggio B, Budakovic A, Perissinotto E, Maggi S, Cantaro S, et al (2005) Atherosclerotic risk factors and renal function in the elderly: the role of hyperfibrinogenaemia and smoking. Results from the Italian Longitudinal Study on Ageing (ILSA). Nephrol Dial Transplant 20(1): 114–123.
18. Hallan S, de Mutsert R, Carlsen S, Dekker FW, Aasarod K, et al. (2006) Obesity, smoking, and physical inactivity as risk factors for CKD: are men more vulnerable? Am J Kidney Dis 47(3): 396–405.
19. Ishani A, Grandits GA, Grimm RH, Svendsen KH, Collins AJ, et al. (2006) Association of single measurements of dipstick proteinuria, estimated glomerular filtration rate, and hematocrit with 25-year incidence of end-stage renal disease in the multiple risk factor intervention trial. J Am Soc Nephrol 17(5): 1444–1452.
20. Shankar A, Klein R, Klein BE (2006) The association among smoking, heavy drinking, and chronic kidney disease. Am J Epidemiol 164(3): 263–271.
21. Yamagata K, Ishida K, Sairenchi T, Takahashi H, Ohba S, et al. (2007) Risk factors for chronic kidney disease in a community-based population: a 10-year follow-up study. Kidney Int 71(2): 159–166.
22. Ejerblad E, Fored CM, Lindblad P, Fryzek J, Dickman PW, et al. (2004) Association between smoking and chronic renal failure in a nationwide population-based case-control study. J Am Soc Nephrol 15(8): 2178–2185.
23. Yamamoto R, Nagasawa Y, Shoji T, Iwatani H, Hamano T, et al. (2010) Cigarette smoking and progression of IgA nephropathy. Am J Kidney Dis 56(2): 313–324.
24. Stengel B, Couchoud C, Cénée S, Hémon D (2000) Age, blood pressure and smoking effects on chronic renal failure in primary glomerular nephropathies. Kidney Int 57(6): 2519–2526.
25. Hofstra JM, Wetzels JF (2012) Management of patients with membranous nephropathy. Nephrol Dial Transplant 27: 6–9.
26. Matsuo S, Imai E, Horio M, Yasuda Y, Tomita K, et al. (2009) Collaborators developing the Japanese equation for estimated GFR. Revised equations for estimated GFR from serum creatinine in Japan. Am J Kidney Dis 53: 982–992.
27. Hallan SI, Orth SR (2011) Smoking is a risk factor in the progression to kidney failure. Kidney Int 80: 516–523.
28. Cattran DC, Appel GB, Hebert LA, Hunsicker LG, Pohl MA, et al; North America Nephrotic Syndrome Study Group (2001) Cyclosporine in patients with steroid-resistant membranous nephropathy: a randomized trial. Kidney Int 59: 1484–1490.
29. Cattran DC, Greenwood C, Ritchie S, Bernstein K, Churchill DN, et al. (1995) A controlled trial of cyclosporine in patients with progressive membranous nephropathy. Canadian Glomerulonephritis Study Group. Kidney Int 47: 1130–1135.
30. Alexopoulos E, Papagianni A, Tsamelashvili M, Leontsini M, Memmos D (2006) Induction and long-term treatment with cyclosporine in membranous nephropathy with the nephrotic syndrome. Nephrol Dial Transplant 21: 3127–3132.
31. KDIGO Working Group (2012) KDIGO clinical practice guideline for glomerulonephritis. Kidney Int Suppl 2: 186–197.
32. Reichert LJ, Koene RA, Wetzels JF (1998) Prognostic factors in idiopathic membranous nephropathy. Am J Kidney Dis 31(1): 1–11.
33. Yu M, Ryu D-R, Kim S-J, Choi K-B, Kang D-H (2010) Clinical implication of metabolic syndrome on chronic kidney disease depends on gender and

menopausal status: results from the Korean National Health and Nutrition Examination Survey. Nephrol Dial Transplant 25: 469–477.
34. Soyoral YU, Aslan M, Emre H, Begenik H, Erdur FM, et al. (2011) Serum paraoxonase activity and oxidative stress in patients with adult nephrotic syndrome. Atherosclerosis 218(1): 243–246.
35. Nagasawa Y, Yamamoto R, Rakugi H, Isaka Y (2012) Cigarette smoking and chronic kidney diseases. Hypertens Res 35(3): 261–265.
36. Amaral S, Oliveira PJ, Ramalho-Santos J (2008) Diabetes and the impairment of reproductive function: possible role of mitochondria and reactive oxygen species. Curr Diabetes Rev 4(1): 46–54.
37. Maiese K, Chong ZZ, Shang YC (2007) Mechanistic insights into diabetes mellitus and oxidative stress. Curr Med Chem 14(16): 1729–1738.
38. Fatehi-Hassanabad Z, Chan CB, Furman BL (2010) Reactive oxygen species and endothelial function in diabetes. Eur J Pharmacol 636(1–3): 8–17.
39. Hua P, Feng W, Ji S, Raij L, Jaimes EA (2010) Nicotine worsens the severity of nephropathy in diabetic mice: implications for the progression of kidney disease in smokers. Am J Physiol Renal Physiol 299: F732–F739.
40. Jaimes EA, Tian RX, Raij L (2007) Nicotine: the link between cigarette smoking and the progression of renal injury? Am J Physiol Heart Circ Physiol 292: H76–H82.
41. Haak T, Jungmann E, Raab C, Usadel KH (1994) Elevated endothelin-1 levels after cigarette smoking. Metabolism 43(3): 267–269.
42. Gambaro G, Verlato F, Budakovic A (1998) Renal impairment in chronic cigarette smokers. J Am Soc Nephrol 9(4): 562–567.
43. Alves SA, Carlos CP, Mendes GEF, Oliveira SM, Luz MAM, et al. (2012) Previous exposure to cigarette smoke aggravates experimental cyclosporine-induced nephrotoxicity. Am J Nephrol 36: 334–341.
44. Sherman BW, Lynch WD (2014) The association of smoking with medical treatment adherence in the workforce of a large employer. Patient Prefer Adherence.8:477–486.
45. Sellers EM (1998) Pharmacogenetics and ethnoracial differences in smoking. JAMA 280: 179–180.

Correlations of *MTHFR* 677C>T Polymorphism with Cardiovascular Disease in Patients with End-Stage Renal Disease: A Meta-Analysis

Xian-Hui Gao[1]*, Guo-Yi Zhang[1], Ying Wang[2], Hui-Ying Zhang[3]

1 Laboratory of Preventive Medicine, School of Public Health, Liaoning Medical University, Jinzhou, China, **2** Department of Toxicology, School of Public Health, Liaoning Medical University, Jinzhou, China, **3** Sleep Monitoring Center, First Affiliated Hospital of Liaoning Medical University, Jinzhou, China

Abstract

Objective: This meta-analysis was conducted to evaluate the correlations of a common polymorphism (677C>T) in the methylenetetrahydrofolate reductase (*MTHFR*) gene with risk of cardiovascular disease (CVD) in patients with end-stage renal disease (ESRD).

Method: The following electronic databases were searched without language restrictions: Web of Science (1945~2013), the Cochrane Library Database (Issue 12, 2013), MEDLINE (1966~2013), EMBASE (1980~2013), CINAHL (1982~2013) and the Chinese Biomedical Database (CBM) (1982~2013). Meta-analysis was performed using STATA statistical software. Odds ratios (ORs) with their 95% confidence intervals (95%CIs) were calculated.

Results: Eight cohort studies met all inclusion criteria and were included in this meta-analysis. A total of 2,292 ESRD patients with CVD were involved in this meta-analysis. Our meta-analysis results revealed that the *MTHFR* 677C>T polymorphism might increase the risk of CVD in ESRD patients (TT vs. CC: OR = 2.75, 95%CI = 1.35~5.59, *P* = 0.005; CT+TT vs. CC: OR = 1.39, 95%CI = 1.09~1.78, *P* = 0.008; TT vs. CC+CT: OR = 2.52, 95%CI = 1.25~5.09, *P* = 0.010; respectively). Further subgroup analysis by ethnicity suggested that the *MTHFR* 677C>T polymorphism was associated with an elevated risk for CVD in ESRD patients among Asians (TT vs. CC: OR = 3.38, 95%CI = 1.11~10.28, *P* = 0.032; CT+TT vs. CC: OR = 1.44, 95%CI = 1.05~1.97, *P* = 0.022; TT vs. CC+CT: OR = 3.15, 95%CI = 1.02~9.72, *P* = 0.046; respectively), but not among Africans or Caucasians (all *P*>0.05).

Conclusion: Our findings indicate that the *MTHFR* 677C>T polymorphism may be associated with an elevated risk for CVD in ESRD patients, especially among Asians.

Editor: Yan Gong, University of Florida, United States of America

Funding: The authors have no support or funding to report.

Competing Interests: The authors have declared that no competing interests exist.

* Email: gaoxianhui16@126.com

Introduction

Hemodialysis (HD) is a common form of dialysis therapy for kidney disease by achieving the extracorporeal removal of waste products such as creatinine, urea and free water from the blood [1]. HD is the most common procedure performed for patients with end-stage renal disease (ESRD), with an estimation of 1.5 million ESRD patients receiving HD worldwide [2]. Despite its important role in treating ESRD, HD also serves as a multiplier for other vascular risk factors, contributing to an increased incidence of cardiovascular disease, such as atrial fibrillation and myocardial ischemia [3,4]. Moreover, it has been reported that mortality caused by cardiovascular disease (CVD) in ESRD patients is 25% higher than that in the general population [5,6]. Therefore, the assessment and prevention of CVD are major considerations for dealing patients with HD [7]. Generally, CVD refers to any disease that affects the cardiovascular system, principally cardiac disease, vascular diseases of the brain and kidney, and peripheral arterial disease [8]. Clinically, traditional CVD risk factors include old age, male sex, diabetes mellitus, and systolic hypertension and so on [9]. Over past few decades, studies have demonstrated that the severity and extent of cardiovascular complications in ESRD patients is disproportionate to the number and severity of traditional risk factors [10,11]. In recent years, nontraditional risk factors such as hemoglobin levels, inflammation, oxidative stress, and particularly epigenetic mechanisms of gene regulation have been emphasized as factors that may play an important role in the development of cardiovascular disease in patients with HD [12]. In addition, genetic polymorphisms have received considerable attention as a competitive candidate for the risk of CVD in ESRD patients [13].

Methylene tetrahydrofolate reductase (MTHFR), encoded by the *MTHFR* gene, is a key enzyme in folate metabolism which plays a critical role in the synthesis and methylation of DNA encoding for an enzyme responsible for re-methylation of homocysteine (Hcy) to methionine [14–16]. Actually, Hazra et al. confirmed that the functional polymorphism in MTHFR

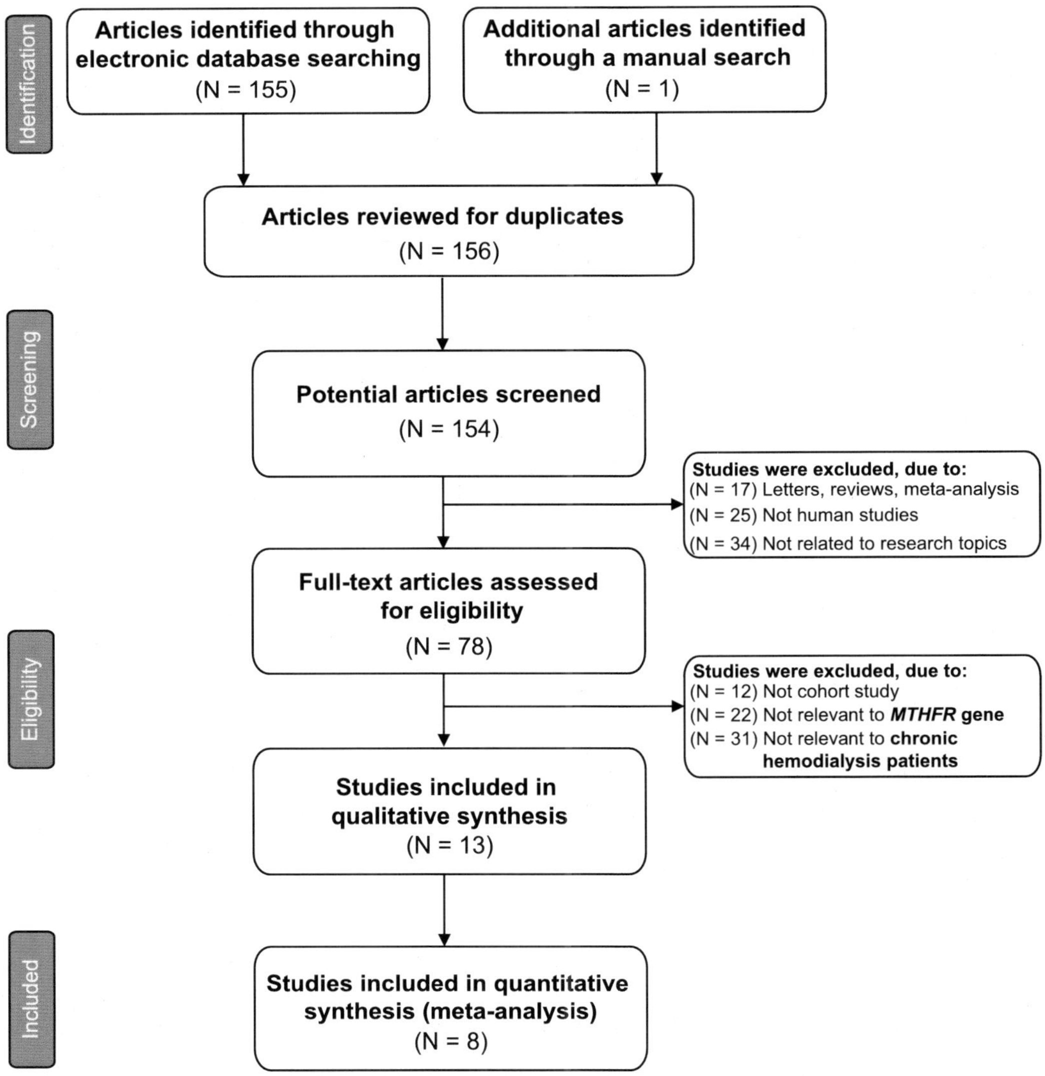

Figure 1. Flow chart shows study selection procedure. Eight cohort studies were included in this meta-analysis.

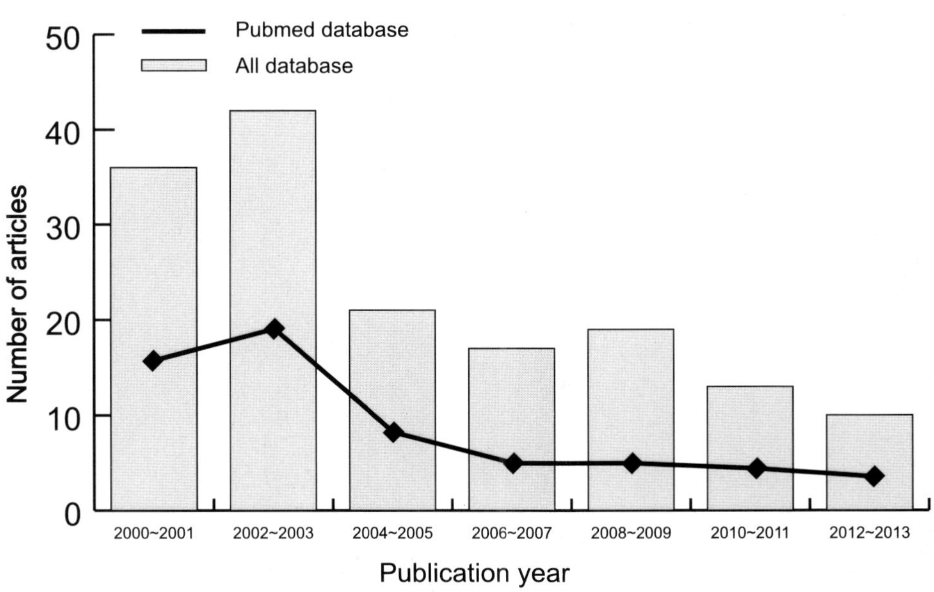

Figure 2. The distribution of the number of topic-related literatures in the electronic database over the last decade.

Table 1. Baseline characteristics and methodological qualities of all included studies.

First author	Year	Country	Ethnicity	Case number	Gender (M/F)	Age (years)	Genotyping method	Genotype frequency			HWE test	NOS score
								CC	CT	TT	(*P* value)	
Lee et al [21]	2011	Korea	Asians	152	83/69	56.8±13.6	PCR-RFLP	44	72	36	0.538	7
Ibrahim et al [30]	2009	Egypt	Africans	50	29/21	41.6±11.8	Direct sequencing	30	16	4	0.385	6
Aucella et al [28]	2005	Italy	Caucasians	461	217/244	58.8±15.6	PCR-RFLP	134	220	86	0.801	8
Fukasawa et al [23]	2003	Japan	Asians	337	196/141	61.5±13.7	Direct sequencing	111	158	68	0.390	8
Morimoto et al [32]	2002	Japan	Asians	168	87/81	60.7±13.1	PCR-RFLP	78	67	23	0.167	7
Haviv et al [29]	2002	USA	Caucasians	120	72/48	48.0±13.0	PCR-RFLP	40	60	19	0.656	7
Wrone et al [24]	2001	USA	Caucasians	459	230/226	-	Direct sequencing	216	184	59	0.049	7
Kimura et al [31]	2000	Japan	Asians	545	319/226	58.7±12.5	PCR-RFLP	199	251	95	0.303	8

Legend: M – male; F – female; SNP - single nucleotide polymorphism; HWE - Hardy-Weinberg equilibrium; NOS - Newcastle-Ottawa Scale; PCR-RFLP - polymerase chain reaction-restriction fragment length polymorphism.

Ala222Val (also reported as MTHFR C677T), rs1801133, on chromosome 1 was associated with plasma homocysteine in a healthy population [17]. The human *MTHFR* gene is located on the short arm of chromosome 1 (1p36.3), is comprised of 11 exons and 10 introns, and is 19.3 kb in length [17]. Currently, multiple researchers have demonstrated that genetic variations in the *MTHFR* gene might alter its production and function, thereby affecting individual prevalence rates of some diseases and even cancers [18,19]. More specifically, multiple polymorphic sites such as 677C>T (rs1801133) and 1298A>C (rs1801131) within the *MTHFR* promoter region have been reported in previous studies, of which 677C>T has been suggested to be implicated in the susceptibility to CVD in ESRD patients [20,21]. It should be noted that plasma Hcy levels have been found to be an important risk factor for the development of CVD in ESRD patients [22]. However, polymorphism at nucleotide 677C>T may reduce the activation and thermo-stability of MTHFR, and subsequently inhibit the generation of 5-Methylenetetrahydrofolate and interfere with the normal metabolism and re-methylation of Hcy, thereby resulting in the accumulation of Hcy and an elevated plasma Hcy concentration in individuals; however, contradictory results have also been reported [23,24]. Given the conflicting evidence on this issue, we conducted a meta-analysis of all available cohort studies to determine whether *MTHFR* genetic polymorphisms contribute to the pathogenesis of CVD in ESRD patients.

Methods

Publication search

The following electronic databases were searched without language restrictions: Web of Science (1945~2013), the Cochrane Library Database (Issue 12, 2013), MEDLINE (1966~2013), EMBASE (1980~2013), CINAHL (1982~2013) and the Chinese Biomedical Database (CBM) (1982~2013). We used the following keywords and MeSH terms in conjunction with a highly sensitive search strategy: ["SNP" or "mutation" or "genetic polymorphism" or "variation" or "polymorphism" or "single nucleotide polymorphism" or "variant"] and ["cardiovascular disease" or "CVD" or "cardiovascular risk" or "Hemodialysis" or "HD"] and ["methylenetetrahydrofolate reductase" or "MTHFR" or "methylene tetrahydrofolate reductase" or "5,10-methylenetetrahydrofolate reductase"]. We also conducted a manual search to find other potential articles based on references identified in retrieved articles.

Inclusion and exclusion criteria

The following criteria were used to determine the eligibility of included studies: (1) the study design must be a clinical cohort study; (2) the study must relate to the relationships of *MTHFR* 677C>T polymorphisms with the risk of CVD in ESRD patients; (3) all patients met the diagnostic criteria for HD; (4) the study must provide sufficient information about the frequencies of the *MTHFR* 677C>T polymorphism. If a study could not meet the inclusion criteria, it was excluded. The most recent or the largest sample size publication was included when the authors published several studies using the same subjects. The supporting PRISMA checklist is available as Checklist S1.

Data extraction

Data were systematically extracted by two authors from each included study using a standardized form. The form used for data extraction documented the most relevant items including publication year, language of publication, the first author's surname,

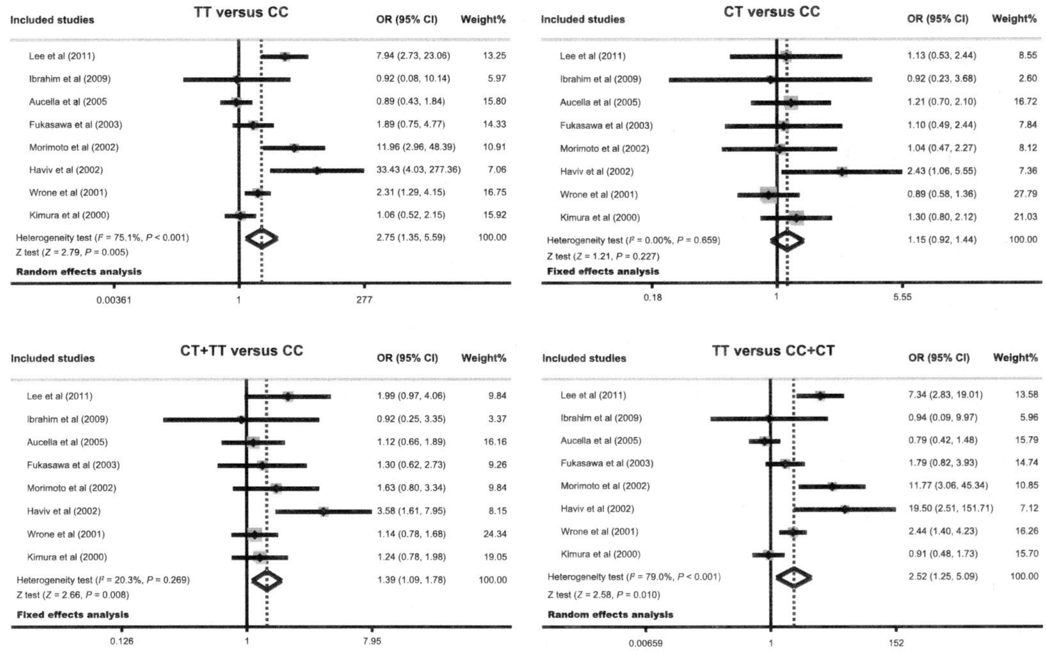

Figure 3. Forest plots for the relationships between the *MTHFR* 677C>T polymorphism and the risk of cardiovascular disease in chronic hemodialysis patients.

geographical location, sample size, design of study, the source of the subjects, source of samples, allele frequencies, genotyping method of SNP, evidence of HWE in healthy controls, etc.

Methodological assessment

Methodological quality was independently assessed by two observers according to the Newcastle-Ottawa Scale (NOS) criteria [25]. The NOS criteria includes three aspects: (1) subject selection: 0~4 points; (2) comparability of subject: 0~2 points; (3) clinical outcome: 0~3 points. NOS scores range from 0 to 9 with a score ≥7 indicating good quality. The supporting NOS score criteria are available in Supplement S1.

Statistical analysis

Meta-analysis was performed with the use of the STATA statistical software (Version 12.0, Stata Corporation, College Station, TX, USA). Odds ratios (ORs) with their 95% confidence intervals (95%CIs) were calculated as estimates of relative risk for CVD in ESRD patients. The *Z* test was used to estimate the statistical significance of pooled ORs. Heterogeneity among studies was estimated by the Cochran's *Q*-statistic and I^2 tests [26]. If a *Q*-test shows a $P<0.05$ or $I^2>50\%$, indicating significant heterogeneity, the random-effects model was conducted; otherwise the fixed-effects model was used. We also explored reasons for heterogeneity using meta-regression and subgroup analyses. In order to evaluate the influence of single studies on the overall estimate, a sensitivity analysis was performed. Funnel plots and Egger's linear regression test were applied to investigate publication bias [27].

Results

Eligible studies

Initially, the highly sensitive search strategy identified 156 articles. After screening the titles and abstracts of all retrieved articles, 78 articles were excluded. Then full texts were reviewed and 65 articles were further excluded. Another 5 studies were also excluded due to lack of data integrity (Figure 1). Finally, 8 cohort studies were included in this meta-analysis [21,23,24,28–32]. Publication years of the eligible studies ranged from 2000 to 2011. Figure 2 shows the distribution of the number of topic-related literatures in electronic databases over the last decade. A total of 2,292 ESRD patients with CVD were involved in this meta-analysis. Four studies were conducted among Asians, three studies among Caucasians, and one study among Africans. The polymerase chain reaction-amplified genes with restriction endonucleases (PCR-RFLP) was performed in 5 studies, while 3 studies used the direct DNA sequencing method. The genotype frequencies of controls were all in HWE (all $P>0.05$). The NOS scores of all included studies were ≥6. The main characteristics of all eligible studies are listed in Table 1.

Quantitative data synthesis

Meta-analysis findings on the relationship between the *MTHFR* 677C>T polymorphism and susceptibility to CVD in ESRD patients is shown in Table 2. The random-effects model was conducted due to significant heterogeneity between studies. Our meta-analysis results revealed that the *MTHFR* 677C>T polymorphism might increase the risk of CVD in ESRD patients (TT vs. CC: OR = 2.75, 95%CI = 1.35~5.59, $P = 0.005$; CT+TT vs. CC: OR = 1.39, 95%CI = 1.09~1.78, $P = 0.008$; TT vs. CC+CT: OR = 2.52, 95%CI = 1.25~5.09, $P = 0.010$; respectively) (Figure 3).

Subgroup and meta-regression analysis were conducted based on ethnicity to investigate potential sources of heterogeneity. Our results suggested that the *MTHFR* 677C>T polymorphism was associated with the incidence of CVD in ESRD patients among Asians (TT vs. CC: OR = 3.38, 95%CI = 1.11~10.28, $P = 0.032$; CT+TT vs. CC: OR = 1.44, 95%CI = 1.05~1.97, $P = 0.022$; TT vs. CC+CT: OR = 3.15, 95%CI = 1.02~9.72, $P = 0.046$; respectively), but not among Africans or Caucasians (all $P>0.05$). Further subgroup analyses based on genotyping method suggested

Table 2. Meta-analysis of the relationships between the *MTHFR* 677 C>T polymorphism and the risk of cardiovascular disease in patients with end-stage renal disease.

	Sample size	TT vs. CC			CT vs. CC			CT+TT vs. CC			TT vs. CC+CT		
		OR	95%CI	P	OR	95%CI	P	OR	95%CI	P	OR	95%CI	P
Overall		2.75	1.35–5.59	0.005	1.15	0.92–1.44	0.227	1.39	1.09–1.78	0.008	2.52	1.25–5.09	0.010
Ethnicity													
Asians (n = 4)	1202	3.38	1.11–10.28	0.032	1.18	0.85–1.65	0.327	1.44	1.05–1.97	0.022	3.15	1.02–9.72	0.046
Africans (n = 1)	50	0.92	0.08–10.14	0.943	0.92	0.23–3.68	0.902	0.92	0.25–3.35	0.895	0.94	0.09–9.97	0.962
Caucasians (n = 3)	1040	2.72	0.76–9.78	0.125	1.25	0.75–2.07	0.389	1.52	0.84–2.73	0.165	2.35	0.69–7.96	0.171
Genotyping method													
PCR-RFLP (n = 5)	1446	4.00	1.19–13.53	0.025	1.31	0.98–1.74	0.065	1.61	1.11–2.32	0.012	3.42	1.04–11.23	0.043
Direct sequencing (n = 3)	846	2.11	1.30–3.42	0.003	0.93	0.65–1.34	0.695	1.16	0.83–1.61	0.394	2.14	1.37–3.33	0.001

Legend: OR - odds ratio; 95%CI - 95% confidence interval; PCR-RFLP - polymerase chain reaction-restriction fragment length polymorphism.

that the *MTHFR* 677C>T polymorphism was closely linked to an increased risk of CVD in the majority of subgroups (as shown in Table 2).

Meta-regression analysis confirmed that none of the considered factors was the main source of heterogeneity (as shown in Table 3). Sensitivity analysis suggested that no single study could influence the overall pooled estimates (Figure 4). We found no evidence of obvious asymmetry in the funnel plots (Figure 5). Egger's test also did not display strong statistical evidence for publication bias (all $P>0.05$).

Discussion

MTHFR can catalyze a rate-limiting reaction in the transformation of methionine into Hcy and back exclusively through the transfer of the methyl group to and from methyl-tetrahydrofolate, separately [33–35]. It is well documented that an elevated level of the sulphur amino-acid Hcy in plasma is an independent risk factor for atherosclerosis, coronary heart disease, stroke and other CVDs [36,37]. Meanwhile, the increased fasting level of total Hcy was found to establish an independent contribution to the excess incidence of fatal and non-fatal cardiovascular outcomes [38]. Indeed, the formation of hyperhomocysteinemia (HHcy) was closely associated with folic acid, Vitamin B_6 and B_{12} supplementation [39], but also correlated with sulfur amino acid metabolism [40]. As for *MTHFR*, since the methyl groups for Hcy mediated DNA-methylation to methionine are related to the provision of 5-methylenetetrahydrofolate, which can be irreversibly transferred from 5 to 10-methylenetetrahydrofolate through MTHFR catalysis, the *MTHFR* gene probably plays a crucial role in the remethylation of Hcy [41]. On the other hand, it has been estimated by statistical data in clinical studies that HD patients suffering from mild to moderate HHcy account for a great proportion of the high-risk population for CVD [42]. Therefore, it was hypothesized that common polymorphisms in the *MTHFR* gene could be functional and associated with the development and progression of CVD in ESRD patients. Recently, the usage of human *MTHFR* gene mutations in predicting the increased Hcy levels and susceptibility to CVD has been widely adopted [13,34]. In particular, a relatively common functional polymorphism in *MTHFR* rs1801133 (677C>T) in exon 4 may influence the plasma Hcy in ESRD patients. Abundant evidence has supported the view that a half reduction in enzymatic capability might lead to a mild Hcy, as well as total elevation of plasma Hcy concentrations in individuals, both of which might contribute to the genetic predisposition to CVD [30,43].

We undertook the present meta-analysis to elucidate the association of genetic mutations in the *MTHFR* gene with the incidence of CVD in ESRD patients. Our meta-analysis results showed that the *MTHFR* 677C>T polymorphism was associated with an increased risk of CVD in ESRD patients, indicating that variants in the *MTHFR* gene may play a pivotal role in the pathology of CVD in ESRD patients. Although the mechanism by which *MTHFR* genetic polymorphisms lead to the development of CVD in ESRD patients still remains partially understood, a possible explanation is that the *MTHFR* 677C>T polymorphism may lead to a mild decrease in MTHFR activity which plays a crucial role in the remethylation of Hcy to methionine, resulting in elevated total plasma Hcy levels which may contribute independently to the excess incidence of fatal and nonfatal CVD. Haviv YS et al. have suggested a major role for plasma Hcy level as a determinant of CVD in ESRD patients, whereby the *MTHFR* variants and low serum folate are important determinants of plasma Hcy level and therefore may also have an indirect impact

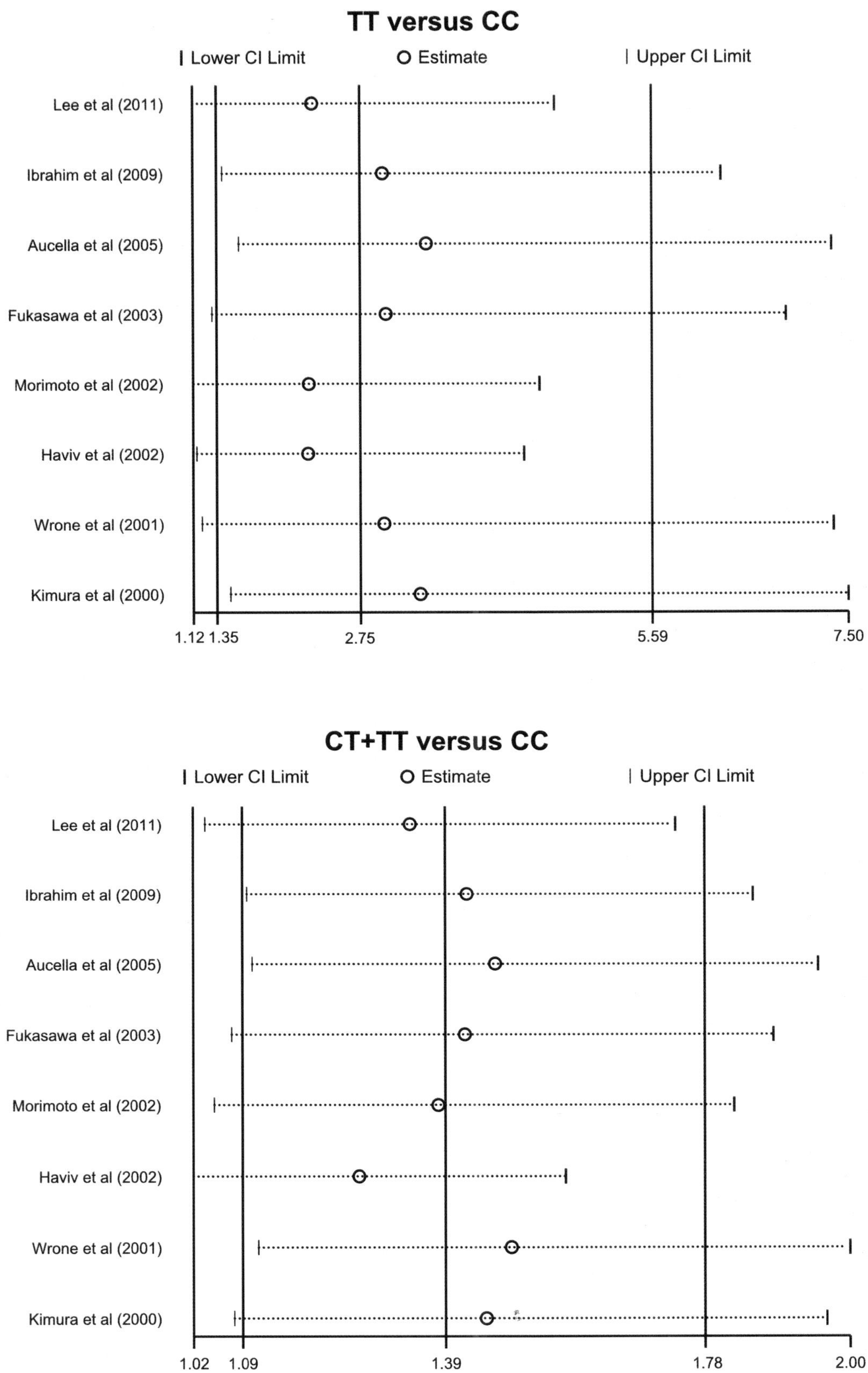

Figure 4. Sensitivity analysis of the summary odds ratio coefficients on the relationships between the *MTHFR* 677C>T polymorphism and the risk of cardiovascular disease in chronic hemodialysis patients.

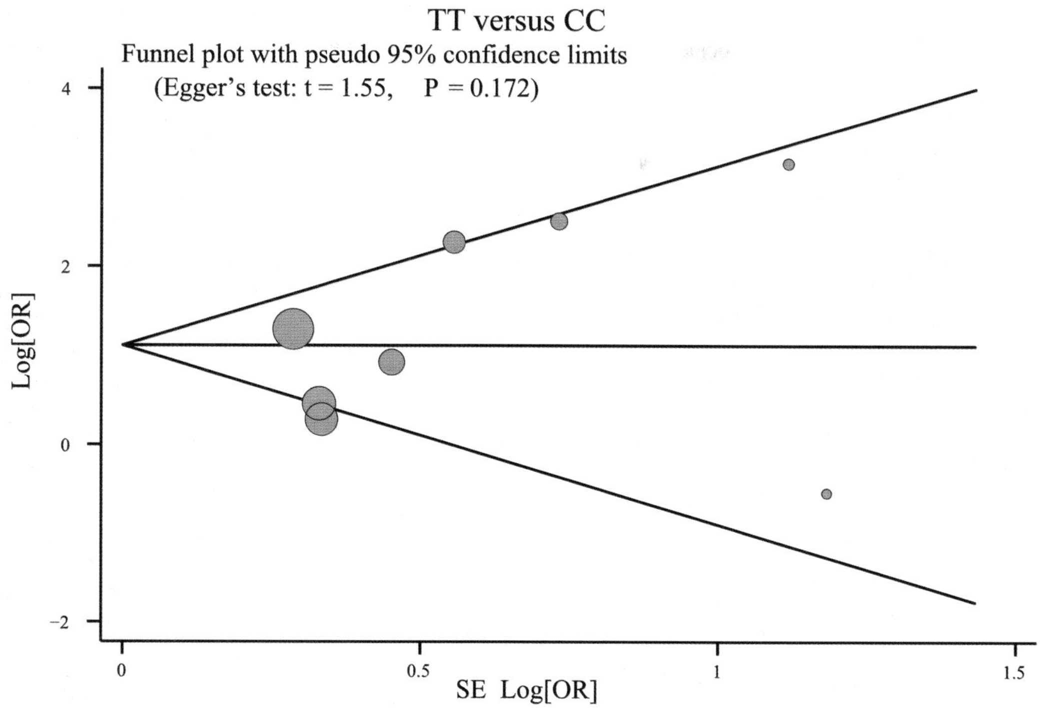

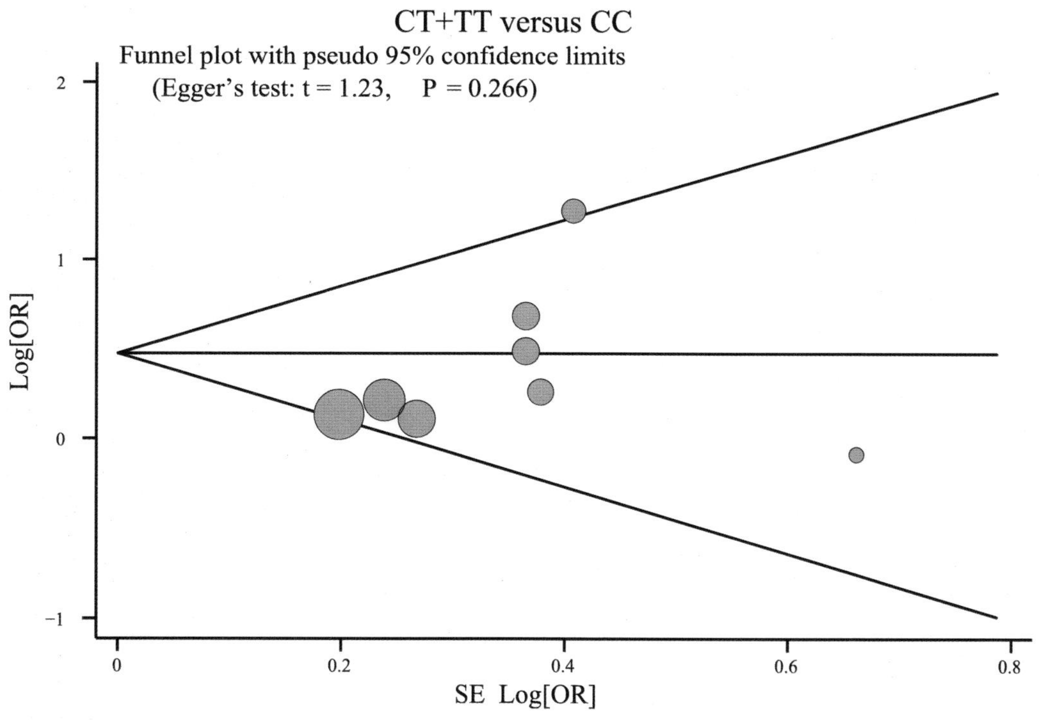

Figure 5. Funnel plot of publication biases on the relationships between the *MTHFR* 677C>T polymorphism and the risk of cardiovascular disease in chronic hemodialysis patients.

on the cardiovascular status [29]. Since heterogeneity obviously existed in our meta-analysis, we performed stratified analyses based on ethnicity and genotyping method. Subgroup analysis by ethnicity indicated that there were marked associations between the *MTHFR* 677C>T polymorphism and an increased risk of CVD in ESRD patients among Asians. In short, our findings were in accordance with previous studies that found that the *MTHFR* 677C>T polymorphism may alter the risk of developing CVD in ESRD patients, suggesting that these polymorphisms may be useful as biomarkers for the early diagnosis of CVD in ESRD patients.

Table 3. Univariate and multivariate meta-regression analyses of potential source of heterogeneity.

Heterogeneity factors	Coefficient	SE	Z	P	95%CI	
					LL	UL
Publication year						
Univariate	0.028	0.122	0.23	0.820	−0.212	0.267
Multivariate	−0.078	0.067	−1.17	0.241	−0.209	0.053
Ethnicity						
Univariate	−0.439	0.697	−0.63	0.528	−1.806	0.927
Multivariate	−0.132	0.339	−0.39	0.697	−0.796	0.532
Genotyping method						
Univariate	−0.769	0.922	−0.83	0.405	−2.577	1.039
Multivariate	0.562	0.372	1.51	0.131	−0.167	1.291

Legend: SE - standard error; 95%CI - 95% confidence interval; UL - upper limit; LL - lower limit.

As the first meta-analysis focused on the relationships between the *MTHFR* 677C>T polymorphism and the risk of CVD in ESRD patients, our study has some limitations. First, our results lacked sufficient statistical power to assess correlations between the *MTHFR* 677C>T polymorphism and susceptibility to CVD in ESRD patients due to a relatively small sample size. Second, as a retrospective study, our meta-analysis may have been influenced by subject selection bias, thereby affecting the reliability of our results. Third, our meta-analysis failed to obtain original data from the included studies, which may have limited further evaluation of the potential roles of the *MTHFR* 677C>T polymorphism in the development and progression of CVD in ESRD patients. Importantly, the inclusion criteria of cases and controls were not well defined in all included studies, which might also have influenced our results.

In conclusion, our findings indicate that the *MTHFR* 677C>T polymorphism may contribute to increased CVD risk in ESRD patients. Thus, the *MTHFR* 677C>T polymorphism may be a useful and promising biomarker for the early detection and prognosis of CVD in ESRD patients. However, due to the limitations mentioned above, more research studies with larger sample sizes are still needed to provide a more representative statistical analysis.

Acknowledgments

We would like to acknowledge the helpful comments on this paper received from our reviewers.

Author Contributions

Conceived and designed the experiments: XHG. Performed the experiments: XHG HYZ. Analyzed the data: XHG YW. Contributed reagents/materials/analysis tools: GYZ YW. Wrote the paper: XHG.

References

1. Mehrotra R, Chiu YW, Kalantar-Zadeh K, Bargman J, Vonesh E (2011) Similar outcomes with hemodialysis and peritoneal dialysis in patients with end-stage renal disease. Arch Intern Med, 171(2): 110–118.
2. Palacio S, Gonzales NR, Sangha NS, Birnbaum LA, Hart RG (2011) Thrombolysis for acute stroke in hemodialysis: international survey of expert opinion. Clin J Am Soc Nephrol, 6(5): 1089–1093.
3. Winkelmayer WC, Patrick AR, Liu J, Brookhart MA, Setoguchi S (2011) The increasing prevalence of atrial fibrillation among hemodialysis patients. J Am Soc Nephrol, 22(2): 349–357.
4. McIntyre CW (2010) Haemodialysis-induced myocardial stunning in chronic kidney disease - a new aspect of cardiovascular disease. Blood Purif, 29(2): 105–110.
5. Weiner DE, Scott TM, Giang LM, Agganis BT, Sorensen EP, et al (2011) Cardiovascular disease and cognitive function in maintenance hemodialysis patients. Am J Kidney Dis, 58(5): 773–781.
6. Matias PJ, Jorge C, Ferreira C, Borges M, Aires I, et al (2010) Cholecalciferol supplementation in hemodialysis patients: effects on mineral metabolism, inflammation, and cardiac dimension parameters. Clin J Am Soc Nephrol, 5(5): 905–911.
7. Shiotsu Y, Mori Y, Nishimura M, Sakoda C, Tokoro T, et al (2011) Plasma S100A12 level is associated with cardiovascular disease in hemodialysis patients. Clin J Am Soc Nephrol, 6(4): 718–723.
8. Anderson JL, May HT, Horne BD, Bair TL, Hall NL, et al (2010) Relation of vitamin D deficiency to cardiovascular risk factors, disease status, and incident events in a general healthcare population. Am J Cardiol, 106(7): 963–968.
9. Stenvinkel P, Carrero JJ, Axelsson J, Lindholm B, Heimburger O, et al (2008) Emerging biomarkers for evaluating cardiovascular risk in the chronic kidney disease patient: how do new pieces fit into the uremic puzzle? Clin J Am Soc Nephrol, 3(2): 505–521.
10. Kendrick J, Chonchol MB (2008) Nontraditional risk factors for cardiovascular disease in patients with chronic kidney disease. Nat Clin Pract Nephrol, 4(12): 672–681.
11. Chonchol M, Kendrick J, Targher G (2011) Extra-skeletal effects of vitamin D deficiency in chronic kidney disease. Ann Med, 43(4): 273–282.
12. Cozzolino M, Biondi ML, Galassi A, Cusi D, Brancaccio D, et al (2010) Vascular calcification and cardiovascular outcome in dialysis patients: the role of gene polymorphisms. Blood Purif, 29(4): 347–351.
13. Fung MM, Salem RM, Lipkowitz MS, Bhatnagar V, Pandey B, et al (2012) Methylenetetrahydrofolate reductase (MTHFR) polymorphism A1298C (Glu429Ala) predicts decline in renal function over time in the African-American Study of Kidney Disease and Hypertension (AASK) Trial and Veterans Affairs Hypertension Cohort (VAHC). Nephrol Dial Transplant, 27(1): 197–205.
14. Spellicy CJ, Northrup H, Fletcher JM, Cirino PT, Dennis M, et al (2012) Folate metabolism gene 5,10-methylenetetrahydrofolate reductase (MTHFR) is associated with ADHD in myelomeningocele patients. PLoS One, 7(12): e51330.
15. Garner JL, Niles KM, McGraw S, Yeh JR, Cushnie DW, et al (2013) Stability of DNA methylation patterns in mouse spermatogonia under conditions of MTHFR deficiency and methionine supplementation. Biol Reprod, 89(5): 125.
16. Field MS, Shields KS, Abarinov EV, Malysheva OV, Allen RH, et al (2013) Reduced MTHFD1 activity in male mice perturbs folate- and choline-

dependent one-carbon metabolism as well as transsulfuration. J Nutr, 143(1): 41–45.
17. Hazra A, Kraft P, Lazarus R, Chen C, Chanock SJ, et al (2009) Genome-wide significant predictors of metabolites in the one-carbon metabolism pathway. Hum Mol Genet, 18(23): 4677–4687.
18. Abbas S, Raza ST, Ahmed F, Ahmad A, Rizvi S, et al (2013) Association of Genetic polymorphism of PPARgamma-2, ACE, MTHFR, FABP-2 and FTO genes in risk prediction of type 2 diabetes mellitus. J Biomed Sci, 20(1): 80.
19. Zhang J, Qiu LX, Wang ZH, Wu XH, Liu XJ, et al (2010) MTHFR C677T polymorphism associated with breast cancer susceptibility: a meta-analysis involving 15,260 cases and 20,411 controls. Breast Cancer Res Treat, 123(2): 549–555.
20. Perna AF, Lanza D, Sepe I, Conzo G, Altucci L, et al (2013) Altered folate receptor 2 expression in uraemic patients on haemodialysis: implications for folate resistance. Nephrol Dial Transplant, 28(5): 1214–1224.
21. Lee SY, Kim HY, Park KM, Hong SG, Kim HJ, et al (2011) MTHFR C677T polymorphism as a risk factor for vascular calcification in chronic hemodialysis patients. J Korean Med Sci, 26(3): 461–465.
22. Heinz J, Kropf S, Luley C, Dierkes J (2009) Homocysteine as a risk factor for cardiovascular disease in patients treated by dialysis: a meta-analysis. Am J Kidney Dis, 54(3): 478–489.
23. Fukasawa M, Matsushita K, Kamiyama M, Mikami Y, Araki I, et al (2003) The methylentetrahydrofolate reductase C677T point mutation is a risk factor for vascular access thrombosis in hemodialysis patients. Am J Kidney Dis, 41(3): 637–642.
24. Wrone EM, Zehnder JL, Hornberger JM, McCann LM, Coplon NS, et al (2001) An MTHFR variant, homocysteine, and cardiovascular comorbidity in renal disease. Kidney Int, 60(3): 1106–1113.
25. Stang A (2010) Critical evaluation of the Newcastle-Ottawa scale for the assessment of the quality of nonrandomized studies in meta-analyses. Eur J Epidemiol, 25(9): 603–605.
26. Zintzaras E, Ioannidis JP (2005) HEGESMA: genome search meta-analysis and heterogeneity testing. Bioinformatics, 21(18): 3672–3673.
27. Peters JL, Sutton AJ, Jones DR, Abrams KR, Rushton L (2006) Comparison of two methods to detect publication bias in meta-analysis. JAMA, 295(6): 676–680.
28. Aucella F, Margaglione M, Grandone E, Vigilante M, Gatta G, et al (2005) The C677T methylenetetrahydrofolate reductase gene mutation does not influence cardiovascular risk in the dialysis population: results of a multicentre prospective study. Nephrol Dial Transplant, 20(2): 382–386.
29. Haviv YS, Shpichinetsky V, Goldschmidt N, Atta IA, Ben-Yehuda A, et al (2002) The common mutations C677T and A1298C in the human methylenetetrahydrofolate reductase gene are associated with hyperhomocysteinemia and cardiovascular disease in hemodialysis patients. Nephron, 92(1): 120–126.
30. Ibrahim S, El Dessokiy O (2009) Prevalence of methylenetetrahydrofolate gene (MTHFR) C677T polymorphism among chronic hemodialysis patients and its association with cardiovascular disease: a cross-sectional analysis. Clin Exp Nephrol, 13(5): 501–507.
31. Kimura H, Gejyo F, Suzuki S, Miyazaki R (2000) The C677T methylenetetrahydrofolate reductase gene mutation in hemodialysis patients. J Am Soc Nephrol, 11(5): 885–893.
32. Morimoto K, Haneda T, Okamoto K, Ishida H, Kikuchi K (2002) Methylenetetrahydrofolate reductase gene polymorphism, hyperhomocysteinemia, and cardiovascular diseases in chronic hemodialysis patients [PMID: 11744804]. Nephron, 90(1): 43–50.
33. Yang Q, Bailey L, Clarke R, Flanders WD, Liu T, et al (2012) Prospective study of methylenetetrahydrofolate reductase (MTHFR) variant C677T and risk of all-cause and cardiovascular disease mortality among 6000 US adults. Am J Clin Nutr, 95(5): 1245–1253.
34. Clarke R, Bennett DA, Parish S, Verhoef P, Dotsch-Klerk M, et al (2012) Homocysteine and coronary heart disease: meta-analysis of MTHFR case-control studies, avoiding publication bias. PLoS Med, 9(2): e1001177.
35. Pereira TV, Rudnicki M, Pereira AC, Pombo-de-Oliveira MS, Franco RF (2006) 5,10-Methylenetetrahydrofolate reductase polymorphisms and acute lymphoblastic leukemia risk: a meta-analysis. Cancer Epidemiol Biomarkers Prev, 15(10): 1956–1963.
36. Yun KU, Ryu CS, Oh JM, Kim CH, Lee KS, et al (2013) Plasma homocysteine level and hepatic sulfur amino acid metabolism in mice fed a high-fat diet. Eur J Nutr, 52(1): 127–134.
37. Benight NM, Stoll B, Chacko S, da Silva VR, Marini JC, et al (2011) B-vitamin deficiency is protective against DSS-induced colitis in mice. Am J Physiol Gastrointest Liver Physiol, 301(2): G249–259.
38. Di Minno MN, Tremoli E, Coppola A, Lupoli R, Di Minno G (2010) Homocysteine and arterial thrombosis: Challenge and opportunity. Thromb Haemost, 103(5): 942–961.
39. Stanger O, Fowler B, Piertzik K, Huemer M, Haschke-Becher E, et al (2009) Homocysteine, folate and vitamin B12 in neuropsychiatric diseases: review and treatment recommendations. Expert Rev Neurother, 9(9): 1393–1412.
40. Stipanuk MH, Ueki I (2011) Dealing with methionine/homocysteine sulfur: cysteine metabolism to taurine and inorganic sulfur. J Inherit Metab Dis, 34(1): 17–32.
41. Safarinejad MR, Shafiei N, Safarinejad S (2011) Genetic susceptibility of methylenetetrahydrofolate reductase (MTHFR) gene C677T, A1298C, and G1793A polymorphisms with risk for bladder transitional cell carcinoma in men. Med Oncol, 28 Suppl 1: S398–412.
42. Shemin D, Bostom AG, Selhub J (2001) Treatment of hyperhomocysteinemia in end-stage renal disease. Am J Kidney Dis, 38(4 Suppl 1): S91–94.
43. Rubino E, Ferrero M, Rainero I, Binello E, Vaula G, et al (2009) Association of the C677T polymorphism in the MTHFR gene with migraine: a meta-analysis. Cephalalgia, 29(8): 818–825.

Role of WNT10A-Expressing Kidney Fibroblasts in Acute Interstitial Nephritis

Akihiro Kuma[1,2], Sohsuke Yamada[3], Ke-Yong Wang[4], Noriaki Kitamura[1], Takahiro Yamaguchi[1], Yoshiko Iwai[1], Hiroto Izumi[5], Masahito Tamura[2], Yutaka Otsuji[2], Kimitoshi Kohno[6]*

1 Department of Molecular Biology, School of Medicine, University of Occupational and Environmental Health, Kitakyushu, Japan, **2** Second Department of Internal Medicine, Cardiology and Nephrology, School of Medicine, University of Occupational and Environmental Health, Kitakyushu, Japan, **3** Department of Pathology and Cell Biology, School of Medicine, University of Occupational and Environmental Health, Kitakyushu, Japan, **4** Bio-information Research Center, University of Occupational and Environmental Health, Kitakyushu, Japan, **5** Department of Occupational Pneumology, Institute of Industrial Ecological Science, University of Occupational and Environmental Health, Kitakyushu, Japan, **6** The President Laboratory, University of Occupational and Environmental Health, Kitakyushu, Japan

Abstract

WNT signaling mediates various physiological and pathological processes. We previously showed that WNT10A is a novel angio/stromagenic factor involved in such processes as tumor growth, wound healing and tissue fibrosis. In this study, we investigated the role of WNT10A in promoting the fibrosis that is central to the pathology of acute interstitial nephritis (AIN). We initially asked whether there is an association between kidney function (estimated glomerular filtration rate; eGFR) and WNT10A expression using kidney biopsies from 20 patients with AIN. Interestingly, patients with WNT10A expression had significantly lower eGFR than WNT10A-negative patients. However, changes in kidney function were not related to the level of expression of other WNT family members. Furthermore, there was positive correlation between WNT10A and α-SMA expression. We next investigated the involvement of WNT10A in kidney fibrosis processes using COS1 cells, a kidney fibroblast cell line. WNT10A overexpression increased the level of expression of fibronectin and peroxiredoxin 5. Furthermore, WNT10A overexpression renders cells resistant to apoptosis induced by hydrogen peroxide and high glucose. Collectively, WNT10A may induce kidney fibrosis and associate with kidney dysfunction in AIN.

Editor: Robert Dettman, Northwestern University, United States of America

Funding: This work was supported by JSPS KAKENHI (Grant Number 22249025) and an UOEH grant for advanced research to Ke-Yong Wang. The funders had no role in study design, data collection and analysis, decision to publish, or preparation of the manuscript.

Competing Interests: The authors have declared that no competing interests exist.

* Email: k-kohno@med.uoeh-u.ac.jp

Introduction

Acute interstitial nephritis (AIN) is a general cause of acute kidney injury (AKI). Patients with AIN can either completely recover or progress to chronic kidney disease (CKD) or end-stage renal disease (ESRD) [1]. Although several antifibrotic strategies have been proposed, there are no effective treatments for kidney fibrosis. Kidney fibrosis is generally considered to result from tissue inflammation and the tissue repair/wound healing responses [2]. Wound healing is a complex process involving several signal transduction systems, and ultimately can result in scar formation. The first phase begins with tissue damage caused by anti-inflammatory cytokines [3]. The next phase is defined by deposition of granulation tissue and new extracellular matrix (ECM) proteins. Acute inflammatory reactions are considered to be a part of early wound healing and play a key role in triggering fibrosis. Since prevention of the initial fibrotic process in AIN may lead to retention of kidney function, we investigated what kinds of signaling systems mediate kidney fibrosis associated with AIN.

There are two major WNT signaling pathways, the canonical (involving β-catenin) [4] and the non-canonical pathways (independent of β-catenin) [5,6]. WNT is a family of highly conserved glycoproteins, and 19 WNT members have been identified so far in humans [7]. The WNT/Frizzled signal transduction system is a highly complex cascade that is fundamental for a wide variety of physiological processes, as well as pathological states. Some WNT proteins were previously investigated in kidney interstitial fibrosis [8,9], but the relation between WNT10A and kidney fibrosis has not been determined. We asked whether WNT10A promotes kidney fibrosis. We previously reported that WNT10A is expressed in dermal fibroblasts, and that α-SMA-positive cells are involved in wound healing [10]. Myofibroblasts, or activated fibroblasts with α-SMA expression, differentiate from diverse sources including local interstitial fibroblasts, vascular pericytes, and endothelial cells [11]. Furthermore, they produce ECM (collagen and fibronectin). Therefore, we hypothesized that WNT10A expression in myofibroblasts may also play an important role in tissue repair and the fibrotic processes associated with AIN.

Here, we discovered that WNT10A is expressed in kidney fibroblasts expressing α-SMA. Patients with WNT10A expression had a significantly lower estimated glomerular filtration rate (eGFR) than WNT10-negative patients. We investigated mechanism of fibroblasts (COS1) behavior with WNT10A expression.

Materials and Methods

Cell culture and conditioned media

COS1 cells (kidney fibroblasts of African green monkey) were purchased from ATCC (VA, USA) and cultured in Dulbecco's

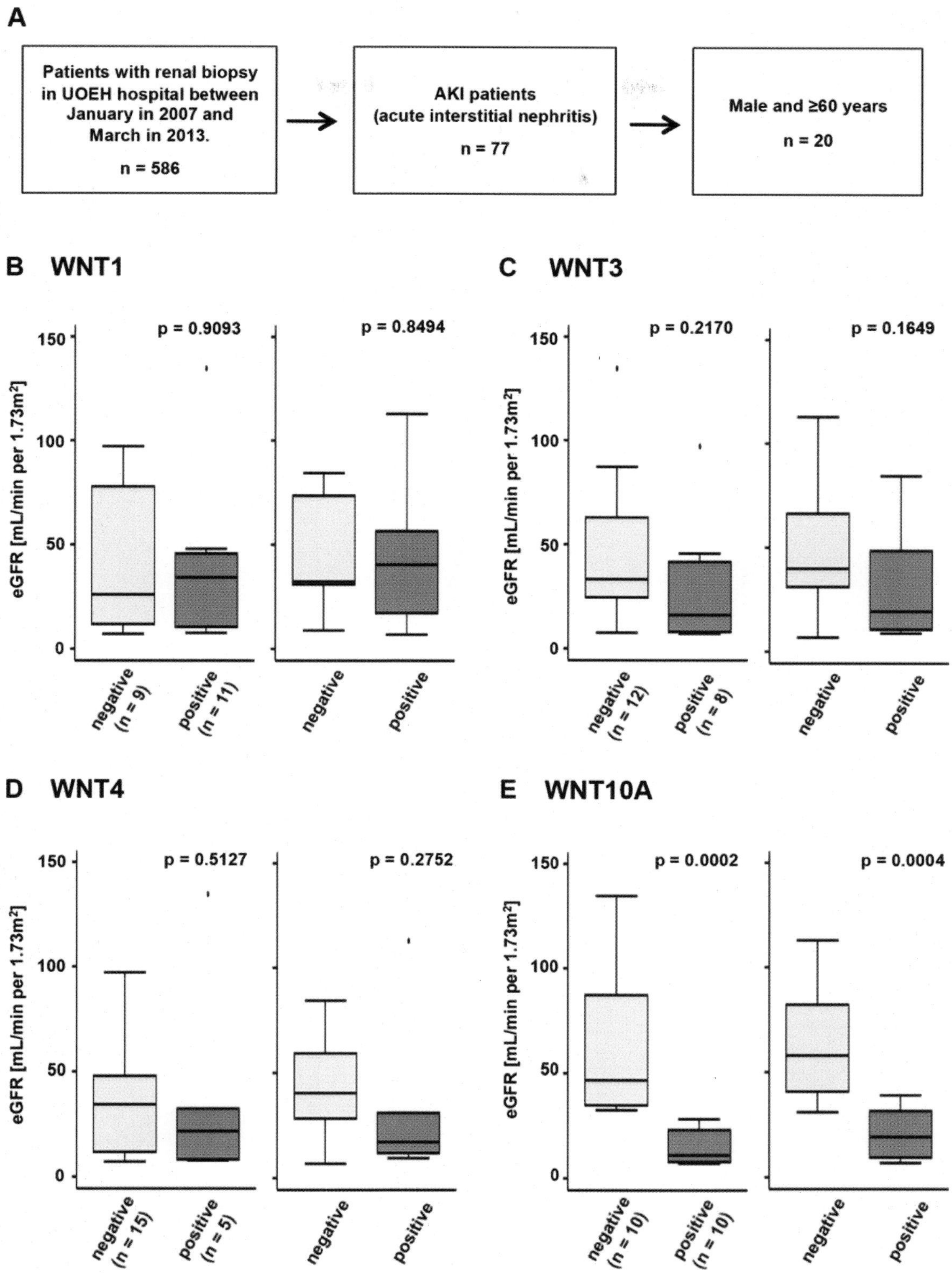

Figure 1. The relationship between WNT family gene expression and kidney function. (A) Patient selection method to evaluate eGFR among AIN patients. eGFR (mL/min per 1.73 m^2) of AIN patients with (B) WNT1, (C) WNT3, (D) WNT4, and (E) WNT10A. (B) WNT1 negative-expression; n = 9, positive-expression; n = 11 (C) WNT3 negative-expression; n = 12, positive-expression; n = 8 (D) WNT4 negative-expression; n = 15, positive-expression; n = 5 (E) WNT10A negative expression; n = 10, positive-expression; n = 10. Light gray box indicates eGFR of patients without WNT protein expression, and dark gray box indicates eGFR of patients with WNT protein expression. The left panels show kidney function on kidney biopsy, and right panels show kidney function on discharge. Data of each category is shown in Table 2.

modified Eagle's medium (Nissui Seiyaku, Tokyo, Japan) containing 10% fetal bovine serum and 5.5 mM glucose. Low glucose medium (LM) contained 5.5 mM glucose, moderate-high glucose medium (MM) contained 11 mM glucose, and high glucose medium (HM) contained 22 mM glucose. Cell lines were maintained in a 5% CO_2 atmosphere at 37°C.

Plasmid construction and transfectants

The WNT10A cDNA expression plasmid was constructed by PCR as described previously [10]. The PCR product was cloned into the pGEM-T easy vector (Promega, WI, USA). The full-length cDNA fragment was recloned into the pEB-Multi vector (Wako). COS1 cells were transfected with either vector (control cells) or pEB-WNT10A (WNT10A-overexpressing cells; COS1-10A) using the X-tremeGENE 9 (Roche, Basel, Switzerland) and cultured with normal medium for three days. After that, medium was changed to 300 μg/ml hygromycin contining medium and cultured for 21 days. The resulting colonies were isolated and the cellular expression levels of WNT10A were confirmed by Western blotting with an anti-WNT10A antibody.

Preparation of human kidney samples

Patients (Japanese) who were hospitalized with AKI in the Department of Nephrology of University of Occupational and Environmental Health (UOEH) hospital in Kitakyushu, Japan, received kidney biopsy to diagnose the cause of AKI between January 2007 and March 2013. Human kidney tissue samples were examined in the department of nephrology and pathology at UOEH. The diagnosis was re-evaluated and confirmed by at least three board-certified nephrologists and one board-certified surgical pathologist. All the intended procedures of the present study, including use of specimens from human subjects, were approved by the Ethics Committee of UOEH in Kitakyushu, Japan. Especially, written consent of next of kin for research use of the materials was obtained according to the guidelines of the Japanese Society of Pathology and also approved by the Ethics Committee of UOEH, where the biopsy was performed.

Histology and Immunohistochemical staining

Deparaffinized and rehydrated 3-μm sequential sections from kidney samples were stained with hematoxylin and eosin (HE) or Masson's trichrome stain, or underwent immunohistochemistry (IHC) preparations. IHC was performed as previously described [12]. For IHC performed by the antibody-linked dextran polymer method (EnVision; DAKO, Glostrup, Denmark), samples were incubated in 10% H_2O_2 for 5 min to block endogenous peroxidase activity. Then, these sections were rinsed and incubated with the indicated antibodies for 30 min, respectively. The second antibody-peroxidase-linked polymers were then applied, and the sections were incubated with a solution consisting of 20 mg of 3.3′-diaminobenzidine tetrahydrochloride, 65 mg of sodium azide, and 20 ml of 30% H_2O_2 in 100 ml of Tris-HCl (50 mM, pH 7.6). After counterstaining with Mayer's haematoxylin, sections were observed under a light microscope. The immune-reactivity with WNT proteins and α-SMA in each case were assessed semi-quantitatively by evaluating the proportion of positive cells over total stromal cells. For WNT proteins or α-SMA expression, positive areas that were equal to or more than 10% or 50% were considered positively stained respectively, in accord with the performance of receiver operating characteristic (ROC) curve analyses. Finally, to assess the co-localization of both proteins in the same or at least in adjacent fibrogenic cells (i.e., myofibroblasts), we stained tissues in consecutive sections with rabbit polyclonal anti-WNT10A antibodies and mouse monoclonal anti-human α-SMA, respectively, as previously described [13]. For fibronectin expression, positive areas that were equal to or more 30% were considered positively stained. All histological and immunohistochemical staining was evaluated by two independent observers (a certified surgical pathologist and a nephrology doctor) using a blind protocol design (observers were blinded to the clinicopathological data).

Immunofluorescence staining

Control and WNT10A-overexpressing cells was cultured on 6 well-plate for 72 hours and fixed with 15% formalin for 10 minutes after washing with PBS. Cells were incubated with 0.2% (v/v) Triton X-100 with PBS for 10 minutes at room temperature. Cells were treated with 4% (w/v) skimmed milk (DS Pharma Biomedical Co., Ltd., Osaka, Japan) in PBS and incubated for 30 minutes at room temperature, washed with PBS, and incubated for 1 hour at room temperature with each primary antibody (anti-WNT10A and anti-fibronectin antibody). Primary antibodies were used at a 1:100 dilution. Cells were reacted with Alexa 488 conjugated anti-rabbit IgG for 45 minutes at room temperature. After washed with PBS containing DAPI, specimens were observed.

Table 1. Patient characteristics.

Characteristics	All	WNT10A(−)	WNT10A(+)	p-value
Number (n)	20	10	10	
Age (years, mean±S.D)	70.6±7.1	71.2±6.5	70.0±8.0	0.717
α-SMA positive (n, %)	10 (50)	1 (5)	9 (45)	0.0005
Fibronectin positive (n, %)	12 (60)	3 (15)	9 (45)	0.0062
Strongly interstitial fibrosis (n, %)	7 (35)	1 (5)	6 (30)	0.0191
Drug induced AIN (n, %)	4 (20)	1 (5)	3 (15)	0.264
Unknown AIN (n, %)	6 (30)	3 (15)	3 (15)	1.000
Crescentic nephritis (n, %)	9 (45)	5 (25)	4 (20)	0.653
MPA (n, %)	1 (5)	1 (5)	0 (0)	0.305
Administer maintenance HD (n, %)	3 (15)	0 (0)	3 (15)	0.060

AIN; acute interstitial nephritis, MPA; microscopic polyangiitis, HD; hemodialysis.
S.D; standard deviation.

Table 2. eGFR according to WNT proteins.

WNT protein	negative	positive	p-value
WNT1	26.06 [11.79–77.82]	34.28 [16.05–41.68]	0.9093
	32.31 [30.90–73.46]	40.40 [19.27–55.58]	0.8494
WNT3	33.29 [25.32–55.43]	16.05 [8.08–39.69]	0.2170
	39.91 [31.31–62.76]	19.27 [11.28–44.44]	0.1649
WNT4	34.28 [17.45–46.81]	21.66 [8.16–32.30]	0.5127
	40.40 [29.82–57.87]	17.14 [11.89–30.90]	0.2752
WNT10A	46.81 [35.45–84.91]	11.12 [7.93–22.74]	0.0002
	57.87 [44.25–79.96]	19.27 [10.05–30.64]	0.0004

eGFR; median [interquartile range] mL/min per 1.73 m^2 above (on biopsy), below (on discharge).

Western blotting analysis

Whole-cell lysates were prepared as previously described [14]. The 50 μg of protein from whole-cell lysates were separated by sodium dodecyl sulfate-polyacrylamide gel electrophoresis and transferred to polyvinylidene difluoride microporous membranes (Millipore, MA, USA). The blotted membranes were treated with 5% (w/v) skimmed milk in 10 mM Tris, 150 mM NaCl and 0.2% (v/v) Tween 20, and incubated for 1 h at room temperature with the primary antibody. anti-β-actin (Santa Cruz, CA, USA) antibody was used as an internal control at a 1:5,000 dilution. The membranes were then incubated for 45 minutes at room temperature with a peroxidase-conjugated secondary antibody, and visualized using an ECL kit (GE Healthcare Bio-Science, Buckinghamshire, UK). The detection was performed with an LAS-4000 mini (Fujifilm, Tokyo, Japan).

Antibodies

For western blotting and IHC, the following antibodies were used: anti-WNT10A (SAB3500393) was purchased from Sigma-Aldrich (MO, USA), anti-WNT1 (PAB11850) and anti-WNT3 (PAB7032) were purchased from Abnova (Taipei, Taiwan), and anti-WNT4 (sc-13962), anti-fibronectin (sc-9068), anti-COL1A1 (sc-25974), anti-COL3A1 (sc-28888), anti-PRDX2 (sc-23967), anti-PRDX4 (sc-23974) and anti-caspase9 (sc-56076) were purchased from Santa Cruz, and anti-caspase-3 (9662), anti-cleaved caspase-3 (9664), and anti-PARP (9532) were purchased from Cell Signaling Technology (MA, USA), anti-αSMA (M851) was purchased from Dako, and anti-PRDX3 (ab16751) was purchased from Abcam (MA, USA). To generate anti-PRDX1 and anti-PRDX5 antibodies, the synthetic peptides PDVQKSKEYFSKQK and GLTCSLAPNIISQL were used as immunogens, respectively, and the antisera obtained from immunized rabbits were affinity purified using the synthetic peptide antigens [15].

PRDX5 siRNA knockdown

Double-stranded RNA oligonucleotides 25 base pairs long were commercially generated (Life technologies, CA, USA): 5′-GGAUGGCAUAGUGAAGGCCCUGAAU-3′ and 5′-AUUCAGGGCCUUCACUAUGCCAUCC-3′ for PRDX5#1; 5′-CCUGAGACGCUCAGCGGGCUAUAUA-3′ and 5′-UAUAUAGCCCGCUGAGCGUCUCAGG-3′ for PRDX5#3. siRNA transfections were performed as previously described [16,17]. A sample of 5 μL of Lipofectamine 2000 (Qiagen, Hilden, Germany) was diluted in 250 μL Opti-MEM medium (Invitrogen, CA, USA) and incubated for 5 minutes at room temperature. Next, 250 pmol of siRNA and Lipofectamine 2000, serving as the control siRNA, were gently mixed in 250 μL Opti-MEM and incubated for 20 minutes at room temperature. Oligomer-Lipofectamine complexes and aliquots of 2×10^5 WNT10A-overexpressing cells in 500 μL culture medium were combined and incubated for 48 hr. Whole cell extracts (50 μg) were prepared from cells after siRNA transfection, and western blotting was performed.

Cytotoxicity analysis

Cytotoxicity analysis (water-soluble tetrazolium salt: WST-8 assay) was performed as described previously [18,19]. Briefly, 2.5×10^3 cells were seeded into 96-well plates. After 24 hours, to induce oxidative stress, cells were incubated with the indicated concentrations of H_2O_2 in the serum-free medium for 4 hours. After 48 hours, surviving cells were analyzed using a Cell Counting Kit −8 (Dojindo, Kumamoto, Japan) for 2 hours at 37°C. The absorbance was then measured at 450 nm.

Cell proliferation assay

Cell lines were seeded into 12-well plates (2×10^4 cells per well). For the purposes of analysis, the 0 hour was taken to be 24 hours after seeding. The cells were harvested with trypsin and counted every 24 hours.

Statistical analysis

Statistical analyses of the data were carried out using STATA SE12 (Stata Co., TX, USA). Comparison between the two groups was performed by Mann-Whitney U-test or Student's t-test. The X^2 test was used for dichotomous variables. A p-value <0.05 was considered significant.

Results

Patients with WNT10A expression had a lower estimated eGFR

A total of 586 patients received kidney biopsy in the hospital of UOEH during a 75-month period starting in 2007. Of these patients, 77 were AKI and diagnosed with AIN. We investigated the relationship between eGFR and the expression of WNT proteins (WNT1, 3, 4, and 10A) in kidney tissue of 20 patients (Fig. 1A). We selected 20 male patients over 60 years of age because patient background was statistically matched. Primary causes of AIN were rapidly progressive glomerulonephritis (50%), drug-induced AIN (20%), and unknown AIN (30%) (Table 1). Interestingly, 10 patients with WNT10A expression had significantly lower eGFR (median; 11.12 mL/min per 1.73 m^2, [interquartile range; 7.93–22.74 mL/min per 1.73 m^2]) than that

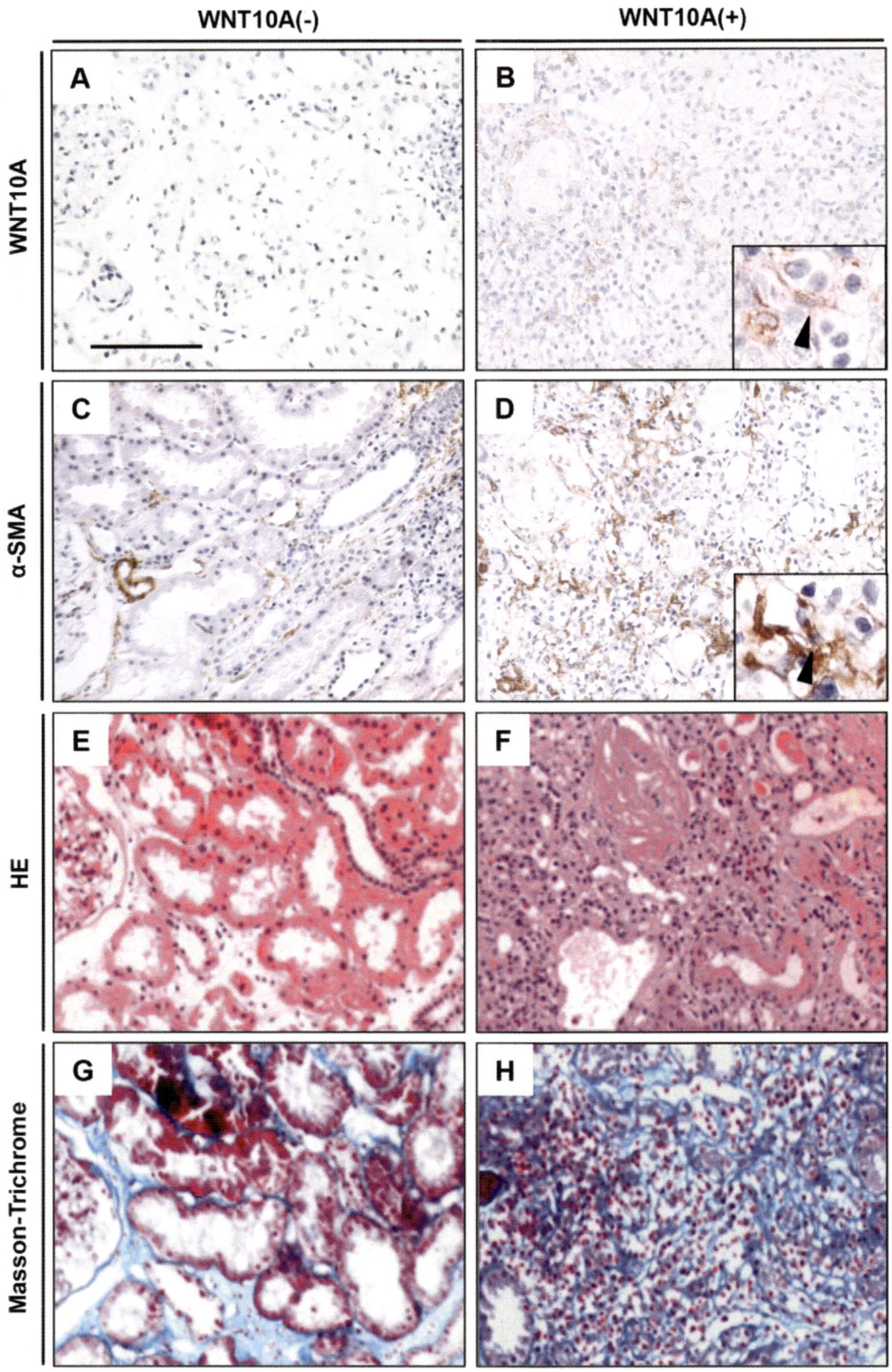

Figure 2. Histopathological analysis of kidney tissue from acute interstitial nephritis patients. Left panels are kidney interstitium without WNT10A expression, and right panels are kidney interstitium with WNT10A expression. (A–B); immunohistochemical staining for WNT10A, (C–D); immunohistochemical staining for α-SMA, (E–F); HE staining, (G–H); Masson-Trichrome staining. Arrow head is spindle cell with WNT10A and α-SMA positive respectively. All photos were taken at 200×. Scale bar is 100 μm.

(46.81 [35.45–84.91]) of the 10 patients without WNT10A expression on kidney biopsy (Fig. 1E left panel). Concerning eGFR on discharge, patients with WNT10A expression also had significantly lower eGFR (19.27 [10.05–30.64] vs 57.87 [44.25–79.96]) (Fig. 1E right panel). However, expression of other WNT proteins (WNT1, 3, and 4) was not correlated with altered kidney function both on biopsy and discharge (Fig. 1B, C and D, Table 2). There was not statistical correlation between high WNT10A

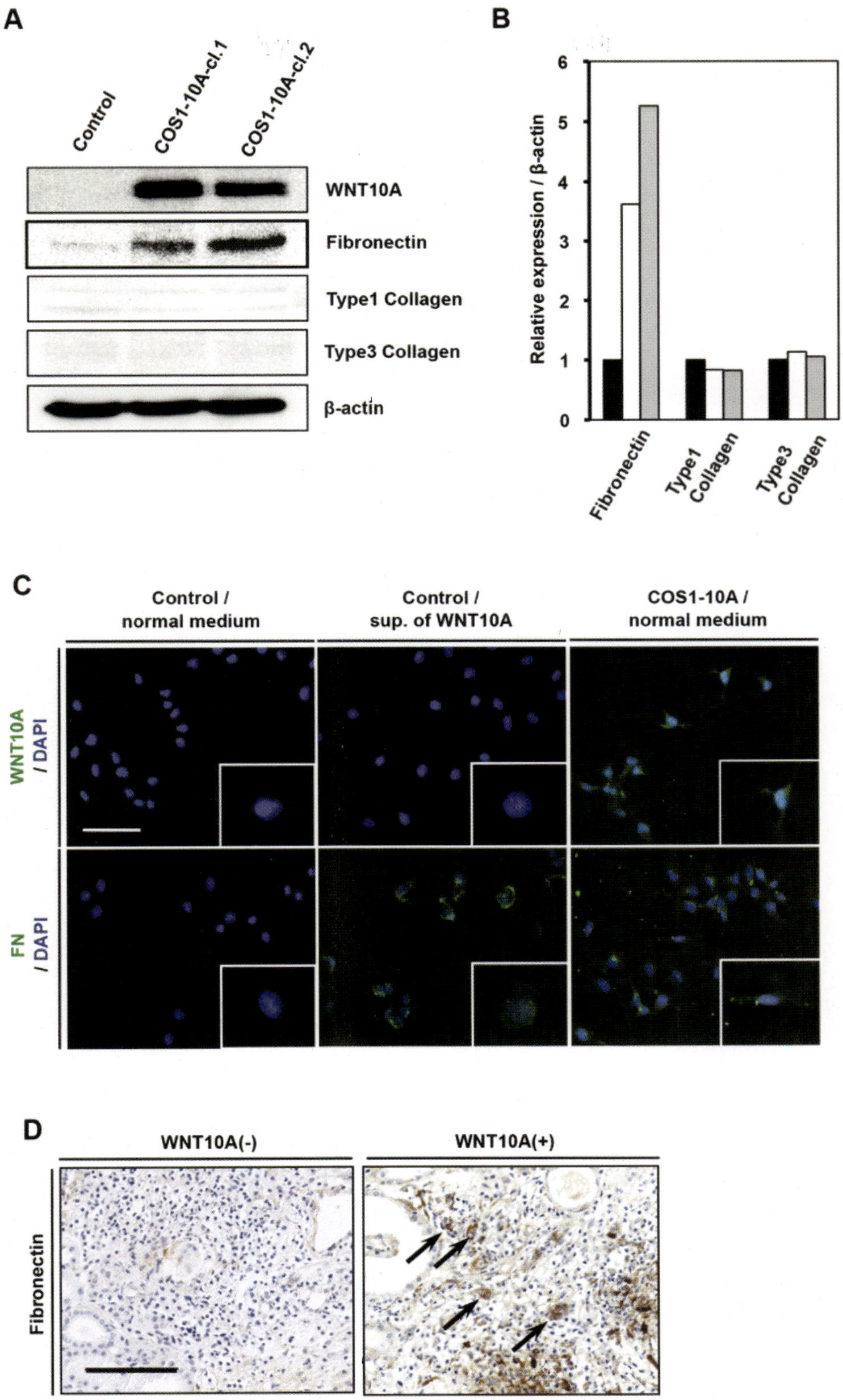

Figure 3. WNT10A overexpression enhances fibronectin expression in COS1 cells. (A) The expression of ECM components in WNT10A-overexpressing cells. Western analysis was performed using whole lysates obtained from control and WNT10A-overexpressing cells (COS1-10A). (B) Relative expression of fibronectin, type 1 collagen, and type 3 collagen, which were normalized to β-actin expression. The black bar shows control cells, white and gray bars showed COS1-10A-cl.1 and COS1-10A-cl.2 respectively. (C) Immunofluorescence staining for WNT10A (green), fibronectin (FN) (green), and DAPI (blue). Control cells treated with normal medium (left panel), control cells treated with supernatant (sup.) of WNT10A-overexpressing cells (middle panel), and COS1-10A cells treated with normal medium (right panel). Each cell was cultured for 72 hours. All photos were taken at 200×. Scale bar is 100 μm. (D) Immunohistochemical staining for fibronectin (brown) in AIN tissues. Kidney tissues from WNT10A-negative (left panel) or -positive (right panel) patients are shown. Arrows indicate fibronectin-positive cells. All photos were taken at 200×. Scale bar is 100 μm.

expression in kidney tissue and low eGFR (data not shown). Furthermore, three patients with WNT10A-positive tissue progressed to ESRD and were administered hemodialysis therapy (Table 1). No patient whose biopsied tissue was negative for WNT10A expression received renal replacement therapy. Thus, WNT10A expression may be correlated with poor prognosis of kidney function.

WNT10A and α-SMA expression in kidney fibroblasts associated with AIN

WNT10A expression in kidney tissues obtained from AIN patient biopsies was much higher than that of samples from chronic kidney disease patients (Fig. 2B and Fig. S1). Inflammatory cells (primarily lymphocytes) were found associated with uriniferous tubules in tissues from patients with AIN (Fig. 2F). Fibroblasts that are α-SMA positive are thought to be myofibroblasts or activated fibroblasts that produce ECM components, such as type 1 collagen, type 3 collagen, and fibronectin. Some α-SMA-expressing cells were present at the interstitium of uriniferous tubules in kidneys without AIN (Fig. S2). Many more α-SMA-positive cells were identified in WNT10A-positive AIN cases (Fig. 2B and D) compared with WNT10A-negetive AIN cases (Fig. 2A and C). The consecutive IHC sections also demonstrated co-localization of both WNT10A and α-SMA in the same or at least in adjacent myofibroblasts/fibroblasts (Fig. 2B and D). Moreover, there was a significantly close positive correlation to the IHC WNT10A-positive and α-SMA-positive expression pattern ($p = 0.0005$) (Table 1). Finally, Masson-Trichrome staining showed that more ECM was found in WNT10A-positive AIN (Fig. 2H) than in WNT10A-negetive AIN (Fig. 2G). WNT10A expression in kidney tissue had significantly strong kidney fibrosis (fibrosis area is equal or more than 20%) compared with WNT10A-negative expression ($p = 0.0191$) (Table 1). However, there was not statistical correlation between high WNT10A expression (positive area is equal or more than 30%) and strong kidney fibrosis ($p = 0.7782$) (data not shown). Thus, WNT10A protein expression in α-SMA-expressing fibroblasts may contribute to the kidney interstitial fibrotic process characteristic of AIN.

Fibroblasts with WNT10A expression produce fibronectin

We investigated the involvement of WNT10A in the kidney fibrosis processes of AIN using COS1 cells, a cell line derived from kidney fibroblasts of the African green monkey. Two WNT10A-overexpressing COS1 cells (COS1-10A) were established (Fig. 3A). Interestingly, WNT10A overexpression enhances the expression of fibronectin (an ECM component) about three to five fold but does not alter the expression of type 1 and type 3 collagen (Fig. 3B). WNT10A is a secreted protein. In contrast to normal medium, supernatant from WNT10A-overexpressin COS1 cells induced fibronectin expression in untransfected COS1 cells (Fig. 3C). As expected, kidney tissues with WNT10A expression also expressed fibronectin (Fig. 3D). Furthermore, there was statistical positive correlation to the IHC WNT10A-positive and fibronectin-positive expression ($p = 0.0062$) in kidney tissues (Table 1). This indicates that WNT10A signaling plays a role in fibronectin synthesis and in activating stromagenic factors to induce fibrosis.

WNT10A protects fibroblasts from oxidative stress

We previously reported that WNT10A expression is induced by treatment with hydrogen peroxide [10], suggesting that WNT10A signaling might induce the expression of antioxidant protein genes to protect cells. In this study, we found that WNT10A overexpression enhanced the expression of peroxiredoxin (PRDX) 5, but not PRDX 1, 2, 3 and 4 (Fig. 4A). COS1-10A cells expressed PRDX5 at approximately twice the level of control cells (Fig. 4B). PRDXs are a ubiquitous family of multifunctional antioxdant thioredoxin-dependent peroxidase that scavenge reactive oxygen species (ROS), suggesting that WNT10A overexpressing cells may be resistant against oxidative stress. As we expected, COS1-10A cells may be resistant to oxidative stress because WNT10A overexpression renders cells resistant to hydrogen peroxide (Fig. 4C). Down regulation of PRDX5 expression by siRNA sensitizes cells to hydrogen peroxide (Fig. 4D and E). COS1-10A cells expressed weakly active caspase-3 than control cells under hydrogen peroxide (Fig. 4F). WNT10A prevented apoptosis from oxidative stress via PRDX5 expression.

WNT10A prevented apoptosis of fibroblasts from high-glucose stress

High glucose triggers cell apoptosis, the generation of free radicals, and oxidative stress [20]. The control COS1 cells demonstrated poor survival following treatment with moderate- and high-glucose (MM and HM) compared with treatment with low-glucose medium (LM). However, COS1-10A cells survived even when treated with MM and HM, indicating that WNT10A overexpression protected fibroblasts from high glucose stress (Fig. 5A). Thus, high glucose stress leads to apoptosis of COS1 cells. As shown in Fig. 5B, control COS1 cells expressed caspase-3, cleaved caspase-3, PARP (poly ADP ribose polymerase), and cleavage-PARP compared with COS1-10A (Fig. 5B). WNT10A also prevented apoptosis from high glucose stress.

Discussion

The kidney is exposed to several kinds of stresses including oxidative stress, high glucose stress, hypoxic stress, and uremic stress. Oxidative stress in the kidney is considered a major cause of kidney injury and inflammation [21]. The pathogenesis and recovery processes of AKI is regulated by a wide variety of pathways in various inflammatory cells that produce cytokines/chemokines and ROS. Tissue-specific fibrosis is differentially regulated by intrinsic and extrinsic mechanisms that involve organ-specific autocrine and paracrine systems. The molecular mechanisms that determine progressive CKD after AKI are largely unknown. A previous report showed that persistently high profibrotic signaling activity induces paracrine signaling that drives fibroblasts proliferation and inflammation [22]. WNT signaling is persistently active in areas exposed to stress. However, following AKI, WNT signaling becomes widely activated in kidney [23]. Since WNT10A induces angio/stromagenesis [10], we considered the possibility that there may be a relationship between WNT10A, tissue fibrosis, and inflammation. In contrast to AIN tissue, WNT10A hardly expressed in kidney of chronic kidney disease (Fig. S1). Therefore, we hypothesized that WNT10A-positive cells are found in proximity to areas of severe tissue injury, and that secreted WNT10A might be involved in fibrotic synthesis on AIN.

Tissue repair and fibrosis from injury involves multiple evolutionarily-conserved processes. Hydrogen peroxide can function as a chemoattractant following injury to transmit an immediate damage signal. After the initial response, angio/stromagenesis occurs leading to formation of new blood vessels, the appearance of (myo) fibroblasts, and the ECM gradually forming granulation tissue. The tissue remodeling after granulation is regulated by contractile fibroblasts called myofibroblasts [24]. The sources of renal myofibroblasts are local resident fibroblasts that arise from proliferation (50%), and nonproliferat-

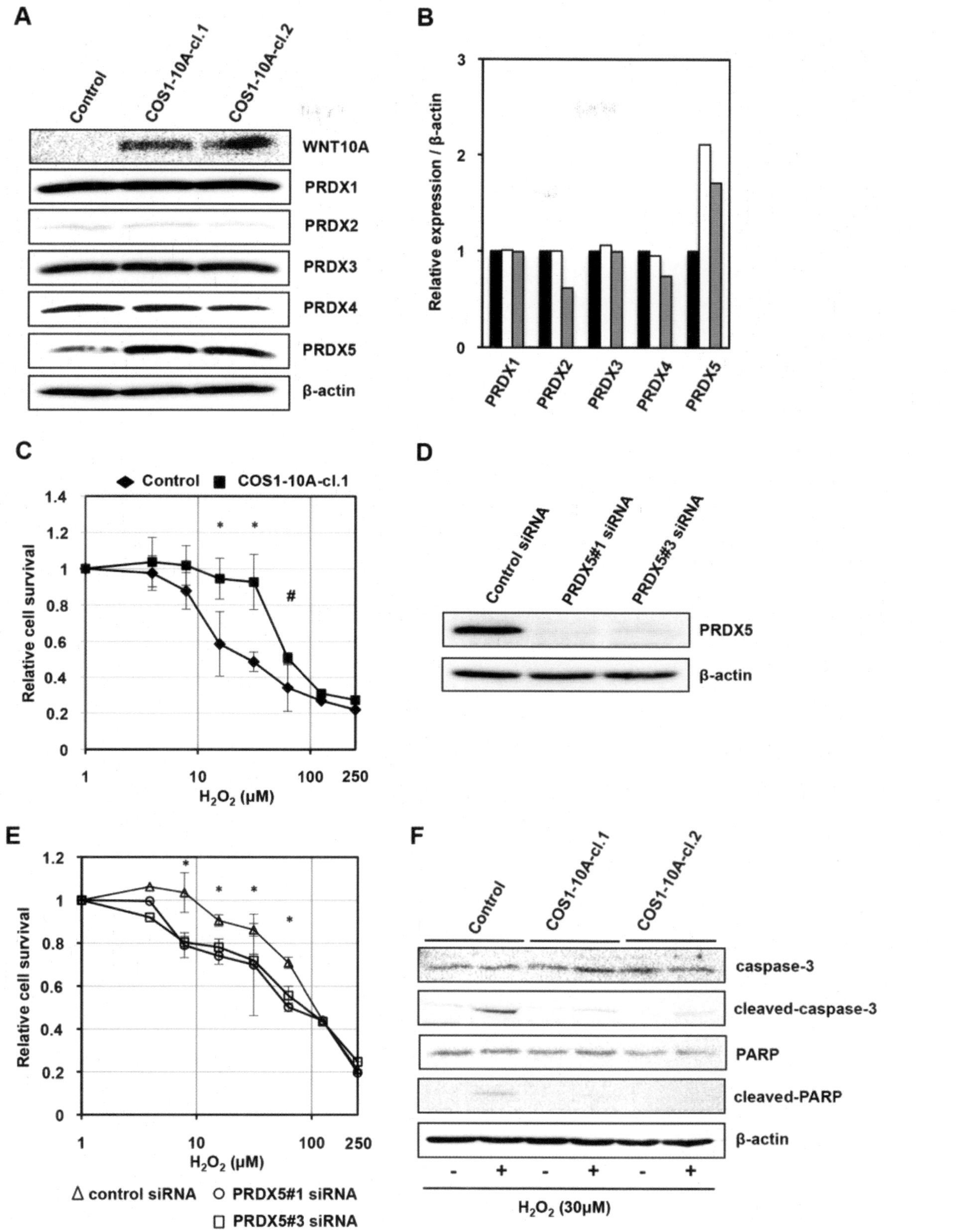

Figure 4. WNT10A protected fibroblasts against oxidative stress. (A) Western blot analysis of peroxiredoxin (PRDX)1, 2, 3, 4, and 5. Western blot analysis was performed using whole lysates obtained from COS1-vector (control) and COS1-10A cells. Only PRDX5 was increased with expression of WNT10A. (B) Relative expression of PRDX1, 2, 3, 4, and 5 normalized to β-actin expression. The black bar shows control cells, white and gray bars show COS1-10A-cl.1 and COS1-10A-cl.2 respectively. (C) The sensitivity of control and WNT10A-overexpressing cells (COS1-10A-cl.1) to H_2O_2. All values are the means of at least three independent experiments. Bars indicate standard deviation. *$p<0.01$ vs control. #$p<0.05$ vs control. (D) Downregulation of PRDX5 in WNT10A-overexpressing cells (COS1-10A-cl.1) by two kinds of siRNA. (E) The sensitivity of siRNA transfected cells to H_2O_2. All values are the means of at least three independent experiments. Bars indicate standard deviation. *$p<0.05$ vs PRDX5#1 and #3 siRNA. (F) Western blot analysis of caspase-3 and PARP expression. Western blot analysis was performed using whole lysates obtained from COS1-vector (control) and COS1-10A. Each cells were cultured in normal medium or medium containing hydrogen peroxide (30 μM) for 4 hours.

ing myofibroblasts derived from bone marrow (35%) [25]. It has been proposed that the remaining progenitor population is derived from circulating fibrocytes, local pericytes, and resident epithelial cells, although this remains to be fully characterized [26,27]. α-SMA expression induces fibroblasts into myofibroblasts [28]. Persistent myofibroblasts activation results in hypertrophic scars including keloid tissue or tissue fibrosis. Local activating fibroblasts express α-SMA and become fibrotic tissue [29]. Activation of WNT-β-catenin signaling has been reported in kidney and skin fibrosis [30,31]. WNT10A expression in kidney tissue associated with α-SMA and fibronectin expression, and interstitial fibrosis (Table 1). The patients with WNT10A expression showed significantly lower eGFR than patients without WNT10A expression on kidney biopsy (Fig. 1 and 2), suggesting that WNT10A may induce persistent myofibroblasts activation leading to tissue fibrosis.

TGF-β and connective tissue growth factor are cytokines that up-regulate fibronectin expression during fibrogenesis [32]. As shown in Fig. 3, WNT10A overexpression enhances the expression of one of the ECM components, fibronectin. This data supports relation between WNT10A and fibronectin expression in AIN kidney tissue (Fig. 3D and Table 1). Consequently, WNT10A increases synthesis of interstitial fibrosis. Fibronectin has two different forms, cellular and plasma fibronectin. Cellular fibronectin is expressed by fibroblasts and is deposited locally into the ECM [33]. In general, locally-produced cellular fibronectin

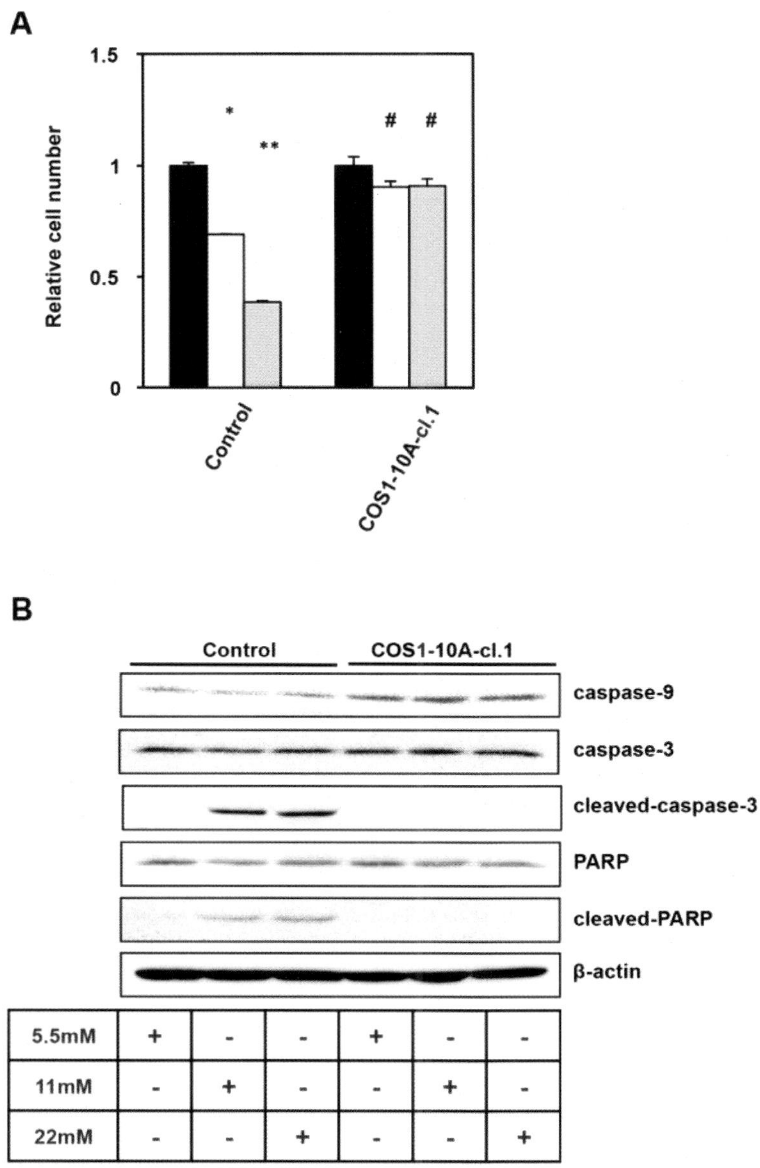

Figure 5. WNT10A protected fibroblasts against high glucose stress. (A) Proliferation assay. Control and WNT10A-overexpressing cells (COS1-10A-cl.1) (2×10^4 cells/well) were seeded into a 12-well plate, and incubated in normal DMEM. After 24 hours, cells (0hr) were harvested, and other cells were cultured in each medium (5.5 mM, 11 mM, and 22 mM of glucose concentration) for 72 hours. Proliferative rates for 72 hours were compared. Black bar (5.5 mM), white bar (11 mM), gray bar (22 mM). All values are the means of at least three independent experiments. Bars indicate standard deviation. *$p<0.001$ vs 5.5 mM, **$p<0.001$ vs 5.5 mM and 11 mM, #$p<0.05$ vs 5.5 mM (B) Caspase and PARP expression. Whole lysates obtained from control and WNT10A-overexpressing cells treated with each medium (5.5 mM, 11 mM, and 22 mM of glucose concentration) were analyzed by western blotting.

appears at the injury site within the early phase after tissue injury [34]. Plasma fibronectin is synthesized by hepatocytes and secreted into the blood plasma. Plasma fibronectin levels have been shown to increase after major trauma resulting in vascular tissue damage and inflammation such as atherosclerosis and ischemic diseases [35,36]. Previous studies suggested that mechanical stress contributes to injury and fibrosis by inducing epithelial-mesenchymal transition (EMT) via a mechanism driven by TGF-β1 and WNT signaling [37,38].

PRDXs are a ubiquitous family of multifunctional antioxidant thioredoxin-dependent peroxidases that scavenge reactive oxygen species (ROS). There are six distinct members located in various subcellular compartments. PRDX1, PRDX2, and PRDX6 are in the cytoplasm, and PRDX3 is in mitochondria. And PRDX4 is in endoplasmic reticulum and secreted. PRDX5 is expressed in mitochondria, the peroxisome, and the cytosol [39]. ROS are involved in initiation and implementation of apoptosis. PRDXs can efficiently eliminate hydrogen peroxide and participate in physiological processes such as apoptosis [40]. WNT10A promotes PRDX5 expression, and protects COS1 cells from oxidative stress (Fig. 4). Our study showed that WNT10A prevented COS1 cells from apoptosis by hydrogen peroxide. So, WNT10A may be helpful of fibroblasts to synthesize ECM under oxidative stress. As mentioned above, AKI is exposed several kinds of stresses including oxidative stress. WNT10A in kidney fibroblasts might play an important role in AKI/AIN.

We also investigated the relation between high glucose and WNT10A in COS1 cells. High glucose induces caspase-3-dependent apoptosis in fibroblasts, and activation of caspase caused by high glucose stress is independent of Fas/FasL signaling pathways system [41]. Activation of caspase-3 requires proteolytic cleavage of its inactive zymogen into active subunits. Cleaved caspase-3 causes apoptosis by degrading PARP. Our results show that WNT10A overexpression COS1 cells weaker expressed cleaved caspase-3 and PARP than control cells (Fig. 5B). WNT10A protected cells from apoptosis caused by high glucose stress. Consequently, a proliferation of WNT10A-overexpressing COS1 cells was small reduction than control cells (Fig. 5A).

3-hydroxy-3-methylglutaryl-coenzyme A (HMG-CoA) reductase inhibitors (statins) are used as therapy for hyperlipidemia. Statins inhibit kidney fibrosis and inflammation in rats [42,43], and inhibits fibronectin expression in human airway fibroblasts [44]. Several studies have reported that statins are anti-inflammatory and block proliferation by G1 arrest of the cell cycle [45,46,47]. Our investigation also indicated that simvastatin suppressed proliferation of COS1 via inducing apoptosis regardless of WNT10A expression (data not shown). Our work suggests that it will be important to study the effects of statins during kidney fibrosis in a clinical setting.

In conclusion, we should point out that WNT10A expression leads to loss of kidney function due to excess tissue fibrosis. WNT10A enhances the synthesis of fibronectin. Furthermore, WNT10A expression in kidney is thought to promote kidney fibrosis following severe kidney dysfunction. COS1 cells with WNT10A expression are not induced to apoptosis against for hydrogen peroxide and high glucose. Thus, these findings might imply kidney fibroblasts with WNT10A-expression maintain their viability and cause kidney fibrosis under several kinds of stresses in AKI. We expect that WNT10A expression in kidney tissue may be a bio-maker of prognosis for AKI. Further studies to validate our conclusions in other model systems such as animal model and 3-D culture system will be critical for understanding the role of WNT10A in kidney fibrosis.

Supporting Information

Figure S1 Expression of WNT10A in the kidney tissues of a chronic kidney disease (CKD) patient (left panel) and AIN patient (right panel). Immunohistochemical staining for WNT10A (brown). CKD patient had taken therapy for IgA nephropathy for a few decades. All photos were taken at 200×. Scale bar is 100 μm.

Figure S2 Expression of α-SMA in the kidney tissues. Each tissue is minor glomerular abnormalities (left panel) and AIN with WNT10A expression (right panel). Few myofibroblasts with α-SMA expression can be seen in the circumference of uriniferous tubule in minor glomerular abnormalities. Immunohistochemical staining for α-SMA (brown). All photos were taken at 200×. Scale bar is 100 μm.

Acknowledgments

We thank Naoko Une, Akiko Matsumura and Michiko Kurihara for their technical assistance.

Author Contributions

Conceived and designed the experiments: AK KK. Performed the experiments: AK SY KYW NK TY YI HI MT YO KK. Analyzed the data: AK SY KYW MT YO KK. Contributed reagents/materials/analysis tools: AK SY KYW HI KK. Wrote the paper: AK KK.

References

1. Eddy AA (2000) Molecular basis of renal fibrosis. Pediatr Nephrol 15: 290–301.
2. Liu Y (2006) Renal fibrosis: new insights into the pathogenesis and therapeutics. Kidney Int 69: 213–217.
3. Wynn TA, Ramalingam TR (2012) Mechanisms of fibrosis: therapeutic translation for fibrotic disease. Nat Med 18: 1028–1040.
4. Moon RT, Kohn AD, De Ferrari GV, Kaykas A (2004) WNT and beta-catenin signalling: diseases and therapies. Nat Rev Genet 5: 691–701.
5. Kohn AD, Moon RT (2005) Wnt and calcium signaling: beta-catenin-independent pathways. Cell Calcium 38: 439–446.
6. Carroll TJ, Das A (2011) Planar cell polarity in kidney development and disease. Organogenesis 7: 180–190.
7. Nusse R (2005) Wnt signaling in disease and in development. Cell Res 15: 28–32.
8. He W, Dai C, Li Y, Zeng G, Monga SP, et al. (2009) Wnt/beta-catenin signaling promotes renal interstitial fibrosis. J Am Soc Nephrol 20: 765–776.
9. Dai C, Stolz DB, Kiss LP, Monga SP, Holzman LB, et al. (2009) Wnt/beta-catenin signaling promotes podocyte dysfunction and albuminuria. J Am Soc Nephrol 20: 1997–2008.
10. Yasuniwa Y, Izumi H, Wang KY, Shimajiri S, Sasaguri Y, et al. (2010) Circadian disruption accelerates tumor growth and angio/stromagenesis through a Wnt signaling pathway. PLoS One 5: e15330.
11. Grande MT, López-Novoa JM (2009) Fibroblast activation and myofibroblast generation in obstructive nephropathy. Nat Rev Nephrol 5: 319–328.
12. Kitada S, Yamada S, Kuma A, Ouchi S, Tasaki T, et al. (2013) Polypeptide N-acetylgalactosaminyl transferase 3 independently predicts high-grade tumors and poor prognosis in patients with renal cell carcinomas. Br J Cancer 109: 472–481.
13. Noguchi H, Yamada S, Nabeshima A, Guo X, Tanimoto A, et al. (2014) Depletion of apoptosis signal-regulating kinase 1 prevents bile duct ligation-induced necroinflammation and subsequent peribiliary fibrosis. Am J Pathol 184: 644–661.
14. Igarashi T, Izumi H, Uchiumi T, Nishio K, Arao T, et al. (2007) Clock and ATF4 transcription system regulates drug resistance in human cancer cell lines. Oncogene 26: 4749–4760.
15. Shiota M, Izumi H, Miyamoto N, Onitsuka T, Kashiwagi E, et al. (2008) Ets regulates peroxiredoxin1 and 5 expressions through their interaction with the high-mobility group protein B1. Cancer Sci 99: 1950–1959.

16. Miyamoto N, Izumi H, Noguchi T, Nakajima Y, Ohmiya Y, et al. (2008) Tip60 is regulated by circadian transcription factor clock and is involved in cisplatin resistance. J Biol Chem 283: 18218–18226.
17. Izumi H, Takahashi M, Uramoto H, Nakayama Y, Oyama T, et al. (2011) Monocarboxylate transporters 1 and 4 are involved in the invasion activity of human lung cancer cells. Cancer Sci 102: 1007–1013.
18. Wakasugi T, Izumi H, Uchiumi T, Suzuki H, Arao T, et al. (2007) ZNF143 interacts with p73 and is involved in cisplatin resistance through the transcriptional regulation of DNA repair genes. Oncogene 26: 5194–5203.
19. Miyamoto N, Izumi H, Miyamoto R, Kubota T, Tawara A, et al. (2009) Nipradilol and timolol induce Foxo3a and peroxiredoxin 2 expression and protect trabecular meshwork cells from oxidative stress. Invest Ophthalmol Vis Sci 50: 2777–2784.
20. Sedeek M, Callera G, Montezano A, Gutsol A, Heitz F, et al. (2010) Critical role of Nox4-based NADPH oxidase in glucose-induced oxidative stress in the kidney: implications in type 2 diabetic nephropathy. Am J Physiol Renal Physiol 299: F1348–1358.
21. Joshi S, Peck AB, Khan SR (2013) NADPH oxidase as a therapeutic target for oxalate induced injury in kidneys. Oxid Med Cell Longev 2013: 462361.
22. Hinz B, Phan SH, Thannickal VJ, Prunotto M, Desmoulière A, et al. (2012) Recent developments in myofiroblast biology: paradigms for connective tissue remodeling. Am J Pathol 180: 1340–1355.
23. Kawakami T, Ren S, Duffield JS (2013) Wnt signalling in kidney diseases: dual roles in renal injury and repair. J Pathol 229: 221–231.
24. Tomasek JJ, Gabbiani G, Hinz B, Chaponnier C, Brown RA (2002) Myofibroblasts and mechano-regulation of connective tissue remodelling. Nat Rev Mol Cell Biol 3: 349–363.
25. LeBleu VS, Taduri G, O'Connell J, Teng Y, Cooke VG, et al. (2013) Origin and function of myofibroblasts in kidney fibrosis. Nat Med 19: 1047–1053.
26. Humphreys BD, Lin SL, Kobayashi A, Hudson TE, Nowlin BT, et al. (2010) Fate tracing reveals the pericyte and not epithelial origin of myofibroblasts in kidney fibrosis. Am J Pathol 176: 85–97.
27. Zeisberg M, Kalluri R (2004) The role of epithelial-to-mesenchymal transition in renal fibrosis. J Mol Med (Berl) 82: 175–181.
28. El Kahi CG, Atiyeh BS, Abdallah Hajj Hussein I, Jurjus R, Dibo SA, et al. (2009) Modulation of wound contracture alpha-smooth muscle actin and multispecific vitronectin receptor integrin alphavbeta3 in the rabbit's experimental model. Int Wound J 6: 214–224.
29. Hinz B, Celetta G, Tomasek JJ, Gabbiani G, Chaponnier C (2001) Alpha-smooth muscle actin expression upregulates fibroblast contractile activity. Mol Biol Cell 12: 2730–2741.
30. Wei J, Melichian D, Komura K, Hinchcliff M, Lam AP, et al. (2011) Canonical Wnt signaling induces skin fibrosis and subcutaneous lipotrophy: a novel mouse model for scleroderma? Arthritis Rheum 63: 1707–1717.
31. Surendran K, Schiavi S, Hruska KA (2005) Wnt-dependent β-catenin signaling is activated after unilateral ureteral obstraction, and recombinant secreted fizzled-related protein 4 alters the progression of renal fibrosis. J Am Soc Nephrol 16: 2373–2384.
32. Leask A, Abraham DJ (2004) TGF-beta signaling and the fibrotic response. FASEB J 18: 816–827.
33. Mao Y, Schwarzbauer JE (2005) Fibronectin fibrillogenesis, a cell-mediated matrix assembly process. Matrix Biol 24: 389–399.
34. Gabbiani G (2003) The myofibroblast in wound healing and fibrocontractive diseases. J Pathol 200: 500–503.
35. Song KS, Kim HK, Shim W, Jee SH (2001) Plasma fibronectin levels in ischemic heart disease. Atherosclerosis 154: 449–453.
36. Claudepierre P, Allanore Y, Belec L, Larget-Piet B, Zardi L, et al. (1999) Increased Ed-B fibronectin plasma levels in spondyloarthropathies: comparison with rheumatoid arthritis patients and a healthy population. Rheumatology (Oxford) 38: 1099–1103.
37. Heise RL, Stober V, Cheluvaraju C, Hollingsworth JW, Garantziotis S (2011) Mechanical stretch induces epithelial-mesenchymal transition in alveolar epithelia via hyaluronan activation of innate immunity. J Biol Chem 286: 17435–17444.
38. Chen JH, Chen WL, Sider KL, Yip CY, Simmons CA (2011) β-catenin mediates mechanically regulated, transforming growth factor-β1-induced myofibroblast differentiation of aortic valve interstitial cells. Arterioscler Thromb Vasc Biol 31: 590–597.
39. Wood ZA, Schröder E, Robin Harris J, Poole LB (2003) Structure, mechanism and regulation of peroxiredoxins. Trends Biochem Sci 28: 32–40.
40. Oláhová M, Taylor SR, Khazaipoul S, Wang J, Morgan BA, et al. (2008) A redox-sensitive peroxiredoxin that is important for longevity has tissue- and stress-specific roles in stress resistance. Proc Natl Acad Sci U S A 105: 19839–19844.
41. Liu J, Jiang Y, Mao J, Gu B, Liu H, et al. (2013) High levels of glucose induces a dose-dependent apoptosis in human periodontal ligament fibroblasts by activating caspase-3 signaling pathway. Appl Biochem Biotechnol 170: 1458–1471.
42. Gianella A, Nobili E, Abbate M, Zoja C, Gelosa P, et al. (2007) Rosuvastatin treatment prevents progressive kidney inflammation and fibrosis in stroke-prone rats. Am J Pathol 170: 1165–1177.
43. Vieira JM Jr, Mantovani E, Rodrigues LT, Dellê H, Noronha IL, et al. (2005) Simvastatin attenuates renal inflammation, tubular transdifferentiation and interstitial fibrosis in rats with unilateral ureteral obstruction. Nephrol Dial Transplant 20: 1582–1591.
44. Schaafsma D, McNeill KD, Mutawe MM, Mutawe MM, Ghavami S, et al. (2011) Simvastatin inhibits TGFβ1-induced fibronectins in human airway fibroblasts. Respir Res 12: 113.
45. Bereswill S, Muñoz M, Fischer A, Plickert R, Haag LM, et al. (2010) Anti-inflammatory effects of resveratrol, curcumin and simvastatin in acute small intestinal inflammation. PLoS One 5: e15099.
46. Yagi H, Kato T, Nagata T, Habu T, Nozaki M, et al. (1995) Regulation of the mouse histone H2A.X gene promoter by the transcription factor E2F and CCAAT binding protein. J Biol Chem 270: 18759–18765.
47. Javanmoghadam-Kamrani S, Keyomarsi K (2008) Synchronization of the cell cycle using lovastatin. Cell Cycle 7: 2434–2440.

The Effects of Super-Flux (High Performance) Dialyzer on Plasma Glycosylated Pro-B-Type Natriuretic Peptide (proBNP) and Glycosylated N-Terminal proBNP in End-Stage Renal Disease Patients on Dialysis

Yasuaki Nakagawa[1], Toshio Nishikimi[1]*, Koichiro Kuwahara[1], Shinji Yasuno[2], Hideyuki Kinoshita[1], Yoshihiro Kuwabara[1], Kazuhiro Nakao[1], Takeya Minami[1], Chinatsu Yamada[1], Kenji Ueshima[2], Yoshihiro Ikeda[3], Hiroyuki Okamoto[4], Kazukiyo Horii[4], Kiyoshi Nagata[4], Kenji Kangawa[5], Naoto Minamino[6], Kazuwa Nakao[1]

1 Department of Medicine and Clinical Science, Kyoto University Graduate School of Medicine, Kyoto, Japan, **2** Department of EBM Research, Kyoto University Hospital, Institute for Advancement of Clinical and Translational Science, Kyoto, Japan, **3** Medical corporation, Ikeda Clinic, Kyoto, Japan, **4** Diagnostics Division, Shionogi & Co., Ltd, Oska, Japan, **5** Department of Biochemistry, National Cerebral and Cardiovascular Center Research Institute, Fujishirodai, Suita, Osaka, Japan, **6** Department of Molecular Pharmacology, National Cerebral and Cardiovascular Center Research Institute, Fujishirodai, Suita, Osaka, Japan

Abstract

Background: Plasma BNP levels are predictive of prognosis in hemodialysis patients. However, recent studies showed that the current BNP immunoassay cross-reacts with glycosylated proBNP, and the NT-proBNP assay underestimates glycosylated NT-proBNP. In addition, the recently developed high performance dialyzer removes medium-sized molecular solutes such as β2-microgloburin. We therefore investigated the effects of high performance dialysis on measured levels of glycosylated proBNP, glycosylated NT-proBNP and other BNP-related peptides in end-stage renal disease (ESRD) patients on hemodialysis.

Method: The relationships between clinical parameters and BNP-related molecule were also investigated. We used our newly developed immunoassay to measure plasma total BNP and proBNP in 105 normal subjects and 36 ESRD patients before and after hemodialysis. Plasma NT-proBNP was measured using Elecsys II after treatment with or without deglycosylating enzymes. We also measured plasma ANP and cGMP using radioimmunoassays.

Results: All the measured BNP-related peptides were significantly higher in ESRD patients than healthy subjects. Total BNP (−38.9%), proBNP (−29.7%), glycoNT-proBNP (−45.5%), nonglycoNT-proBNP (−53.4%), ANP (−50.4%) and cGMP (−72.1%) were all significantly reduced after hemodialysis, and the magnitude of the reduction appeared molecular weight-dependent. Both the proBNP/total BNP and glycoNT-proBNP/nonglycoNT-proBNP ratios were increased after hemodialysis. The former correlated positively with hemodialysis vintage and negatively with systolic blood pressure, while the latter correlated positively with parathyroid hormone levels.

Conclusion: These results suggest that hemodialysis using super-flux dialyzer removes BNP-related peptides in a nearly molecular weight-dependent manner. The ProBNP/total BNP and glycoNT-proBNP/nonglycoNT-proBNP ratios appear to be influenced by hemodialysis-related parameters in ESRD patients on hemodialysis.

Editor: Emmanuel A. Burdmann, University of Sao Paulo Medical School, Brazil

Funding: This study was supported in part by Scientific Research Grants-in-Aid 20590837 and 23591041 from the Ministry of Education, Culture, Sports, Science and Technology of Japan (to T. Nishikimi); a grant (AS 232Z01302F) from the Japan Science and Technology Agency (to T. Nishikimi); and a grant from the Suzuken Memorial Foundation (to T. Nishikimi). The funders had no role in study design, data collection and analysis, decision to publish, or preparation of the manuscript.

Competing Interests: HO, KH, and KN are employees of Shionogi & Co., Ltd. Shionogi Company previously developed the BNP kit used in this study (Patent name: monoclonal antibody recognizing for C-terminal region of BNP and Patent number: 665850) and intend to develop a new assay kit for proBNP. There are no further patents, products in development or marketed products to declare.

* E-mail: nishikim@kuhp.kyoto-u.ac.jp

Introduction

Hemodialysis patients exhibit a greatly heightened risk of cardiovascular morbidity and mortality. For example, these patients experience an extremely high prevalence of left ventricular hypertrophy and heart failure. Consequently, there is a great need for a good clinical biomarker enabling early identification of dialysis patients at risk of cardiovascular events and mortality, as well as earlier aggressive intervention.

B-type natriuretic peptide (BNP; also termed brain natriuretic peptide) is a cardiac hormone produced and secreted mainly by the ventricles; another cardiac hormone, atrial natriuretic peptide (ANP), is produced and secreted by the atria. [1] Ventricular wall stress and/or ischemia stimulate expression of the BNP precursor proBNP [2,3], which is thought to be cleaved to BNP-32 (BNP or mature BNP) and N-terminal proBNP (NT-proBNP) prior to its secretion [4]. Plasma levels of BNP, NT-proBNP and ANP are elevated in patients with cardiac hypertrophy or heart failure. [5] They are also elevated in patients with chronic kidney disease, especially those receiving dialysis. [6] This is likely related to left ventricular dysfunction as well as to reduced clearance and increased plasma volume. It is widely recognized that cardiac function is a major confounder influencing levels of these peptides in dialysis patients. Thus, even in dialysis patients with end-stage renal disease (ESRD), BNP is used for diagnosis and evaluation of the severity of heart failure and is predictive of patient prognosis. [7].

Recent studies have shown that unprocessed precursor proBNP circulates in healthy individuals [8], and that its levels in plasma are increased in patients with severe heart failure. This is noteworthy in part because the immunoassay system currently being used to measure BNP also detects proBNP (the anti-BNP antibody cross-reacts with proBNP). In fact, it appears that about 70% of the plasma BNP measured using the BNP immunoassay system is proBNP in healthy human subjects. [9] In addition, it was recently shown that recombinant proBNP derived from mammalian cells has seven sites capable of *O*-linked oligosaccharide attachment within the N-terminal portion of the peptide, [10] and that both proBNP and NT-proBNP are glycosylated in human plasma. [11] [12].

The latest dialyzer membranes used for hemodialysis have the ability to remove large solutes, like β2-microglobulin. The function of these "super-flux" membranes is to remove larger and protein-bound uremic toxins. Earlier reports showed that plasma BNP and ANP levels are reduced after hemodialysis using a "low-flux" membrane, most likely due to body fluid volume removal and/or dialyzer membrane-mediated removal. However, the effect of super-flux membranes on BNP and BNP-related molecules, such as glycosylated proBNP and glycosylated NT-proBNP, remains unknown. In the present study, therefore, we examined the levels of total BNP, proBNP, mature BNP, glycosylated NT-proBNP, nonglycosylated NT-proBNP, ANP and cGMP in ESRD patients, before and after hemodialysis using a super-flux membrane.

Subjects and Methods

Patients

105 healthy subjects and 36 ESRD patients attending routine outpatient hemodialysis sessions were included in the study. Ethical approval was granted by the Kyoto University Hospital Ethical Committee. The aims of study were explained to each participant, and written consent was obtained. All clinical investigations were conducted according to the principles expressed in the Declaration of Helsinki.

In the ESRD group, all the patients underwent regular hemodialysis three times a week. The clinical characteristics of the healthy subjects and ESRD patients in this study are listed in Table 1. In the ESRD group, all the patients were dialyzed using super-flux polysulphonedialyzers: PES-19SEa eco in 4 cases, PES-21SEa eco in 8 cases, PES25SEa eco in 3 cases (Nipro, Tokyo, Japan), PS-15EL in 4 cases, APS18EL in 4 cases, APS-21EL in 11 cases and KF-20C in 2 cases (Asahikasei, Tokyo Japan). The mean dialysis session time was 3.96±0.30 h, and the QB was 209±25.1 ml/h. Cardiac function, heart size and blood pressure were relatively well controlled. Total body fluid volume was estimated using the equation: body weight×0.6 [13]. The percent changes in total body fluid volume were calculated as: body weight change/calculated total body weight before hemodialysis.

Blood Sampling

Venous blood was collected before and immediately after dialysis for measurement of total BNP, proBNP, mature BNP, nonglycoNT-proBNP, glycoNT-proBNP, ANP and cGMP. Blood samples were transferred to chilled glass tubes containing disodium EDTA (1 mg/ml) and aprotinin (500 U/ml) and immediately centrifuged at 4°C, after which the resultant plasma was frozen and stored at −80°C until used. We also measured levels of hemoglobin, serum c-reactive protein, albumin and parathyroid hormone, among others.

Biochemical Analyses

Measurement of plasma ANP, cGMP, total BNP, proBNP, and mature BNP. Plasma ANP levels were measured using a specific immunoradiometric assay, while levels of cGMP were measured using a radioimmunoassay, as previously described.[10]

Plasma total BNP and proBNP levels were measured using an immunochemiluminescent assay, as previously described. [9] All BNP assays, regardless of the source (e.g., Shionogi, Biosite), cross-react with proBNP, because the two antibodies used in the assays recognize epitopes common to BNP and proBNP. For that reason, total BNP means the sum of proBNP plus mature BNP, most of which is BNP[1–32]. In the present study, we measured total BNP and proBNP separately and calculated the mature BNP as follows: mature BNP = total BNP − proBNP. [9].

Measurement of plasma glycoNT-proBNP and nonglycoNT-proBNP in HD patients. ProBNP is post-translationally glycosylated to varying degrees in its N-terminal region, at Thr36, Ser37, Ser44, Thr48, Ser53, Thr58 and Thr71. [10] NT-proBNP is similarly glycosylated. The Elecsys proBNP II system (Roche Diagnostics, Germany) is comprised of a capture monoclonal antibody that recognizes NT-proBNP[27–31] and a monoclonal signal antibody that recognizes NT-proBNP[42–46], which contains a glycosylation site at amino acid residue 44. [14] Notably, *O*-linked oligosaccharide attachment inhibits the binding of the signal antibody to NT-proBNP. [15,16] We therefore postulated that NT-proBNP measured using Elecsys proBNP II is actually only nonglycoNT-proBNP. To measure total NT-proBNP, plasma samples were incubated for 24 h at 37°C with or without a cocktail of deglycosylating enzymes, included *O*-glycosidase (Roche Diagnostics) and neuraminidase (Roche Diagnostics) at final concentrations of 4.25 and 42.5 mU/ml, respectively, as described previously. [10] [14] NT-proBNP levels were then measured using Elecsys proBNP II, after which the glycoNT-proBNP level was calculated as: total NT-proBNP − nonglycoNT-proBNP.

Echocardiographic measurements. An experienced echocardiographer without knowledge of the clinical features of the patients performed the echocardiography using a cardiac ultra-

Table 1. Clinical profiles of the healthy subjects and ESRD patients enrolled in this study.

	Healthy subjects (N = 105)	ESRD patients (N = 36)	p
Age, years	51.3±12.1	64.0±11.7	<0.0001
Sex, m/f	50/55	20/16	0.2663
BMI, kg/m^2	22.2±3.0	20.2±2.4	0.0005
HD vintage, year	(−)	11.2±8.9	
Before HD			
Systolic BP, mmHg	115.4±17.3	142.2±22.4	<0.0001
Diastolic BP, mmHg	73.9±13.0	71.4±10.8	0.3016
Mean BP, mmHg	87.7±14.0	95.0±13.1	0.0071
After HD			
Systolic BP, mmHg		128.5±19.9	
Diastolic BP, mmHg		69.9±9.4	
Mean BP, mmHg		89.5±11.2	
Inter-dialysis weight gain, kg		2.67±0.92	
CTR,%	44.4±4.6	49.7±5.0	<0.0001
BUN, mg/dl	14.0±3.1	59.3±17.2	<0.0001
Cre, mg/dl	0.76±0.14	10.59±1.27	<0.0001
Alb, g/dl	4.3±0.2	3.60±0.35	<0.0001
Hemoglobin, g/dl	14.0±1.3	10.62±1.15	<0.0001
Ht, %	43.1±3.6	32.1±3.6	<0.0001
Diabetes mellitus	(−)	27.8 (10)	
Anti-hypertensive drug	(−)		
Calcium channel blocker		44.4%(16)	
Alpha blocker		2.8%(1)	
Beta blocker		38.9%(14)	
ACEI		2.8%(1)	
ARB		36.1%(13)	
Nitrate		5.6.%(2)	
Digoxin		2.8%(1)	
Statin		25.0%(9)	
Aspirin		30.6%(11)	
Insulin		2.8%(1)	
Echocardiographic data	Not examined		
IVS thickness, mm		10.8±1.9	
PW thickness, mm		11.35±2.0	
LV mass index, g/m^2		131.7±37.0	
Left atrium diameter, mm		37.9±5.3	
LV end-diastolic diameter, mm		43.8±5.8	
LV end-systolic diameter, mm		26.6±6.1	
Ejection fraction, %		64.2±11.5	

sound unit (Logic 500 MD; GE Healthcare, England) before hemodialysis in the ESRD group. Left atrial diameter, interventricular thickness, posterior wall thickness, left ventricular end-diastolic diameter and left ventricular end-systolic diameter were all measured. Fractional shortening (FS), left ventricular mass index (LVMI) and left ventricular ejection fraction (LVEF) were calculated using standard formulae according to the recommendations of the American Society of Echocardiography.

Gel filtration chromatography. We analyzed immunoreactive proBNP levels in plasma to determine whether it is glycosylated in hemodialysis patients. Eluate lyophilized after extraction on a Sep-Pak C18 column (Waters, Milford, MA, USA) was dissolved in phosphate buffer and incubated with or without a cocktail of deglycosylation enzymes for 24 h at 37°C, as described above. The eluate was then lyophilized again and dissolved in 30% acetonitrile containing 0.1% TFA. The resultant solution was separated by gel filtration high-performance liquid chromatography (HPLC) on a Superdex 75 10/300 GL column (10×300 mm×2, GE Healthcare) using the same buffer at a flow rate of 0.4 mL/min. The column effluent was fractionated every minute into polypropylene tubes containing bovine serum albumin (100 mg), after which each fraction was analyzed using our recently developed total BNP and proBNP immunochemiluminescent assay [9].

Statistical Analyses

All values are expressed as means±SE. The statistical significance of differences between two groups was evaluated using Fisher's exact test or paired Student's t test, as appropriate. The distribution of plasma peptide levels was normalized by log transformation, when appropriate. The statistical significance of differences among three or more groups was evaluated using one-way analysis of variance followed by Bonferroni's multiple comparison test. Correlation coefficients were calculated using linear regression analysis. Values of $p<0.05$ were considered significant.

Results

The clinical profiles of the healthy subjects and ESRD patients enrolled in this study are shown in Table 1. The healthy subjects received no medication. Among the ESRD patients, 86% were prescribed antihypertensive medication (Table 1). The average percentage weight loss during hemodialysis was 4.9% (2.2% to 8.4%), with a post-dialysis relative extracellular fluid volume of 20.2% (11.1% to 31.5%). Standard two-dimensional transthoracic echocardiography revealed an average cardiac ejection fraction of 64% (36% to 92%), and the cardiothoracic ratio measured on posterior-anterior chest X-rays was 50±5%.

Plasma Concentrations of Total BNP, proBNP, Mature BNP, nonglycoNT-proBNP, glycoNT-proBNP, ANP and cGMP in Healthy Subjects and ESRD Patients Before Hemodialysis

Plasma levels of total BNP, proBNP, mature BNP, nonglycoNT-proBNP, glycoNT-proBNP, ANP and cGMP in healthy subjects and ESRD patients before hemodialysis are shown in Table 2. All seven parameters were significantly higher in the hemodialysis patients than the healthy subjects ($p<0.0001$). In addition, glycoNT-proBNP levels was significantly higher than nonglycoNT-proBNP in both groups. There was no significant difference in the glycoNT-proBNP/nonglycoNT-proBNP ratio (healthy subject vs. ESRD patients: 4.6±1.8 vs. 4.4±1.7; n.s.) between the two groups.

Differences in the Plasma Concentrations of Total BNP, proBNP, Mature BNP, nonglycoNT-proBNP, glycoNT-proBNP, ANP and cGMP before and after Hemodialysis

We next focused on the profile of natriuretic peptide-related molecules in ESRD patients. We initially evaluated the changes in plasma levels of total BNP, proBNP, mature BNP, nonglycoNT-proBNP, glycoNT-proBNP, ANP and cGMP associated with hemodialysis. As shown in Figure 1A, B, C, D, E, F and G, levels of all seven parameters were significantly lower after hemodialysis ($p<0.001$).

As shown in Figure 1H, the reduction ratios were calculated using the formula $(A-B)/A$, where A and B were the plasma concentrations before and after hemodialysis, and the values obtained give the relative magnitudes of the reductions. The reduction ratio for proBNP was smaller than the others, whereas the ratio for cGMP, which had the smallest molecular weight (MW = 523), was the largest among the molecules tested. The reduction ratio for mature BNP (MW = 3500) was significantly greater than that for proBNP, but was about the same as those for ANP (MW = 3000) and nonglycoNT-proBNP (MW = 8500). And not surprisingly, the reduction ratio for total BNP, which includes proBNP plus mature BNP, was between the ratios for mature BNP and proBNP.

It is well known that decreasing cardiac load reduces circulating levels of BNP and ANP, and that decreasing total body fluid volume could reduce cardiac preload. We therefore evaluated the relationship between dialysis-induced loss of body weight and total body fluid volume and the plasma levels of total BNP, proBNP, nonglycoNT-proBNP, glycoNT-proBNP and ANP. However, we found no significant correlation between the percent body weight change or percent total body fluid volume loss and the percent reduction of any of these peptides (Table 3).

Gel-filtration Chromatography Before and after Deglycosylation Procedure

Figure 2A shows two immunoreactive BNP peaks detected using the total BNP assay with gel filtration fractions. The first peak appeared in fractions 52–55 and the second peak in fractions 72–75. When subjected to gel filtration, recombinant proBNP, glycosylated proBNP and BNP were eluted mainly in fractions 53, 56 and 74, respectively. Treating the same plasma sample with an enzyme cocktail catalyzing deglycosylation shifted the first peak to fractions 54–56, which is consistent with the proBNP peak. These results suggest the major molecular form of proBNP in the plasma of hemodialysis patients is glycosylated proBNP.

Table 2. Natriuretic peptide-related molecules in healthy subjects and ESRD patients.

	Healthy subjects (n = 105)	ESRD patients (n = 36)	p
Total BNP, pM	1.8±22.0	35.7±34.4	<0.0001
proBNP, pM	1.2±1.2	22.6±22.7	<0.0001
Mature BNP, pM	0.6±0.8	13.1±12.9	<0.0001
Nonglyco-NT-proBNP, pM	44.8±64.5	600.3±779.1	<0.0001
Glyco-NT-proBNP, pM	173.0±157.3	1934.2±1829.5	<0.0001
ANP, pM	21.1±12.4	44.3±30.9	<0.0001
cGMP, nM	2.9±1.3	20.2±13.0	<0.0001

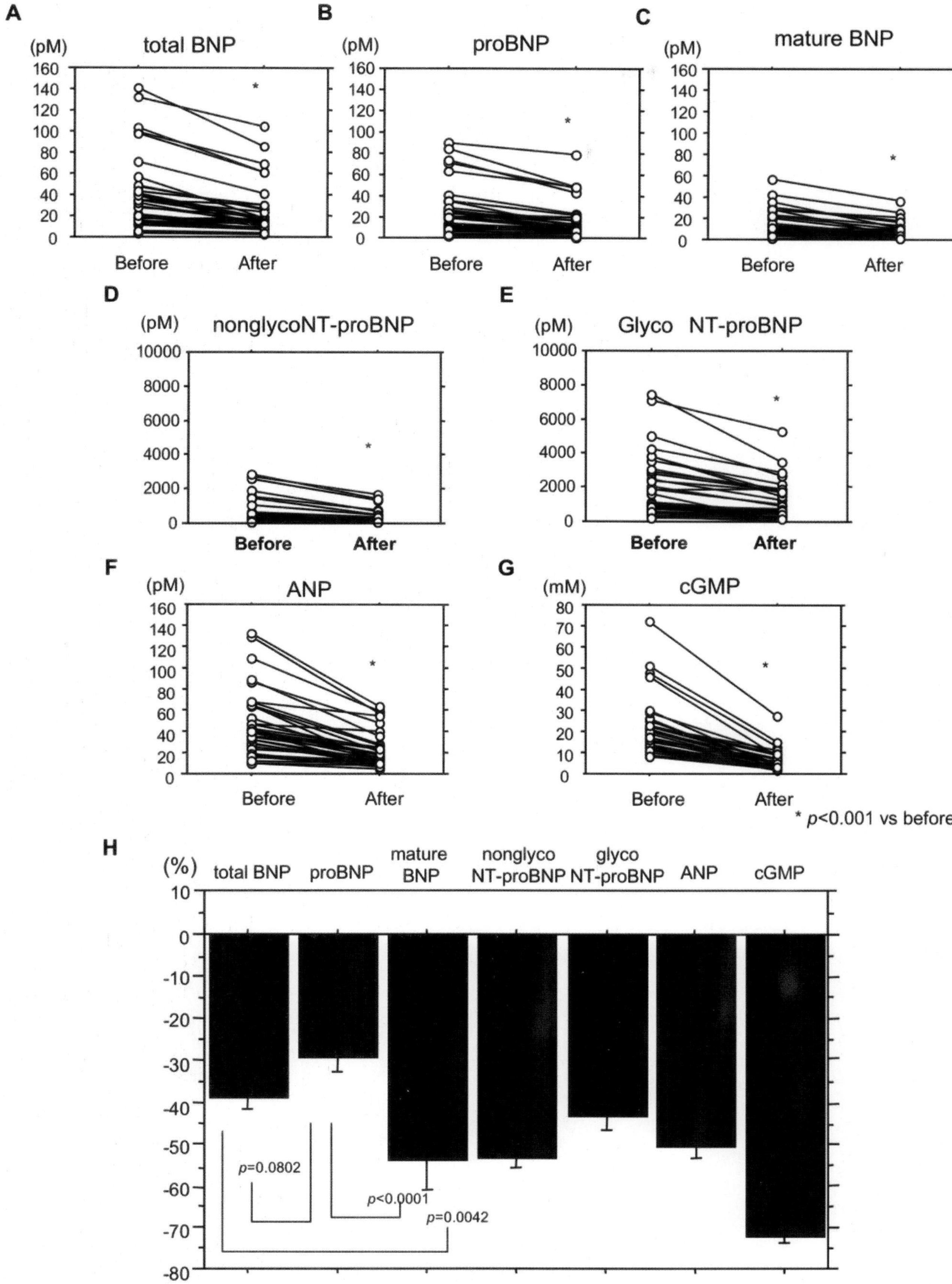

Figure 1. Changes in plasma levels of individual parameters during hemodialysis. (A–G) Individual changes in the levels of total BNP (A), proBNP (B), mature BNP (C), nonglycoNT-proBNP (D), glycoNT-proBNP (E), ANP (F) and cGMP (G) in ESRD patients during hemodialysis. Values are

means ± SE. *p<0.001 vs. before hemodialysis. Before, before hemodialysis; After, after hemodialysis. (H) Reduction ratios for total BNP, proBNP, mature BNP, nonglycoNT-proBNP, glycoNT-proBNP, ANP and cGMP in ESRD patients during hemodialysis. Values are means ± SE.

Relationship between proBNP and Total BNP, Mature BNP, nonglycoNT-proBNP, glycoNT-proBNP and ANP

We next evaluated the relationships between proBNP and the other natriuretic peptide molecules in hemodialysis patients (Figure 2B, C, D, E and F). We found that levels of proBNP significantly correlated with those of total BNP, mature BNP, nonglycoNT-proBNP, glycoNT-proBNP and ANP, most of which are established biomarkers.

Relationship between cGMP and Total BNP, proBNP, Mature BNP, nonglycoNT-proBNP, glycoNT-proBNP and ANP in ESRD Patients before and after Hemodialysis

When we evaluated the correlation between the levels of cGMP and those of natriuretic peptide-related molecules, we found that levels of total BNP, proBNP, mature BNP, nonglycoNT-proBNP, glycoNT-proBNP and ANP all correlated significantly with cGMP, both before and after hemodialysis (Figure 3). In particular, proBNP appeared to correlate more strongly with cGMP before hemodialysis than did the other molecules. After hemodialysis, ANP showed the highest correlation with cGMP among the natriuretic peptide-related molecules.

ProBNP/Total BNP Ratios, Biochemical Parameters and Patient Profiles

It was previously suggested that the ratio of proBNP to total BNP varied widely, depending on the patient's heart failure status. [8] We next evaluated proBNP/total BNP ratios in ESRD patients. As shown in Figure 4, ProBNP/total BNP ratios were significantly increased after hemodialysis, which could, in part, reflect the fact that the relative reduction in proBNP was smaller than that for total BNP. There was also a significant (but weak) positive correlation with hemodialysis vintage. Upon examination of the patient profiles, we found no significant correlation between the proBNP/total BNP ratios and any other biochemical parameter. ProBNP/total BNP ratios showed weak but significant negative correlations with systolic and mean blood pressures ($R = -0.358$, $P = 0.014$, $R = -0.350$, $P = 0.036$), and tended toward a negative correlation with left atrial diameter ($R = -0.302$, $p = 0.073$).

NonglycoNT-proBNP and glycoNT-proBNP in Hemodialysis Patients

We also compared the levels of glycoNT-proBNP with those of nonglycoNT-proBNP in hemodialysis patients. We found that levels of glycoNT-proBNP were several times higher than those of nonglycoNT-proBNP in the patients before hemodialysis; nonetheless, the glycoNT-proBNP/nonglycoNT-proBNP ratio was significantly larger after hemodialysis than before it (Figure 5). This is in part because the relative reduction in nonglycoNT-proBNP during hemodialysis was significantly greater than that for glycoNT-proBNP. We then evaluated the correlations between the glycoNT-proBNP/nonglycoNT-proBNP ratios and other biochemical parameters, which revealed the ratio correlated significantly with serum parathyroid hormone levels in the patients, but not with serum calcium or phosphate levels (data not shown).

Discussion

Plasma BNP and NT-proBNP levels are elevated in patients with heart failure, [17] [18] [19] correlate strongly with LV filling pressure, and increase with increasing severity of heart failure evaluated based on New York Heart Association Class [20] [21], functional capacity [22], or systolic and diastolic dysfunction [23,24]. Even in patients with chronic kidney disease and ESRD, left ventricular end-diastolic wall stress remains a strong determinant of circulating BNP levels [25]. Moreover, in ESRD patients receiving long-term dialysis, BNP and NT-proBNP levels are strongly associated with the severity of LV hypertrophy and systolic dysfunction [6] [26,27,28,29,30], and their elevation also reflects the presence of myocardial ischemia and is indicative of the severity of coronary artery disease [31]. Finally, BNP and NT-proBNP are highly predictive of subsequent cardiac events and mortality in hemodialysis patients. [32].

It was once thought that proBNP is cleaved to BNP and NT-proBNP within cardiac myocytes and then secreted into the circulation. However, recent studies have shown that circulating levels of unprocessed precursor proBNP are elevated in heart failure. In addition, proBNP and NT-proBNP contain seven sites suitable for *O*-linked oligosaccharide attachment within their N-terminal regions. In the present study, therefore, we measured plasma levels of proBNP, total BNP, mature BNP, nonglycoNT-

Table 3. Correlation coefficients and p values relating changes in percent body weight or total body fluid volume to the percent reduction in natriuretic peptide-related molecules.

	% body weight change		% total body fluid volume change	
% Reduction rate	**r**	**p**	**r**	**p**
total BNP	−0.086	0.621	−0.096	0.580
mature BNP	−0.130	0.452	−0.124	0.474
proBNP	−0.039	0.823	−0.054	0.756
ANP	−0.117	0.500	0.119	0.493
nonglyco- NT-proBNP	−0.120	0.488	−0.122	0.483
glyco- NT-proBNP	−0.208	0.224	−0.209	0.222
cGMP	−0.047	0.785	−0.034	0.846

r is the correlation coefficient.

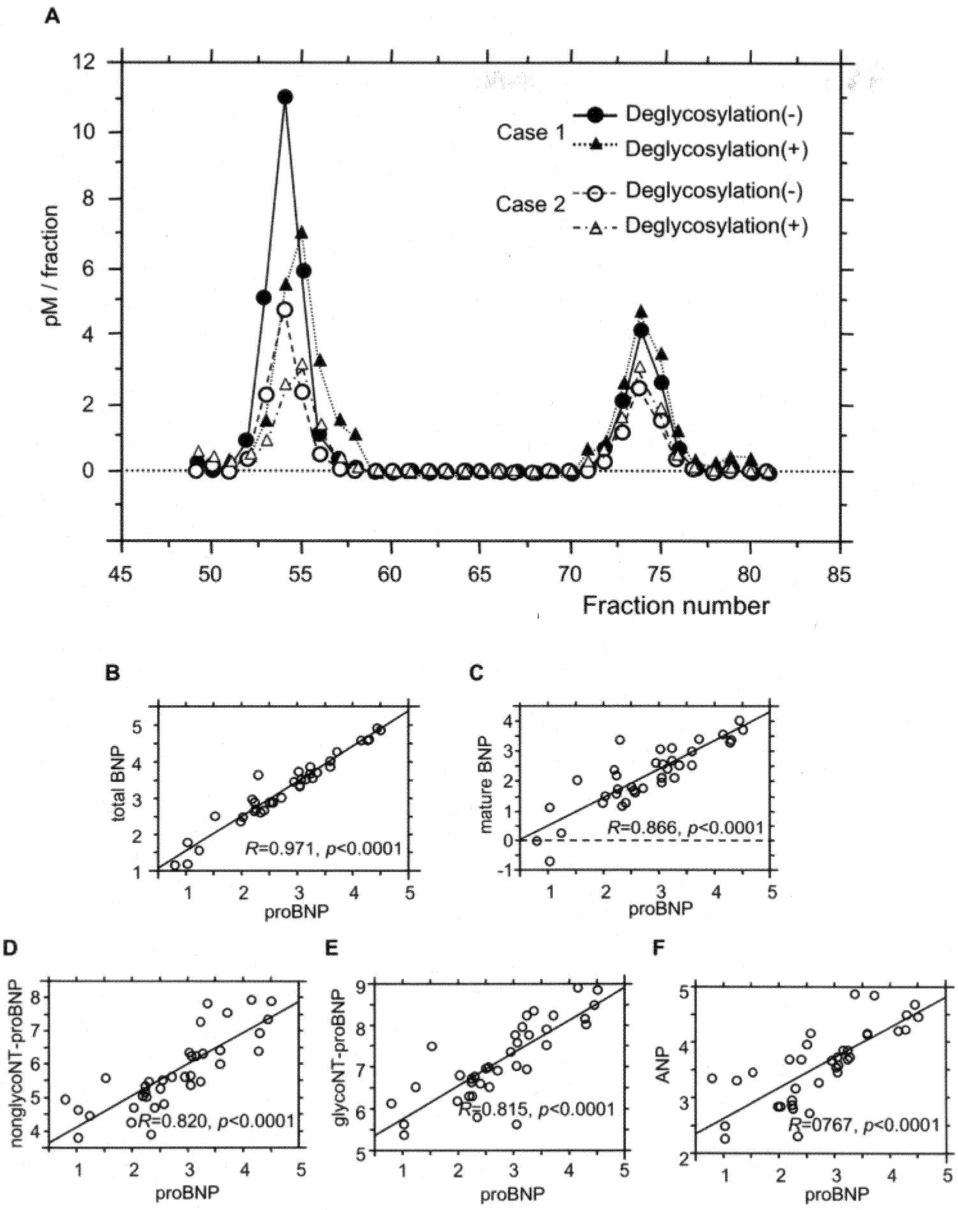

Figure 2. Gel filtration analysis of total BNP and proBNP in hemodialysis patients. (A) Fractions were assayed using total BNP systems. The first and second peaks show proBNP and BNP-32, respectively. (B–F) Correlations between proBNP and other natriuretic peptide-related molecules in ESRD patients before hemodialysis. *R* is the correlation coefficient. Values are expressed as $\log_{10}$ of each level of the indicated molecules.

proBNP, glycoNT-proBNP, ANP and cGMP, in healthy subjects and ESRD patients, and found that all of them were higher in ESRD patients, most of whom had preserved cardiac systolic function (Table 1), than in healthy persons. These increases in ESRD patients can be explained by reductions in their clearance due to the renal failure, increased plasma volume, and diastolic dysfunction caused by left ventricular hypertrophy, among others. Moreover we also found that all of these molecules declined during hemodialysis, though the magnitudes of the reductions did not correlate with any indices of body fluid volume. These results may be explained in part by dialyzer membrane-mediated removal. The so-called super-flux membranes currently in use are able to remove medium-sized molecular solutes, such as β2-microglobulin (MW = 12,000), which enables removal of larger and protein-bound uremic toxins. The pore size for the membranes used in the present study was 78–84 Å, and the sieving coefficient for β2-microglobulin was 0.99. It is therefore likely that the super-flux membranes removed a great deal of BNP and BNP-related molecules during hemodialysis.

Consistent with that idea, the reduction ratio for cGMP, which has a molecular weight of about 500, was the largest, while the reduction ratio for proBNP, which has a molecular weight of about 20,000~25,000, was the smallest. The reduction ratio for mature BNP (MW: 3,500) was similar to that of ANP (MW 3,000), reflecting the similarity of their molecular weights. The reduction ratio for total BNP was comparatively modest, because it is the mean of the ratios for mature BNP and proBNP. It thus appears that the magnitudes of the reductions in peptide concentration associated with hemodialysis depends on their molecular weights.

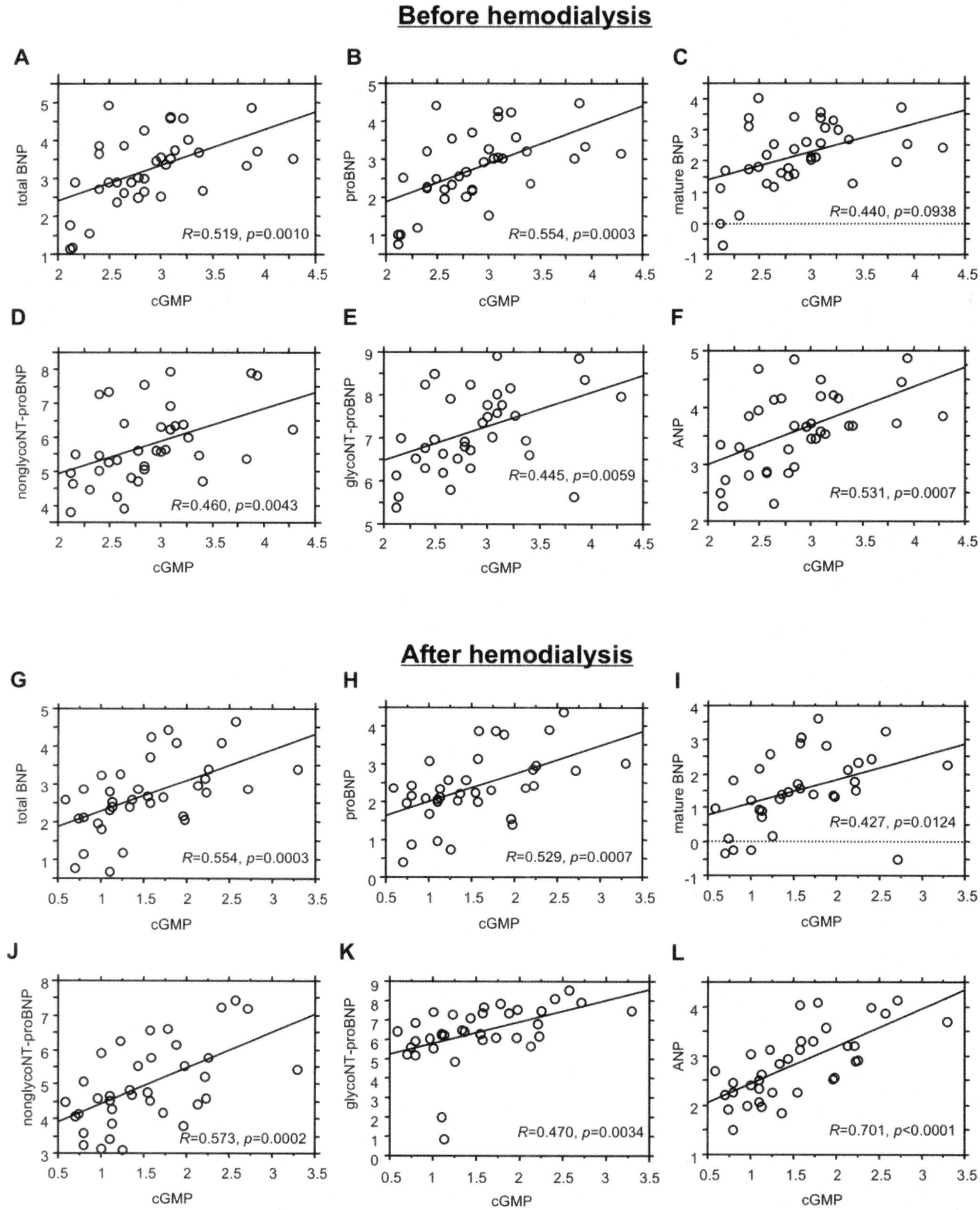

Figure 3. Correlations between cGMP and natriuretic peptide-related molecules in ESRD patients before and after hemodialysis. *R* is the correlation coefficient. Values are expressed as $\log_{10}$ of each level of the indicated molecules.

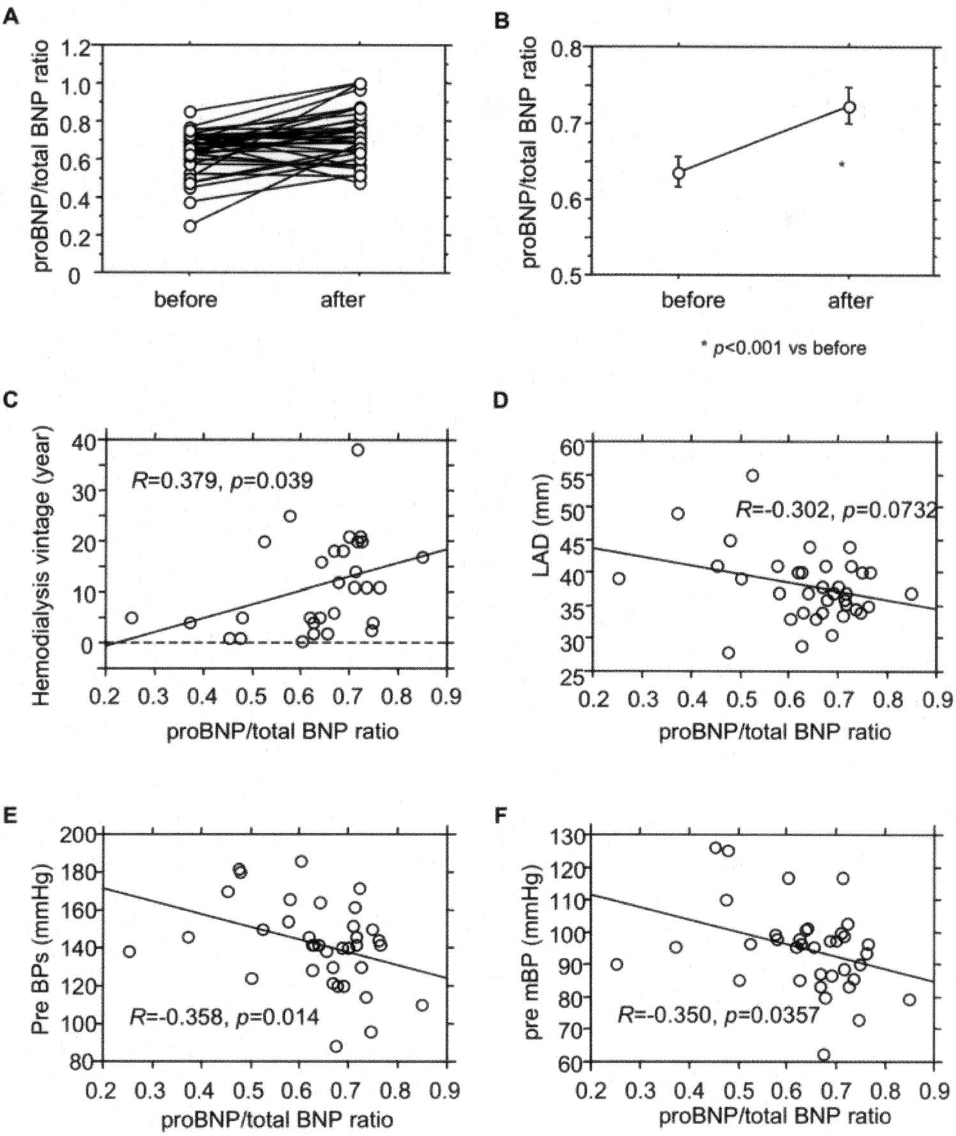

Figure 4. ProBNP/total BNP ratios and their correlation with the indicated clinical parameters. (A) Individual changes in proBNP/total BNP ratios in ESRD patients during hemodialysis: Before, before hemodialysis; After, after hemodialysis. (B) ProBNP/total BNP ratios in ESRD patients during hemodialysis expressed as means ± SE. (C–F) Correlation between proBNP/total BN ratios and hemodialysis vintage (C), left atrial diameter (LAD) (D), systolic blood pressure before hemodialysis (preBPs) (E) and mean blood pressure before hemodialysis (pre mBP) (F). *R* is the correlation coefficient between the indicated parameters.

Previously, we also reported the plasma levels of BNP, nonglycoNT-proBNP, glycoNT-proBNP, ANP and cGMP in patients with chronic renal failure before and after hemodialysis. [14] In that study, patients were hemodialyzed using older generation dialyzers that removed less of the large solutes like β2-microglobulin than the super-flux membrane we used in the present study. In that earlier study the calculated reduction ratio for each parameter during hemodialysis was as follows: BNP 37.9%, nonglycoNT-proBNP 23.0%, glycoNT-proBNP 4.4%, ANP 61.0%, and cGMP 75.0%. The reduction ratio for nonglycoNT-proBNP and glycoNT-proBNP, which are higher molecular weight molecules, was much smaller than in the present study, most likely due to the difference in the membrane's ability to remove large molecules.

In the present study, we used the Elecsys proBNP II assay (Roche Diagnostics, Indianapolis, IN, USA) to measure non-glycoNT-proBNP and glycoNT-proBNP, with and without deglycosylation enzyme treatment. This assay is the most frequently used NT-proBNP assay in the world and contains a capture monoclonal and a signal monoclonal antibody that recognizes NT-proBNP[27–31] and NT-proBNP[42–46], respectively. Notably, NT-proBNP[42–46] has a glycosylation site at amino acid 44, and a recent study demonstrated that *O*-linked oligosaccharide attachment markedly inhibits binding of the antibody to its antigen peptide [16]. Consequently, Elecsys proBNP II is thought to measure only nonglycoNT-proBNP. We found that nonglycoNT-proBNP was greatly elevated in ESRD patients and that levels of glycoNT-proBNP were 4–5 times higher than those of nonglycoNT-proBNP. The remarkable increase of nonglycoNT-proBNP in hemodialysis patients is thought to reflect the following conditions: (1) NT-proBNP does not bind to the natriuretic peptide receptor-A or -C; (2) NT-proBNP is not

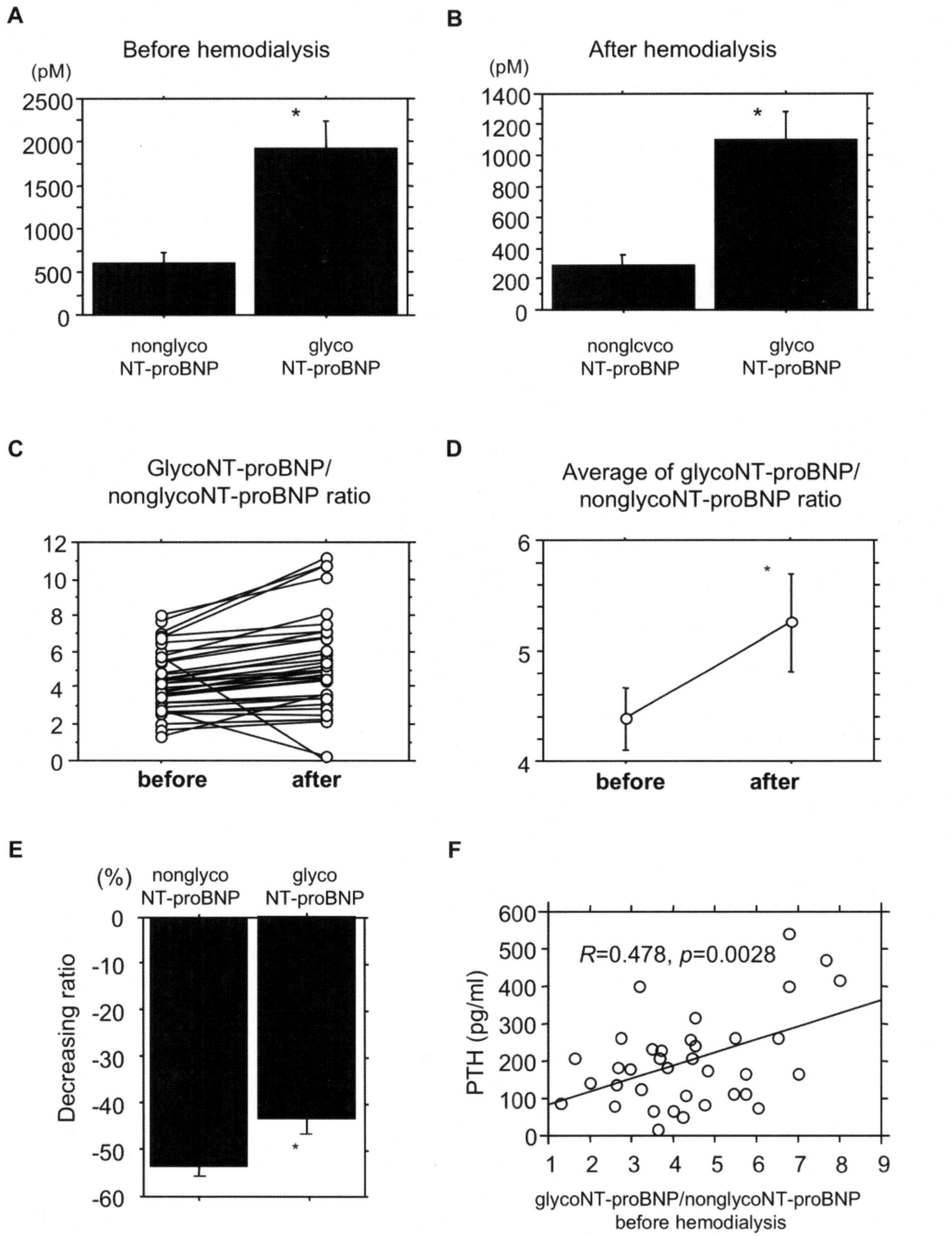

Figure 5. NonglycoNT-proBNP and glycoproBNP levels, glycoNT-proBNP/nonglycoNT-proBNP ratios and correlations between glycoNT-proBNP/nonglycoNT-proBNP ratios and clinical parameters. (A, B) Circulating levels of nonglycoNT-proBNP and glycoNT-proBNP in

ESRD patients before (A) and after (B) hemodialysis. Values are expressed means ± SE. (C, D) Individual changes and values of glycoNT-proBNP/nonglycoNT-proBNP ratios in ESRD patients during hemodialysis. Values are expressed as mean ± SE. *$p<0.001$ vs. before hemodialysis. before, before hemodialysis; after, after hemodialysis. (E) Reduction ratios for nonglycoNT-proBNP and glycoNT-proBNP during hemodialysis. *$p<0.001$ vs. nonglycoNT-proBNP. (F) Correlation between the glycoNT-proBNP/nonglycoNT-proBNP ratio and the serum parathyroid hormone (PTH) levels. *R* is the correlation coefficient.

metabolized by neutral endopeptidase; and (3) clearance of NT-proBNP is largely dependent on excretion from the kidney. The glycoNT-proBNP/nonglycoNT-proBNP ratio was larger after hemodialysis than before it. This is most likely because the molecular weight of glycoNT-proBNP is much larger than that of nonglycoNT-proBNP, so it is less likely to be affected by membrane-dependent removal than nonglycoNT-proBNP.

Using gel-filtration HPLC combined with direct chemiluminescent immunoassay, in the present study we showed that the major molecular form of proBNP in the plasma of hemodialysis patients is glycosylated proBNP. Similarly, recent studies have also shown that the major molecular form of plasma proBNP in patients with heart failure and control is glycosylated proBNP [9]. It is thus possible that proBNP in human plasma is glycosylated. We found that proBNP levels were closely correlated with those of total BNP, mature BNP, nonglycoNT-proBNP, glycoNT-proBNP and ANP. This suggests proBNP may also be a useful biomarker of cardiovascular disease, like BNP and NT-proBNP, two well-established biomarkers of cardiovascular disease in ESRD patients. In addition, levels of proBNP correlated significantly with cGMP before hemodialysis, suggesting proBNP may be a good marker of the biological action of natriuretic peptides. After hemodialysis, proBNP still correlated significantly with cGMP, but the correlation coefficient was modest. This may be because the reduction ratio for proBNP is small, while that for cGMP is large.

Interestingly, the proBNP/total BNP ratio correlated positively with hemodialysis vintage and correlated negatively with LAD and blood pressure. Longer hemodialysis vintage may lead to accumulation of the glycosylated proBNP, and diastolic dysfunction and/or increased afterload may alter the processing of glycosylated proBNP to BNP and glycoNT-proBNP. Notably, the glycoNT-proBNP/nonglycoNT-proBNP ratio correlated positively with parathyroid hormone levels in hemodialysis patients. Given that parathyroid hormone induces cardiac hypertrophy via its receptor on myocytes [33], its signal may influence glycosylation within cardiac myocytes and thus the glycoNT-proBNP/nonglycoNT-proBNP ratio. Further studies will be needed to elucidate the mechanism involved.

It has been suggested that hemodialysis reduces natriuretic peptide levels through dialytic clearance or by improving volume control, which results in decreased cardiac overload and reduced secretion from the heart [34]. A limitation of the present study is that we evaluated changes in volume status during hemodialysis based only on changes in body weight or estimated total body fluid volume. No other methods (e.g., bioimpedance analysis) were used. In addition, we did not perform echocardiography after hemodialysis. Had we evaluated changes in cardiac load during hemodialysis using different methods, perhaps some relationship might have been found between changes of the levels of natriuretic peptide-related molecules during hemodialysis and the magnitude of the reduction in cardiac load. Nonetheless, our results suggest that the reduction in the natriuretic peptide-related molecules after hemodialysis is due not only to the reduction in atrial overload, but also to removal via the super-flux dialyzer.

In conclusion, this is a first report showing the hemodialysis-associated changes of natriuretic peptide-related molecules, including proBNP, in ESRD patients in the super-flux dialyzer era. With the development of the super-flux dialysis membrane, there has been a marked change in the kinetics of molecules before and after hemodialysis. In addition, recent studies have shown that glycosylated proBNP is a major molecular form in human plasma and that glycosylated NT-proBNP is underestimated by the NT-proBNP assay system currently being used. Under these conditions, correct interpretation of the peptide levels in the plasma of ESRD patients undergoing hemodialysis and their clinical application may require careful consideration. Further study will be necessary to determine which BNP-related peptides, including proBNP, are most indicative of cardiac complications and predictive of prognosis in hemodialysis patients.

Acknowledgments

We thank Ms. Aoi Fujishima for her excellent technical assistance and Ms. Yukari Kubo and Ms. Mieko Seto for her excellent secretarial work.

Author Contributions

Conceived and designed the experiments: YN TN. Performed the experiments: YN TN K. Kuwahara SY HK YK Kazuhiro Nakao TM. Analyzed the data: CY KU YI. Contributed reagents/materials/analysis tools: HO KH K. Nagata K. Kangawa NM. Wrote the paper: TN YN. Supervision: Kazuwa Nakao.

References

1. Yasue H, Yoshimura M, Sumida H, Kikuta K, Kugiyama K, et al. (1994) Localization and mechanism of secretion of B-type natriuretic peptide in comparison with those of A-type natriuretic peptide in normal subjects and patients with heart failure. Circulation 90: 195–203.
2. Nishikimi T, Kuwahara K, Nakao K (2011) Current biochemistry, molecular biology, and clinical relevance of natriuretic peptides. J Cardiol 57: 131–140.
3. Nishikimi T, Maeda N, Matsuoka H (2006) The role of natriuretic peptides in cardioprotection. Cardiovasc Res 69: 318–328.
4. Weber M, Dill T, Deetjen A, Neumann T, Ekinci O, et al. (2006) Left ventricular adaptation after atrial septal defect closure assessed by increased concentrations of N-terminal pro-brain natriuretic peptide and cardiac magnetic resonance imaging in adult patients. Heart 92: 671–675.
5. Nishikimi T, Yoshihara F, Morimoto A, Ishikawa K, Ishimitsu T, et al. (1996) Relationship between left ventricular geometry and natriuretic peptide levels in essential hypertension. Hypertension 28: 22–30.
6. Nishikimi T, Futoo Y, Tamano K, Takahashi M, Suzuki T, et al. (2001) Plasma brain natriuretic peptide levels in chronic hemodialysis patients: influence of coronary artery disease. Am J Kidney Dis 37: 1201–1208.
7. Daniels LB, Maisel AS (2007) Natriuretic peptides. J Am Coll Cardiol 50: 2357–2368.
8. Nishikimi T, Minamino N, Ikeda M, Takeda Y, Tadokoro K, et al. (2010) Diversity of molecular forms of plasma brain natriuretic peptide in heart failure—different proBNP-108 to BNP-32 ratios in atrial and ventricular overload. Heart 96: 432–439.
9. Nishikimi T, Okamoto H, Nakamura M, Ogawa N, Horii K, et al. (2013) Direct immunochemiluminescent assay for proBNP and total BNP in human plasma proBNP and total BNP levels in normal and heart failure. PLoS One 8: e53233.
10. Schellenberger U, O'Rear J, Guzzetta A, Jue RA, Protter AA, et al. (2006) The precursor to B-type natriuretic peptide is an O-linked glycoprotein. Arch Biochem Biophys 451: 160–166.
11. Liang F, O'Rear J, Schellenberger U, Tai L, Lasecki M, et al. (2007) Evidence for functional heterogeneity of circulating B-type natriuretic peptide. J Am Coll Cardiol 49: 1071–1078.
12. Seferian KR, Tamm NN, Semenov AG, Tolstaya AA, Koshkina EV, et al. (2008) Immunodetection of glycosylated NT-proBNP circulating in human blood. Clin Chem 54: 866–873.

13. Jackson S (1985) Anatomy & Physiology for Nurses. Nurses' Aids Series (9th ed.).
14. Nishikimi T, Ikeda M, Takeda Y, Ishimitsu T, Shibasaki I, et al. (2012) The effect of glycosylation on plasma N-terminal proBNP-76 levels in patients with heart or renal failure. Heart 98: 152–161.
15. Luckenbill KN, Christenson RH, Jaffe AS, Mair J, Ordonez-Llanos J, et al. (2008) Cross-reactivity of BNP, NT-proBNP, and proBNP in commercial BNP and NT-proBNP assays: preliminary observations from the IFCC Committee for Standardization of Markers of Cardiac Damage. Clin Chem 54: 619–621.
16. Hammerer-Lercher A, Halfinger B, Sarg B, Mair J, Puschendorf B, et al. (2008) Analysis of circulating forms of proBNP and NT-proBNP in patients with severe heart failure. Clin Chem 54: 858–865.
17. Cowie MR, Struthers AD, Wood DA, Coats AJ, Thompson SG, et al. (1997) Value of natriuretic peptides in assessment of patients with possible new heart failure in primary care. Lancet 350: 1349–1353.
18. Davis M, Espiner E, Richards G, Billings J, Town I, et al. (1994) Plasma brain natriuretic peptide in assessment of acute dyspnoea. Lancet 343: 440–444.
19. Januzzi JL Jr, Camargo CA, Anwaruddin S, Baggish AL, Chen AA, et al. (2005) The N-terminal Pro-BNP investigation of dyspnea in the emergency department (PRIDE) study. Am J Cardiol 95: 948–954.
20. Maisel AS, Krishnaswamy P, Nowak RM, McCord J, Hollander JE, et al. (2002) Rapid measurement of B-type natriuretic peptide in the emergency diagnosis of heart failure. N Engl J Med 347: 161–167.
21. Hunt PJ, Richards AM, Nicholls MG, Yandle TG, Doughty RN, et al. (1997) Immunoreactive amino-terminal pro-brain natriuretic peptide (NT-PROBNP): a new marker of cardiac impairment. Clin Endocrinol (Oxf) 47: 287–296.
22. Jourdain P, Funck F, Bellorini M, Guillard N, Loiret J, et al. (2003) Bedside B-type natriuretic peptide and functional capacity in chronic heart failure. Eur J Heart Fail 5: 155–160.
23. Yamamoto K, Burnett JC Jr, Jougasaki M, Nishimura RA, Bailey KR, et al. (1996) Superiority of brain natriuretic peptide as a hormonal marker of ventricular systolic and diastolic dysfunction and ventricular hypertrophy. Hypertension 28: 988–994.
24. Troughton RW, Prior DL, Pereira JJ, Martin M, Fogarty A, et al. (2004) Plasma B-type natriuretic peptide levels in systolic heart failure: importance of left ventricular diastolic function and right ventricular systolic function. J Am Coll Cardiol 43: 416–422.
25. Niizuma S, Iwanaga Y, Yahata T, Tamaki Y, Goto Y, et al. (2009) Impact of left ventricular end-diastolic wall stress on plasma B-type natriuretic peptide in heart failure with chronic kidney disease and end-stage renal disease. Clin Chem 55: 1347–1353.
26. Wang AY, Lam CW, Yu CM, Wang M, Chan IH, et al. (2007) N-terminal pro-brain natriuretic peptide: an independent risk predictor of cardiovascular congestion, mortality, and adverse cardiovascular outcomes in chronic peritoneal dialysis patients. J Am Soc Nephrol 18: 321–330.
27. Mallamaci F, Zoccali C, Tripepi G, Benedetto FA, Parlongo S, et al. (2001) Diagnostic potential of cardiac natriuretic peptides in dialysis patients. Kidney Int 59: 1559–1566.
28. Madsen LH, Ladefoged S, Corell P, Schou M, Hildebrandt PR, et al. (2007) N-terminal pro brain natriuretic peptide predicts mortality in patients with end-stage renal disease in hemodialysis. Kidney Int 71: 548–554.
29. Satyan S, Light RP, Agarwal R (2007) Relationships of N-terminal pro-B-natriuretic peptide and cardiac troponin T to left ventricular mass and function and mortality in asymptomatic hemodialysis patients. Am J Kidney Dis 50: 1009–1019.
30. Cataliotti A, Malatino LS, Jougasaki M, Zoccali C, Castellino P, et al. (2001) Circulating natriuretic peptide concentrations in patients with end-stage renal disease: role of brain natriuretic peptide as a biomarker for ventricular remodeling. Mayo Clin Proc 76: 1111–1119.
31. Niizuma S, Iwanaga Y, Yahata T, Goto Y, Kita T, et al. (2009) Plasma B-type natriuretic peptide levels reflect the presence and severity of stable coronary artery disease in chronic haemodialysis patients. Nephrol Dial Transplant 24: 597–603.
32. Sivalingam M, Suresh M, Farrington K (2011) Comparison of B-type natriuretic peptide and NT proBNP as predictors of survival in patients on high-flux hemodialysis and hemodiafiltration. Hemodial Int 15: 359–365.
33. Schluter KD, Piper HM (1998) Cardiovascular actions of parathyroid hormone and parathyroid hormone-related peptide. Cardiovasc Res 37: 34–41.
34. Sheen V, Bhalla V, Tulua-Tata A, Bhalla MA, Weiss D, et al. (2007) The use of B-type natriuretic peptide to assess volume status in patients with end-stage renal disease. Am Heart J 153: 244 e241–245.

Quantitative Trait Loci for Resistance to the Congenital Nephropathy in Tensin 2-Deficient Mice

Hayato Sasaki[1], Nobuya Sasaki[2]*, Tomohiro Nishino[1], Ken-ichi Nagasaki[3], Hiroshi Kitamura[4], Daisuke Torigoe[1], Takashi Agui[1]

1 Laboratory of Laboratory Animal Science and Medicine, Department of Disease Control, Graduate School of Veterinary Medicine, Hokkaido University, Sapporo, Japan, **2** Laboratory of Laboratory Animal Science and Medicine, Faculty of Veterinary Medicine, Kitasato University, Towada, Japan, **3** Section of Biological Safety Research, Chitose Laboratory, Japan Food Research Laboratories, Chitose, Japan, **4** Department of Veterinary Physiology, School of Veterinary Medicine, Rakuno Gakuen University, Ebetsu, Japan

Abstract

The ICR-derived glomerulonephritis (ICGN) mouse is a chronic kidney disease (CKD) model that is characterized histologically by glomerulosclerosis, vascular sclerosis and tubulointerstitial fibrosis, and clinically by proteinuria and anemia, which are common symptoms and pathological changes associated with a variety of kidney diseases. Previously, we performed a quantitative trait locus (QTL) analysis to identify the causative genes for proteinuria in ICGN mice, and found a deletion mutation of the tensin 2 gene (*Tns2^{nph}*, MGI no: 2447990). Interestingly, the congenic strain carrying the *Tns2^{nph}* mutation on a C57BL/6J (B6) genetic background exhibited milder phenotypes than did ICGN mice, indicating the presence of several modifier genes controlling the disease phenotype. In this study, to identify the modifier/resistant loci for CKD progression in *Tns2*-deficient mice, we performed QTL analysis using backcross progenies from susceptible ICGN and resistant B6 mice. We identified a significant locus on chromosome (Chr) 2 (LOD = 5.36; 31 cM) and two suggestive loci on Chrs 10 (LOD = 2.27; 64 cM) and X (LOD = 2.65; 67 cM) with linkage to the severity of tubulointerstitial injury. One significant locus on Chr 13 (LOD = 3.49; approximately 14 cM) and one suggestive locus on Chr 2 (LOD = 2.41; 51 cM) were identified as QTLs for the severity of glomerulosclerosis. Suggestive locus in BUN was also detected in the same Chr 2 region (LOD = 2.34; 51 cM). A locus on Chr 2 (36 cM) was significantly linked with HGB (LOD = 4.47) and HCT (LOD = 3.58). Four novel epistatic loci controlling either HGB or tubulointerstitial injury were discovered. Further genetic analysis should lead to identification of CKD modifier gene(s), aiding early diagnosis and providing novel approaches to the discovery of drugs for the treatment and possible prevention of kidney disease.

Editor: Christos Chatziantoniou, Institut National de la Santé et de la Recherche Médicale, France

Funding: This work was supported by the Ministry of Education, Culture, Sports, Science and Technology (MEXT), Glant-in-Aid for Scientific Research, KAKENHI (20302614) to N.S. H.S. was a research assistant of the Program of Leading Graduate School supported by MEXT. The funders had no role in study design, data collection and analysis, decision to publish, or preparation of the manuscript.

Competing Interests: The authors have declared that no competing interests exist.

* Email: nobsasa@vmas.kitasato-u.ac.jp

Introduction

ICR-derived glomerulonephritis (ICGN) mice are an inbred strain that exhibit glomerulosclerosis characterized by marked glomerular hypertrophy, mesangial expansion, foot process effacement of podocytes and thickening of the glomerular basement membrane. The ICGN mouse is also a chronic kidney disease (CKD) model that presents common symptoms and pathological changes associated with a variety of kidney diseases, such as albuminuria, hypoproteinemia, hyperlipidemia, anemia and systemic edema and eventual end-stage renal failure [1,2]. In ICGN mice, nephrotic syndrome occurs at the suckling stage, which is unique in spontaneously nephropathic strains of mice or rats [3]. Although glomerular alteration is observed from two weeks after birth, renal function is preserved until three to four months after birth, when ICGN mice begin to show tubulointerstitial fibrosis [4]. This pathological process in ICGN mice conforms well with the clinical presentation of glomerular disease in humans [5].

Proteinuria is intimately involved in the dysfunction of podocytes or slit diaphragm, and glomerulosclerosis (GS) sequentially starts with podocytopenia. A line of evidence suggests that podocytes act as the main component of this barrier as mutations in a number of podocyte-specific genes (*NPHS1, NPHS2, CD2AP, ACTN4, TRPC6, PLCE1, MYH9*) responsible for GS have been identified [6,7]. Therefore, podocyte loss is a common determining factor for progression toward many types of kidney disease [8,9]. Previously, we performed a QTL analysis to isolate the causative genes for ICGN phenotypes, and identified a major QTL on chromosome (Chr) 15 that is identical to a single recessive locus causing albuminuria, and found a deletion mutation of the tensin 2 gene (*Tns2*, also known as *Tenc1*). This mutation (*Tns2^{nph}*, MGI no: 2447990) leads to the loss of tensin 2 in podocytes, parietal epithelial cells and tubular epithelial cells [10]. The tensin (Tns) family of multidomain scaffold proteins (including Tns1, Tns2, Tns3 and Tns4) bind to the cytoplasmic tail of β-integrins, and localize to adhesions that anchor stress fibers in cells [11]. Therefore, Tns2 is thought to be a component of the actin cytoskeletal structures linking actin filaments with focal adhesions

Table 1. QTL identified for nephropathic traits.

Chr	Peak (cM)	Nearest marker	LOD	Phenotype	ICGN/ICGN[a]	B6/ICGN[a]	Resistance allele
2	31	*D2Mit369*	5.36	Tubule	1.0	0.4	B6[b**]
2	36	*D2Mit380*	4.47	HGB (g/dL)	12.6	13.2	B6[c]
			3.58	HCT (%)	43.1	45.2	B6[c]
2	51	*D2Mit66*	2.41	Glomeruli	30.2	25.9	B6[b**]
			2.34	BUN (mg/dL)	38.2	31.3	B6[c]
10	64	*D10Mit271*	2.27	Tubule	0.8	0.4	B6[b*]
13	14	*D13Mit60*	3.49	Glomeruli	30.4	24.9	B6[b**]
X	67	*DXMit186*	2.65	Tubule	0.8	0.4	B6[b*]

[a]Data resent the mean of the phenotype.
[b]Mann-Whitney's U test,
**$P<0.001$;
*$P<0.01$.
[c]Student's T test, $P<0.001$.

and plays a role as an intracellular signal transduction mediator through integrin [11]. It has been reported that Tns2 may be involved in the expression of nephrin (*Nphs1*) and synaptopodin (*Synpo*) in podocytes [12]. However, the mechanism by which *Tns2* deficiency leads to CKD is unclear.

In humans, the prevalence rates of CKD vary considerably by race, sex and age [13]. Multiple studies, such as genome-wide association studies, have identified many genetic factors that participate in kidney disease, although it is estimated that a vast amount of genetic factors for CKD remain to be identified [14]. CKD has a complex etiology resulting from the combination of multiple genetic and environmental factors, each with small effects. Epistatic interactions among susceptibility modifier loci make many of the loci difficult to detect in genome-wide association studies [15,16]. Several reports using mouse models of nephropathy have demonstrated similar phenomena in that the effects of nephropathy-inducing factors were attenuated in other genetic backgrounds [17,18,19]. Recently, we have shown that congenic strains carrying the $Tns2^{nph}$ mutation on a B6 or 129×1/SvJ (129) genetic background exhibited milder phenotypes than do ICGN mice [20,21]. In contrast, other researchers have reported DBA/2J (D2) congenic mice with $Tns2^{nph}$ were susceptible to CKD at a level similar to ICGN mice [22]. This suggests that B6 and 129 mice have resistant genes to CKD induced by $Tns2^{nph}$. In the present study, we performed a genome-wide linkage analysis in (B6×ICGN) F_1 ×ICGN backcross mice carrying $Tns2^{nph}$ to identify the CKD resistance genes and elucidate the mechanism by which *Tns2* deficiency leads to CKD.

Materials and Methods

Animals

ICGN mice were purchased from Osaka National Institute of Biomedical Innovation. C57BL/6J (B6: Charles River) mice were backcrossed to ICGN mice. *Tns2* (*nph*/*nph*) N_2 backcross progenies were obtained by mating ICGN male mice to *Tns2* (+/*nph*) F_1 hybrid female mice heterozygous for $Tns2^{nph}$. Backcross mice homozygous for $Tns2^{nph}$ were born in accordance with Mendelian inheritance and at an equal sex ratio. B6-$Tns2^{nph}$ congenic mice were generated as described previously [20]. The animal room was air-conditioned at 22±4°C, maintained at 40–60% relative humidity, and mice were maintained under a 12 hr light-dark cycle. A standard laboratory diet, CE-2 (Nihon Clea, Tokyo, Japan), and tap water were available *ad libitum*. In this study, 16-week-old mice were selected for all analyses as the ICGN mice show severe albuminuria and anemia, which are the end stages of a variety of pathological conditions. A humane end point was applied when the mice with severe anemia became moribund.

Ethical Statement

All research and experimental protocols were adhered to the Regulation for the Care and Use of Laboratory Animals, Hokkaido University and approved by the President of Hokkaido University following to the review of the Institutional Animal Care and Use Committee (Approval ID: No. 110226).

Phenotypic Analysis

Blood samples were collected from the postcava under isoflurane anesthesia. Hemoglobin concentration (HGB), hematocrit (HCT) and blood urea nitrogen (BUN) were measured as described previously [20].

Formalin-fixed and paraffin-embedded kidney blocks were sectioned at a thickness of 2 μm, and stained with Periodic acid-Schiff (PAS). In this study, two types of histopathological scores

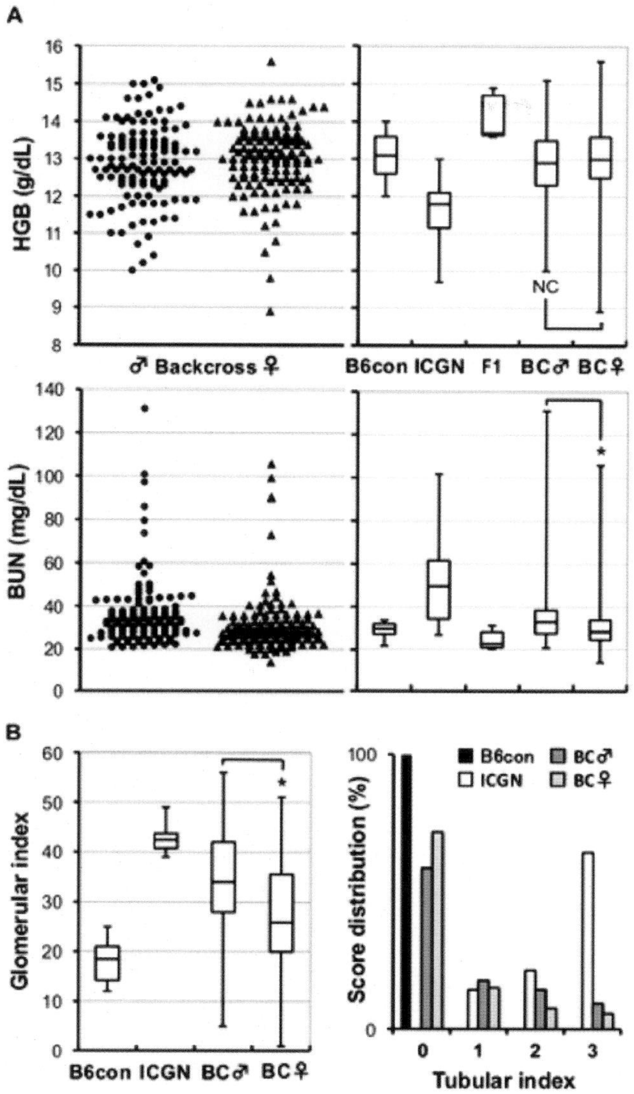

Figure 1. Hemoglobin concentration and BUN and kidney injury in backcross mice. (A, left) Distributions of HGB and BUN in (ICGN×B6) F_1×ICGN backcross progenies. (A, right) Distributions of HGB and BUN in B6-*Tns2^{nph}*, ICGN, (ICGN×B6) F_1, backcross mice. (B) Glomerular index and tubular index distributions in (ICGN×B6) F_1×ICGN backcross progenies. B6con, B6-*Tns2^{nph}*; BC, backcross mice; NS, no significant; asterisk, $P<0.001$.

were adopted to quantitate the severities of renal damage. A glomerular index, in which the severities were based on glomerular injury, was calculated from the scores for twenty glomeruli randomly selected from each sample. The severity of glomerular injury was scored as follows: 0, no abnormality or nearly normal; 1, expansion of the mesangial matrix; 2, severe expansion of the mesangial matrix; 3, hyalinosis or collapse (Fig. S1). First, the highest and lowest scores were removed to exclude bias in random selection. The sum of the eighteen glomerular scores was then taken as the glomerular index. However, if there were glomeruli that scored 3 points, the index was the sum of 36 and the number of glomeruli that scored 3 points. This calculation method means that a kidney with hyalinosis or collapse has a more severe glomerular injury than a kidney with only mesangial expansion. The tubular index was the sum of two histopathological parameters, urinary cast and tubule dilation. The severity of tubule dilation was performed using scale 0 to 2:0, no abnormality; 1, mild; 2, severe. One point was then added to the tubular index if a urinary cast was detected (Fig. S2). These analyses were performed by two independent observers. There were remarkable congruences in both blinded scores [the interclass correlation coefficients (ICCs) = 0.96].

Genotyping Analysis

We used 246 (male = 124, female = 122) *Tns2* (*nph/nph*) N2 backcross mice for a genome-wide scan. Extraction of genomic DNA from tail tips was performed by a standard method. *Tns2* genotypes were determined by PCR using genomic DNA from the tail tips. *Tns2^{nph}* homozygous mice were identified using the primers AGACACCACCAGCACCTTCT and CGATC-CAGCTCCTGTCTTTC, which distinguish the *Tns2^{nph}* allele by the 8-base deletion in exon 18 of *Tns2* [10]. For QTL analysis, a total of 92 informative microsatellite markers and coat color were used for the genotyping analysis, as listed in Table S1. The map positions of the microsatellite markers were based on information from the Mouse Genome Informatics of Jackson Laboratory (MGI; http://www.informatics.jax.org/, MGI_4.41). PCR was carried out with a cycling sequence of 95°C for 5 min (one cycle), followed by 35 cycles consisting of denaturation at 95°C for 30 sec, primer annealing at 55°C for 30 sec, and extension at 72°C for 30 sec. Amplified samples were electrophoresed with 12% polyacrylamide gels and stained with ethidium bromide. The stained gels were then visualized and photographed under an ultraviolet lamp.

QTL Analysis and Statistics

QTL analysis was performed using the Map Manager QTXb20 software program that uses a maximum likelihood algorithm with "interval mapping" and "simultaneous search", and permits better localization of loci and exclusion mapping [23]. Recombination frequencies (%) were converted into genetic distance (cM) using the Kosambi map function. This program provides linkage data as a likelihood ratio statistic (LRS) score. For each Chr, the LRS values were calculated by 10000 random permutations of the trait values relative to the genotypes of the marker loci. Genome-wide significance thresholds were calculated in terms of LRS by 10000 random permutation tests based on the established guidelines. The logarithm of odds (LOD) score was calculated by dividing the LRS value by 4.61. LOD values of the suggestive and significant thresholds for each trait are summarized in Table 1. Significant linkage was determined according to the traditional threshold (LOD score >3.3) [24]. Statistical analyses were performed using the Stat-View program (SAS Institute Inc. Cary, USA). Spearman's rank correlation analysis was used to find the correlation between two sets of tested traits.

Results

1. Phenotypic Characterization of *Tns2^{nph}* Backcross Mice

To verify the effect of genetic background on susceptibility to CKD induced by *Tns2^{nph}*, we produced a total of 246 (ICGN×B6) F_1×ICGN backcross mice and performed blood testing and histopathological analysis at the beginning of a genome-wide linkage analysis. Blood samples collected at 16 weeks old were analyzed. In CKD, a high BUN level and low HGB signify renal impairment and renal anemia, respectively, which is also a common symptom in ICGN mice (Fig. 1A, right). In backcross progenies, wide spectrums of BUN and HGB were observed from the various degrees of B6 type to that of ICGN types (Fig. 1A).

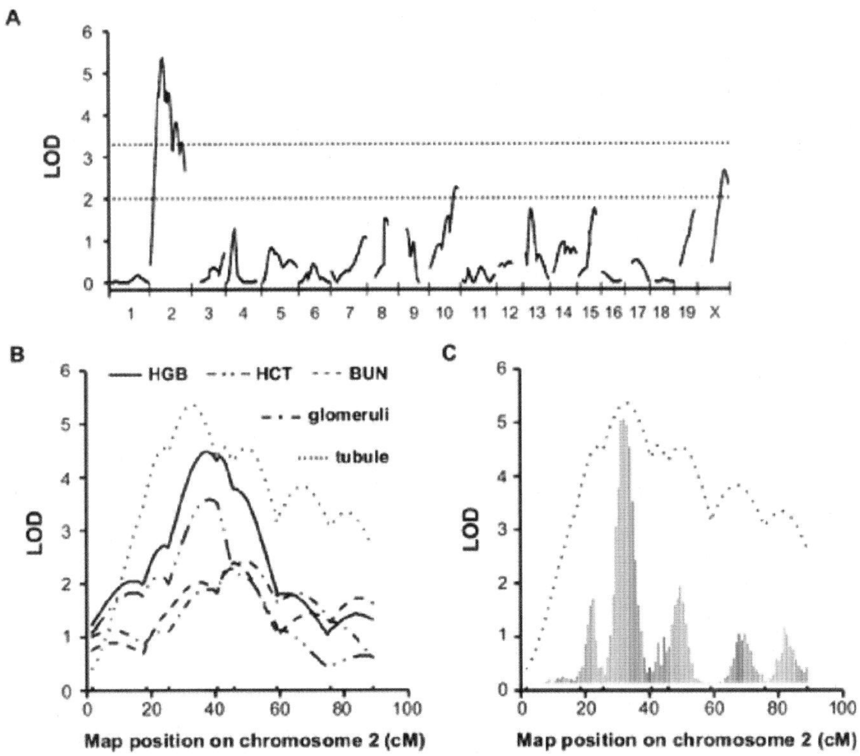

Figure 2. Linkage of nephropathy to chromosome 2. (A) Genome-wide linkage analysis of the tubular index. (B) LOD plots show the linkage of nephropathic traits to chromosome 2. HGB (solid line) and tubular index (dotted line) yielded significant LOD scores. The approximate 95% confidential intervals: 19.6–56.4 cM (tubule), 26–73 cM (glomeruli), 26–55 cM (HGB), 23–59 cM (HCT), 27–72 cM (BUN). (C) LOD curve and bootstrap histogram of the QTL on chromosome 2 for tubular index.

These results imply the existence of multiple modifier loci for CKD caused by *Tns2*^{nph}. In addition, the distribution of BUN in backcross males, as compared with females, was statistically more severe ($P<0.001$, Mann-Whitney's U test).

Figure 1B shows the box plot for glomerular index and the histogram for tubular index. The scores histologically evaluate glomerular injury and tubulointerstitial injury, respectively. The backcross mice showed wide range of the histopathological severity, from B6 types to ICGN types (see also Fig. S1, S2, S3). There were also significant sexual dimorphism in both scores, with males exhibiting a higher level of severity than females (glomerular index $P<0.001$, tubular index $P<0.05$, Mann-Whitney's U test).

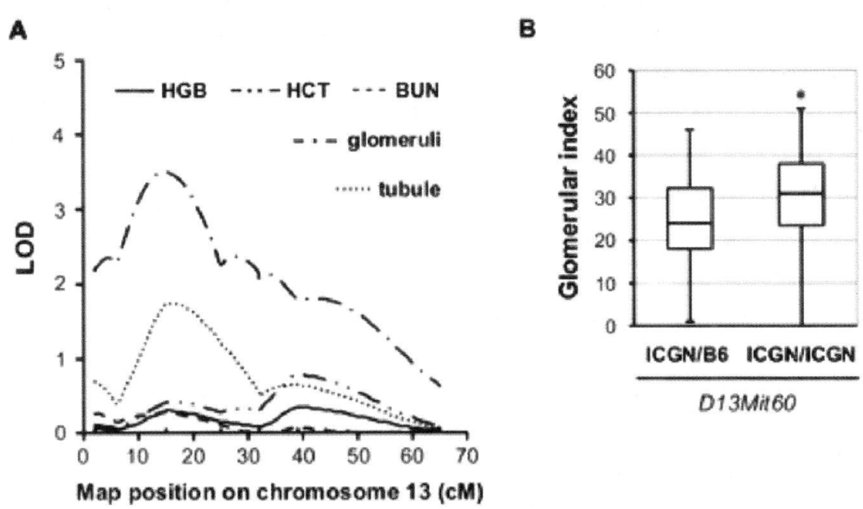

Figure 3. LOD score curves on chromosome 13. (A) A significant QTL for glomerular index was detected on chromosome 13. The approximate 95% confidential intervals: 0–31.5 cM. (B) Glomerular index at the peak LOD score (*D13Mit60*). The resistance phenotype associated with ICGN/B6 genotype ($P<0.001$, Mann-Whitney's U test).

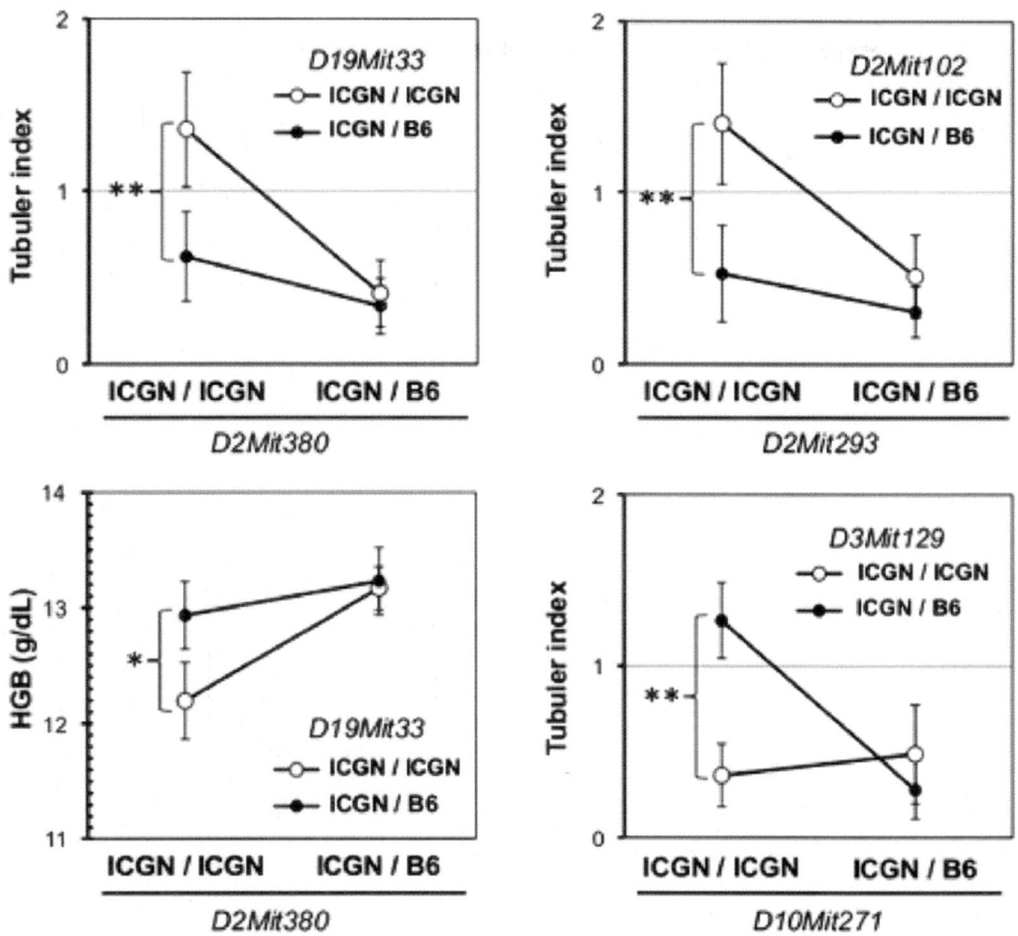

Figure 4. Epistasis associated with QTLs. Epistatic interactions were detected associated with the markers on chromosome 2 and 10. Open circles and closed circles represent homozygous and heterozygous variants for the tested markers, respectively. Asterisks signify significant differences between the two genotypes (**$P<0.001$; *$P<0.01$; Mann-Whitney's U test).

These differences were presumably due to the protective effect of estrogen in the female glomeruli [25].

The symptom severity of all tested traits exhibited significant correlations with each other according to Spearman's rank correlation analysis ($P<0.01$). However, the Spearman's rank correlation coefficients were comparatively smaller for BUN combinations ($|r| = 0.27 \sim 0.48$) than for the other sets ($|r| = 0.4 \sim 0.65$).

2. Genome-wide Linkage Analysis for the Mapping of CKD-Resistant Genes in Backcross Mice

To identify the modifier genes for CKD, we carried out a genome-wide linkage analysis using *Tns2*^{nph} backcross mice. HGB, HCT, BUN, glomerular index and tubular index at 16 weeks of age were used as indicators for CKD. Table 1 summarizes the microsatellite markers linked to the phenotype, LOD score, interval and phenotypic values of each genotype. The QTL analysis of the tubular index, which shows the intensity of tubulointerstitial injury, identified one significant locus on Chr 2 and two suggestive loci on Chrs 10 and X, respectively (Fig. 2A, Table 1). The significant QTL had a peak LOD score of 5.36 and explained 10% of the variance. Regarding the other nephropathic traits (HGB, HCT, BUN and glomerular index), significant or suggestive loci were also detected on Chr 2 (Fig. 2B, Table 1). Within these QTLs, each trait exhibited CKD resistance associated with the ICGN/B6 genotype.

The QTL analysis of the glomerular index, which shows the severity of GS, identified one significant locus (peak LOD = 3.49) on Chr 13 (Fig. 3A). Grouping backcross mice by their genotype at the marker near the linkage peak, *D13Mit60* (14.44 cM), ICGN/B6 heterozygous mice showed statistically milder glomerular injury than did ICGN/ICGN homozygous mice ($P<0.001$, Mann-Whitney's U test, Fig. 3B). Although the linkage of the tubular index to Chr 13 was similar to that of glomerular index, the peak LOD score was only 1.73. No suggestive linkages were observed for hematological phenotypes on Chr 13 (Fig. 3A).

Epistatic interactions were searched between all of the tested markers by MapManager QTXb20 ($P<0.000001$). We detected three significant interactions in the tubular index associated with markers on Chrs 2 and 10, which showed significant or suggestive linkages to tubular index ($P<0.01$, ANOVA test, Fig. 4). Genotype variations in the tubular index at *D2Mit380* (40.89 cM), *D2Mit293* (17.24 cM) and *D10Mit271* (72.31 cM) were only expressed in the presence of the ICGN/ICGN genotype at *D19Mit33* (51.76 cM), the ICGN/ICGN genotype at *D2Mit102* (57.65 cM) and the ICGN/B6 genotype at *D3Mit129* (80.49 cM), respectively. The B6 allele at *D19Mit33* also suppressed the genotypic effect of *D2Mit380* in HGB. *D2Mit293* (17.24 cM), which lies outside the

Table 2. Podocyte-related genes on Chr 2 QTL.

Candidate genes	Interacting proteins (XPodNet)
Enkur	Pak1, Pik3r2
Apbb1ip	Enah, Vasp
Pax8	Paxip1, Wt1 (Chr 2:55 cM)
Grin1	Ctnnb1, Src (Chr 2:78 cM), Actb, Spnb2, Prkce, Camk2a, Camk2b, Dnm1 (Chr 2:22 cM), Ppp3ca
Notch1	Wwp1, Psen1, Psen2, Ep300, Rbpj, Wdr12, Fbxw7, Kat2a, Kat2b, Smarcd3
Vav2	Lcp2, Rac1, Nckipsd, Ptpn6, Src (Chr 2:78 cM)
Rxra	Trim24, Rarb, Rara, Ppara, Thra, Thrb, Zfp423, Nsd1, Med25
Olfm1	N.D.
Tsc1	Ezr, Ywhab (Chr 2:85 cM)
Abl1	Nck1, Pxn
Lamc3	Nid1, Nid2, Lama5 (Chr 2:103 cM)
Dnm1	Atp9a (Chr 2:89 cM), Grin1 (Chr 2:17 cM), Grin2b, Sh3gl2, Itsn1, Pfn2, Prnp (Chr 2:64 cM), Ctsl, Ap2a2, Kif2a, Kif5a, Tuba1a
Eng	Tgfbr1, Tgfbr2
Cdk9	Cdkn1a, Cdkn1b
Angptl2	N.D.
Lmx1b	Ldb1, Tcf3, Bmpr2
Mapkap1	Akt1
Crb2	N.D.
Lrp1b	Pick1
Zeb2	Smad2
Prpf40a	Wasl
Pkp4	Ctnnb1
Pla2r1	N.D.
Itga6	Lama5 (Chr.2:103 cM), Itgb1, Itgb4, Nisch
Wipf1	Cttn
Hoxd1	Ldb1 (Chr.19:38.75 cM)
Itgav	Itgb1, Itgb3, Itgb5, Spp1, Plaur, Col4a3
Ctnnd1	Yes, Cdh2, Cdh4 (Chr.2:102 cM), Cdh22 (Chr.2:85 cM)
Lrp4	Pick1
Syt13	Nrxn1
Wt1	Pawr, Wtip, Fhl2, Fhl3, Pax2 (Chr.19:38 cM), Pax8 (Chr.2:16 cM)
Pax6	Paxip1

N.D.: not detected.

95% confidence interval for the QTL of the tubular index (19.6–56.4 cM), showed a significant epistatic interaction with *D2Mit102*, whereas the inner marker *D2Mit369* (24.51 cM) did not, although both markers exhibited significant LOD scores of 3.6 and 4.4, respectively. On the other hand, *D2Mit380* (40.89 cM) showed a significant epistatic interaction with *D19Mit33*, as did *D2Mit66* (49.45 cM) and *D2Mit102* (57.65 cM) (data not shown). These results suggest multiple QTLs for tubular index on Chr 2. The bootstrap analysis also supports this hypothesis (Fig. 2C). Next, to identify the candidate genes, we screened the QTLs on Chrs 2 and 13 for podocyte-related genes using XPodNet, and protein-protein interactions in the podocytes [19]. In total, 46 candidate genes are listed (Table 2 and 3).

We also detected seven genetic loci associated with blood cell traits (Table S2). These loci (except for Chr 2) were not linked to the histopathological traits, so that the loci only influenced hematological parameters between the two mice, independent of CKD. Correspondingly, numerous genetic loci of this kind have been identified in recent genome-wide linkage analyses of humans and other mouse strains [26,27,28,29].

Discussion

In this study, we report the mapping of genetic loci responsible for the resistance to congenital nephropathy caused by *Tns2* deficiency in a B6 genetic background. Analysis of backcrossing between resistant B6 mice and susceptible ICGN mice identified significant QTLs on Chrs 2 and 13. Among the tested traits, tubulointerstitial injury (tubular index) and anemia (HGB and HCT) were strongly associated with the same locus on Chr 2. In patients with CKD, anemia develops due to decreased renal erythropoietin synthesis resulting from tubulointerstitial damage. A significant locus for tubular index, ranging approximately from 19.6 to 56.4 cM on Chr 2, which overlaps the QTLs of the other tested traits, appears to be separated into three QTLs with peaks at 22, 31 and 50 cM (Fig. 2). The proximal QTL (22 cM) has

Table 3. Podocyte-related genes on Chr 13 QTL.

Candidate genes	Interacting proteins (XPodNet)
Net1	Magi1
Actn2	Camk2a
Nid1	Lama2, Lamc1, Lamc2, Lamc3, Hspg2, Eln
E2f3	Ccnd1
Agtr1a	Agtrap
Ripk1	Atg5
Nm1	N.D.
Bmp6	Bmpr1a
Nedd9	Src, Nck2, Ptk2
Gadd45g	Cdkn1a
Nsd1	Rxra
Slc34a1	Itgav
Dbn1	Gja1, Lrrk2
Ntrk2	Cdk5, Cdk5r1

N.D.: not detected.

epistatic interactions with *D2Mit102* and *D2Mit282* (Fig. 4, data not shown). The region between the two markers exhibiting a peak LOD score of 3.8 in tubular index includes the syntenic locus for albuminuria previously reported in humans, rats and mice [30,31]. The middle QTL (31 cM) maps to the same region that was found in a (B6×D2) F_2 intercross and in a (B6×A/J) F_2 intercross as a second QTL for albuminuria on Chr 2 [30,31]. The distal QTL (50 cM), where the glomerular score and BUN showed a suggestive linkage, maps to the same region as the suggestive locus for proteinuria that was found in an HIV-associated nephropathy (HIVAN) model mouse on a mixed genetic background of B6 and FVB [32]. The syntenic human region (2q32.1) is associated with the early onset of end-stage renal disease in black families enriched for nondiabetic nephropathy [33]. Taken together, the resistance to CKD in Tns2-deficient B6 mice can be mainly exerted in combination with the multiple loci on Chr 2.

While *Tns2* mRNA is broadly expressed in the kidney and other organs, significant abnormalities (i.e., podocytopenia) were only observed in the kidney of ICGN mice [1]. In the glomeruli, Tns2 expression is localized in podocytes [10,34]. Therefore, the dysfunction of Tns2 in podocytes has been speculated to cause renal dysfunction. Tns is an actin-binding protein that is present in focal adhesions and has been suggested to play an important role in the actin cytoskeleton and integrin-mediated signaling [11]. Recently, it has been reported that Tns2 may bind to integrin β1, and regulate the activity of the integrin β1 downstream effector molecule, integrin-linked kinase (ILK), which is known to play an essential role in GBM assembly and podocyte function [22]. In addition, ILK expression is stimulated in podocytes by renal injury and induces podocyte epithelial-mesenchymal transition [35]. Interestingly, the podocyte-specific knockout of ILK induces progressive focal segmental GS with increased mesangial matrix deposition and downregulation of *Nphs1* and *Synpo* with age, as observed in ICGN mice [12,36,37]. Activation of FAK, another effector molecule of the integrin β1 signaling pathway, is also observed in the glomeruli of *Tns2* mutant mice and conditional *Ilk* knockout mice [22,37]. This upregulation of FAK activity is considered to compensate for the ILK abnormality structurally, but not functionally [22,37]. It is notable that the *Ilk* knockout genetic background is derived from B6 (*NPHS2* promoter-Cre transgenic mice) and 129 ($ILK^{flox/flox}$ mice) [36,37]. That is, the genetic backgrounds of B6 and 129 are resistant to *Tns2*-deficiency, but their resistance has no effect on *Ilk*-deficiency. Hence, it is assumed that the resistance effects are exhibited by functionally regulating the disorders in the integrin β1-ILK signaling pathway or structurally reinforcing the fragility of the actin cytoskeleton and slit diaphragm induced by aberrant ILK activity in *Tns2*-deficient podocytes.

Under this assumption, we screened QTLs mapped on Chr 2 for podocyte-related genes using XPodNet and identified 32 candidate genes (Table 2). Among these, we were especially interested in *Notch1*, *Dnm1*, *Lmx1b*, *Zeb2* and *Wt1*. NOTCH1 (18.91 cM) is a transmembrane receptor protein whose signaling pathway correlates with GS and renal function [38]. DNM1 (22.09 cM), dynamin1, participates in endocytosis in the podocyte foot process and contributes to maintenance of the slit diaphragm [39]. WT1 (55.06 cM) and LMX1B (22.48 cM) are transcription factors that regulate podocyte-specific structural genes, *Nphs1* and *Podxl*, and *Nphs2* respectively, and play a key role in the development and maintenance of the actin cytoskeleton and slit diaphragm in podocytes [40,41,42]. ZEB2 (27.31 cM), a transcriptional repressor of E-cadherin, is upregulated by the integrin β1-ILK signaling pathway downstream target SNAIL and induces the epithelial–mesenchymal transition [43].

In the same way, 14 candidate genes of the Chr 13 QTL are listed in Table 3. This locus partially overlaps the HIVAN susceptibility locus, *HIVAN2*, that was found in an (HIV-1 transgenic FVB×B6) F_2 intercross [32]. An expression quantitative trait locus (eQTL) analysis has revealed that *HIVAN2* influences the transcript abundance of *Nphs2*, a membrane protein linking the slit diaphragm to the cytoskeleton [32]. However, *HIVAN2* includes none of transcription factors known to regulate *Nphs2* expression. In our cross, the locus was not linked to anemia, so that it is not considered to be essential for susceptibility to CKD induced by $Tns2^{nph}$.

Our genomic analysis of CKD in a cross between B6 and ICGN assumes that the Chr 2 loci critically contribute to resistance in

Tns2-deficient mice. The Chr 2 QTLs identified in crosses for proteinuria between resistant B6 and susceptible D2 or A/J or HIV-1 transgenic FVB are similar to ours [30,31,32]. This suggests that our QTL is not limited to resistance to the CKD induced by $Tns2^{nph}$, but is generally associated with resistance to CKD. Although this locus has not been noted in previous reports due to the absence of a homologous human QTL, we believe that this locus also plays an important role in resistance to CKD. Identification of resistant genes on this locus would help reveal the mechanism by which *Tns2* deficiency leads to CKD and provide a novel insight into susceptibility to CKD, leading to the development of treatment strategies for CKD.

Supporting Information

Figure S1 Representative examples of glomerular score.

Figure S2 Representative examples of tubular score.

Figure S3 Histopathological severity, resistant strain vs. susceptible strain.

Table S1 Genotyping markers.

Table S2 QTLs identified for hematological phenotypes.

Author Contributions

Conceived and designed the experiments: NS. Performed the experiments: HS TN KN NS. Analyzed the data: HS HK DT NS. Contributed reagents/materials/analysis tools: NS TA. Wrote the paper: HS NS.

References

1. Ogura A, Asano T, Matsuda J, Takano K, Nakagawa M, et al. (1989) Characteristics of mutant mice (ICGN) with spontaneous renal lesions: a new model for human nephrotic syndrome. Lab Anim 23: 169–174.
2. Mizuno S, Matsumoto K, Kurosawa T, Mizuno-Horikawa Y, Nakamura T (2000) Reciprocal balance of hepatocyte growth factor and transforming growth factor-beta 1 in renal fibrosis in mice. Kidney Int 57: 937–948.
3. Mizuno S, Mizuno-Horikawa Y, Yue BF, Okamoto M, Kurosawa T (1999) Nephrotic mice (ICGN strain): a model of diffuse mesangial sclerosis in infantile nephrotic syndrome. Am J Nephrol 19: 73–82.
4. Ogura A, Fujimura H, Asano T, Koura M, Naito I, et al. (1995) Early ultrastructural glomerular alterations in neonatal nephrotic mice (ICGN strain). Vet Pathol 32: 321–323.
5. Mizuno S, Yue BF, Okamoto M, Horikawa Y, Kurosawa T (1997) Diffuse glomerulosclerosis without tubular injury does not directly manifest renal dysfunction in nephrotic mice (ICGN strain). Exp Nephrol 5: 498–507.
6. Mundel P, Schwarz K, Reiser J (2001) Podocyte biology: a footstep further. Adv Nephrol Necker Hosp 31: 235–241.
7. Wiggins RC (2007) The spectrum of podocytopathies: a unifying view of glomerular diseases. Kidney Int 71: 1205–1214.
8. Pavenstadt H, Kriz W, Kretzler M (2003) Cell biology of the glomerular podocyte. Physiol Rev 83: 253–307.
9. Warsow G, Endlich N, Schordan E, Schordan S, Chilukoti RK, et al. (2013) PodNet, a protein-protein interaction network of the podocyte. Kidney Int 84: 104–115.
10. Cho AR, Uchio-Yamada K, Torigai T, Miyamoto T, Miyoshi I, et al. (2006) Deficiency of the tensin 2 gene in the ICGN mouse: an animal model for congenital nephrotic syndrome. Mamm Genome 17: 407–416.
11. Lo SH (2004) Tensin. Int J Biochem Cell Biol 36: 31–34.
12. Kato T, Mizuno S, Taketo MM, Kurosawa TM (2008) The possible involvement of tensin 2 in the expression and extension of nephrin by glomerular podocytes in mice. Biomed Res 29: 279–287.
13. Stevens LA, Claybon MA, Schmid CH, Chen J, Horio M, et al. (2011) Evaluation of the Chronic Kidney Disease Epidemiology Collaboration equation for estimating the glomerular filtration rate in multiple ethnicities. Kidney Int 79: 555–562.
14. Kottgen A, Pattaro C, Boger CA, Fuchsberger C, Olden M, et al. (2010) New loci associated with kidney function and chronic kidney disease. Nat Genet 42: 376–384.
15. Manolio TA, Collins FS, Cox NJ, Goldstein DB, Hindorff LA, et al. (2009) Finding the missing heritability of complex diseases. Nature 461: 747–753.
16. Boger CA, Heid IM (2011) Chronic kidney disease: novel insights from genome-wide association studies. Kidney Blood Press Res 34: 225–234.
17. Andrews KL, Mudd JL, Li C, Miner JH (2002) Quantitative trait loci influence renal disease progression in a mouse model of Alport syndrome. Am J Pathol 160: 721–730.
18. Hartner A, Cordasic N, Klanke B, Veelken R, Hilgers KF (2003) Strain differences in the development of hypertension and glomerular lesions induced by deoxycorticosterone acetate salt in mice. Nephrol Dial Transplant 18: 1999–2004.
19. Roselli S, Heidet L, Sich M, Henger A, Kretzler M, et al. (2004) Early glomerular filtration defect and severe renal disease in podocin-deficient mice. Mol Cell Biol 24: 550–560.
20. Nishino T, Sasaki N, Nagasaki K, Ahmad Z, Agui T (2010) Genetic background strongly influences the severity of glomerulosclerosis in mice. J Vet Med Sci 72: 1313–1318.
21. Nishino T, Sasaki N, Nagasaki K, Ichii O, Kon Y, et al. (2012) The 129 genetic background affects susceptibility to glomerulosclerosis in tensin 2-deficient mice. Biomed Res 33: 53–56.
22. Uchio-Yamada K, Sawada K, Tamura K, Katayama S, Monobe Y, et al. (2013) Tenc1-deficient mice develop glomerular disease in a strain-specific manner. Nephron Exp Nephrol 123: 22–33.
23. Manly KF, Cudmore RH, Jr., Meer JM (2001) Map Manager QTX, cross-platform software for genetic mapping. Mamm Genome 12: 930–932.
24. Kruglyak L, Lander ES (1995) A nonparametric approach for mapping quantitative trait loci. Genetics 139: 1421–1428.
25. Elliot SJ, Karl M, Berho M, Potier M, Zheng F, et al. (2003) Estrogen deficiency accelerates progression of glomerulosclerosis in susceptible mice. Am J Pathol 162: 1441–1448.
26. van der Harst P, Zhang W, Mateo Leach I, Rendon A, Verweij N, et al. (2012) Seventy-five genetic loci influencing the human red blood cell. Nature 492: 369–375.
27. Peters LL, Shavit JA, Lambert AJ, Tsaih SW, Li Q, et al. (2010) Sequence variation at multiple loci influences red cell hemoglobin concentration. Blood 116: e139–149.
28. Davis RC, van Nas A, Bennett B, Orozco L, Pan C, et al. (2013) Genome-wide association mapping of blood cell traits in mice. Mamm Genome 24: 105–118.
29. Kelada SN, Aylor DL, Peck BC, Ryan JF, Tavarez U, et al. (2012) Genetic analysis of hematological parameters in incipient lines of the collaborative cross. G3 (Bethesda) 2: 157–165.
30. Sheehan S, Tsaih SW, King BL, Stanton C, Churchill GA, et al. (2007) Genetic analysis of albuminuria in a cross between C57BL/6J and DBA/2J mice. Am J Physiol Renal Physiol 293: F1649–1656.
31. Doorenbos C, Tsaih SW, Sheehan S, Ishimori N, Navis G, et al. (2008) Quantitative trait loci for urinary albumin in crosses between C57BL/6J and A/J inbred mice in the presence and absence of Apoe. Genetics 179: 693–699.
32. Papeta N, Chan KT, Prakash S, Martino J, Kiryluk K, et al. (2009) Susceptibility loci for murine HIV-associated nephropathy encode trans-regulators of podocyte gene expression. J Clin Invest 119: 1178–1188.
33. Freedman BI, Langefeld CD, Rich SS, Valis CJ, Sale MM, et al. (2004) A genome scan for ESRD in black families enriched for nondiabetic nephropathy. J Am Soc Nephrol 15: 2719–2727.
34. Nishino T, Sasaki N, Chihara M, Nagasaki K, Torigoe D, et al. (2012) Distinct distribution of the tensin family in the mouse kidney and small intestine. Exp Anim 61: 525–532.
35. Kang YS, Li Y, Dai C, Kiss LP, Wu C, et al. (2010) Inhibition of integrin-linked kinase blocks podocyte epithelial-mesenchymal transition and ameliorates proteinuria. Kidney Int 78: 363–373.
36. El-Aouni C, Herbach N, Blattner SM, Henger A, Rastaldi MP, et al. (2006) Podocyte-specific deletion of integrin-linked kinase results in severe glomerular basement membrane alterations and progressive glomerulosclerosis. J Am Soc Nephrol 17: 1334–1344.
37. Kanasaki K, Kanda Y, Palmsten K, Tanjore H, Lee SB, et al. (2008) Integrin beta1-mediated matrix assembly and signaling are critical for the normal development and function of the kidney glomerulus. Dev Biol 313: 584–593.
38. Murea M, Park JK, Sharma S, Kato H, Gruenwald A, et al. (2010) Expression of Notch pathway proteins correlates with albuminuria, glomerulosclerosis, and renal function. Kidney Int 78: 514–522.
39. Soda K, Balkin DM, Ferguson SM, Paradise S, Milosevic I, et al. (2012) Role of dynamin, synaptojanin, and endophilin in podocyte foot processes. J Clin Invest 122: 4401–4411.

40. Harendza S, Stahl RA, Schneider A (2009) The transcriptional regulation of podocin (NPHS2) by Lmx1b and a promoter single nucleotide polymorphism. Cell Mol Biol Lett 14: 679–691.
41. Burghardt T, Kastner J, Suleiman H, Rivera-Milla E, Stepanova N, et al. (2013) LMX1B is essential for the maintenance of differentiated podocytes in adult kidneys. J Am Soc Nephrol 24: 1830–1848.
42. Guo JK, Menke AL, Gubler MC, Clarke AR, Harrison D, et al. (2002) WT1 is a key regulator of podocyte function: reduced expression levels cause crescentic glomerulonephritis and mesangial sclerosis. Hum Mol Genet 11: 651–659.
43. Beltran M, Puig I, Pena C, Garcia JM, Alvarez AB, et al. (2008) A natural antisense transcript regulates Zeb2/Sip1 gene expression during Snail1-induced epithelial-mesenchymal transition. Genes Dev 22: 756–769.

11

The Relationship between Renal Function and Plasma Concentration of the Cachectic Factor Zinc-Alpha2-Glycoprotein (ZAG) in Adult Patients with Chronic Kidney Disease

Caroline C. Pelletier[1,2,3¶], Laetitia Koppe[1,2,3¶], Pascaline M. Alix[1,2,3¶], Emilie Kalbacher[1,2,3], Marine L. Croze[1,2], Aoumeur Hadj-Aissa[1,4], Denis Fouque[1,2,5], Fitsum Guebre-Egziabher[1,2,3], Christophe O. Soulage[1,2]*

1 Université de Lyon, F-69600, Oullins, France, **2** INSERM, U1060, CarMeN, INSA-Lyon, Univ. Lyon-1, Villeurbanne, France, **3** Hospices Civils de Lyon, Service de Néphrologie, Hôpital E Herriot, Lyon, France, **4** Hospices Civils de Lyon, Exploration Fonctionnelle Rénale et Métabolique, Hôpital E Herriot, Lyon, France, **5** Hospices Civils de Lyon, Service de Néphrologie, Centre Hospitalier Lyon-SUD, Pierre-Bénite, France

Abstract

Zinc-α2-glycoprotein (ZAG), a potent cachectic factor, is increased in patients undergoing maintenance dialysis. However, there is no data for patients before initiation of renal replacement therapy. The purpose of the present study was to assess the relationship between plasma ZAG concentration and renal function in patients with a large range of glomerular filtration rate (GFR). Plasma ZAG concentration and its relationship to GFR were investigated in 71 patients with a chronic kidney disease (CKD) stage 1 to 5, 17 chronic hemodialysis (HD), 8 peritoneal dialysis (PD) and 18 non-CKD patients. Plasma ZAG concentration was 2.3-fold higher in CKD stage 5 patients and 3-fold higher in HD and PD patients compared to non-CKD controls ($P<0.01$). The hemodialysis session further increased plasma ZAG concentration (+39%, $P<0.01$). An inverse relationship was found between ZAG levels and plasma protein ($r_s = -0.284$; $P<0.01$), albumin ($r_s = -0.282$, $P<0.05$), hemoglobin ($r_s = -0.267$, $P<0.05$) and HDL-cholesterol ($r_s = -0.264$, $P<0.05$) and a positive correlation were seen with plasma urea ($r_s = 0.283$; $P<0.01$). In multiple regression analyses, plasma urea and HDL-cholesterol were the only variables associated with plasma ZAG ($r^2 = 0.406$, $P<0.001$). In CKD-5 patients, plasma accumulation of ZAG was not correlated with protein energy wasting. Further prospective studies are however needed to better elucidate the potential role of ZAG in end-stage renal disease.

Editor: Leighton R. James, University of Florida, United States of America

Funding: This study was supported by two governmental institutions from France, INSERM and INSA-Lyon, and by the Fédération Nationale d'Aide aux Insuffisants Rénaux (FNAIR). CC.PELLETIER and PM. ALIX held grants from "Société Française de Néphrologie," E KALBACHER was the recipient of a grant from "Académie de Médecine" and L. KOPPE held a fellowship from "Fondation pour la Recherche Médicale". ML CROZE held a grant from the French "Ministère de l'Enseignement Supérieur et de la Recherche." The authors have no competing financial interests to disclose. The funders had no role in study design, data collection and analysis, decision to publish, or preparation of the manuscript.

Competing Interests: The authors have declared that no competing interests exist.

* Email: Christophe.Soulage@insa-lyon.fr

¶ These authors contributed equally to this work.

Introduction

Chronic kidney disease (CKD) and especially end-stage renal disease (ESRD) are associated with increased plasma concentration of numerous adipokines presumably as the result of a decreased glomerular filtration and/or a blunted renal degradation. Indeed, plasma concentrations of leptin [1], adiponectin [2,3], fibroblast growth factor 21 (FGF-21) [4], retinol binding protein 4 (RBP-4) [5], chemerin [6] were found to be increased in ESRD patients. Zinc-α2-glycoprotein (thereafter referred to as ZAG) is a 43-kDa soluble glycoprotein first isolated from human plasma [7] and proposed as a tumour-derived cancer cachexia factor [8,9]. Indeed, ZAG is overexpressed in many malignant tumours and is strongly associated with adipose tissue atrophy in cancer cachexia [10]. ZAG is however also produced by many non-malignant tissues, including white adipose tissue (WAT) and epithelia cells from liver, breast, gastrointestinal tract as well as sweat glands [11]. ZAG is described as a lipid-mobilizing factor in adipose tissue [12]. The biological activity of ZAG is linked to a cyclic AMPc-mediated signalling system through interaction with a β3/β2 adrenoreceptors [9,10,13,14]. ZAG displays both lipolytic and antilipogenic effects on adipose tissue [9,15] and stimulates uncoupling protein-1 (UCP-1) expression in brown adipose tissue, increasing thermogenesis and lipid utilization [16]. Currently, only few data are available on ZAG metabolism in kidney disease. Philipp et al [17] and Leal et al [18,19] recently showed an increased plasma ZAG concentration in chronic hemodialysis patients, suggesting a defect of its renal clearance. However, there is no data regarding the actual plasma level of ZAG in CKD patients before initiation of renal replacement therapy. It therefore remains unclear whether the plasma accumulation of ZAG simply results from the decrease in glomerular filtration rate (GFR). The purpose of this cross-sectional study was therefore to prospectively assess the relationship between plasma ZAG concentration and GFR in patients with a large range of renal function. Plasma ZAG concentration was measured in a cohort of 71 CKD patients from stage 1 to 5, 18 non-CKD patients and correlations were explored with clinical and biochemical markers of renal function and metabolism. Plasma ZAG was further measured in 17 hemodialysis (HD) and 8 peritoneal dialysis (PD) patients.

Materials and Methods

Ethic statement

This research was approved by the local institutional review committee (reference D-09-17, Comité de Protection des Personnes - Recherche Biomédicale, CPP Lyon Sud-Est IV) and conducted in accordance with its ethical standards and the principles of the Declaration of Helsinki. All subjects involved in the research signed written informed consent forms prior to enrolment.

Subjects

From November 2010 to March 2013, a total of 89 subjects (43 men and 46 women), among which 18 non-CKD subjects, were recruited from Nephrology department and Unité de Jour d'Exploration Rénale et Néphrologie (UJERN) (E. Herriot University hospital Lyon, France). Glomerular filtration rate (eGFR) was estimated using the CKD EPI formula [20,21] and CKD stages were determined according to K/DOQI guidelines [22]. Seventeen chronic HD and 8 PD patients on renal replacement therapy for more than 6 months were further recruited at the Nephrology/Hemodialysis unit (E. Herriot University hospital, Lyon, France). Patients with severe conditions including systemic inflammation or known malignant active diseases were excluded from the study. People were classified into 8 groups: Healthy volunteers, CKD stage 1, CKD stage 2, CKD stage 3, CKD stage 4, CKD stage 5 - no renal replacement therapy, CKD stage 5 - hemodialysis, CKD stage 5 - peritoneal dialysis.

Anthropometric and clinical measurements

Body weight was measured in light clothing without shoes to the nearest 100 g on a digital scale, corresponding to dry weights for HD patients. Height was measured in standard position with a portable stadiometer. Body mass index (BMI) was calculated as body weight divided by squared height. Body fat mass was calculated according to Deurenberg et al (1991) using the following formula: Body fat (%) = (1.20×BMI)+(0.23×Age)−(10.8×Gender) where male gender = 1, female gender = 0 [23]. CKD patients were considered having PEW if they presented at least 3 out of 4 of the following criterions, BMI<23 kg/m^2, Albumin<38 g/L (bromcresol green assay), Pre-albumin < 300 mg/L or Protein intake<0.6 g/kg.24 h according to Fouque et al (2008) [24].

Blood sampling

After an overnight fast, blood samples were obtained by venipuncture, except for HD blood samples that were obtained immediately before and after dialysis from arterial line of the mechanical bloodstream. Blood samples were centrifuged at 3500×g for 10 min to isolate plasma supernatant which was snap frozen in liquid nitrogen and stored at −20°C until use.

Glomerular filtration rate measurements (mGFR)

In a subset of 42 CKD stage 1 to 4 subjects, GFR was measured by the gold standard method, i.e. the urinary inulin clearance (ml/min per 1.73 m^2), as described previously [25]. Briefly, inulin (Polyfructosan[inutest], Laevosan, Linz, Austria) was infused continuously for 4 hours after a priming dose. Blood and urine were collected every 30 minutes by peripheral venous catheter and spontaneous voiding, respectively. Inulin was measured by the enzymatic method [26]. GFR was calculated with the UV/P formula with U = urine inulin concentration, V = urinary volume and P = plasma inulin concentration.

ZAG immunoassay

Plasma ZAG concentrations were determined with a commercially available ZAG Enzyme Immunoassay (RayBiotech Inc, Tebu-Bio, Le-Perray-en-Yvelines, France) according to the manufacturer's instructions. The detection limit was 21 pg/ml and intra and inter-assay coefficient was 3.6% and 3.2% respectively. Measurements were performed at least in duplicate. Post-dialysis ZAG concentrations were corrected for hemoconcentration using plasma protein concentrations assayed according to the method of Bradford [27] with bovine serum albumin as standard. The correction was performed using the following equation: $[ZAG]_{Corrected} = ([Proteins]_{pre\text{-}HD}/[Proteins]_{post\text{-}HD}) \times [ZAG]_{post\text{-}HD}$ with $[Proteins]_{pre\text{-}HD}$, plasma protein concentration before haemodialysis session, $[Proteins]_{post\text{-}HD}$ and $[ZAG]_{post\text{-}HD}$, plasma protein and plasma ZAG concentrations after haemodialysis session, respectively.

Other biochemical measurements

Plasma urea, bicarbonate, hemoglobin, protein, glucose, HDL and LDL cholesterol, triglycerides, and C-reactive protein (CRP) were measured by standard laboratory methods in a certified laboratory. Albumin was measured by immunonephelometry. Creatinine assay was performed by enzymatic method (Roche, Meylan, France), with calibrators assigned by an isotope-dilution mass spectrometry. Plasma glycerol concentration (an index of white adipose tissue lipolysis) was measured using a colorimetric enzymatic assay (Glycerol assay, R-Biopharm, Saint-Didier, France) and normalized to body fat mass as described by Axelsson et al (2011) [28].

Statistical analysis

Data were analysed using Graphpad Prism 5.0 (GraphPad softwares, La Jolla, USA) and Statview 4.5 (Abacus concept, Berkeley, USA) softwares. The data are expressed as mean±1 standard deviation (SD) or as median (interquartile range [IQR]) when variable were not normally distributed. Distributions were tested for normality using d'Agostino-Pearson test. Differences between groups were assessed by Kruskall & Wallis test followed when appropriate by Dunn tests. Simple comparisons were made using Mann & Whitney U test. Sex ratio and medications between groups were compared using Chi-square test. Univariate analysis was performed using the Spearman rank correlation method. A multivariate linear regression analysis was used to define the variables most predictive of circulating ZAG concentration after selection of the measures found to be associated with ZAG by univariate analysis (i.e. urea, plasma proteins, hemoglobin and HDL-cholesterol). A $P<0.05$ was considered as statistically significant in all analysis.

Table 1. Baseline characteristics of non CKD, CKD, hemodialysis and peritoneal dialysis patients involved in the study (N = 114).

	Non CKD	CKD stage					HD	PD	P-value
		1	2	3	4	5			
Sex, male/female	9/9	2/6	8/12	11/7	7/5	6/7	8/9	4/4	P = 0.777
Age, y	52 (28–63)	31 (20–48)	59(48–70)	69 (58–76)	67 (54–76)	61 (58–66)	66 (53–86)	58 (46–71)	P = 0.001
Weight, kg	67.0 (53.0–73.8)	59.5 (48.2–74.5)	65.0 (58.5–76.3)	75.0 (64.5–92.3)	74.0 (64.0–85.8)	71.0 (60.0–87.5)	65.0 (55.0–77.8)	63.9 (55.5–76.8)	P = 0.156
BMI, kg/m^2	23.4 (21.2–25.6)	20.8 (18.5–25.6)	25.3 (22.1–27.2)	26.7 (23.4–32.9)	26.2 (24.3–31.8)	24.0 (22.9–30.8)	25.8 (21.9–30.3)	23.9 (20.7–29.5)	P = 0.100
Creatinine, μM	58.5 (50.8–62.3)	53.5 (42.0–72.0)	82.5 (72.5–93.5)	137 (122–171)	301 (198–368)	456 (382–639)	643 (450–815)	641 (498–846)	P<0.001
eGFR, ml/min.1.73 m^2	109 (99–138)	124 (94–134)	75 (68–88)	43 (33–45)	16 (14–24)	9 (8–12)	N/A	N/A	P<0.001
Urea, mM	4.7 (3.9–5.7)	4.2 (3.6–6.8)	6.1 (5.0–7.7)	13.6 (9.5–15.3)	20.7 (14.3–24.5)	24.0 (17.2–28.5)	21.4 (18.3–28.2)	16.6 (14.7–21.2)	P<0.001
Bicarbonates, mM	25.0 (23.2–27.1)	25.9 (23.9–30.5)	26.8 (24.5–28.3)	23.3 (22.1–25.8)	21.9 (18.6–25.8)	24.8 (21.8–26.8)	24.1 (22.5–25.0)	26.9 (24.4–28.7)	P = 0.002
Proteins, g/L	70.0 (65.8–76.5)	70.5 (54.3–75.8)	70.0 (66.5–75.8)	73.0 (70.3–79.3)	73.5 (70.3–75.0)	72.0 (65.0–76.0)	68.0 (66.0–72.0)	74.5 (65.5–78.0)	P = 0.385
Albumin, g/L	41.5 (37.0–42.9)	37.0 (17.0–41.0)	41.8 (37.0–43.7)	36.9 (35.0–42.5)	38.0 (33.0–40.0)	32.0 (26.5–34.5)	38.0 (33.5–40.5)	35.0 (27.0–36.0)	P = 0.009
Hemoglobin, g/L	127 (117–144)	126 (107–140)	130 (122–138)	119 (102–134)	112 (101–122)	118 (102–122)	116 (102–122)	125 (104–136)	P = 0.003
Glucose, mM	4.8 (4.3–5.4)	4.8 (4.2–5.4)	5.0 (4.5–5.7)	5.9 (4.4–7.0)	5.3 (4.8–6.3)	5.6 (4.8–6.9)	5.4 (4.4–5.8)	4.9 (4.7–8.1)	P = 0.129
Triacylglycerols, mM	0.76 (0.55–1.33)	1.74 (1.44–3.02)	1.30 (1.00–1.97)	1.46 (1.08–2.21)	1.37 (1.21–2.60)	1.61 (1.33–2.16)	1.87 (1.04–2.38)	1.32 (0.71–2.84)	P = 0.038
HDL cholesterol, mM	1.10 (0.95–1.32)	1.10 (0.91–1.57)	1.29 (0.98–1.86)	1.19 (1.00–1.36)	1.14 (0.90–1.24)	1.01 (0.87–1.1)	1.18 (0.99–1.56)	1.48 (0.69–4.03)	P = 0.449
LDL cholesterol, mM	2.38 (1.87–3.22)	2.25 (1.73–5.02)	2.83 (2.20–3.84)	1.61 (1.33–2.01)	1.44 (1.26–2.79)	2.18 (1.64–2.67)	2.02 (1.42–3.68)	2.18 (1.68–2.52)	P = 0.044
CRP, mg/L	2.9 (2.9–3.2)	3.0(2.9–7.2)	2.9 (2.9–3.1)	4.5 (2.9–7.0)	2.9 (2.9–9.6)	3.2 (2.9–11.3)	4.4 (2.9–9.2)	2.9 (2.9–2.9)	P = 0.067
Anti diabetic therapy,%	0.0	12.5	5.0	50.0	77.7	23.1	17.6	50.0	P<0.001
Lipid-lowering therapy,%	5.9	12.5	30.0	66.7	80.0	38.5	47.0	50.0	P = 0.001
RAA inhibitors,%	11.8	37.5	25.0	88.9	60.0	77.0	41.2	62.5	P<0.001
Beta blockers, %	0	0	22.2	47.1	27.3	30.8	58.8	37.5	P = 0.005

Continuous data are expressed as median (interquartile range) and compared using Kruskall & Wallis test. Categorical data are expressed as the frequency (%) and compared using Chi square test. Abbreviations: CKD, chronic kidney disease, BMI, body mass index, eGFR estimated glomerular filtration rate, HD, hemodialysis, N/A, not applicable, PD, peritoneal dialysis, RAA, renin angiotensin aldosterone. eGFR was calculated using CKD EPI formula. Differences were considered significant at P<0.05.

Table 2. Dialysis adequacy for HD and DP patients.

	Hemodialysis	Peritoneal Dialysis
Dialysis modality	9 HD/8 HDF	5 CAPD/3 CCPD
Catheter/Fistula/not documented, n =	3/12/2	NA
Time of dialysis (h/week)	12.27±0.61	NA
Blood flow (ml/mn)	340.91±24.27	NA
Kt/V	1.67±0.31	NA
Weekly Kt/V urea	NA	2.43±0.51
Weekly peritoneal clearance (L/week/1.73 m^2)	NA	89.18±22.53
Residual renal fonction (L/week/1.73 m^2)	NA	48.3±25.01

Data are expressed as means ± one standard deviation. Abbreviations: CAPD, continuous ambulatory peritoneal dialysis, CCPD continuous cyclic peritoneal dialysis, HD, hemodialysis; HDF, hemodiafiltration, NA, not applicable.

Results

Patient data

We recruited 71 patients with CKD from stage 1 to end-stage 5 (aged 57±17 years), 18 non-CKD patients (aged 48±19 years), 17 HD patients (aged 66±17 years) and 8 PD patients (aged 58±14 years). Their renal diseases were glomerulonephritis (N = 32 including 19 diabetes), renovascular disease (N = 22, including 14 nephroangiosclerosis), 9 tubulointerstitial disease, 5 cystic kidney diseases and of other or unknown aetiologies in 28 patients. Non-CKD patients were referred of renal function evaluation for urinary lithiasis exploration or before kidney donation. Out of the 96 CKD, HD and PD patients, 54 were on antihypertensive drugs (56.8%), 45 on lipid lowering drugs (47.3%), 32 were on beta-

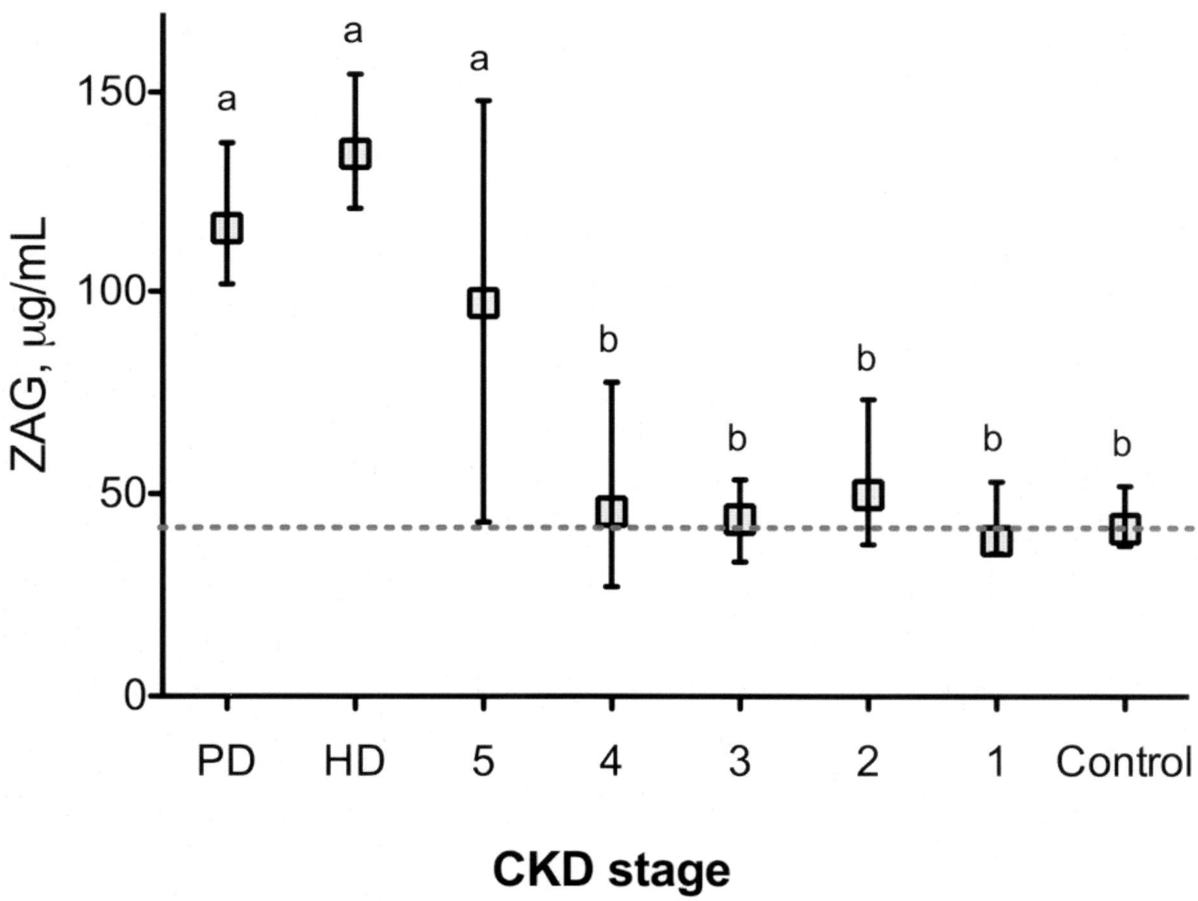

Figure 1. Plasma ZAG concentration is increased in end stage renal disease patients. ZAG concentration was quantified in plasma from non-CKD subjects (N = 18), chronic kidney disease (CKD stage 1 to 5, N = 71), hemodialysis (HD, N = 17) and peritoneal dialysis (PD, N = 8) patients by enzyme immunoassay. eGFR was estimated using CKD EPI formula as described in methods. Data are presented as median (interquartile range). Different letters indicate a significant difference at the $P<0.05$ level.

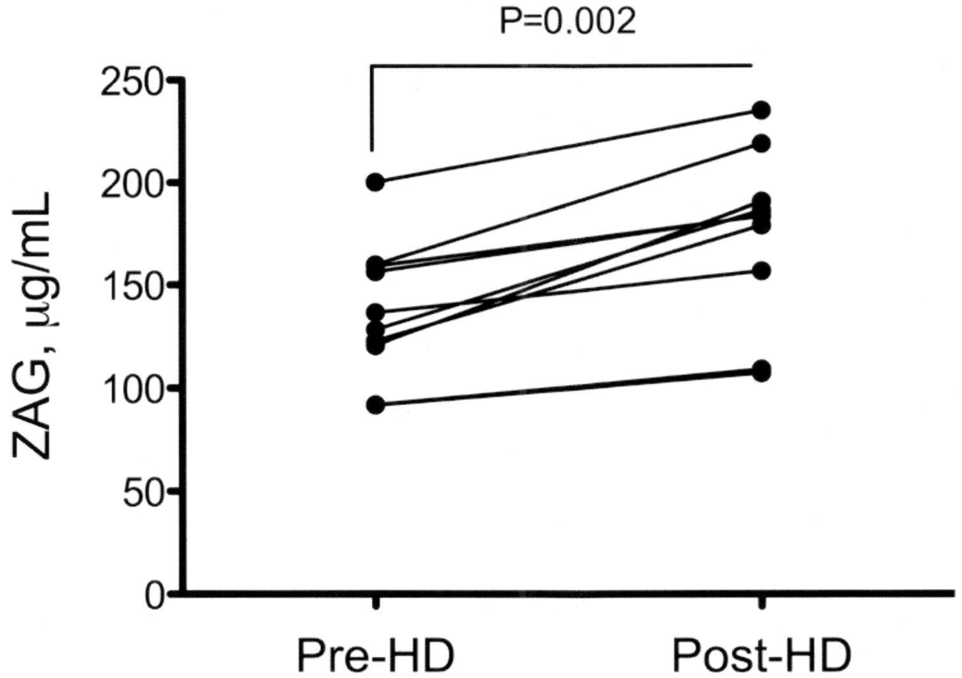

Figure 2. Plasma ZAG concentration increases during hemodialysis session. ZAG concentration was quantified by enzyme immunoassay before and after an hemodialysis session in ESRD patients (N = 8). ZAG concentrations were corrected for hemoconcentration as described in methods. Differences between pre and post dialysis concentrations were considered significant at the $P<0.05$ level (Wilcoxon test for paired samples). Abbreviation: HD, hemodialysis.

blockers (33.3%) and 30 on antidiabetic drugs (31.5%, amongst which 24 used insulin and 6 oral antidiabetics). The main clinical, anthropometric and biochemical characteristics of the cohort are summarized in **Table 1** and dialysis adequacy is described in **Table 2**. As expected, eGFR (estimated by CKD EPI, $P<0.001$), plasma creatinine ($P<0.001$) and urea ($P<0.001$) were different between groups.

Plasma ZAG concentration increases in ESRD patients

Surprisingly, plasma ZAG concentration did not gradually increase from CKD stage 1 to CKD stage 4 when compared to non-CKD patients (**Figure 1**). Plasma ZAG concentration was however 2.3-fold higher in CKD 5 (ESRD) patients as compared with non-CKD patients or CKD stage 1 to 4 patients (Kruskall & Wallis test, $P<0.005$). The plasma ZAG concentration was 41.5 (interquartile range (IQR), 37.3–52.0) µg/ml for non-CKD

Table 3. Univariate correlations with ZAG concentrations.

	rho	P-value	
Age, y	0.103	0.340	
BMI, $kg.m^{-2}$	0.112	0.296	
CRP, mg L^{-1}	0.088	0.507	
Protein, $g.L^{-1}$	−0.284	0.008	**
Albumin, $g.L^{-1}$	−0.282	0.016	*
Hemoglobin, $g.L^{-1}$	−0.264	0.015	*
Bicarbonate, mM	−0.001	0.905	
Urea, mM	0.283	0.008	**
Creatinine, µM	0.274	<0.01	**
Proteinuria, $g.24\ h^{-1}$	0.257	0.061	
Glucose, mM	0.138	0.200	
HDL-cholesterol, mM	−0.265	0.034	*
LDL-cholesterol, mM	−0.097	0.448	
Triacylglycerols, mM	0.119	0.340	

Abbreviations: BMI: Body mass index, CRP: C-reactive protein, eGFR: estimated glomerular filtration rate. Correlations were significant at P<0.05 level.

Table 4. Multiple linear regression showing association with plasma ZAG concentration ($r^2 = 0.406$, $P < 0.001$).

Dependent variable: plasma ZAG				
Independent variable	**β coefficient**	**Standard error**	**P-value**	
Urea	2.024	0.583	<0.005	***
Proteins	−1.346	0.571	0.023	*
Hemoglobin	−0.195	0.264	0.465	
HDL-cholesterol	−27.217	11.739	0.025	*
Intercept	181.182	54.338		

Correlations were significant at P<0.05 level.

patients and 97.2 (43.1–147.9) µg/ml for CKD 5 subjects (P< 0.01). No significant difference in ZAG concentration could be demonstrated depending on gender (male vs female: 56 (33–126) vs 40 (31–100) µg/ml, P = 0.096) or diabetic status (non diabetes mellitus *vs* diabetes mellitus, 46 (33–115) vs 48 (27–110) µg/ml, P = 0.908). Plasma ZAG concentration was not significantly different from non-dialyzed CKD 5 patients neither in HD patients (134.6 (120.7–154.7) µg/ml) nor in PD patients (134.6 (98.2–137.3) µg/ml). To get further insight, GFR was measured in a subset of patients (CKD 1 to CKD 5, N = 42) by the gold standard method, i.e. the urinary inulin clearance. In good agreement, no correlation was found between GFR assessed by inulin clearance and plasma ZAG concentration in patients with CKD stage 1 to 4 (Spearman $r_s = 0.174$, P = 0.283).

HD patients exhibited a further increase in plasma ZAG concentration after the dialysis session. The mean plasma ZAG concentration was 132.3 (113.3–159.2) µg/ml before and 196.1 (168.8–217.9) µg/ml after haemodialysis session (+48%, P = 0.002). Hemodialysis resulted in a significant hemoconcentration evidenced by the increased plasma protein concentration (68.3±6.1 vs 74.8±7.8 g/L, before and after HD, respectively, + 9%, P = 0.015). However, the post-dialysis increase in ZAG concentration did not only result from hemoconcentration since normalization of ZAG concentration to plasma protein concentration did not abolish this difference (**Figure 2**). Corrected ZAG concentration after haemodialysis session was 183.7 (144.7–197.7) µg/ml (+39%, P = 0.008).

Table 5. Characteristics of CKD-5 patients with PEW.

	No PEW	**PEW**	
Sex, male/female	14/12	6/5	P = 0.969
Age, y	63 (54–73)	62 (47–84)	P = 0.947
Weight, kg	68.0 (57–78)	55 (51–77)	P = 0.122
BMI, kg/m^2	27.4 (23.0–30.0)	21.8 (19.2–24.0)	P = 0.021*
Creatinine, µM	589.5 (443.3–822.5)	613.0 (407.0–683.0)	P = 0.921
Urea, mM	21.0 (17.0–27.8)	18.5 (17.1–26.9)	P = 0.642
Bicarbonates, mM	24.5 (22.8–26.0)	24.0 (22.0–25.0)	P = 0.393
Proteins, g/L	69.5 (66.8–76.3)	64.0 (59–77.0)	P = 0.079
Albumin, g/L	36.0 (33.5–39.2)	27.0 (26.0–33.1)	P = 0.001***
Prealbumin, mg/L	0.31 (0.28–0.39)	0.22 (0.18–0.32)	P = 0.013*
Hemoglobin, g/L	116.5 (103.5–123.3)	116.0 (103.0–121.0)	P = 0.907
Glucose, mM	5.5 (4.8–6.6)	5.4 (4.5–6.0)	P = 0.505
Triacylglycerols, mM	1.75 (1.29–1.56)	1.45 (1.01–1.39)	P = 0.290
HDL cholesterol, mM	1.13 (0.86–1.32)	1.04 (0.98–1.57)	P = 0.816
LDL cholesterol, mM	2.15 (1.69–3.59)	1.76 (1.32–2.56)	P = 0.113
CRP, mg/L	3.2 (2.9–9.1)	2.9 (2.9–12.0)	P = 0.912
Anti diabetic therapy, %	30.8	18.2	P = 0.668
Lipid-lowering therapy, %	45.5	46.2	P = 1.000
RAA, %	45.4	57.7	P = 0.860
Beta blocking agents, %	45.4	42.3	P = 1.000

Continuous data are expressed as median (interquartile range) and compared using Mann & Whitney U test. Categorical data are expressed as the frequency (%) and compared using Chi square test. Abbreviations: CKD, chronic kidney disease, CRP, C-reactive protein, BMI, body mass index, PEW, protein-energy wastng, RAA, renin angiotensin aldosterone.

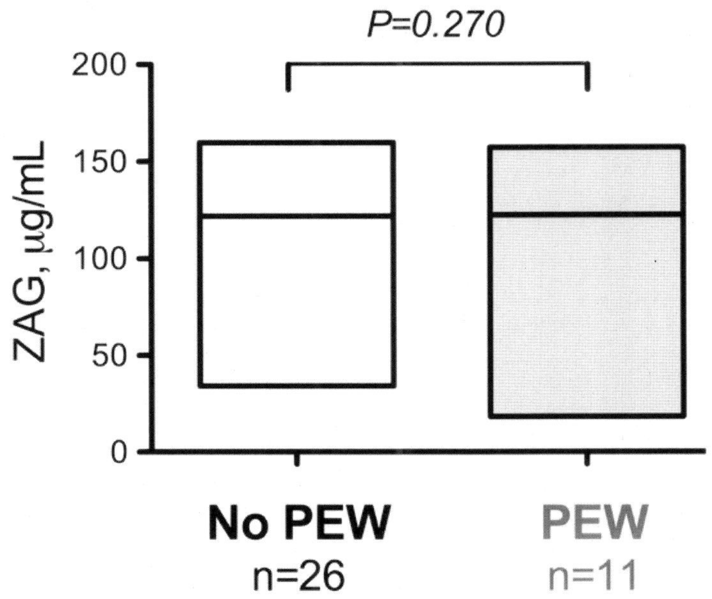

Figure 3. Plasma ZAG concentration in CKD-5 patients with a diagnostic of protein-energy wasting. The boxes indicate the range (i.e. min to max) and the line indicate the median. Note that no difference was found to be significant at the P<0.05 level. Abbreviation: PEW, protein-energy wasting.

Relationships between plasma ZAG Concentration and clinical or biochemical parameters

The results of the univariate correlation analysis are summarized in **Table 3**. In CKD patients stage 1 to 5, plasma ZAG concentrations negatively correlated with plasma protein concentration ($r_s = -0.284$, $P<0.01$), albumin ($r_s = -0.282$, $P<0.05$) hemoglobin ($r_s = -0.264$, $P<0.05$), urea ($r_s = 0.283$, $P<0.01$) and HDL-cholesterol ($r_s = -0.265$, $P<0.05$). Multiple regression analysis (**Table 4**) including urea, protein, haemoglobin and HDL-cholesterol indicated that only urea ($P<0.005$) and HDL-cholesterol ($P<0.05$) were associated with ZAG plasma concentration. Urea, proteins, haemoglobin and HDL-cholesterol explained 41% of the variance of plasma ZAG concentration ($P<0.001$). Out of the 38 patients CKD-5, HD or PD, 11 (29%) presented PEW according to the criterions described in the method section (see patient characteristics in **Table 5**). We therefore re-analyzed the plasma ZAG concentrations of CKD-5, HD and PD patients presenting or not PEW. No significant difference in plasma ZAG concentration was noticed between these 2 sub-groups (**Figure 3**) suggesting that ZAG accumulates in CKD but does not have any relation with PEW. Since ZAG was described to exert potent lipolytic activity, plasma glycerol was measured in a subset of 39 patients (17 non CKD and 22 CKD) as an index of lipolysis. We did not observe any difference in plasma glycerol concentration between HV and CKD patients (**Figure 4**). Additionally, no significant correlation was found between ZAG and plasma glycerol concentration.

Discussion

Zinc alpha2-glycoprotein is a soluble glycoprotein acting as a cachexia factor through its activity on adipose tissue. Few studies [17–18,19] recently demonstrated that plasma ZAG concentration was increased in chronic hemodialysis patients, suggesting a defect of its renal clearance. However, there is no data reporting the actual concentration of ZAG in CKD patients before initiation of renal replacement. We report in the present study that plasma ZAG concentration sharply increases in CKD 5 patients, as in patients with renal replacement therapy, but is poorly correlated to the decrease in GFR.

The CKD stage 5 patients included in the present investigation exhibited a marked elevation of plasma ZAG concentration (2.3-fold, $p<0.005$) that was also observed for PD patients, pre- and post-dialysis HD patients. ZAG accumulation in CKD 5 can result from a decrease of its renal clearance, an increased secretion rate by epithelia cells or both. In a pioneering work, Eckman et al suggested that the kidney could play a key role in the catabolism of ZAG [29]. Because of its rather small molecular weight (43 kDa) and size (Stokes radius 3.24 nm), a fraction of plasma ZAG normally passes through the glomerular membrane after which it is totally reabsorbed at the tubular level. They reported that impairment of renal function, with either decreased GFR or decreased tubular reabsorption, results in a rise in ZAG/creatinine clearance ratio [29]. In the present study, we did not find a strong correlation between plasma ZAG and GFR since ZAG concentration only rises in CKD stage 5. It is well known that glomerular filtration rate estimated by the CKD EPI formula may not accurately reflect renal function [30]. We therefore confirmed these findings with the direct measurement of GFR using the gold standard method of inulin clearance that yielded similar results.

To the best of our knowledge there is only scarce data in the literature regarding the fate of ZAG in the body. The actual turnover rate of ZAG in plasma is to date unknown. Many works documented the increase in plasma concentration of cytokines and hormones such as adiponectin and leptin in ESRD subjects [1–3,31]. Indeed, leptin is cleared from the bloodstream by the kidney through glomerular filtration followed by metabolic degradation in the renal tubules [32]. Normal renal function removes 12% of circulating leptin while in patients with CKD, there is virtually no renal uptake of leptin [32]. If ZAG breakdown occurs as it has been described for leptin in renal tubules, a decrease in GFR and/ or tubular reabsorption could explain the rise of plasma ZAG concentration observed in CKD patients. An alternative hypothesis is that ZAG secretion could be specifically increased in uremic

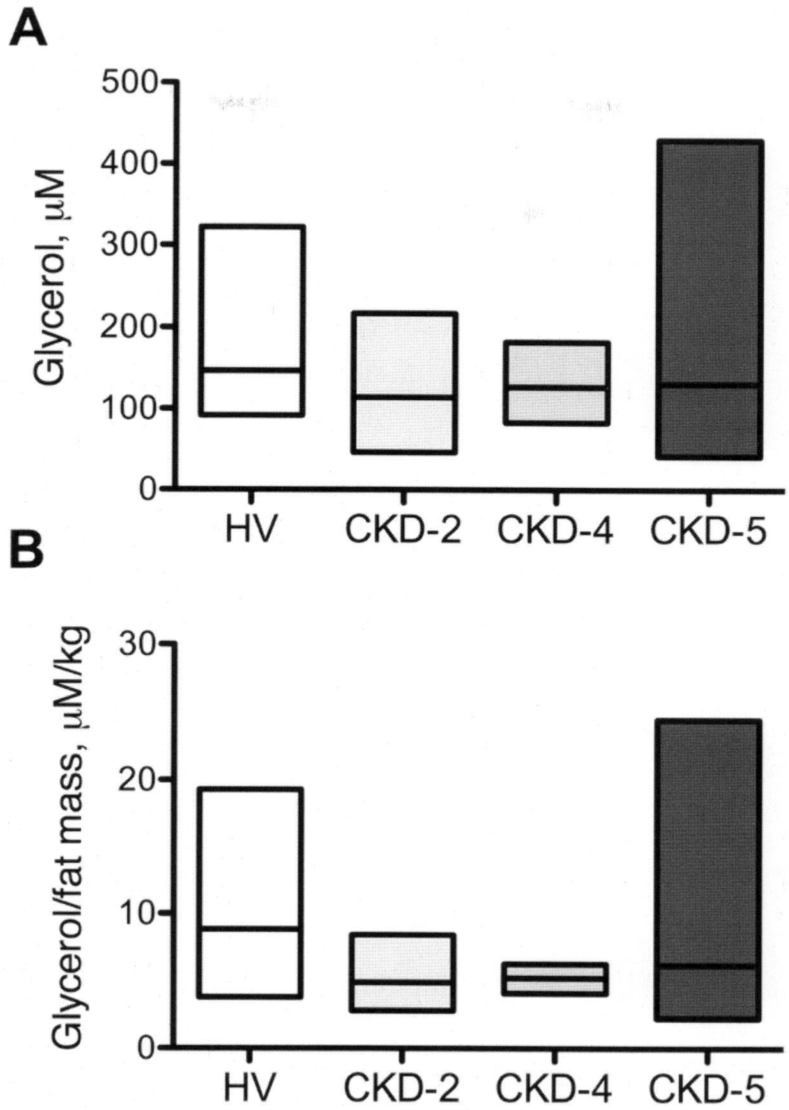

Figure 4. Plasma glycerol concentration in non-CKD and CKD patients. Plasma glycerol was measured as an index of lipolysis in 17 non-CKD patients, 6 CKD-2, 4 CKD-4 and 12 CKD-5 patients. **A)** plasma glycerol concentration **B)** Plasma glycerol, concentration normalized to body fat mass as described in methods. No difference was found to be significant at the $P<0.05$ level using Kruskall & Wallis test.

subjects. Supporting this idea, we recently demonstrated that uremic plasma stimulates ZAG production by adipocytes *in vitro* and that 5/6 nephrectomized rodents exhibited a significantly increased ZAG protein content in WAT associated with a significant decrease in WAT deposition [33]. We further showed that subcutaneous white adipose tissue biopsies from patients with end-stage renal disease exhibited a higher content of ZAG (5.7 folds) than age-matched controls [33], raising the hypothesis that deregulation of ZAG secretion could also contribute to the increased plasma ZAG concentration reported ESRD patients. Although Ryden et al reported that there was no significant contribution of WAT to the circulating levels of ZAG [34], we can hypothesize that an up-regulation of ZAG production by some tissues could contribute to the increased plasma ZAG concentration. We noticed that plasma ZAG concentration increased during HD independently of hemoconcentration (**Figure 3**) suggesting that additional ZAG is secreted in the organism during HD process. Inflammation, shear stress, oxidative stress, catecholamine secretion or lack of biocompatibility, associated with HD could enhance ZAG secretion. In good agreement, we found a significant increase in plasma ZAG concentration in post-HD patient compared to PD patients ($P = 0.004$). This result suggests that the increase in circulating ZAG that occurs during HD process is related to factors that are lacking in PD. Glucocorticoids are described to increase ZAG secretion [35,36]. And cortisol level has been shown to be increased by hemodialysis session [37] suggesting that glucocorticoids could enhance ZAG secretion and contribute to the perdialytic increase in plasma ZAG concentration. In contrast, inflammatory cytokines such as TNF-alpha were shown to decreased ZAG secretion [38–40]. The hemodialysis procedure has been associated with enhanced sympathetic activity (recently reviewed in [41]). When the plasma concentration of norepinephrine (NE) was used as a measure of sympathetic outflow, plasma NE was shown to be increased above values in 45% of hemodialysis patients [42]. Beta agonists were described to increase ZAG secretion in white adipose tissue, sympathetic overactivity/catecholamine release could therefore contribute to the perdialytic increase in ZAG. Tedeschi et al (2012) indeed reported a relationship between plasma norepinephrine and ZAG in heart failure patients [43].

The physiological consequences of increased ZAG concentration in renal failure remain to be elucidated. Axelsson et al [28] reported that plasma glycerol concentration (normalized to body fat mass) was increased in CKD stage 5 suggesting an increased lipolytic activity from their white adipose tissue (WAT). In contrast, we failed to show any increase of plasma glycerol in CKD patients (with or without normalization to body fat mass) or any relationship between plasma glycerol and ZAG concentrations. From our data, there is therefore no line of evidence that ZAG accumulation could contribute to PEW in CKD patients as observed in patients with cancer cachexia. ZAG could however contribute to metabolic disturbances since Philipp et al [17] reported that ZAG serum levels negatively correlated with fasting insulin and homeostasis model assessment of insulin resistance (HOMA-IR). Olofsson et al [44] also noticed that ZAG serum levels correlated with serum levels of cholesterol in healthy subjects. Thus, as described in patients with cancer [45], ZAG could contribute to CKD-associated metabolic disturbances, such as insulin resistance and dyslipidemia.

A negative correlation was found between ZAG concentration and plasma albumin ($r_s = -0.282$, $p<0.05$) and positive correlation between ZAG and urea ($r_s = 0.283$, $P<0.01$). We however failed to find a significant correlation between plasma albumin level and urea ($r_s = -0.005$, $P = 0.953$) that does not support an association with wasting. The significant correlation found between plasma ZAG and urea could be explained by the fact that level of urea reflects the accumulation of many uremic toxins that could stimulate ZAG production in CKD [33]. In an animal study, ZAG was further described to exert antiproliferative activity on epithelial tubular cells after acute kidney injury [46] suggesting that accumulation of ZAG could maybe compound renal dysfunction. Further studies are however needed to decipher the pathophysiological role of ZAG in ESRD.

In conclusion, in this study, we report that ZAG protein accumulates in plasma in ESRD and hemodialysis patients but this increase is not directly correlated to the decrease in GFR. In our study, plasma ZAG concentration was not associated with PEW. The main limitation of the present study is however that it is observational and therefore that it is difficult to make causal inference. Further prospective studies are needed to better elucidate the potential role of ZAG in end-stage renal disease.

Acknowledgments

The authors gratefully acknowledge Dr Bertrand CARE, PhD and Assoc. Prof. Hédi A SOULA, PhD (CarMeN Lab, INSERM U1060, Lyon, France) for mathematical and statistical assistance.

Author Contributions

Conceived and designed the experiments: CCP LK DF COS. Performed the experiments: CCP LK PA MLC EK. Analyzed the data: CCP FGE AHA DF COS. Wrote the paper: CCP FGE COS. Recruited patients and collected clinical data: CCP LK EK AHA FGE. Discussed, reviewed and edited the manuscript: LK PA EK MLC FGE AHA DF.

References

1. Merabet E, Dagogo-Jack S, Coyne DW, Klein S, Santiago JV, et al (1997) Increased plasma leptin concentration in end-stage renal disease. J Clin Endocrinol Metab 82: 847–850.
2. Zoccali C, Mallamaci F, Tripepi G, Benedetto FA, Cutrupi S, et al (2002) Adiponectin, metabolic risk factors, and cardiovascular events among patients with end-stage renal disease. J Am Soc Nephrol 13: 134–141.
3. Guebre-Egziabher F, Bernhard J, Funahashi T, Hadj-Aissa A, Fouque D (2005) Adiponectin in chronic kidney disease is related more to metabolic disturbances than to decline in renal function. Nephrol Dial Transplant 20: 129–134.
4. Stein S, Bachmann A, Lössner U, Kratzsch J, Blüher M, et al (2009) Serum levels of the adipokine FGF21 depend on renal function. Diabetes Care 32: 126–128.
5. Ziegelmeier M, Bachmann A, Seeger J, Lossner U, Kratzsch J, et al (2007) Serum levels of adipokine retinol-binding protein-4 in relation to renal function. Diabetes Care 30: 2588–2592.
6. Pfau D, Bachmann A, Lössner U, Kratzsch J, Blüher M, et al (2010) Serum levels of the adipokine chemerin in relation to renal function. Diabetes Care 33: 171–173.
7. Burgi W, Schmid K (1961) Preparation and properties of Zn-alpha 2-glycoprotein of normal human plasma. J Biol Chem 236: 1066–1074.
8. Sánchez LM, Chirino AJ, Bjorkman Pj (1999) Crystal structure of human ZAG, a fat-depleting factor related to MHC molecules. Science 283: 1914–1919.
9. Russell ST, Zimmerman TP, Domin BA, Tisdale MJ (2004) Induction of lipolysis in vitro and loss of body fat in vivo by zinc-alpha2-glycoprotein. Biochim Biophys Acta 1636: 59–68.
10. Bing C (2011) Lipid mobilization in cachexia: mechanisms and mediators. Curr Opin Support Palliat Care 5: 356–360.
11. Tada T, Ohkubo I, Niwa M, Sasaki M, Tateyama H, et al (1991) Immunohistochemical localization of Zn-alpha 2-glycoprotein in normal human tissues. J Histochem Cytochem 39: 1221–1226.
12. Hirai K, Hussey HJ, Barber MD, Price SA, Tisdale MJ (1998) Biological evaluation of a lipid-mobilizing factor isolated from the urine of cancer patients. Cancer Res 58: 2359–2365.
13. Russell ST, Tisdale MJ (2012) Role of β-adrenergic receptors in the anti-obesity and anti-diabetic effects of zinc-α2-glycoprotien (ZAG). Biochim Biophys Acta 1821: 590–599.
14. Russell ST, Hirai K, Tisdale MJ (2002) Role of beta3-adrenergic receptors in the action of a tumour lipid mobilizing factor. Br J Cancer 86: 424–428.
15. Gong F-Y, Zhang S-J, Deng J-Y, Zhu H-J, Pan H, et al (2009) Zinc-alpha2-glycoprotein is involved in regulation of body weight through inhibition of lipogenic enzymes in adipose tissue. Int J Obes (Lond) 33: 1023–1030.
16. Sanders PM, Tisdale MJ (2004) Effect of zinc-alpha2-glycoprotein (ZAG) on expression of uncoupling proteins in skeletal muscle and adipose tissue. Cancer Lett 212: 71–81.
17. Philipp A, Kralisch S, Bachmann A, Lossner U, Kratzsch J, et al (2011) Serum levels of the adipokine zinc-α2-glycoprotein are increased in chronic hemodialysis. Metab Clin Exp 60: 669–672.
18. Leal VO, Lobo JC, Stockler-Pinto MB, Farage NE, Abdalla DSP, et al (2012) Is zinc-α2-glycoprotein a cardiovascular protective factor for patients undergoing hemodialysis? Clin Chim Acta 413: 616–619.
19. Leal VO, Lobo JC, Stockler-Pinto MB, Farage NE, Velarde GC, et al (2012) Zinc-α2-glycoprotein: is there association between this new adipokine and body composition in hemodialysis patients? Ren Fail 34: 1062–1067.
20. Levey AS, Bosch JP, Lewis JB, Greene T, Rogers N, et al (1999) A more accurate method to estimate glomerular filtration rate from serum creatinine: a new prediction equation. Modification of Diet in Renal Disease Study Group. Ann Intern Med 130: 461–470.
21. Stevens LA, Schmid CH, Greene T, Zhang YL, Beck GJ, et al (2010) Comparative performance of the CKD Epidemiology Collaboration (CKD-EPI) and the Modification of Diet in Renal Disease (MDRD) Study equations for estimating GFR levels above 60 mL/min/1.73 m2. Am J Kidney Dis 56: 486–495.
22. K/DOQI clinical practice guidelines for chronic kidney disease: evaluation, classification, and stratification (2002). Am J Kidney Dis 39: S1–266.
23. Deurenberg P, Weststrate JA, Seidell JC (1991) Body mass index as a measure of body fatness: age- and sex-specific prediction formulas. Br J Nutr 65: 105–114.
24. Fouque D, Kalantar-Zadeh K, Kopple J, Cano N, Chauveau P, et al (2008) A proposed nomenclature and diagnostic criteria for protein-energy wasting in acute and chronic kidney disease. Kidney Int 73: 391–398.
25. Buron F, Hadj-Aissa A, Dubourg L, Morelon E, Steghens J-P, et al (2011) Estimating glomerular filtration rate in kidney transplant recipients: performance over time of four creatinine-based formulas. Transplantation 92: 1005–1011.
26. Dubourg L, Hadj-Aïssa A, Ferrier B (2010) Adaptation of an enzymatic polyfructosan assay to clinical practice. Anal Biochem 405: 266–268.
27. Bradford MM (1976) A rapid and sensitive method for the quantitation of microgram quantities of protein utilizing the principle of protein-dye binding. Anal Biochem 72: 248–254.
28. Axelsson J, Aström G, Sjölin E, Qureshi AR, Lorente-Cebrián S, et al (2011) Uraemic sera stimulate lipolysis in human adipocytes: role of perilipin. Nephrol Dial Transplant 26: 2485–2491.
29. Ekman R, Johansson BG, Ravnskov U (1976) Renal handling of Zn-alpha2-glycoprotein as compared with that of albumin and the retinol-binding protein. J Clin Invest 57: 945–954.
30. Cirillo M, Anastasio P, De Santo NG (2005) Relationship of gender, age, and body mass index to errors in predicted kidney function. Nephrol Dial Transplant 20: 1791–1798.

31. Guebre-Egziabher F, Bernhard J, Geelen G, Malvoisin E, Hadj-Aissa A, et al (2005) Leptin, adiponectin, and ghrelin dysregulation in chronic kidney disease. J Ren Nutr 15: 116–120.
32. Cumin F, Baum HP, de Gasparo M, Levens N (1997) Removal of endogenous leptin from the circulation by the kidney. Int J Obes Relat Metab Disord 21: 495–504.
33. Pelletier CC, Koppe L, Croze ML, Kalbacher E, Vella RE, et al (2013) White adipose tissue overproduces the lipid-mobilizing factor zinc α2-glycoprotein in chronic kidney disease. Kidney Int 83: 878–886.
34. Rydén M, Agustsson T, Andersson J, Bolinder J, Toft E, et al (2012) Adipose zinc-α2-glycoprotein is a catabolic marker in cancer and noncancerous states. J Intern Med 271: 414–420.
35. Russell ST, Tisdale MJ (2005) The role of glucocorticoids in the induction of zinc-alpha2-glycoprotein expression in adipose tissue in cancer cachexia. Br J Cancer 92: 876–881.
36. Hassan MI, Waheed A, Yadav S, Singh TP, Ahmad F (2008) Zinc alpha 2-glycoprotein: a multidisciplinary protein. Mol Cancer Res 6: 892–906.
37. Letizia C, Mazzaferro S, De Ciocchis A, Cerci S, Morabito S, et al (1996) Effects of haemodialysis session on plasma beta-endorphin, ACTH and cortisol in patients with end-stage renal disease. Scand J Urol Nephrol 30: 399–402.
38. Bao Y, Bing C, Hunter L, Jenkins JR, Wabitsch M, et al (2005) Zinc-alpha2-glycoprotein, a lipid mobilizing factor, is expressed and secreted by human (SGBS) adipocytes. FEBS Lett 579: 41–47.
39. Gao D, Trayhurn P, Bing C (2010) Macrophage-secreted factors inhibit ZAG expression and secretion by human adipocytes. Mol Cell Endocrinol 325: 135–142.
40. Mracek T, Gao D, Tzanavari T, Bao Y, Xiao X, et al (2010) Downregulation of zinc-{alpha}2-glycoprotein in adipose tissue and liver of obese ob/ob mice and by tumour necrosis factor-alpha in adipocytes. J Endocrinol 204: 165–172.
41. Rubinger D, Backenroth R, Sapoznikov D (2013) Sympathetic nervous system function and dysfunction in chronic hemodialysis patients. Semin Dial 26: 333–343.
42. Zoccali C, Mallamaci F, Parlongo S, Cutrupi S, Benedetto FA, et al (2002) Plasma norepinephrine predicts survival and incident cardiovascular events in patients with end-stage renal disease. Circulation 105: 1354–1359.
43. Tedeschi S, Pilotti E, Parenti E, Vicini V, Coghi P, et al (2012) Serum adipokine zinc α2-glycoprotein and lipolysis in cachectic and noncachectic heart failure patients: relationship with neurohormonal and inflammatory biomarkers. Metab Clin Exp 61: 37–42.
44. Olofsson LE, Olsson B, Lystig T, Jacobson P, Jernås M, et al (2010) Preliminary report: Zn-alpha2-glycoprotein genotype and serum levels are associated with serum lipids. Metab Clin Exp 59: 1316–1318.
45. Mracek T, Stephens NA, Gao D, Bao Y, Ross JA, et al (2011) Enhanced ZAG production by subcutaneous adipose tissue is linked to weight loss in gastrointestinal cancer patients. Br J Cancer 104: 441–447.
46. Schmitt R, Marlier A, Cantley LG (2008) Zag expression during aging suppresses proliferation after kidney injury. J Am Soc Nephrol 19: 2375–2383.

12

A Meta-Analysis of Mortality in End-Stage Renal Disease Patients Receiving Implantable Cardioverter Defibrillators (ICDs)

Tien-Hsing Chen[1,2]*, Hung-Ta Wo[1], Po-Cheng Chang[1], Chun-Chieh Wang[1], Ming-Shien Wen[1], Chung-Chuan Chou[1]

1 Department of Cardiology, Chang-Gung Memorial Hospital, Linko, Taiwan, **2** Department of Cardiology, Chang-Gung Memorial Hospital, Xiamen, China, Chang Gung University College of Medicine, Kaohsiung, Taiwan

Abstract

Data on the effectiveness of implantable implantable cardioverter defibrillators (ICDs) with respect to reducing mortality in patients with chronic kidney disease (CKD) and end-stage renal disease (ESRD) are lacking. The purpose of this meta-analysis was to compare the mortality of patients with ESRD who have received and not received an ICD. A search was conducted on January 31, 2013 of Medline, Cochrane, EMBASE, and Google Scholar. Studies were selected for inclusion based on the following criteria. 1) Randomized controlled trial. 2) ESRD patients with heart failure. 3) Device therapy (ICD, CRT-defibrillator [CRT-D]) used to treat heart failure. 4) Primary outcome is survival analysis. 5) Retrospective study if survival analysis was performed. The primary outcome was overall survival (OS), and the secondary outcome was 2-year survival. Odds ratios (ORs) with 95% confidence intervals (CI) were calculated, and a χ^2-based test of homogeneity was performed. Three studies were included in the analysis. The combined OR for OS was 2.245 (95% CI 1.871 to 2.685, $P<0.001$), indicating that patients with an ICD had a significantly higher OS than those without an ICD. The combined OR for 2-year survival was 2.312 (95% CI 1.921 to 2.784, $P<0.001$), indicating that patients with an ICD had a significantly higher 2-year survival rate than those without an ICD. The use of ICD in patients with ESRD is associated with an increase in the OS and the 2-year survival rate.

Editor: Thomas Berger, Medical University Innsbruck, Austria

Funding: The authors have no support or funding to report.

Competing Interests: The authors have declared that no competing interests exist.

* Email: skyheart0826@gmail.com

Introduction

The number of patients with end-stage renal disease (ESRD) receiving dialysis is increasing worldwide. It is estimated that in the United States alone more than 2 million people will be receiving dialysis by 2020 [1]. Patients receiving dialysis have approximately 8-fold greater all-cause mortality as compared to the general population, with cardiovascular disease accounting for approximately 43% of the mortality [1,2]. Individuals with chronic kidney disease (CKD) are at a markedly increased risk of death from cardiovascular causes, including sudden cardiac death (SCD) due to arrhythmias [3,4].

Implantable implantable cardioverter defibrillators (ICDs) have been shown to reduce mortality and the risk of SCD in patients with severe heart failure as a result of ischemic and nonischemic cardiomyopathy, and in patients with arrhythmias [5–8]. However, data on the effectiveness of ICDs in patients with CKD and ESRD are lacking, and sometimes conflicting [9–14]. This is in part because patients with renal disease were often excluded from ICD studies [15,16]. It has been proposed that the survival advantage of ICDs in patients with renal disease as suggested by some studies may be negated as a result of comorbidities such as anemia, diabetes, and hypertension in these patients [15].

Tompkins et al. [17] reported that bleeding and ICD device-related complications were significantly more common in patients with ESRD. Alsheikh-Ali et al. [18] categorized patients by New York Heart Association (NYHA) class and estimated glomerular filtration rate (eGFR). The analysis suggested that the benefits of ICDs in patients with more advanced disease may be limited by the greater frequency of deaths due to causes other than arrhythmias. Bilchick et al. [19] found that CKD was associated with increased mortality rate in patients undergoing ICD implantation for the primary prevention of SCD (hazard ratio [HR] = 2.33). Similarly, a meta-analysis performed by Korantzopoulos et al. [20] in 2009 suggested that CKD is associated with increased mortality in patients who receive ICD therapy.

Given the increase in mortality rate of patients with CKD and ESRD, and the paucity of data regarding the outcome of ICD implantation in this group of patients, further investigation is warranted. The purpose of this study was to perform a meta-analysis to compare the mortality of ESRD patients receiving device therapy (ICD) with those who did not received device therapy.

Methods

Literature Search Strategy

A search was conducted of Medline, Cochrane, EMBASE, and Google Scholar using combinations of the search terms: chronic kidney disease, end-stage renal disease, dialysis, heart failure,

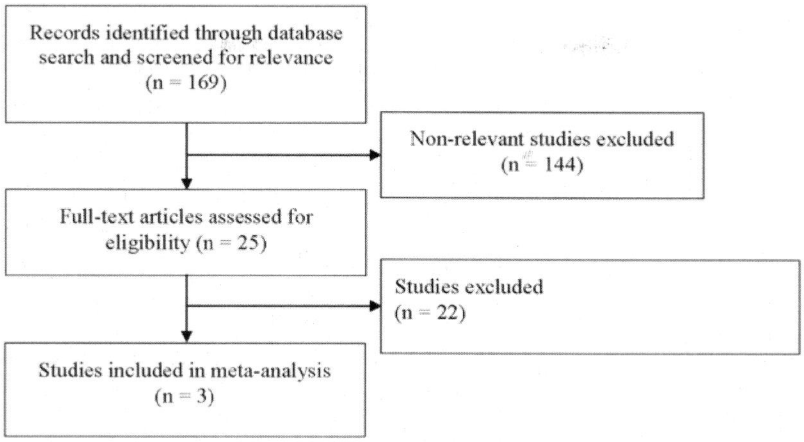

Figure 1. Flow diagram of study selection.

mortality, survival, device therapy, implantable cardioverter-defibrillator/ICD, cardiac resynchronization therapy defibrillator/CRT-D. The search date was January 31, 2013. Each publication was carefully examined, including the names of all authors, to avoid duplication of data.

Selection criteria

Studies were selected for analysis based on the following inclusion criteria. 1) Randomized controlled trial. 2) ESRD patients with heart failure. 3) Device therapy (ICD, CRT-defibrillator [CRT-D]) used to treat heart failure. 4) Primary outcome is survival analysis. 5) Retrospective study if the survival analysis was performed. Exclusion criteria for this analysis were as follows. 1) Study participants were not ESRD patients. 2) The study was not designed for ESRD patients with/without device therapy. 3) Studies that investigated if ESRD is risk factor/predictor of the prognosis for heart failure patients with device therapy (ICD, CRT-D). 4) Survival rate was not part of the analysis.

Data extraction

Studies were identified by two independent reviewers using the aforementioned search strategy. A third reviewer was consulted when there was uncertainty regarding eligibility.

The following data were extracted from studies that met the inclusion criteria: name of the first author, year of publication, study design, number of participants in each treatment group, participants' age and gender, overall survival (OS) rate, median OS time, 2-year survival rate, rate of comorbidities related to heart failure

Data analysis

The primary outcome was OS, and the secondary outcome was 2-year survival rate. The primary outcome, OS was used to evaluate treatment efficacy. Odds ratios (ORs) with 95% confidence intervals (CI) were calculated for binary outcomes and compared between patients with and without device therapy. A χ^2-based test of homogeneity was performed, and the inconsistency index (I^2) statistic was determined. If I^2 was >50% or >75%, the trials were considered to be heterogeneous or highly heterogeneous, respectively. An $I^2<25\%$ indicated homogeneity among the studies. When heterogeneity existed between studies ($I^2>50\%$) a random-effects model was calculated. Otherwise, fixed-effects models were calculated. Pooled summary statistics for ORs of the individual studies were reported. Sensitivity analysis was performed based on the leave-one-out approach. Publication bias analysis was not performed because the number of studies was too few to detect an asymmetric funnel [21]. All analyses were performed using Comprehensive Meta-Analysis statistical software, version 2.0 (Biostat, Englewood, NJ). A value of $P<0.05$ was considered to indicate statistical significance.

Results

Literature search

After applying the inclusion and exclusion criteria, a total of 3 studies were included in this meta-analysis [22–24]. A flowchart of the study selection is shown in Figure 1. The 3 studies included in the meta-analysis are summarized in Table 1. Two studies included only ESRD patients [22,24], whereas one study included both CKD and ESRD patients [23]. For the purposes of this analysis, only data of ESRD patients from the study by Khan et al. [23] were used in the analysis.

Study characteristics and clinical outcomes

The ORs for OS of the 3 studies ranged from 1.164 to 2.317 (Fig. 2). There was homogeneity in the combined OR among the 3 studies ($Q=1.976$, $I^2=0\%$, $P=0.372$); therefore a fixed-effects model of analysis was used. Examination of the combined OR revealed a significant difference between ICD and no-ICD therapy. The combined OR was 2.245 (95% CI 1.871 to 2.685, $P<0.001$), indicating that patients with an ICD had a significantly higher OS than those without ICD therapy.

The ORs for the 2-year survival rate of the 3 studies ranged from 1.688 to 3.500 (Fig. 3). There was homogeneity in the 2-year survival rate between the studies when the data were pooled for analysis ($Q=1.067$, $I^2=0.00\%$, $P=0.586$); therefore a fixed-effects model of analysis was used. Examination of the combined OR revealed a significant difference between ICD and no-ICD therapy. The combined OR was 2.312 (95% CI 1.921 to 2.784, $P<0.001$), indicating that patients with an ICD had a significantly higher 2-year survival rate than those without ICD therapy.

Table 1. Summary of the 3 studies included in the meta-analysis.

1st Author	Year of Publication	Study Type	Group	Number of Patients	Age (y)	Sex (male)	OS rate	Median OS time	2-year Survival Rate	Rate of heart failure-related comorbidity
Hiremath[22]	2010	Retrospective	ICD	50	70.3±10.0	84%	60%	8 years	84%	ND
			Non-ICD	50	69.9±9.7	84%	42%	3.1 years	60%	ND
Khan*[23]	2010	Retrospective	ICD	14	64±12	93%	35.7%	ND	55%	100%
			Non-ICD	31	63±15	68%	32.3%	ND	42%	100%
Herzog[24]	2005	Retrospective	ICD	460	63.1±13.1	57%	51%	ND	53%	60.4%
			Non-ICD	5582	63.1±14.2	46%	31%	ND	33%	55.8%

Age data are presented as mean ± standard deviation.
OS, overall survival; ND, not derived.
*Only data of patients with end-stage renal disease were used in the analysis.

Figure 4 shows the results of the meta-analysis of OS with one study removed in turn. The results indicate that the direction and magnitude of the combined estimates did not have a large variation. This finding indicates that the results of the meta-analysis exhibits good reliability.

Discussion

The results of this meta-analysis indicate that the use of ICD in patients with ESRD is associated with an increase in the OS and the 2-year survival rate.

Data from prospective, randomized studies examining the effect of ICD therapy in patients with CKD/ESRD are lacking, and thus there is no general consensus on the use of device therapy in these patients. An ongoing trial (ICD2 trail) is randomizing dialysis patients, regardless of left ventricular function, to receive ICD therapy or not; however, study results are not expected until 2017 [25]. Most small retrospective studies have failed to show that patients with CKD or ESRD derive any survival benefit from ICD implantation [9,11–14]. A subgroup analysis of data from the MADIT-II study showed a survival benefit of ICD implantation in patients with an eGFR >35 mL/min, but not in those in which the eGFR was ≤35 mL/min [9,10]. Studies have reported a 1-year survival of patients with CKD with ICD implantation of 61% [12] and median survival of 6.3 years [14], and a median survival of ESRD patients with an ICD of 1.1 to 3.2 years [12,13].

Three studies were included in this meta-analysis. Herzog et al. [24] examined dialysis patients hospitalized from 1996 to 2001 for ventricular fibrillation/cardiac arrest who received ICD implantation within 30 day of admission. In the cohort, there were 460 patients (7.6%) who received ICD implantation and 5,582 (92.4%) that did not. The estimated 1-, 2-, 3-, 4-, and 5-year survival rates in the ICD group were 71%, 53%, 36%, 25%, and 22%, respectively, and in the no-ICD group were 49%, 33%, 23%, 16%, and 12% ($P<0.0001$). Analysis of the data showed that ICD implantation was independently associated with a 42% reduction in the risk of death (relative risk [RR] = 0.58). The authors concluded that in addition to the improvement in survival, ICD therapy was underutilized in this population. Khan et al. [23] studied 78 patients with moderate to severe CKD (45 patients with ESRD) with a left ventricular ejection fraction (LVEF) ≤35%, of whom 32 had an ICD, for an average follow-up of 2.7±2.3 years. In the group receiving dialysis (n = 45), ICD placement did not impact survival. In the patients with CKD who were not receiving dialysis (n = 33), survival was significantly better in patients with an ICD (2-year survival 80% vs. 54%, $P = 0.027$) after adjustment for sex, race, GFR, digoxin use, and presence of coronary disease, heart failure, or hypertension (OR = 0.23). Hiremath et al. [22] compared the outcomes of 50 patients with ESRD who had received ICD implantation with 50 patients with ESRD who did not have ICDs. The mean LVEF was similar between the 2 groups (approximately 29%). Median OS in the full cohort was 4.7 years with 20 deaths in the ICD group and 29 deaths in the no-ICD group. The median survival in the ICD group was 8.0 years, and 3.1 years in the no-ICD group. The multivariable analysis indicated that all-cause mortality was significantly less in the ICD group than in the no-ICD group (HR = 0.40).

The benefits of ICDs have been shown to be reduced in patients with advanced renal disease [9,10,26]. Furthermore, the complication rate of ICD implantation is higher in patients with ESRD than in patients without ESRD [27-29]. Patients with CKD have increased mortality from non-cardiac causes, cardiac non-SCD, SCD, and infections and while ICD implantation may decrease the risk of SCD it will not affect the risk of death from non-cardiac

Study (year)	Statistics for each study					Relative weight
	Odds ratio	Lower limit	Upper limit	*Z* value	*P* value	
Hiremath (2010)	2.071	0.933	4.597	1.790	0.073	5.25
Khan (2010)	1.164	0.449	3.013	0.312	0.755	3.69
Herzog (2005)	2.317	1.913	2.805	8.603	0.000	91.06
Total (Fixed)	2.245	1.871	2.695	8.680	0.000	

Q value=1.976, I-square=0%, *P* value=0.372

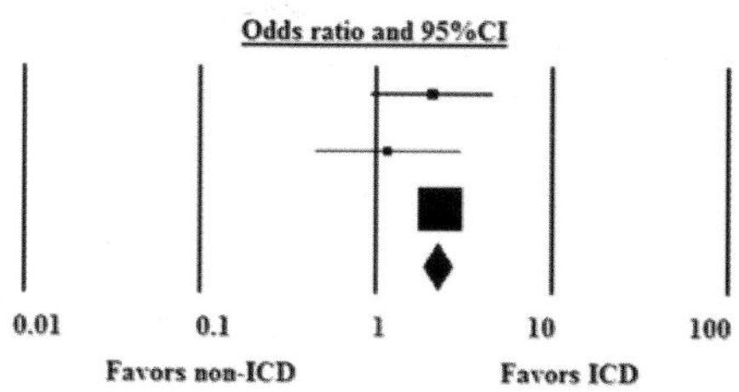

Figure 2. Forest plot of odds ratios (ORs) with 95% confidence intervals (CIs) for overall survival (OS) of the included studies. P<0.05 indicates a statistically significant difference.

causes such as infection, and there is increased risk of complications from device placement. The risk of SCD increases as renal function deteriorates, and this increase in risk is multifactorial in origin. The incidences of coronary artery disease, left ventricular hypertrophy, and left ventricular dysfunction are all increased in patients with ESRD. In addition, dialysis can lead to the development of interstitial fibrosis, endothelial dysfunction, and atheroma formation, which all can worsen the aforementioned conditions. The above highlight the competing causes of death in patients with CKD; conditions that are not affected by ICD placement.

The difference in survival between patients receiving dialysis and those not receiving dialysis as reported by Khan et al. [23] may be because in CKD patients ventricular arrhythmias can be terminated with ICD therapy [30]. In patients receiving dialysis, however, comorbidities which are not affected by ICD therapy may be present [31,32]. It has also been suggested that the defibrillation threshold may be increased in patients with ESRD, and thus optimal conversion of arrhythmias may not occur [33]. Despite the use of an ICD, the OS of patients with CKD is lower as compared to patients with normal kidney function [34]. On the other hand, CKD patients with an ICD still benefit from improved survival with ICD placement. For example, Amin et al. [35] showed in patients with stage 1 and 2 CKD, ICD implantation reduces mortality; however, in more advanced stages of CKD the benefit is less significant and age dependent. The authors attribute this finding to the fact that patients with more advanced CKD having a higher procedural risk and decreased life expectancy. When average procedural mortality was taken into account, the authors found that ICD implantation is favored at <80 years of age for stage 3 CKD, at <75 years of age for stage 4 CKD, and at <65 years of age for ESRD.

ICD therapy appears to be underutilized in patients with CKD, although patients with ESRD are at high risk for ventricular arrhythmias and SCD. Herzog et al. [24] reported a 42% reduction in overall death risk in dialysis patients, yet only 8% of eligible patients received an ICD. Other data [1] and studies [36] have also indicated that the use of ICD therapy in patients with CKD and ESRD is low. Therapies such as aspirin, beta blockers, and angiotensin converting enzyme inhibitors are used less frequently in patients with more severe renal failure [37], and thus physicians may be less likely to use other therapies (i.e., ICD) as well. There is also the concern of increased complications of ICDs in patients with renal failure [17]. Finally, as previously discussed; there is lack of data from well-designed clinical studies for this group of patients. Interestingly, the 2013 American College of Cardiology Foundation (ACCF) guidelines for the use of implantable ICDs and CRT include patients with CKD and ESRD [38].

The primary limitation of this meta-analysis is the small number of included studies. However, the inclusion criteria were strict by design to include only studies that were high quality and relevant to addressing the research question. In addition, only patients with ESRD were included. It remains to be determined if the results are also applicable to patients with CKD, but not ESRD.

Conclusions

In conclusion, the results of this meta-analysis indicate that the use of an ICD in patients with ESRD is associated with an increase in the OS and the 2-year survival rate. Based on these results, the use of ICD therapy in these patients is warranted.

Study (year)	Statistics for each study					Relative weight
	Odds ratio	Lower limit	Upper limit	*Z* value	*P* value	
Hiremath (2010)	3.500	1.361	8.999	2.600	0.009	3.86
Khan (2010)	1.688	0.473	6.021	0.807	0.420	2.13
Herzog (2005)	2.289	1.891	2.772	8.482	0.000	94.01
Total (Fixed)	2.312	1.921	2.784	8.853	0.000	

Q value=1.067, I-square=0%, *P* value=0.586

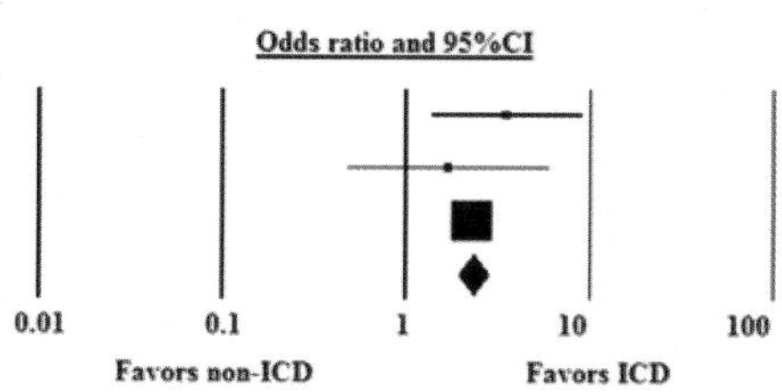

Figure 3. Forest plot of odds ratios (ORs) with 95% confidence intervals (CIs) for 2-year survival of the included studies. P<0.05 indicates a statistically significant difference.

Removed Study (year)	Statistics with study removed				
	Odds ratio	Lower limit	Upper limit	Z value	P value
Hiremath S (2010)	2.255	1.870	2.721	8.495	0.000
Khan (2010)	2.303	1.912	2.774	8.783	0.000
Herzog (2005)	1.633	0.886	3.008	1.573	0.116
Total (Fixed)	2.245	1.871	2.695	8.680	0.000

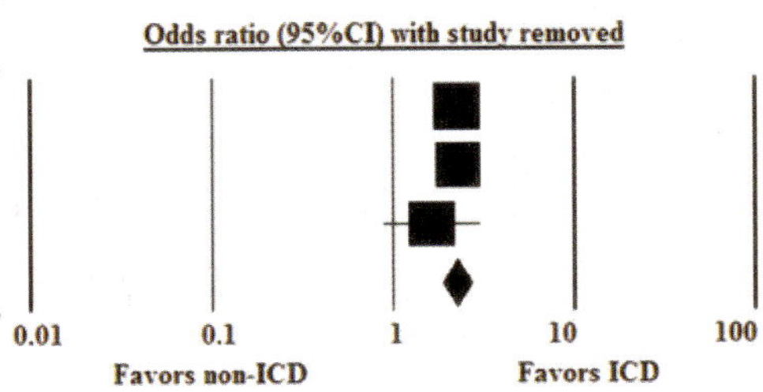

Figure 4. Sensitivity analysis for the influence of individual studies on pooled estimates by the leave-one-out approach for overall survival (OS). Data are presented as odds ratio (OR) with the 95% confidence interval (CI). $P<0.05$ indicates a statistically significant difference.

Author Contributions

Conceived and designed the experiments: T-HC C-CW. Performed the experiments: T-HC H-TW P-CC. Analyzed the data: T-HC M-SW C-CC. Contributed reagents/materials/analysis tools: T-HC. Wrote the paper: T-HC.

References

1. US Renal Data System 2012 Annual Data Report: Atlas of Chronic Kidney Disease and End-Stage Renal Disease in the United States. Bethesda, National Institutes of Health, National Institute of Diabetes and Digestive and Kidney Diseases, 2012. Available at: http://www.usrds.org/atlas.aspx. Accessed August 1, 2013.
2. Herzog CA, Mangrum JM, Passman R (2008) Sudden cardiac death and dialysis patients. Semin Dial 21:300–307.
3. Eknoyan G, Beck GJ, Cheung AK, Daugirdas JT, Greene T, et al. (2002) Effect of dialysis dose and membrane flux in maintenance hemodialysis. N Engl J Med 347:2010–2019.
4. Wanner C, Krane V, Marz W, Olschewski M, Mann JF, et al. (2005) Atorvastatin in patients with type 2 diabetes mellitus undergoing hemodialysis. N Engl J Med 53:238–248.
5. Bardy GH, Lee KL, Mark DB, Poole JE, Packer DL, et al. (2005) Amiodarone or an implantable cardioverter-defibrillator for congestive heart failure. N Engl J Med 352:225–237.
6. Kadish A, Dyer A, Daubert JP, Quigg R, Estes NA, et al. (2004) Prophylactic defibrillator implantation in patients with nonischemic dilated cardiomyopathy. N Engl J Med 350:2151–2158.
7. Moss AJ, Hall WJ, Cannom DS, Daubert JP, Higgins SL, et al. (1996) Improved survival with an implanted defibrillator in patients with coronary disease at high risk for ventricular arrhythmia. Multicenter Automatic Defibrillator Implantation Trial Investigators. N Engl J Med 335:1933–1940.
8. Moss AJ, Zareba W, Hall WJ, Klein H, Wilber DJ, et al. (2002) Prophylactic implantation of a defibrillator in patients with myocardial infarction and reduced ejection fraction. N Engl J Med 346:877–883.
9. Goldenberg I, Moss AJ, McNitt S, Zareba W, Andrews ML, et al. (2006) Relations among renal function, risk of sudden cardiac death, and benefit of the implanted cardiac defibrillator in patients with ischemic left ventricular dysfunction. Am J Cardiol 98:485–490.
10. (2002) K/DOQI Clinical Practice Guidelines for Chronic Kidney Disease: Evaluation, Classification, and Stratification Part 4. Definition and classification of stages of chronic kidney disease. Am J Kidney Dis 39:S46–S75.
11. Chen-Scarabelli C, Scarabelli TM (2007) Chronic renal insufficiency is an independent predictor of mortality in implantable cardioverterdefibrillator recipients. Pacing Clin Electrophysiol 30:371–376.
12. Cuculich PS, Sanchez JM, Kerzner R, Greenberg SL, Sengupta J, et al. (2007) Poor prognosis for patients with chronic kidney disease despite ICD therapy for the primary prevention of sudden death. Pacing Clin Electrophysiol 30:207–213.
13. Robin J, Weinberg K, Tiongson J, Carnethon M, Reddy M, et al. (2006) Renal dialysis as a risk factor for appropriate therapies and mortality in implantable cardioverter-defibrillator recipients. Heart Rhythm 3:1196–1201.
14. Turakhia MP, Varosy PD, Lee K, Tseng ZH, Lee R, et al. (2007) Impact of renal function on survival in patients with implantable cardioverter- defibrillators. Pacing Clin Electrophysiol 30:377–384.
15. O'Shaughnessy MM, Lappin DW, Reddan DN (2012) Sudden cardiac death in dialysis: do current guidelines for implantable cardioverter defibrillator therapy apply to patients with end-stage kidney disease? Semin Dial 25:272–276.
16. Cannizzaro LA, Piccini JP, Patel UD, Hernandez AF (2011) Device therapy in heart failure patients with chronic kidney disease. J Am Coll Cardiol 58:889–896.
17. Tompkins C, McLean R, Cheng A, Brinker JA, Marine JE, et al. (2011) End-stage renal disease predicts complications in pacemaker and ICD implants. J Cardiovasc Electrophysiol 22:1099–1104.
18. Alsheikh-Ali AA, Trikalinos TA, Ruthazer R, Terrin N, Wong JB, et al. (2011) Risk of arrhythmic and nonarrhythmic death in patients with heart failure and chronic kidney disease Am Heart J 161:204–209.e1.
19. Bilchick KC, Stukenborg GJ, Kamath S, Cheng A (2012) Prediction of mortality in clinical practice for medicare patients undergoing defibrillator implantation for primary prevention of sudden cardiac death. J Am Coll Cardiol 60:1647–155.
20. Korantzopoulos P, Liu T, Li L, Goudevenos JA, Li G (2009) Implantable cardioverter defibrillator therapy in chronic kidney disease: a meta-analysis. Europace 11:1469–175.
21. Sutton AJ, Duval SJ, Tweedie RL, Abrams KR, Jones DR (2000) Empirical assessment of effect of publication bias on meta-analyses. BMJ 320:1574–1577.
22. Hiremath S, Punnam SR, Brar SS, Goyal SK, Gardiner JC, et al. (2010) Implantable defibrillators improve survival in end-stage renal disease: results from a multi-center registry. Am J Nephrol 32:305–310.
23. Khan F, Adelstein E, Saba S (2010) Implantable cardioverter defibrillators confer survival benefit in patients with renal insufficiency but not in dialysis-dependent patients. J Interv Card Electrophysiol 28:117–123.
24. Herzog CA, Li S, Weinhandl ED, Strief JW, Collins AJ, et al. (2005) Survival of dialysis patients after cardiac arrest and the impact of implantable cardioverter defibrillators. Kidney Int 68:818–825.
25. de Bie MK, Lekkerkerker JC, van Dam B, Gaasbeek A, van Buren M, et al. (2008) Prevention of sudden cardiac death: rationale and design of the Implantable Cardioverter Defibrillators in Dialysis Patients (ICD2) Trial – a prospective pilot study. Curr Med Res Opin 24:2151–2157.
26. Williams ES, Shah SH, Piccini JP, Sun AY, Koontz JI, et al. (2011) Predictors of mortality in patients with chronic kidney disease and an implantable defibrillator: an EPGEN substudy. Europace 13:1717–122.
27. Aggarwal A, Wang Y, Rumsfeld JS, Curtis JP, Heidenreich PA (2009) Clinical characteristics and in-hospital outcome of patients with end-stage renal disease on dialysis referred for implantable cardioverter-defibrillator implantation. Heart Rhythm 6:1565–1571.
28. Dasgupta A, Montalvo J, Medendorp S, Lloyd-Jones DM, Ghossein C, et al. (2007) Increased complication rates of cardiac rhythm management devices in ESRD patients. Am J Kidney Dis 49:656–663.
29. Teruya TH, Abou-Zamzam AM Jr, Limm W, Wong L, Wong L (2003) Symptomatic subclavian vein stenosis and occlusion in hemodialysis patients with transvenous pacemakers. Ann Vasc Surg 17:526–529.
30. Hreybe H, Ezzeddine R, Bedi M, Barrington W, Bazaz R, et al. (2006) Renal insufficiency predicts the time to first appropriate defibrillator shock. Am Heart J151:852–856.
31. Grothe C, Belasco A, Bettencourt A, Diccini S, Vianna L, et al. (2009) Lethality of endocarditis due to S. aureus among patients on hemodialysis. Nephrol Nurs J 36: 613–619.
32. Thomson P, Stirling C, Traynor J, Morris S, Mactier R (2010) A prospective

observational study of catheter-related bacteraemia and thrombosis in a haemodialysis cohort: Univariate and multivariate analyses of risk association. Nephrol Dial Transplant 25:1596–1604.

33. Wase A, Basit A, Nazir R, Jamal A, Shah S, et al. (2004) Impact of chronic kidney disease upon survival among implantable cardioverter-defibrillator recipients. J Interv Card Electrophysiol 11:199–204.
34. Cuculich PS, Sánchez JM, Kerzner R, Greenberg SL, Sengupta J, et al. (2007) Poor prognosis for patients with chronic kidney disease despite ICD therapy for the primary prevention of sudden death. Pacing Clin Electrophysiol 30:207–213.
35. Amin MS, Fox AD, Kalahasty G, Shepard RK, Wood MA, et al. (2008) Benefit of primary prevention implantable cardioverter-defibrillators in the setting of chronic kidney disease: a decision model analysis. J Cardiovasc Electrophysiol 19:1275–1280.
36. Voigt A, Ezzeddine R, Barrington W, Obiaha-Ngwu O, Ganz LI, et al. (2004) Utilization of implantable cardioverter-defibrillators in survivors of cardiac arrest in the United States from 1996 to 2001. J AmColl Cardiol 44:855–858.
37. Berger AK, Duval S, Krumholz HM (2003) Aspirin, beta-blocker, and angiotensin-converting enzyme inhibitor therapy in patients with end-stage renal disease and an acute myocardial infarction. J Am Coll Cardiol 42:201–208.
38. Russo AM, Stainback RF, Bailey SR, Epstein AE, Heidenreich PA, et al. (2013) ACCF/HRS/AHA/ASE/HFSA/SCAI/SCCT/SCMR 2013 appropriate use criteria for implantable cardioverter-defibrillators and cardiac resynchronization therapy: a report of the American College of Cardiology Foundation appropriate use criteria task force, Heart Rhythm Society, American Heart Association, American Society of Echocardiography, Heart Failure Society of America, Society for Cardiovascular Angiography and Interventions, Society of Cardiovascular Computed Tomography, and Society for Cardiovascular Magnetic Resonance. J Am Coll Cardiol 61:1318–1368.

P Wave Dispersion and Maximum P Wave Duration Are Associated with Renal Outcomes in Chronic Kidney Disease

Jiun-Chi Huang[1,3], Shu-Yi Wei[6,7], Szu-Chia Chen[1,3,4], Jer-Ming Chang[1,3,4], Chi-Chih Hung[1,4], Ho-Ming Su[2,3,4]*, Shang-Jyh Hwang[1,5], Hung-Chun Chen[1,5]

1 Division of Nephrology, Department of Internal Medicine, Kaohsiung Medical University Hospital, Kaohsiung Medical University, Kaohsiung, Taiwan, **2** Division of Cardiology, Department of Internal Medicine, Kaohsiung Medical University Hospital, Kaohsiung Medical University, Kaohsiung, Taiwan, **3** Department of Internal Medicine, Kaohsiung Municipal Hsiao-Kang Hospital, Kaohsiung Medical University, Kaohsiung, Taiwan, **4** Faculty of Medicine, College of Medicine, Kaohsiung Medical University, Kaohsiung, Taiwan, **5** Faculty of Renal Care, College of Medicine, Kaohsiung Medical University, Kaohsiung, Taiwan, **6** Department of Internal Medicine, Kaohsiung Municipal United Hospital, Kaohsiung, Taiwan, **7** Yuh-Ing Junior College of Health Care & Management, Kaohsiung, Taiwan

Abstract

P wave parameters measured by 12-lead electrocardiogram (ECG) are commonly used as a noninvasive tool to evaluate left atrial enlargement. This study was designed to assess whether P wave parameters were associated with renal outcomes in chronic kidney disease (CKD) patients. This longitudinal study enrolled 439 patients with CKD stages 3–5. Renal end points were defined as the commencement of dialysis or death. Change in renal function was measured using the estimated glomerular filtration rate (eGFR) slope. We measured two ECG P wave parameters corrected for heart rate, i.e., corrected P wave dispersion and corrected maximum P wave duration. The values of P wave dispersion and maximum P wave duration were 88.8±21.7 ms and 153.3±21.7 ms, respectively. During the follow-up period (mean, 25.2 months), 95 patients (21.6%) started hemodialysis and 30 deaths (6.8%) were recorded. Multivariate Cox regression analysis identified that increased P wave dispersion [hazard ratio (HR), 1.020; 95% confidence interval (CI), 1.009–1.032; $P<0.001$] and maximum P wave duration (HR, 1.013; 95% CI, 1.003–1.024; $P=0.012$) were associated with progression to renal end points. Furthermore, increased P wave dispersion (unstandardized coefficient $\beta=-0.016$; $P=0.037$) and maximum P wave duration (unstandardized coefficient $\beta=-0.014$; $P=0.040$) were negatively associated with the eGFR slope. We demonstrated that increased P wave dispersion and maximum P wave duration were associated with progression to the renal end points of dialysis or death and faster renal function decline in CKD patients. Screening CKD patients on the basis of P wave dispersion and maximum P wave duration may help identify patients at high risk for worse renal outcomes.

Editor: Martin H. de Borst, University Medical Center Groningen and University of Groningen, Netherlands

Funding: The authors have no support or funding to report.

Competing Interests: The authors have declared that no competing interests exist.

* Email: cobeshm@seed.net.tw

Introduction

Both traditional risk factors, such as hypertension, diabetes, and dyslipidemia, and non-traditional risk factors, such as cardiovascular disease contribute to the risk of progressive renal function loss [1,2]. Faster renal function decline has been significantly associated with high cardiovascular morbidity and mortality in patients with chronic kidney disease (CKD) [3,4]. It is therefore essential to identify those CKD patients with faster renal function decline in order to initiate aggressive treatment interventions and improve survival.

Echocardiographic measures of left ventricular function and structure as well as left atrial size have been reported to predict adverse renal outcomes [5–7]. This implies that patients with cardiac dysfunction and left atrial enlargement might have faster renal function decline and adverse renal outcome. However, structural and functional abnormalities of the heart are frequently evaluated using echocardiography, which may preclude its application if echocardiography or experienced operators are not available. 12-lead electrocardiogram (ECG) is a simple, inexpensive, and noninvasive clinical tool to assess structural and functional abnormalities of the heart [8]. P wave parameters measured by 12-lead ECG have been reported to be useful tools for assessing the risk of left atrial enlargement, left ventricular hypertrophy (LVH), and left ventricular diastolic dysfunction [9–17]. Furthermore, P wave parameters have been independently associated with increased risk of both atrial fibrillation and recurrent transient ischemic attacks [18,19]. However, there are limited studies evaluating whether P wave parameters are associated with progression to end-stage renal disease, decline in renal function, or death in CKD patients. The aim of this study in a cohort of patients with CKD stages 3–5 were to assess whether P wave parameters were associated with progression to the commencement of dialysis or death and whether these parameters were associated with the rate of renal function decline.

Subjects and Methods

Ethics statement

The study protocol was approved by the Institutional Review Board of the Kaohsiung Medical University Hospital (KMUH-IRB-20130305). Informed consent was obtained in written form from patients and all clinical investigations were conducted according to the principles of the Declaration of Helsinki. The patients gave consent for the publication of the clinical details.

Study patients

The study was conducted in a regional hospital in southern Taiwan. From January 2007 to May 2010, we consecutively enrolled 505 pre-dialysis patients with CKD stages 3–5, according to the National Kidney Foundation-Kidney Disease Outcomes Quality Initiative (K/DOQI) guidelines [20] from our Outpatient Department of Internal Medicine. Patients with evidence of kidney damage lasting for more than 3 months were classified as CKD stages 3, 4, and 5, on the basis of an estimated glomerular filtration rate (eGFR) level (mL/min/1.73 m^2) of 30–59, 15–29, and <15 respectively. Patients with atrial fibrillation, significant mitral valve disease, and inadequate ECG image visualization were excluded. Twenty-seven patients with less than three eGFR measurements during the follow-up period were excluded. Those patients who died (n = 9) or entered dialysis therapy (n = 30) within 3 months after enrollment were also excluded to avoid incomplete observation of changes in renal function. Finally, 439 patients (mean age, 66.0±12.0 years, 274 males) were included in this study.

Assessment of P wave parameters

A standard 12-lead surface ECG (25-mm/s, 1-mV/cm, and 100-Hz) was performed in all study patients. An image analysis software system (Image Tool 3.0) was used to perform quantitative assessments. We assessed the correlation of two P wave parameters, corrected P wave dispersion and corrected maximum P wave duration, with progression to dialysis or death and decline in renal function. P wave dispersion was calculated as the difference between maximum and minimum P wave duration [21]. Both the P wave measurements were corrected for heart rate using Bazett's formula, i.e., the corrected P wave parameters were equal to P wave parameters/$(RR)^{1/2}$ [22].

Definition of LVH

LVH was defined as Sokolow-Lyon voltage criteria via 12-lead ECG (sum of the amplitude of the S wave in lead V_1 and the R wave in lead V_5 or V_6 greater than 3.5 mV) [23].

Collection of demographic, medical, and laboratory data

Demographic and medical data including age, gender, smoking history (ever *versus* never), and comorbid conditions were obtained from medical records or patient interviews. The body mass index (BMI) was calculated as the ratio of weight in kilograms divided by square of height in meters. Laboratory data were measured from fasting blood samples using an autoanalyzer (Roche Diagnostics GmbH, D-68298 Mannheim COBAS Integra 400). Serum creatinine was measured by the compensated Jaffé (kinetic alkaline picrate) method in a Roche/Integra 400 Analyzer (Roche Diagnostics, Mannheim, Germany) using a calibrator traceable to isotope-dilution mass spectrometry [24]. The value of eGFR was calculated using the 4-variable equation in the Modification of Diet in Renal Disease (MDRD) study [25]. Dipsticks (Hema-Combistix, Bayer Diagnostics) were used to evaluate proteinuria. A dipstick test result of 1+ or more was defined as positive. Blood and urine samples were obtained within 1 month of study enrollment.

Definition of renal end points

Renal end points were defined as the commencement of dialysis or death. In patients reaching study end points, renal function data were censored at the start of renal replacement therapy or death. The remaining patients were followed until March 2011. The commencement of dialysis was determined according to the regulations of the National Health Insurance for dialysis therapy based on laboratory data, nutritional status, and uremic symptoms and signs. Renal end points-free survival was defined as the time from study enrollment to the commencement of dialysis or death.

Assessment of the rate of renal function decline

The rate of renal function decline was assessed by the eGFR slope, defined as the regression coefficient between eGFR and time in units of mL/min/1.73 m^2/year. At least three eGFR measurements following 12-lead ECG examination were required to estimate the eGFR slope. Faster renal function decline was defined as a greater value of decline in the eGFR slope.

Reproducibility

Thirty-five patients were randomly selected for evaluation of the interobserver variability of P wave dispersion and maximum P wave duration measurements by two independent observers. The same measurement was repeated twice, 1 week apart, to calculate the intraobserver variability. Mean percent error was calculated as the absolute difference divided by the average of the two observations.

Statistical analysis

Statistical analysis was performed using SPSS version 17.0 (SPSS Inc., Chicago, IL, USA) for Windows. Data were expressed as percentages, mean ± standard deviation, mean ± standard error of the mean for the eGFR slope, or median (25th–75th percentile) for triglycerides and number of serum creatinine measurements. The differences between groups were analyzed using the Chi-square test for categorical variables and using the independent *t*-test for continuous variables. Time to renal end points and covariates of risk factors were modeled using the Cox proportional hazards model. The survival curve for renal end points was derived using Kaplan–Meier analysis. Linear regression analysis was used to identify the factors associated with the eGFR slope. The association of P wave parameters with renal end points and the eGFR slope was assessed using a modified stepwise procedure in two modeling steps. The first model consisted of age and sex. In the second model, clinical and biochemical risk factors were added. A significant improvement in model prediction was found by calculating the improvement in −2 log likelihood or adjusted R square values. A difference was considered significant if the P value was less than 0.05.

Results

Four hundred and thirty-nine non-dialyzed CKD patients were included. The mean age was 66.0±12.0 years and there were 274 males and 165 females. The average number of serum creatinine measurements during the follow-up period was eight (25th–75th percentile: 6–12). The values of P wave dispersion and maximum P wave duration were 88.8±21.7 ms and 153.3±21.7 ms, respectively. The eGFR slope for all patients was −1.60±0.15 mL/min/1.73 m^2/year. The underlying etiology of CKD in our patients was diabetic kidney disease in 232 (52.8%), non-diabetic glomerular diseases in 128 (29.2%), tubulointerstitial diseases in 46 (10.5%), hypertension in 23 (5.2%), and other diseases in 10 (2.3%). The clinical characteristics of patients with and without renal end points are shown in Table 1. Compared with patients without renal end points, patients with renal end points were found to have higher P wave dispersion, higher maximum P wave duration, higher prevalence of LVH, females outnumbered males, higher prevalence of diabetes mellitus (DM) and hypertension, higher systolic blood pressure, lower BMI, more advanced CKD stage, lower albumin, higher fasting glucose, lower hemoglobin, lower baseline eGFR, higher calcium-phosphorus product, higher uric acid, and higher prevalence of proteinuria.

Risk of progression to renal end points

The mean follow-up period was 25.2±12.7 months (range, 3.3–50.0 months). During the follow-up period, ninety-five patients (21.6%) started hemodialysis and 30 deaths were recorded in the 439 patients. Causes of death included fatal cardiovascular events (n = 13), infectious disease (n = 13), and other (n = 4). Among the 13 fatal cardiovascular events, 4 were myocardial infarction, 3 were pulseless electrical activity, 3 were ventricular fibrillation and 3 were heart failure. The multivariate Cox proportional hazards regression analyses of P wave dispersion and maximum P wave duration for renal end points are shown in Table 2. In the first analysis, P wave dispersion was associated with progression to renal end points in the multivariable model after adjustment for age and sex [hazard ratio (HR), 1.024; 95% confidence interval (CI), 1.014–1.034; $P<0.001$). The relationship remained significant after further adjustment for smoking, DM, hypertension, coronary artery disease, cerebrovascular disease, LVH, systolic and diastolic blood pressure, BMI, albumin, fasting glucose, log triglycerides, total cholesterol, hemoglobin, baseline eGFR, calcium-phosphorus product, uric acid, and proteinuria (HR, 1.020; 95% CI, 1.009–1.032; $P<0.001$). In the second analysis, there was also a significant prognostic value of maximum P wave duration in relation to renal end points (HR, 1.013; 95% CI, 1.003–1.024; $P=0.012$) in multivariate analysis after adjustment for demographic, clinical, and biochemical factors. In addition, the commencement of dialysis and death were competitive risks for composite end points in this study. We also performed competing risk analysis and found that P wave dispersion ($P=0.046$) remained significantly associated with progression to dialysis after multivariate analysis, but maximum P wave duration did not ($P=0.14$).

Table 1. Comparison of baseline characteristics between patients with and without renal end points.

Characteristics	All patients (n = 439)	Patients without renal end points (n = 314)	Patients with renal end points (n = 125)	*P*
Electrocardiogram data				-
P wave dispersion (ms)	90 (76.5–100.8)	88.5 (73.7–97)	93.9 (84.1–105.9)	<0.001
Maximum P wave duration (ms)	154 (140.4–166.8)	151.5 (138–164)	157.3 (144.7–171.7)	0.002
LVH (%)	4.3	2.9	8.0	0.017
Age (year)	67.6 (57.1–76.3)	65.9 (56.9–76.2)	67.5 (57.6–76.4)	0.768
Male gender (%)	62.4	65.9	53.6	0.016
Smoking history (%)	31.0	30.6	32.0	0.770
Diabetes mellitus (%)	56.7	52.9	66.4	0.010
Hypertension (%)	82.2	79.0	90.4	0.005
Coronary artery disease (%)	11.6	10.8	13.6	0.413
Cerebrovascular disease (%)	15.3	14.0	18.7	0.249
Systolic BP (mmHg)	140 (129.5–153)	140 (126.5–150)	149 (130–163.8)	<0.001
Diastolic BP (mmHg)	80 (70–89)	80 (70–88)	79 (69–90)	0.397
Body mass index (kg/m^2)	25.2 (22.8–27.5)	25.4 (23.3–27.7)	24.4 (22.1–26.9)	0.020
CKD stage				<0.001
Stage 3 (%)	38.7	51.0	8.0	
Stage 4 (%)	31.4	36.0	20.0	
Stage 5 (%)	29.8	13.1	72.0	
Laboratory parameters				
Albumin (g/dL)	4.1 (3.9–4.2)	4.1 (4.0–4.3)	3.8 (3.5–4.1)	<0.001
Fasting glucose (mg/dL)	107 (93–139)	104 (91–138)	114 (97–142.8)	0.024
Triglyceride (mg/dL)	138.5 (97–201)	139 (99–199.5)	135 (96–221.75)	0.449
Total cholesterol (mg/dL)	189 (162–220)	188 (162–219)	190.5 (160.8–230.3)	0.693
Hemoglobin (g/dL)	11.6 (9.8–13.3)	12.2 (10.7–13.7)	9.6 (8.5–10.9)	<0.001
Baseline eGFR (mL/min/1.73 m^2)	25.2 (13.1–37.4)	30.4 (21.3–40.7)	11.1 (7.6–16.6)	<0.001
Calcium-phosphorus product (mg^2/dL^2)	37.4 (32.7–42.4)	36.2 (31.8–40.7)	41.9 (34.7–48.3)	<0.001
Uric acid (mg/dL)	7.9 (6.8–9.3)	7.8 (6.8–9.1)	8.4 (6.9–10.1)	0.001
Proteinuria (%)	65.2	55.1	90.4	<0.001

Abbreviations: LVH, left ventricular hypertrophy; BP, blood pressure; CKD, chronic kidney disease; eGFR, estimated glomerular filtration rate.

Table 2. Predictors of progression to renal end points of dialysis or death using Cox proportional hazards model.

	P wave dispersion		Maximum P wave duration	
	HR (95% CI)	*P*	HR (95% CI)	*P*
Unadjusted	1.024 (1.014–1.034)	<0.001	1.016 (1.008–1.025)	<0.001
Age and sex adjusted	1.024 (1.014–1.034)	<0.001	1.017 (1.008–1.025)	<0.001
Multivariate adjusted	1.020 (1.009–1.032)	<0.001	1.013 (1.003–1.024)	0.012

Values express as hazard ratios (HR) and 95% confidence interval (CI).
Multivariate model: adjusted for age, sex, smoking history, diabetes mellitus, hypertension, and coronary artery disease, cerebrovascular disease, left ventricular hypertrophy, systolic and diastolic blood pressure, body mass index, albumin, fasting glucose, log triglycerides, total cholesterol, hemoglobin, baseline eGFR, calcium-phosphorus product, uric acid, and proteinuria.

Figure 1 illustrates the Kaplan-Meier curves for renal end points-free survival in patients subdivided according to the tertiles of P wave dispersion (<83.2, 83.3–96.0, >96.0 ms; log-rank $P<0.001$). The unadjusted HR for tertile 2 *versus* tertile 1 was 1.834 (95% CI, 1.113–3.023, $P=0.017$) and for tertile 3 *versus* tertile 1 was 2.842 (95% CI, 1.173–4.555, $P<0.001$). Figure 2 illustrates the Kaplan–Meier curves for renal end points-free survival in patients subdivided according to the tertiles of maximum P wave duration (<145.0, 145.0–162.0, >162.0 ms; log-rank $P=0.003$). The unadjusted HR for tertile 2 *versus* tertile 1 was 1.385 (95% CI, 0.861–2.226, $P=0.179$) and for tertile 3 *versus* tertile 1 was 2.115 (95% CI, 1.350–3.314, $P=0.001$).

The addition of P wave dispersion and maximum P wave duration to a basic model (including age, sex, DM, hypertension, coronary artery disease, cerebrovascular disease, LVH, systolic and diastolic blood pressure, BMI, albumin, fasting glucose, log triglycerides, total cholesterol, hemoglobin, baseline eGFR, calcium-phosphorus product, uric acid, and proteinuria) significantly improved the prediction value for renal end points (difference in the −2 log likelihood value: 13.531, $P<0.001$ and 6.335, $P=0.012$, respectively).

Patients with CKD stage 5 (n = 131) were at an extremely high risk of reaching end-stage renal disease in a very short term. Therefore, we performed subgroup analysis after excluding those patients. The results were similar, i.e., patients with increased P wave dispersion (HR, 1.060; 95% CI, 1.031–1.089; $P<0.001$) and maximum P wave duration (HR, 1.048; 95% CI, 1.022–1.074; $P<0.001$) were significantly associated with progression to renal end points after multiple adjustments for demographic, clinical, and biochemical factors.

Risk of faster renal function decline

Table 3 shows the determinants of the eGFR slope. In the first multivariate analysis, P wave dispersion was negatively associated with the eGFR slope after adjustment for age and sex (unstandardized coefficient $\beta=-0.020$, $P=0.015$) and, further adjustment for smoking, DM, hypertension, coronary artery disease, cerebrovascular disease, LVH, systolic and diastolic blood pressure, BMI,

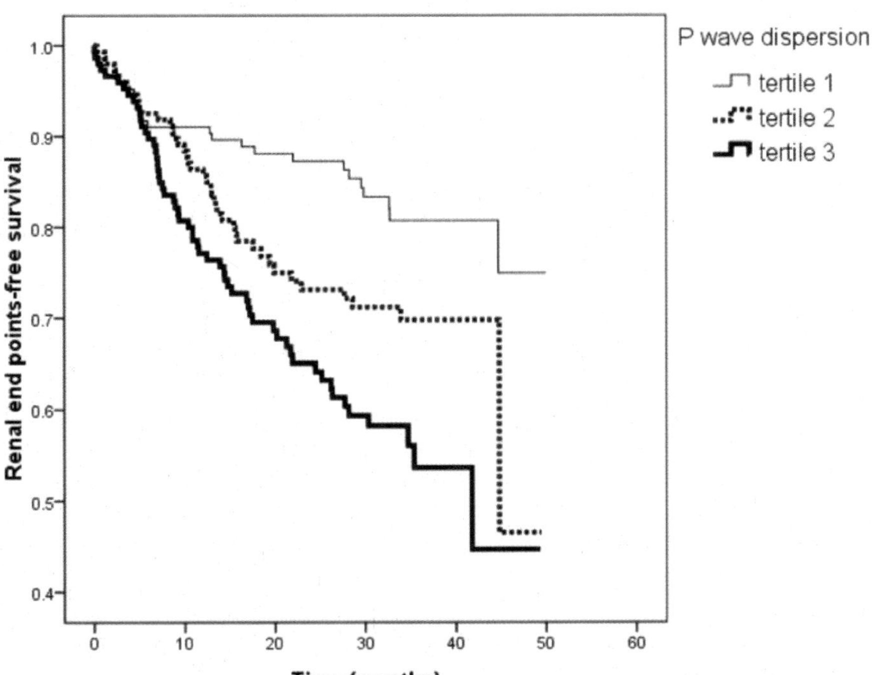

Figure 1. Kaplan-Meier analysis of renal end points-free survival according to the tertiles of P wave dispersion (log-rank $P<0.001$). The group with the highest two tertiles had a worse renal end points-free survival than that with the lowest tertile of P wave dispersion.

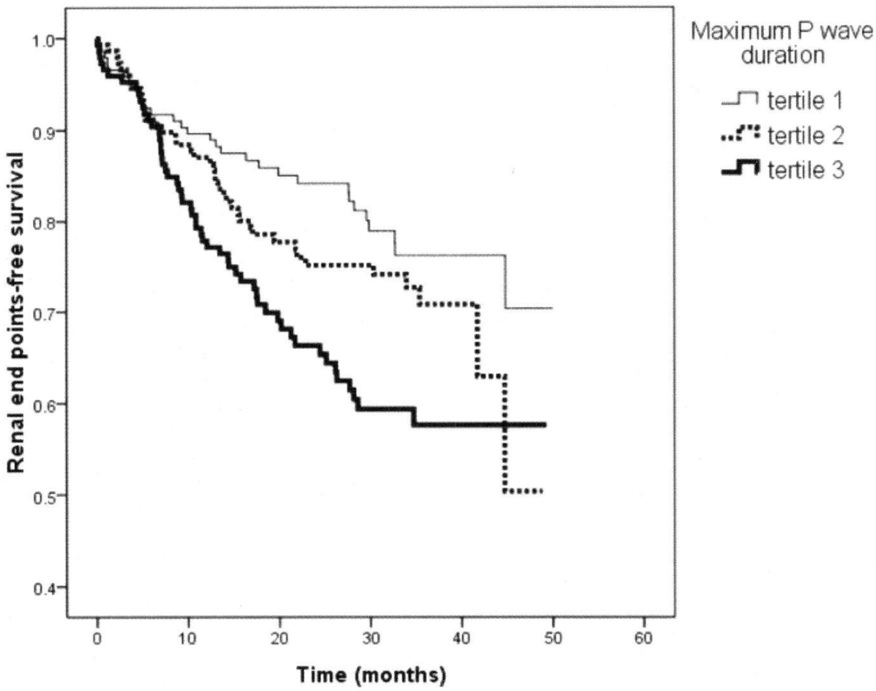

Figure 2. Kaplan-Meier analysis of renal end points-free survival according to the tertiles of maximum P wave duration (log-rank *P* = 0.003). The group with the highest tertile had a worse renal end points-free survival than that with the lowest tertile of maximum P wave duration.

albumin, fasting glucose, log triglycerides, total cholesterol, hemoglobin, baseline eGFR, calcium-phosphorus product, uric acid, and proteinuria (unstandardized coefficient $\beta = -0.016$, $P = 0.037$). In the second multivariate analysis, maximum P wave duration was also negatively associated with the eGFR slope (unstandardized coefficient $\beta = -0.014$, $P = 0.040$) after adjustment for demographic, clinical, and biochemical factors.

The addition of P wave dispersion and maximum P wave duration to a basic model (including age, sex, DM, hypertension, coronary artery disease, cerebrovascular disease, LVH, systolic and diastolic blood pressure, BMI, albumin, fasting glucose, log triglycerides, total cholesterol, hemoglobin, baseline eGFR, calcium-phosphorus product, uric acid, and proteinuria) significantly improved the prediction value for renal function decline (difference in the adjusted R square value: 0.01, $P = 0.037$ and 0.009, $P = 0.040$, respectively).

Determinants of P wave dispersion and maximum P wave duration

In univariate analysis, P wave dispersion had a significant positive correlation with DM (unstandardized coefficient $\beta = 4.366$, $P = 0.020$). In addition, maximum P wave duration had a significant positive correlation with DM, fasting glucose, log triglycerides, and proteinuria. In multivariate analysis, maximum P wave duration was independently correlated with DM (unstandardized coefficient $\beta = 5.635$, $P = 0.015$).

Reproducibility of P wave measurements

The intraobserver mean percent errors for P wave dispersion and maximum P wave duration measurements were 8.6±7.8% and 4.0±3.0%, respectively. The interobserver mean percent errors for P wave dispersion and maximum P wave duration measurements were 10.4±7.3% and 5.0±3.5%, respectively.

Table 3. Determinants of the eGFR slope.

	P wave dispersion		Maximum P wave duration	
	unstandardized coefficient β (95% CI)	*P*	unstandardized coefficient β (95% CI)	*P*
Unadjusted	−0.020 (−0.036, −0.004)	0.017	−0.021 (−0.036, −0.007)	0.003
Age and sex adjusted	−0.020 (−0.036, −0.004)	0.015	−0.021 (−0.035, −0.006)	0.005
Multivariate adjusted	−0.016 (−0.031, 0)	0.037	−0.014 (−0.028, 0)	0.040

Abbreviations: eGFR, estimated glomerular filtration rate.
Values expressed as unstandardized coefficient β and 95% confidence interval (CI).
Multivariate model: adjusted for age, sex, smoking history, diabetes mellitus, hypertension, and coronary artery disease, cerebrovascular disease, left ventricular hypertrophy, systolic and diastolic blood pressure, body mass index, albumin, fasting glucose, log triglycerides, total cholesterol, hemoglobin, baseline eGFR, calcium-phosphorus product, uric acid, and proteinuria.

Discussion

In the present study, we evaluated the association of P wave parameters with kidney disease progression to dialysis or death and the rate of renal function decline in patients with CKD stages 3–5. Increased P wave dispersion and maximum P wave duration were associated with progression to dialysis or death and faster renal function decline. Furthermore, the addition of P wave dispersion and maximum P wave duration to a model of clinical features significantly improved the prediction value for progression to dialysis or death and faster renal function decline.

Paoletti et al. [26] studied the role of LVH in the prediction of progression to dialysis in 144 patients with CKD stages 3–4. They found that increased left ventricular mass index was independently associated with CKD progression to dialysis and with combined end points of dialysis or death. Shlipak et al. [27] demonstrated that decreased left ventricular systolic function was an independent predictor of rapid renal function decline (defined as an annual eGFR loss >3 mL/min/1.73 m^2) in the elderly. We recently reported that concentric LVH, increased left atrial diameter, and decreased left ventricular ejection fraction were associated with adverse renal outcomes [5,6]. This suggested that patients with structural or functional abnormalities of the heart might have a faster renal function decline and worse renal outcomes. The mechanisms of faster renal function decline in patients with cardiac abnormalities are multi-factorial, including chronic renal hypoperfusion, subclinical inflammation, endothelial dysfunction, accelerated atherosclerosis, increased renal vascular resistance, systemic neurohormonal factors, pharmacotherapies, and anemia [28,29]. Previous studies have reported that increased P wave dispersion and maximum P wave duration were correlated with left atrial enlargement, LVH, and left ventricular systolic and diastolic dysfunction [12,16,17]. Furthermore, we have previously reported that increased P wave dispersion and maximum P wave duration were associated with progression to the renal end point of ≥ 25% decline in eGFR in 166 patients with a mean eGFR of 57.0±17.2 mL/min/1.73 m^2 [17]. The present study also revealed that increased P wave dispersion and maximum P wave duration were associated with progression to dialysis or death and faster renal function decline in CKD stages 3–5 patients with a mean eGFR of 26.1±14.2 mL/min/1.73 m^2.

Diabetic nephropathy is one of the major complications of DM and one of the major causes of renal replacement therapy [30]. Cardiovascular disease is the leading cause of morbidity and mortality in patients with diabetic nephropathy [31]. This amplified cardiovascular risk is partly attributable to increased traditional risk factors among diabetic patients, along with the non-traditional risk factors among CKD patients, such as proteinuria, fluid retention, anemia, oxidative stress, and the presence of a chronic inflammatory state [31–33]. There are a number of hemodynamic and metabolic disturbances that affect the structure and function of the heart in patients with diabetic nephropathy. The major factors that contribute to further heart failure in diabetic patients include cardiac microangiopathy, neuropathy of the cardiac autonomic nervous system, disturbed metabolism, and fatty degeneration of the myocardium [34]. These patients were reported to have a high prevalence of decreased left ventricular systolic function and increased left ventricular mass index due to pressure and volume overload [35–37]. Our results demonstrated a significant association between P wave parameters and DM, which might be partially explained by ischemic or non-ischemic diabetic cardiomyopathy.

Our study had some limitations. The number and interval of serum creatinine measurements varied in each patient. We therefore excluded patients with less than three eGFR measurements during the follow-up period and those patients with a follow-up period of <3 months, in order to decrease the chance of not completely observing a change in renal function. In addition, P wave parameters cannot completely replace echocardiography because they do not provide a comprehensive examination of the heart. However, they can provide a simple and inexpensive method for detecting patients at risk of left atrial enlargement and left ventricular diastolic and systolic dysfunction.

In conclusion, our results demonstrated that increases in P wave dispersion and maximum P wave duration were independently associated with progression to the renal end points of dialysis or death and faster renal function decline in patients with CKD stages 3–5. Beyond conventional clinical features, measurement of P wave dispersion and maximum P wave duration offers an extra benefit in predicting the renal end points of dialysis or death and faster renal function decline. Screening CKD patients on the basis of P wave dispersion and maximum P wave duration, measured by 12-lead ECG, may help identify patients at high risk for worse renal outcomes.

Author Contributions

Conceived and designed the experiments: J-CH H-MS. Performed the experiments: J-CH S-YW S-CC H-MS. Analyzed the data: J-CH S-YW S-CC J-MC. Contributed reagents/materials/analysis tools: J-CH S-YW S-CC J-MC C-CH H-MS S-JH H-CC. Wrote the paper: J-CH H-MS.

References

1. Go AS, Chertow GM, Fan D, McCulloch CE, Hsu CY (2004) Chronic kidney disease and the risks of death, cardiovascular events, and hospitalization. N Engl J Med 351: 1296–1305.
2. Tonelli M, Wiebe N, Culleton B, House A, Rabbat C, et al. (2006) Chronic kidney disease and mortality risk: a systematic review. J Am Soc Nephrol 17: 2034–2047.
3. Kovesdy CP (2010) Rate of kidney function decline associates with increased risk of death. J J Am Soc Nephrol 21: 1814–1816.
4. Perkins RM, Bucaloiu ID, Kirchner HL, Ashouian N, Hartle JE, et al. (2011) GFR decline and mortality risk among patients with chronic kidney disease. Clin J Am Soc Nephrol 6: 1879–1886.
5. Chen SC, Lin TH, Hsu PC, Chang JM, Lee CS, et al. (2011) Impaired left ventricular systolic function and increased brachial-ankle pulse-wave velocity are independently associated with rapid renal function progression. Hypertens Res 34: 1052–1058.
6. Chen SC, Su HM, Hung CC, Chang JM, Liu WC, et al. (2011) Echocardiographic Parameters are Independently Associated with Rate of Renal Function Decline and Progression to Dialysis in Patients with Chronic Kidney Disease. Clin J Am Soc Nephrol 6: 2750–2758.
7. Furukawa M, Io H, Tanimoto M, Hagiwara S, Horikoshi S, et al. (2011) Predictive factors associated with the period of time before initiation of hemodialysis in CKD stages 4 and 5. Nephron Clin Pract 117: c341–347.
8. Alpert MA, Munuswamy K (1989) Electrocardiographic diagnosis of left atrial enlargement. Arch Intern Med 149: 1161–1165.
9. Birkbeck JP, Wilson DB, Hall MA, Meyers DG (2006) P-wave morphology correlation with left atrial volumes assessed by 2-dimensional echocardiography. J Electrocardiol 39: 225–229.
10. Kim DH, Kim GC, Kim SH, Yu HK, Choi WG, et al. (2007) The relationship between the left atrial volume and the maximum P-wave and P-wave dispersion in patients with congestive heart failure. Yonsei Med J 48: 810–817.
11. Truong QA, Charipar EM, Ptaszek LM, Taylor C, Fontes JD, et al. (2011) Usefulness of electrocardiographic parameters as compared with computed tomography measures of left atrial volume enlargement: from the ROMICAT trial. J Electrocardiol 44: 257–264.
12. Gunduz H, Binak E, Arinc H, Akdemir R, Ozhan H, et al. (2005) The relationship between P wave dispersion and diastolic dysfunction. Tex Heart Inst J 32: 163–167.
13. Yilmaz R, Demirbag R, Durmus I, Kasap H, Baykan M, et al. (2004) Association of Stage of Left Ventricular Diastolic Dysfunction with P Wave

Dispersion and Occurrence of Atrial Fibrillation after First Acute Anterior Myocardial Infarction. Ann Noninvasive Electrocardiol 9: 330–338.
14. Buxton AE, Josephson ME (1981) The role of P wave duration as a predictor of postoperative atrial arrhythmias. Chest 80: 68–73.
15. Soliman EZ, Prineas RJ, Case LD, Zhang Z-m, Goff DC, Jr (2009) Ethnic Distribution of ECG Predictors of Atrial Fibrillation and Its Impact on Understanding the Ethnic Distribution of Ischemic Stroke in the Atherosclerosis Risk in Communities (ARIC) Study. Stroke 40: 1204–1211.
16. Dagli N, Karaca I, Yavuzkir M, Balin M, Arslan N (2008) Are maximum P wave duration and P wave dispersion a marker of target organ damage in the hypertensive population? Clin Res Cardiol 97: 98–104.
17. Su HM, Tsai WC, Lin TH, Hsu PC, Lee WH, et al. (2012) P wave dispersion and maximum P wave duration are independently associated with rapid renal function decline. PloS one 7: e42815.
18. Koz C, Uzun M, Yokusoglu M, Ulas UH, Baysan O, et al. (2008) Echocardiographic, electrocardiographic, and clinical correlates of recurrent transient ischemic attacks: a follow-up study. South Med J 101: 246–251.
19. Magnani JW, Johnson VM, Sullivan LM, Gorodeski EZ, Schnabel RB, et al. (2011) P wave duration and risk of longitudinal atrial fibrillation in persons >/ = 60 years old (from the Framingham Heart Study). Am J Cardiol 107: 917–921 e911.
20. (2002) K/DOQI clinical practice guidelines for chronic kidney disease: evaluation, classification, and stratification. Am J Kidney Dis 39: S1–266.
21. Dilaveris PE, Gialafos EJ, Sideris SK, Theopistou AM, Andrikopoulos GK, et al. (1998) Simple electrocardiographic markers for the prediction of paroxysmal idiopathic atrial fibrillation. Am Heart J 135: 733–738.
22. Bazett HC (1920) The time relations of the blood-pressure changes after excision of the adrenal glands, with some observations on blood volume changes. J Physiol 53: 320–339.
23. Sokolow M, Lyon TP (1949) The ventricular complex in left ventricular hypertrophy as obtained by unipolar precordial and limb leads. Am Heart J 37: 161–186.
24. Vickery S, Stevens PE, Dalton RN, van Lente F, Lamb EJ (2006) Does the ID-MS traceable MDRD equation work and is it suitable for use with compensated Jaffe and enzymatic creatinine assays? Nephrol Dial Transplant 21: 2439–2445.
25. Levey AS, Bosch JP, Lewis JB, Greene T, Rogers N, et al. (1999) A more accurate method to estimate glomerular filtration rate from serum creatinine: a new prediction equation. Modification of Diet in Renal Disease Study Group. Ann Intern Med 130: 461–470.
26. Paoletti E, Bellino D, Gallina AM, Amidone M, Cassottana P, et al. (2011) Is left ventricular hypertrophy a powerful predictor of progression to dialysis in chronic kidney disease? Nephrol Dial Transplant 26: 670–677.
27. Shlipak MG, Katz R, Kestenbaum B, Siscovick D, Fried L, et al. (2009) Rapid decline of kidney function increases cardiovascular risk in the elderly. J Am Soc Nephrol 20: 2625–2630.
28. Bock JS, Gottlieb SS (2010) Cardiorenal syndrome: new perspectives. Circulation 121: 2592–2600.
29. Ronco C (2010) Cardiorenal syndromes: definition and classification. Contrib Nephrol 164: 33–38.
30. Ritz E (2006) Diabetic nephropathy. Saudi J Kidney Dis Transpl 17: 481–490.
31. Ritz E (2006) Heart and kidney: fatal twins? Am J Med 119: S31–39.
32. Levin A, Singer J, Thompson CR, Ross H, Lewis M (1996) Prevalent left ventricular hypertrophy in the predialysis population: identifying opportunities for intervention. Am J Kidney Dis 27: 347–354.
33. Levin A, Thompson CR, Ethier J, Carlisle EJ, Tobe S, et al. (1999) Left ventricular mass index increase in early renal disease: impact of decline in hemoglobin. Am J Kidney Dis 34: 125–134.
34. Veves A, Akbari CM, Primavera J, Donaghue VM, Zacharoulis D, et al. (1998) Endothelial dysfunction and the expression of endothelial nitric oxide synthetase in diabetic neuropathy, vascular disease, and foot ulceration. Diabetes 47: 457–463.
35. Glowinska I, Grochowski J, Malyszko J (2008) Cardiovascular complications in patients with diabetic nephropathy receiving pharmacological versus renal replacement therapy. Pol Arch Med Wewn 118: 404–412.
36. Mataradzija A, Resic H, Rasic S, Kukavica N, Masnic F (2010) Risk factors for development of cardiovascular complications in patients with chronic renal disease and diabetic nephropathy. Bosn J Basic Med Sci 10 Suppl 1: S44–50.
37. Chen SC, Chang JM, Liu WC, Tsai YC, Tsai JC, et al. (2012) Stepwise increases in left ventricular mass index and decreases in left ventricular ejection fraction correspond with the stages of chronic kidney disease in diabetes patients. Exp Diabetes Res 2012: 789325.

Does Swimming Exercise Affect Experimental Chronic Kidney Disease in Rats Treated with Gum Acacia?

Badreldin H. Ali[1]*, Suhail Al-Salam[2], Mohammed Al Za'abi[1], Khalid A. Al Balushi[1], Aishwarya Ramkumar[1], Mostafa I. Waly[3], Javid Yasin[4], Sirin A. Adham[5], Abderrahim Nemmar[6]

1 Department of Pharmacology and Clinical Pharmacy, College of Medicine and Health Sciences, Sultan Qaboos University, Alkhod, Muscat, Oman, **2** Department of Pathology, College of Medicine and Health Sciences, United Arab Emirates, Alin, United Arab Emirates, **3** Department of Food Sciences and Nutrition, College of Agricultural and Marine Sciences, Sultan Qaboos University, Alkhod, Muscat, Oman, **4** Department of Medicine, College of Medicine and Health Sciences, United Arab Emirates, Alin, United Arab Emirates, **5** Department of Biology, College of Science, Sultan Qaboos University, Sultan Qaboos University, Alkhod, Muscat, Oman, **6** Department of Physiology, College of Medicine and Health Sciences, United Arab Emirates, Alin, United Arab Emirates

Abstract

Different modes of exercise are reported to be beneficial in subjects with chronic kidney disease (CKD). Similar benefits have also been ascribed to the dietary supplement gum acacia (GA). Using several physiological, biochemical, immunological, and histopathological measurements, we assessed the effect of swimming exercise (SE) on adenine –induced CKD, and tested whether SE would influence the salutary action of GA in rats with CKD. Eight groups of rats were used, the first four of which were fed normal chow for 5 weeks, feed mixed with adenine (0.25% w/w) to induce CKD, GA in the drinking water (15% w/v), or were given adenine plus GA, as above. Another four groups were similarly treated, but were subjected to SE during the experimental period, while the first four groups remained sedentary. The pre-SE program lasted for four days (before the start of the experimental treatments), during which the rats were made to swim for 5 to 10 min, and then gradually extended to 20 min per day. Thereafter, the rats in the 5th, 6th, 7th, and 8th groups started to receive their respective treatments, and were subjected to SE three days a week for 45 min each. Adenine induced the typical signs of CKD as confirmed by histopathology, and the other measurements, and GA significantly ameliorated all these signs. SE did not affect the salutary action of GA on renal histology, but it partially improved some of the above biochemical and physiological analytes, suggesting that addition of this mode of exercise to GA supplementation may improve further the benefits of GA supplementation.

Editor: Utpal Sen, University of Louisville, United States of America

Funding: This work was financially supported by a grant from the Research Council of Oman (RC/Med/Phar/10/01), and the Sultan Qaboos University (SQU). The funders had no role in study design, data collection and analysis, decision to publish, or preparation of the manuscript.

Competing Interests: The authors have declared that no competing interests exist.

* Email: alibadreldin@hotmail.com

Introduction

Chronic kidney disease (CKD) is a major public health concern in both developed and developing countries because of the high prevalence of morbidity and mortality associated with it, mainly due to cardiovascular dysfunction [1,2]. It has been suggested that CKD leads to reduced physical activity and an increased risk of cardiovascular disease (CVD) [2,3]. A sedentary lifestyle increases the risk of CVD, but CVD can be ameliorated by physical fitness [3,4,5].

Aerobic exercise has been shown to improve renal and cardiac function in individuals with CKD [6] and in overweight rats with metabolic and cardiac dysfunction [7], and exercise has gained more attention as a possible tool for preventing, reducing or delaying CKD progression [3,4,5,6,7]. It has been suggested that appropriate exercise may improve a patient's physical strength and quality of life [8,9]. Swimming has been increasingly prescribed as a non-pharmacological treatment for arterial hypertension, obesity and coronary heart disease [10,11]. Thus, improving our knowledge of the effects of swimming training in animal models is relevant for CKD patients [5,6,12,13,14].

Because of the rise in recent decades of CKD incidence and its associated cardiovascular risks and damage [15], we thought it of importance to assess the effect of swimming exercise on a relevant rodent model of human CKD [16], and further, to evaluate the effect of co- administration of a natural product, gum acacia, which has recently been shown to ameliorate CKD in patients [17,18] and rats [19,20,21,22,23].

Methods

Animals

Male Wistar rats (9–10 weeks old, weighing 249±10 g) were housed in a room at a temperature of 22±2°C, relative humidity of about 60%, with a 12 h light–dark cycle (lights on 6 00), and free access to standard pellet chow diet containing 0.85% phosphorus, 1.12% calcium, 0.35% magnesium, 25.3% crude protein and 2.5 IU/g vitamin D3 (Oman Flour Mills, Muscat, Oman) and water. Ethical approval of this work was obtained

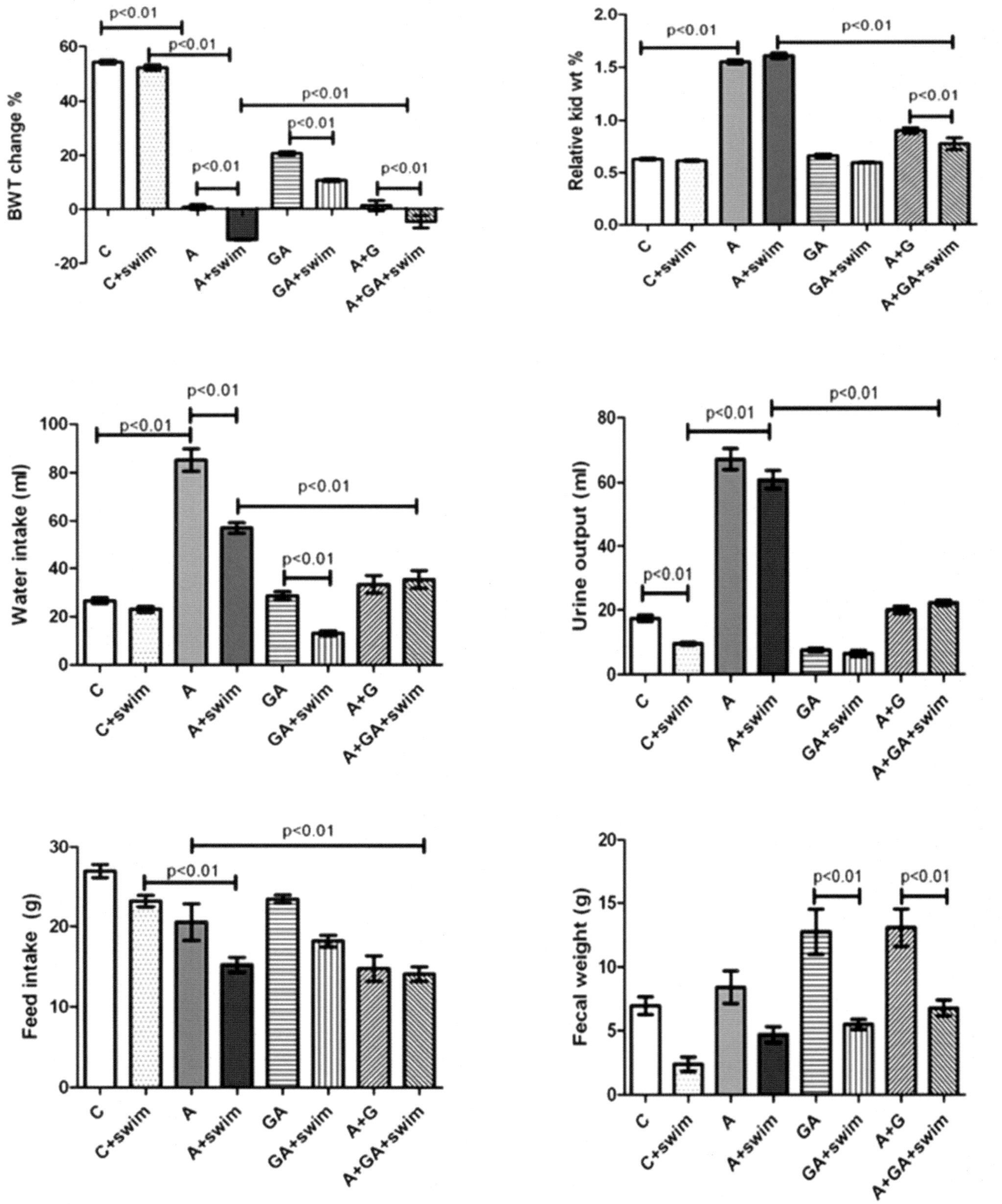

Figure 1. Body weight change (%), relative kidney weight (%), water intake, urine volume, feed intake, and fecal weight in rats treated with saline (C); saline + swimming exercise, (C + swim); adenine (A); A + swim; gum acacia (GA); GA + swim; A + GA; and A + G + swim. Each column is mean ± SEM (n = six rats). Statistical analysis by ANOVA followed by Newman– Keuls test.

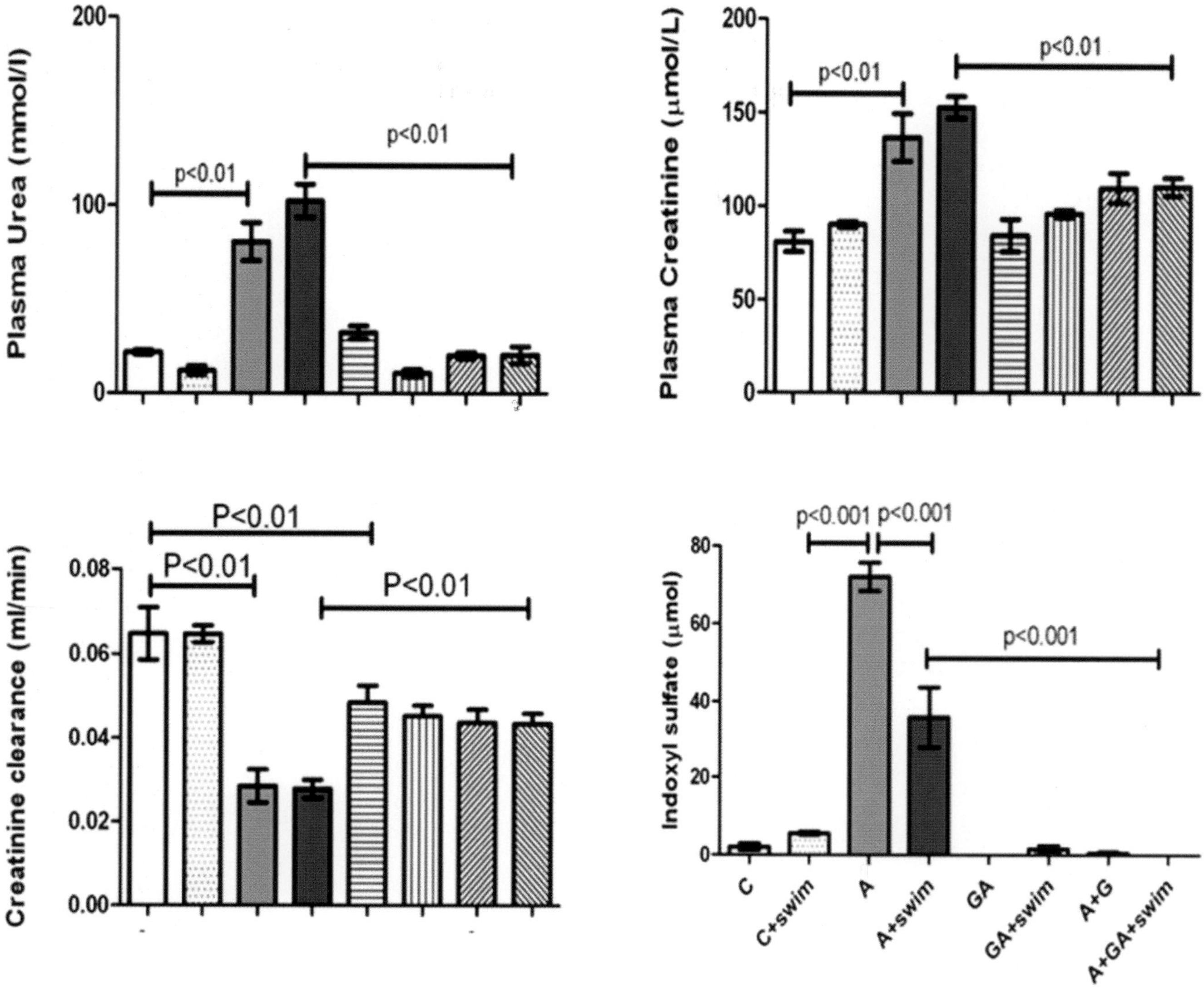

Figure 2. The plasma concentrations of urea, creatinine and indoxyl sulfate, and the creatinine clearance in rats treated with saline (C); saline + swimming exercise, (C + swim); adenine (A); A + swim; gum acacia (GA); GA + swim; A + GA; and A + G + swim. Each column is mean ± SEM (n = six rats). Statistical analysis by ANOVA followed by Newman–Keuls test.

from our University Animal Research Ethics committee, and all procedures involving animals and their care were carried out in accordance with international laws and policies (EEC Council directives 86/609, OJL 358, 1 December, 12, 1987; NIH Guide for the Care and Use of Laboratory Animals, NIH Publications No. 85–23, 1985), and ethical clearance was obtained from the Small Animal Research Ethics Committee of Sultan Qaboos University.

Experimental Design

After an acclimatization period of one week, rats (n = 48) were randomly divided into eight equal groups and treated for five consecutive weeks. The 1st group continued to receive the same diet without treatment until the end of the study (control group). The 2nd group was switched to a powder diet containing adenine (0.25%w/w in feed for 5 weeks). The 3rd group was given normal food and GA in drinking water at a concentration of 15% w/v for 5 weeks. The 4th group was given adenine in the feed as in group two, plus GA in drinking water at a concentration of 15% w/v. The dose of adenine was chosen from previous reports [19–21]. The 5th, 6th, 7th and 8th groups were treated in the same manner as the 1st, 2nd, 3rd and 4th group, respectively, except that these latter four groups were also subjected to swimming exercise (SE) (see below)

Swimming Exercise (SE) Training Protocol

Rats were subjected first to a pre-SE for acclimation in an experimental swimming pool (~30°C, water depth: 30 cm; radius 120 cm), as described by others [14,22,24]. The pre SE program lasted for an acclimation period of four days (before the start of the experimental treatments), during which the rats were made to swim for 5 to 10 min, and then gradually extended to 20 min per day. After the acclimation to swimming, the rats in the 5th, 6th, 7th and 8th groups started to receive their respective treatments, and were subjected to SE three days a week for 45 min each.

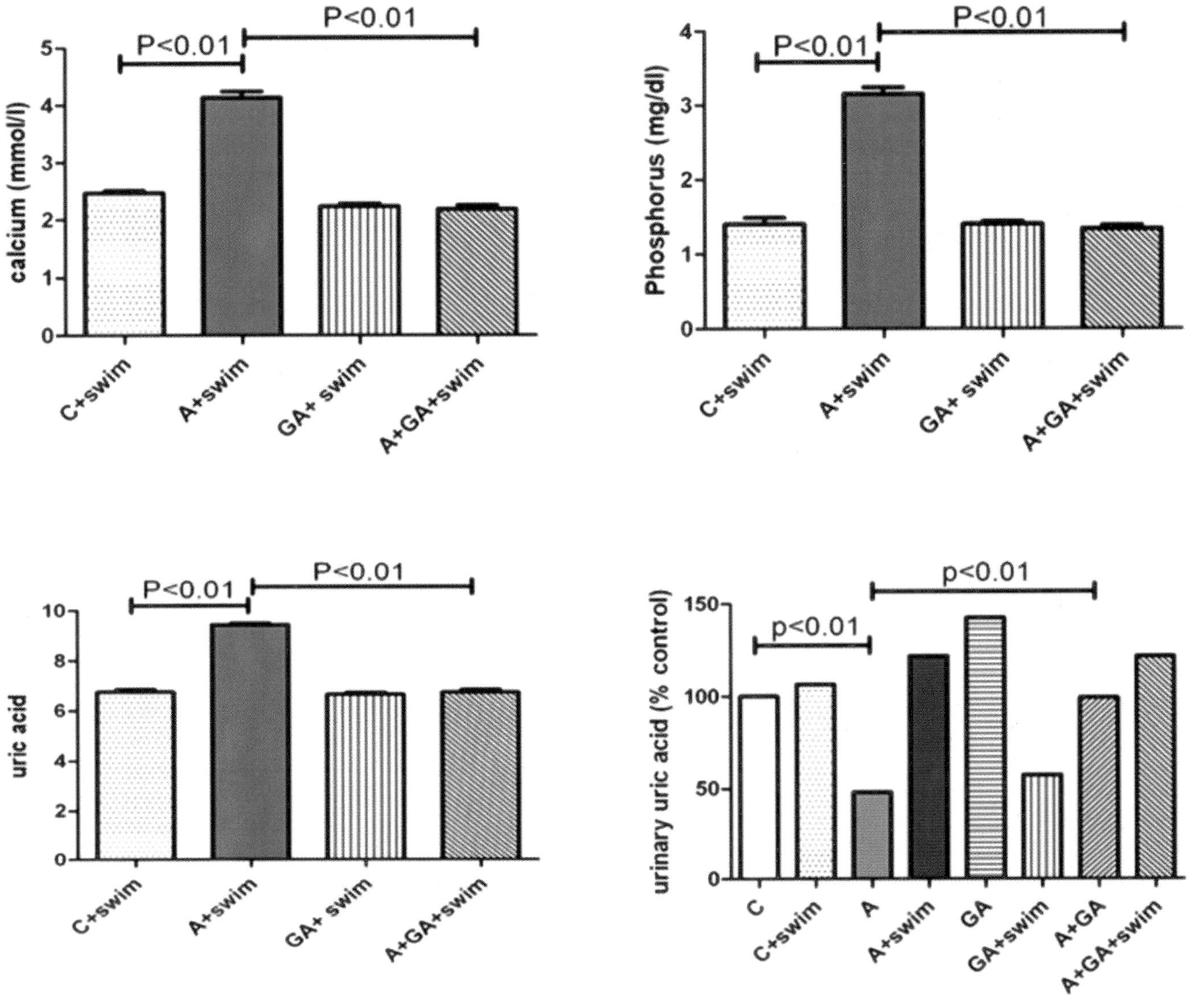

Figure 3. The effect of treatment with saline (C); saline + swimming exercise (C + swim); adenine (A); A + swim; gum acacia (GA); GA + swim; A + GA; and A + G + swim on urinary uric acid concentration, and the plasma concentration of calcium, phosphorus and uric acid in treated with saline, A, GA and A + GA in rats subjected to swimming exercise. Each column is mean ± SEM (n = six rats). Statistical analysis by ANOVA followed by Newman–Keuls test.

Treatments

During the treatment period, the rats were weighed weekly. For the collection of urine, they were placed individually in metabolic cages for 24 h, after the 35 days treatment period. On the morning after the metabolic sampling, the rats were anesthetized with an intraperitoneal injection of ketamine (75 mg/kg) and xylazine (5 mg/kg), and blood (about 4 mL) was collected from the anterior vena cava and placed into heparinized tubes. The blood and urine were centrifuged at 900 *g* at 4°C for 15 min. The plasma obtained, together with the urine specimens, was stored at −80°C to await analysis within 4 weeks after the end of the treatment. The two kidneys were excised, blotted on filter paper and weighed. A part of the right kidney was placed in formalin, awaiting histopathological studies. The rest of the kidneys were kept frozen at −80°C pending biochemical analysis within three days. The left kidney was homogenized in ice-cold Tris buffer (pH 7.4) to give a 10% w/v homogenate. The latter was centrifuged at 1500 *g* at 4°C for 15 min, and the supernatant obtained was used to measure superoxide dismutase (SOD) and catalase (CAT) activities, the concentrations of glutathione (GSH), and total antioxidant capacity (TAC).

Biochemical and Physiological Measurements

Traditional and novel biochemical urinary, plasma and renal biomarkers were measured. Creatinine, urea, uric acid, calcium (Ca), phosphorus (P) and protein concentrations in plasma and/or urine were measured spectrophotometrically using commercial kits. In renal cortex homogenates, protein concentration was measured by Lowry's method using albumin as a standard. TAC, and GSH concentration, as well as CAT and SOD activities in plasma, and urinary 8-oxo-2'-deoxyguanosine(8-OHDG) were measured using ELISA kits, as described before [19–22].

In plasma, nephrin, tumor necrosis factor α (TNFα), 8-isoprostane, adiponectin and cystatin C were measured using

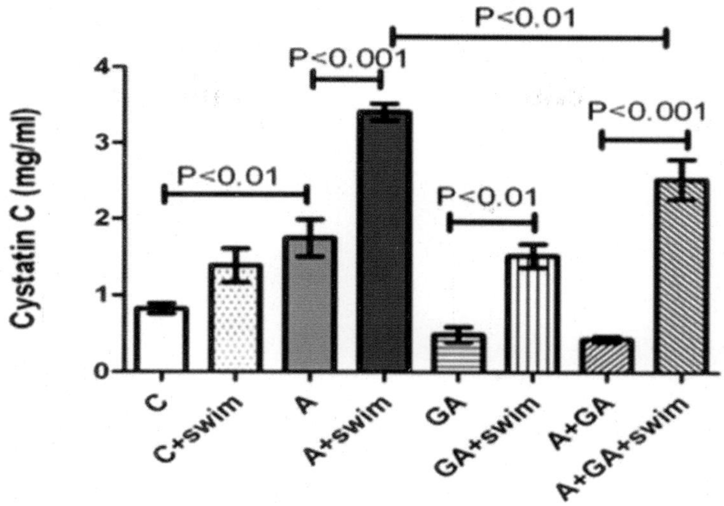

Cystatin C (mg/ml)
0
1
2
3
4
P<0.01
P<0.001
P<0.01
P<0.01
P<0.001
C
C+swim
A
A+swim
GA
GA+swim
A+GA
A+GA+swim

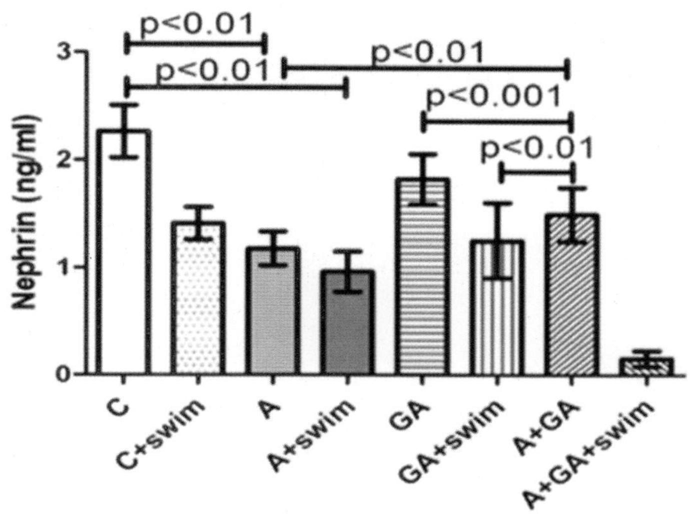

Nephrin (ng/ml)
0
1
2
3
p<0.01
p<0.01
p<0.01
p<0.001
p<0.01
C
C+swim
A
A+swim
GA
GA+swim
A+GA
A+GA+swim

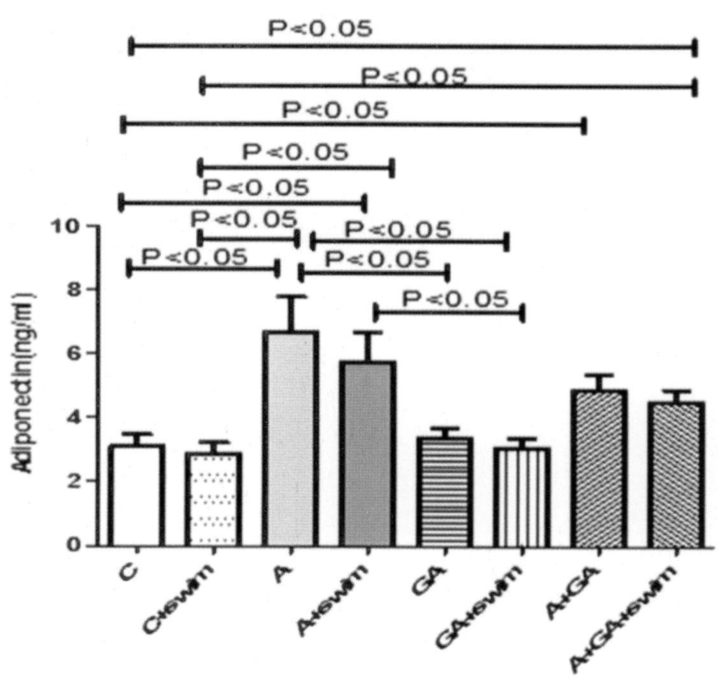

Adiponectin (ng/ml)
0
2
4
6
8
10
P<0.05
P<0.05
P<0.05
P<0.05
P<0.05
P<0.05
P<0.05
P<0.05
P<0.05
P<0.05
C
C+swim
A
A+swim
GA
GA+swim
A+GA
A+GA+swim

Figure 4. The concentrations of cystatin C, nephrin and adiponectinin plasma of rats treated with saline (C); saline + swimming exercise (C + swim); adenine (A); A + swim; gum acacia (GA); GA + swim; A + GA; and A + G + swim. Each column is mean ± SEM (n = six rats). Statistical analysis by ANOVA followed by Newman–Keuls test.

ELISA - based commercial kits. The uremic toxin indoxyl sulfate was measured by a validated HPLC method developed in this laboratory [25].

Histopathology

After weighing, the kidneys were sampled and fixed in 10% neutral-buffered formalin for 24–48 hrs, dehydrated in increasing concentrations of ethanol, cleared with xylene and embedded in paraffin. Four micrometer (μm) sections were prepared from kidney paraffin blocks and stained with hematoxylin and eosin (H & E). The microscopic scoring of the kidney sections was carried out in a blinded fashion by a pathologist who was unaware of the treatment groups, and assigned a score, as described before [19], which represents the approximate extent of the necrotic area in the cortical and medullary tubules, and assigned a score on a scale of 0–4 (0, no necrosis; 1, a few focal necrotic areas of ≤25% of the kidney; 2, necrotic area was about 26–50% of kidney; 3, necrotic area was 51–75% of kidney; 4, nearly the entire area was necrotic, necrotic area was 76–100% of kidney).

The size of the necrosis was also estimated, and values were presented as means ± SEM.

Four-μm sections were prepared from paraffin blocks and stained with Masson trichrome stain to assess the degree of interstitial fibrosis. Image J software (NIH, USA) was used to measure the extent of necrosis and fibrosis.

Staining for apoptosis was performed with a signal stain-cleaved caspase-3immuno-histochemical detection kit. This was used to detect the activation of caspase using the avidin–biotin immuno-peroxidase method to detect intracellular caspase-3 protein. Staining was performed on 5 μm paraffin sections from the left kidney by a standard technique using rabbit anti-cleaved caspase 3 (clone Asp175, 1:50) [16]. Known positive control sections for apoptosis were used. For negative control, primary antibody was replaced with normal rabbit serum. The apoptotic index was calculated by dividing the number of positive tubular epithelial cells for anti-casapase-3 per 100 tubular epithelial cells. The calculation was repeated in at least 10 random high power fields and the total was divided by 10 to get the apoptotic index.

Western blot analysis for caspase-3 and its cleaved isoform

Since caspase cascade activation is a known feature of apoptosis which is associated with CKD [16], we measured here the proteolytic activity of caspase-3 in the rat kidneys collected from the eight different groups. The kidneys were homogenized by crushing 0.5 μg of the tissue using a micro size mortar and pistol in cold lysis buffer (Cell Signaling Technologies, USA) containing protease inhibitor cocktail (Sigma, Aldrich, USA). Kidney lysates were centrifuged and quantified using BCA protein assay system (Pierece, USA). Aliquots of total protein from each sample (100 μg) were loaded into a 15% SDS-PAGE gel. Protein was transferred to PVDF membrane (Millipore, Belgium). The membranes were blocked with 5% nonfat milk in TBST (10 mM Tris, pH 7.5, 150 mM NaCl, 0.05% Tween 20) and probed with 1:1000 dilution of caspase-3 primary monoclonal rabbit antibody which was prepared to detect both caspase-3 bands, not cleaved (37 KDa) and cleaved band (25 KDa) (Cell Signaling Technology, USA) in the same blot. The antibody was added to 5% nonfat milk/TBST solution. Immunoblots were then processed with horseradish–peroxidase-conjugated anti-rabbit immunoglobulin G (IgG) (secondary antibody using the enhanced BM Chemiluminescence Western Blotting Kit (Mouse/Rabbit) (Roche, USA). The membranes were stripped off and re- blotted using beta Actin primary antibody (Cat # 4970 from Cell Signaling Technology, USA). The blots were exposed to X-ray film (Roche, U.S.A) at room temperature. Densitometery was carried out on the scanned X-ray film using Image J software which measures the relative intensity of the test band in respect to the loading control beta actin.

Drugs, Chemicals and Kits

GA used was SUPERGUMTMEM10, Lot 101008, 1.1.11 (San – Ei Gen F. F. I.; Sanwa-Cho, Toyonaka, Osaka, Japan); aqueous solutions were prepared freshly every day. The chemical properties of GA have been fully reported before [20,21]. The SUPERGUMTM EM 10 used was characterized by size

Table 1. The effect of swimming exercise (SE) on some cytokines, antioxidant markers and proteins in plasma or urine from rats with chronic kidney disease induced by feeding adenine (A) [0.25% w/w, 5 weeks], and the influence of gum acacia (GA) [15% w/v in drinking water, 5 weeks] thereon.

Groups	Plasma TNFα (pg/mL)	Plasma 8-isoprostone (pg/mL)	Urine OHdG (ng/mL)	Plasma adiponectin (ng/L)	Plasma cystatin C (pg/L)	Plasma nephrin (pg/mL)
Control (C)	49.3±3.2[a]	51.0±3.9[a]	181.2±14.7[a]	3.7±0.2[a]	0.55±0.03[a]	0.47±0.02[a]
C + SE	47.7±4.0[a]	47.2±3.8[a]	178.9±15.9[a]	3.3±0.2[a]	0.57±0.03[a]	0.45±0.03[a]
A	66.9±6.1[a]	83.4±7.5[a]	223.1±19.2[a]	6.1±0.4[b]	0.87±0.06[a]	0.70±0.05[b]
A + SE	54.0±4.2[a]	61.2±4.3[a]	190.1±15.3[a]	5.7±0.3[b]	0.64±0.05[a]	0.65±0.02[c]
GA	48.3±4.0[a]	50.7±5.2[a]	172.3±16.3[a]	3.9±0.3[a]	0.48±0.04[a]	0.46±0.02[a]
GA + SE	45.9±4.2[a]	47.9±5.0[a]	169.9±17.1[a]	3.6±0.3[a]	0.5±0.05[a]	0.44±0.03[a]
A + GA	56.1±4.8[a]	59.2±4.7[a]	188.1±15.3[a]	4.7±0.4[c]	0.66±0.06[a]	0.6±0.05[c]
A + GA + SE	52.1±4.9[a]	55.2±4.1[a]	179.2±15.4[a]	4.0±0.3[a]	0.59±0.05[a]	0.55±0.04[d]

Values in the table are means ± SEM (n = 6 rats). Values with similar superscripts are not statistically different (level of significance set at $P<0.05$).
TNFα = Tumor necrosis factor alpha; 8- OHdg = 8 – hydroxo – 2- deoxyguanisone;

Table 2. The effect of swimming exercise (SE) on some antioxidant indices in kidney homogenates from rats with chronic kidney disease induced by feeding adenine (A) [0.25% w/w, 5 weeks], and the influence of gum acacia (GA) [15% w/v in drinking water, 5 weeks] with or without SE thereon.

Groups	SOD μmol/min/mg protein	CAT μmol/min/mg protein	GSH nmol/mg protein	TAC nmol/mg protein
Control (C)	66.6±4.1	90.7±6.3	27.6±1.8	118.2±6.4
C + SE	77.7±4.9*	115.2±5.1	31.6±2.0	136.3±7.5
A	35.2±0.6**	28.4±4.8**	11.7±3.4**	68.3±3.9**
A + SE	37.8±1.4**	35.8±1.5**	13.6±1.3**	76.9±2.8**
GA	69.7±3.1	108.3±7.1	29.8±2.2	123.6±5.9
GA + SE	73.3±4.0	110.4±6.0	30.7±1.9	133.9±5.3*
A + GA	65.3±4.3	88.9±3.1	27.1±1.9	117.9±5.1
A + GA + SE	69.2±3.0	96.3±4.9	28.4±1.5	124.0±4.5

Values in the table are means ± SEM (n = 6 rats).
SOD = Superoxide dismutase; CAT = catalase; GSH = reduced glutathione and TAC = total antioxidant capacity.
**P* less than 0.05.
***P* less than 0.01 (Compared to control for the same index).

fractionation followed by multiple angle laser light scattering (GPC-MALLS) to give its molecular profile. The average molecular weight was 3.43×106, and the content of arabinogalactan protein (AGP) 26.4%. Adenine was obtained from Sigma (St. Louis, MO, USA). Creatinine, urea and protein kits were bought from Human GmbH (Mannheim, Germany) and SOD, CAT and AO kits from Randox (Antrim, UK). TAC kits were from Cayman Chemical, Ann Arbor, MI, USA. Nephrin was obtained from Novatein Biosciences, Cambridge, MA, USA, tumor necrosis factor α (TNF α) from Cayman Chemical, Ann Arbor, MI, USA, 8-isoprostane and 8-oxo-2'-deoxyguanosine (8-OHDG) from Statok Kino, Shizuoka, Japan, adiponectin from Cayman Chemical, Ann Arbor, MI, USA, and cystatin C from R &D Systems, Abingdon, UK.

Statistical Analysis

All data were analyzed with GraphPad Prism Version 4.01 for Windows software (Graphpad Software Inc., San Diego, CA). Data were analyzed for normal distribution using the D'Agostino and Pearson omnibus normality test. Data are expressed as means ± SEM.

Comparisons between groups were performed by one-way ANOVA, followed by Newman- Keuls test for comparing treated with control data; *P* values of less than 0.05 are considered significant.

Results

Physiological Results

Rats that had undergone SE in the different groups appeared more active than their sedentary counterparts. As shown in Fig 1, SE did not significantly change body weight of control rats, but it significantly reduced that of rats with CKD. Treatment with GA reduced the body weight, an effect that was potentiated by SE. When GA treatment was combined with SE and adenine, the body weight of rats was depressed even further.

The weights of the kidneys relative to the final body weight of adenine –treated rats were significantly higher than those of the control rats. This action was not significantly affected by the SE.

Water intake and urine volume in the adenine –treated rats were significantly higher than in control rats ($P<0.05$), and this was significantly abated by SE and GA treatment.

Feed intake but not fecal weight was reduced by adenine treatment. In all groups SE reduced both the feed intake and fecal weight.

Biochemical Results

Fig 2 shows the plasma concentrations of indoxyl sulfate, creatinine and urea, as well as the creatinine clearance in the eight groups. Adenine treatment significantly increased the concentrations of indoxyl sulfate, creatinine and urea, and decreased that of the creatinine clearance. This effect was significantly but not completely reversed by GA treatment. Concomitant SE did not significantly affect any of the above analytes.

Adenine treatment significantly decreased Ca, but increased P and uric acid concentrations (data not shown). However, as shown in Fig 3, in rats similarly treated but subjected to SE, Ca and uric acid concentrations were significantly increased, and P remained higher than the control (sedentary and subjected to SE). SE in control rats had no significant effect on urinary uric acid excretion, but in adenine –treated rats SE induced a significant rise ($P<0.01$). The adenine – induced significant decrease in urinary uric acid excretion was significantly ($P<0.01$) but not completely antagonized by GA treatment.

The effects of SE and GA treatments in adenine –treated rats on Cystatin C, nephrin and adiponectin concentrations in plasma are shown in Fig 4. Adenine treatment significantly increased the concentration of cystatin C, while GA caused the opposite effect. However, in all the treated groups, SE significantly increased the concentration of cystatin C. The plasma nephrin concentration was significantly reduced by adenine treatment, an effect which was further enhanced by SE in all groups. Adenine treatment significantly increased adiponectin concentration, and this was not significantly affected by SE in any of the groups (Fig 4).

The effect of SE and GA treatments in adenine –treated rats on the concentration of some proteins, cytokines and antioxidants in plasma is shown in Table 1.

The effect of SE and GA treatment in adenine –treated rats on indices of oxidative damage is shown in Table 2. Compared with control sedentary rats, SE raised the four indices of oxidative damage measured, which was only statistically significant in the case of SOD activity (where it was raised by 17%, $P<0.5$). Adenine treatment significantly decreased the four indices, and SE in adenine –treated rats insignificantly and incompletely reversed

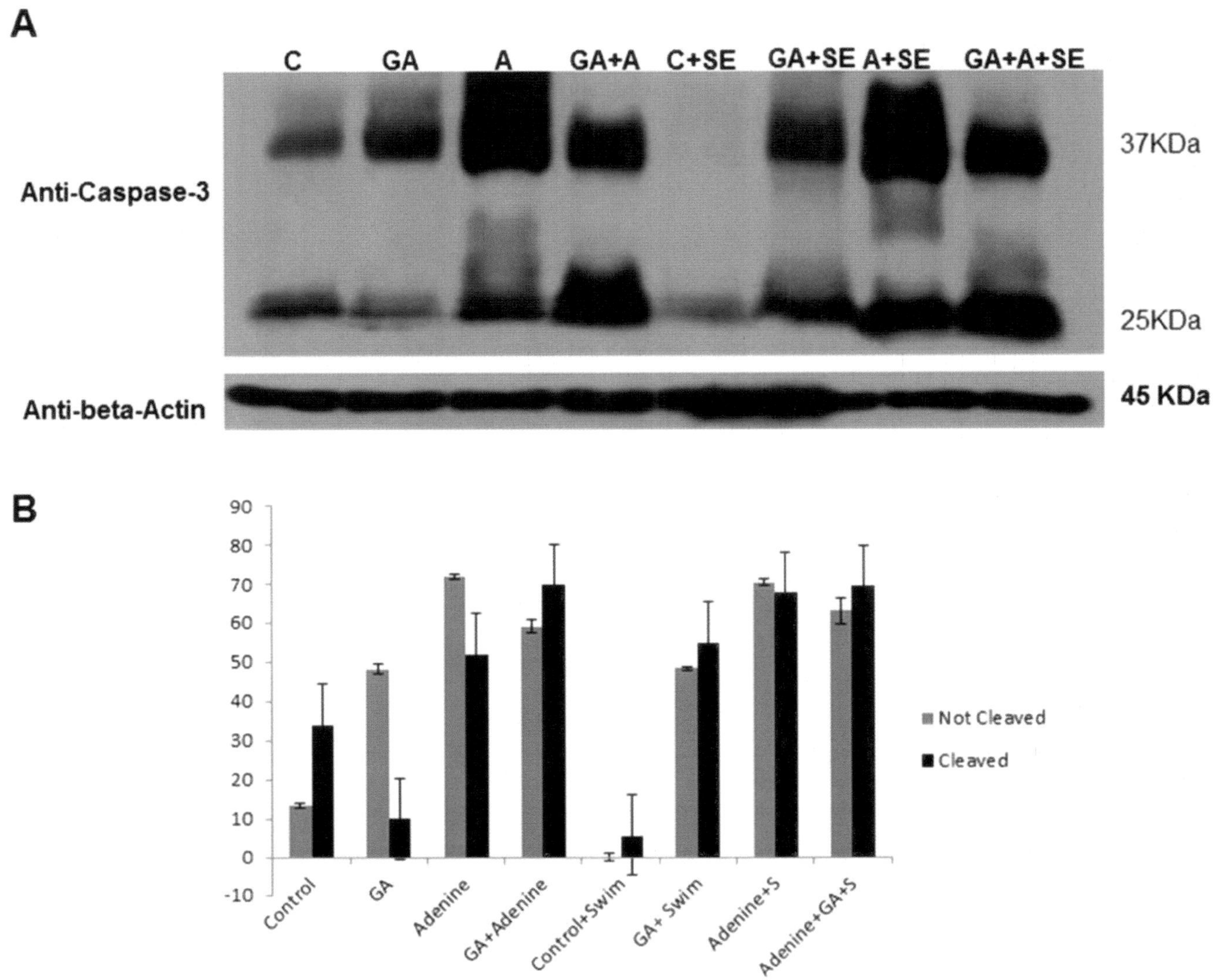

Figure 5. Representative photograph and quantification of apoptosis and caspase 3 cleavage in kidney tissue lysates of rats treated with saline (1); saline + swimming exercise, SE (2); adenine (3); adenine + SE (4);gum acacia, GA (5); GA + SE (6); adenine (3), adenine + GA (7); and adenine + GA + SE (8). Columns and vertical bars represent means ± SEM of relative intensity of cleaved and uncleaved bands. Western blotting is depicted for caspase-3, cleaved caspase-3 and β-Actin loading protein.

that action. Treatment of rats with either GA alone or together with SE had no significant effect on any of the indices of oxidative damage. GA treatment significantly restored these indices to near normal levels, and this action was not significantly affected by SE.

Western Blotting Results

Western blot densitometric quantitation (Fig 5) showed that SE significantly decreased the activity of caspase-3 cleavage only in the control and not in the treated rats ($P = 0.004$). However, SE significantly increased caspase-3 activity in animals treated with either adenine alone, or GA alone ($P = 0.0016$, $P = 0.0004$). SE did not result in any significant difference in caspase-3 cleavage in the group that had been treated with both adenine and GA.

Histopathological and Immunohistochemical Results

The kidneys of both sedentary and exercised control and GA – treated rats had normal kidney architecture and histology and were given a score of 0 for necrosis, using H &E staining (Fig 6 A - D). Using the Masson trichrome stain, there was no evidence of fibrosis in these groups (Fig 7, A –D). There was also no evidence of apoptotic cells in the examined sections (Fig 8, A – D).

Fig 6 I and J, Masson trichrome staining showed that in the adenine – treated rats there was a diffuse tubular necrosis in 71.1±7.3% of the examined tissue areas (score 3), tubular distention with necrotic material, loss of brush border of proximal tubules, dilatation of large number of tubules, mixed inflammatory cells infiltration of the interstitium and focal tubular atrophy.

Fig. 1 I &J, Masson trichrome staining showed foci of interstitial fibrosis involving 41.3±5.6% of the examined surface area. The adenine + swimming group showed diffuse acute tubular necrosis in 69.8±9.1% of the examined tissue areas (score 3) showing tubular distention with necrotic material, loss of brush border of proximal tubules, dilatation of a large number of tubules, mixed inflammatory cells infiltration of the interstitium, and focal tubular atrophy (Fig. 6 K and L).

Masson trichrome staining showed foci of interstitial fibrosis involving 42.1±4.9% of the examined surface area (score 2)

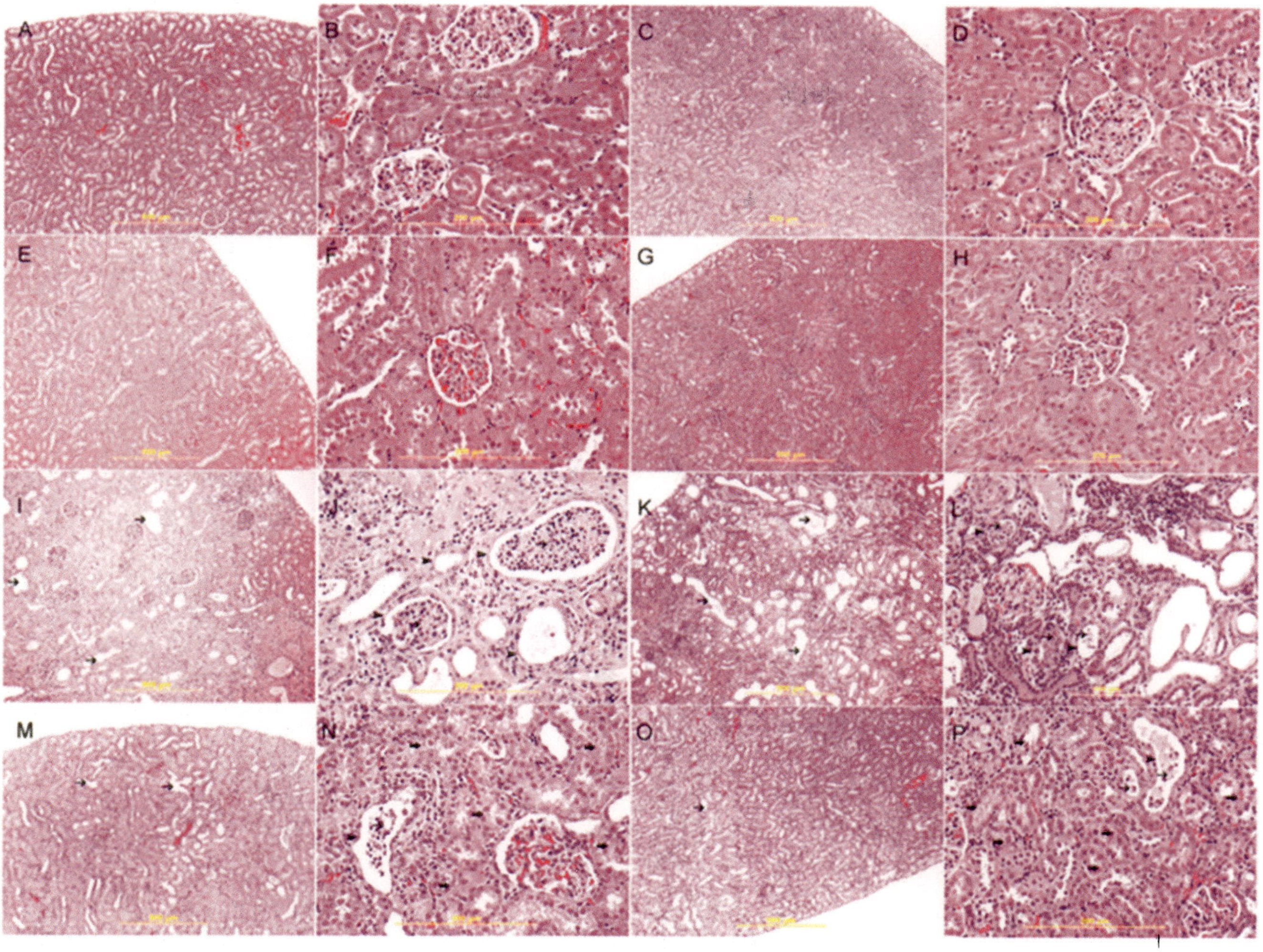

Figure 6. Representative photograph of sections of renal tissue of rats treated with saline (A), saline + swimming exercise, SE (B), gum acacia, GA (C), GA + SE (D), adenine (E), adenine + SE (F), adenine + GA (G) and adenine + GA + SE (H), and stained with hematoxylin & eosin (H&E) stain. Sections **A, B, C,** and **D** showed normal kidney architecture and histology. Sections **E** and **F** showed acute tubular necrosis (arrow head) with tubular distention with necrotic material (thin arrows), and many apoptotic cells (thin arrows). Sections G and F showed similar improvement in histological appearance with focal areas of acute tubular necrosis (arrow head), and less dilated tubules (thin arrow).

(Fig. 2F). Many apoptotic cells were seen in Fig.3F. There was no significant histological improvement in necrosis and fibrosis following SE.

The group treated with adenine +GA showed dramatic improvement in the histological appearance when compared with the group treated with adenine alone. There were focal areas of acute tubular necrosis involving 18.2±2.4% of the examined areas (score 1), few tubules showing dilatation, less interstitial inflammatory cells infiltration, less tubular atrophy (Fig.1 M&N), minimal fibrosis of 3.35±0.24%, a score of 1 (Fig.2 G), and few apoptotic cells (Fig. 3G).

The adenine-GA-swimming - treated group showed dramatic improvement in the histological appearance when compared with the adenine –treated group, and showed no significant histological difference from the adenine-GA- treated group (Table 3). There were focal areas of acute tubular necrosis involving 17.8±4.9% of the examined areas (score 1), few tubules showing dilatation, less interstitial inflammatory cells infiltration, less tubular atrophy (Fig.1 O&P), minimal fibrosis of 3.42±0.16% (score 1) (Fig.2 H), and few apoptotic cells(Fig. 3H).

Discussion

CKD is known to be a long –term condition that is associated in most cases with physical and psychological symptoms. The former include fatigue, muscle weakness and reduced stamina. It is conceivable that various forms of appropriate exercise can improve these signs and symptoms. It has previously been shown that GA can ameliorate CKD experimentally in rats and mice [16] and clinically in humans [17]. It was of interest, therefore, to find out if there is any interaction between these two variables.

Our results indicated that the body weight of exercised rats did not increase compared with that of sedentary control rats when both were given free access to food. Such exercise is considered of moderate intensity [28]. In the present work we have confirmed an earlier observation that treatment with GA decreases body weight [16,20] in rats, and also in humans [29]. SE in control rats did not significantly affect the body weight, but it enhanced further the drop in body weights of adenine – treated and GA – treated healthy rats. The body growth depressive action of SE in our rats may be due to a lower intake of feed, although it has previously

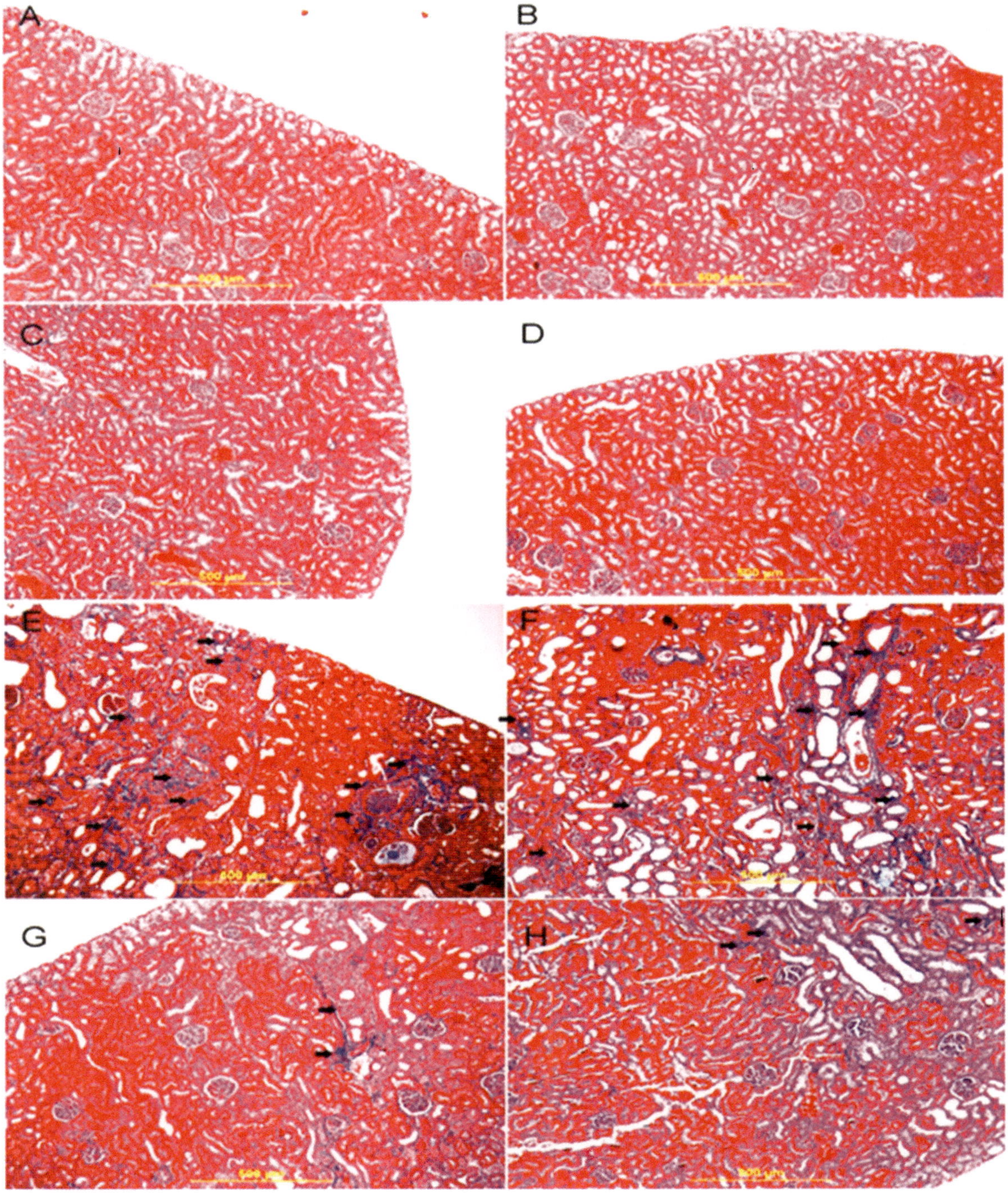

Figure 7. Representative photograph of sections of renal tissue of rats treated with saline (A), saline + swimming exercise, SE (B), gum acacia, GA (C), GA + SE (D), adenine (E), adenine + SE (F), adenine + GA (G) and adenine + GA + SE (H), and stained with Masson trichrome stain. Sections A, B, C, and D showed normal kidney architecture and histology and no evidence of fibrosis. Sections E and F showed large areas of interstitial fibrosis (thick arrows). Sections G and F showed similar improvements in histological appearance with dramatic decrease in fibrosis (thick arrows).

been reported that energy intake in the hemodialysis patients of Koufaki et al [30] was slightly (5%) but significantly increased.

In this work, the adenine – treated rats exhibited the urinary and plasma profile of several traditional and novel markers of renal damage, as reported by us and others [20,36,37]. Most of these were improved in rats given either GA or SE, and even more so in rats given GA and subjected to SE at the same time, supporting our hypothesis that the ameliorative action of GA on adenine- induced CRF is further enhanced by SE. The use of novel urinary and plasma biomarkers has been recently highlighted as being able to detect subtle and early renal changes in both chronic and acute renal injury [38]. In this work, both traditional and novel biomarkers measured in urine and plasma were nearly all in full agreement. Examples of these novel biomarkers used included

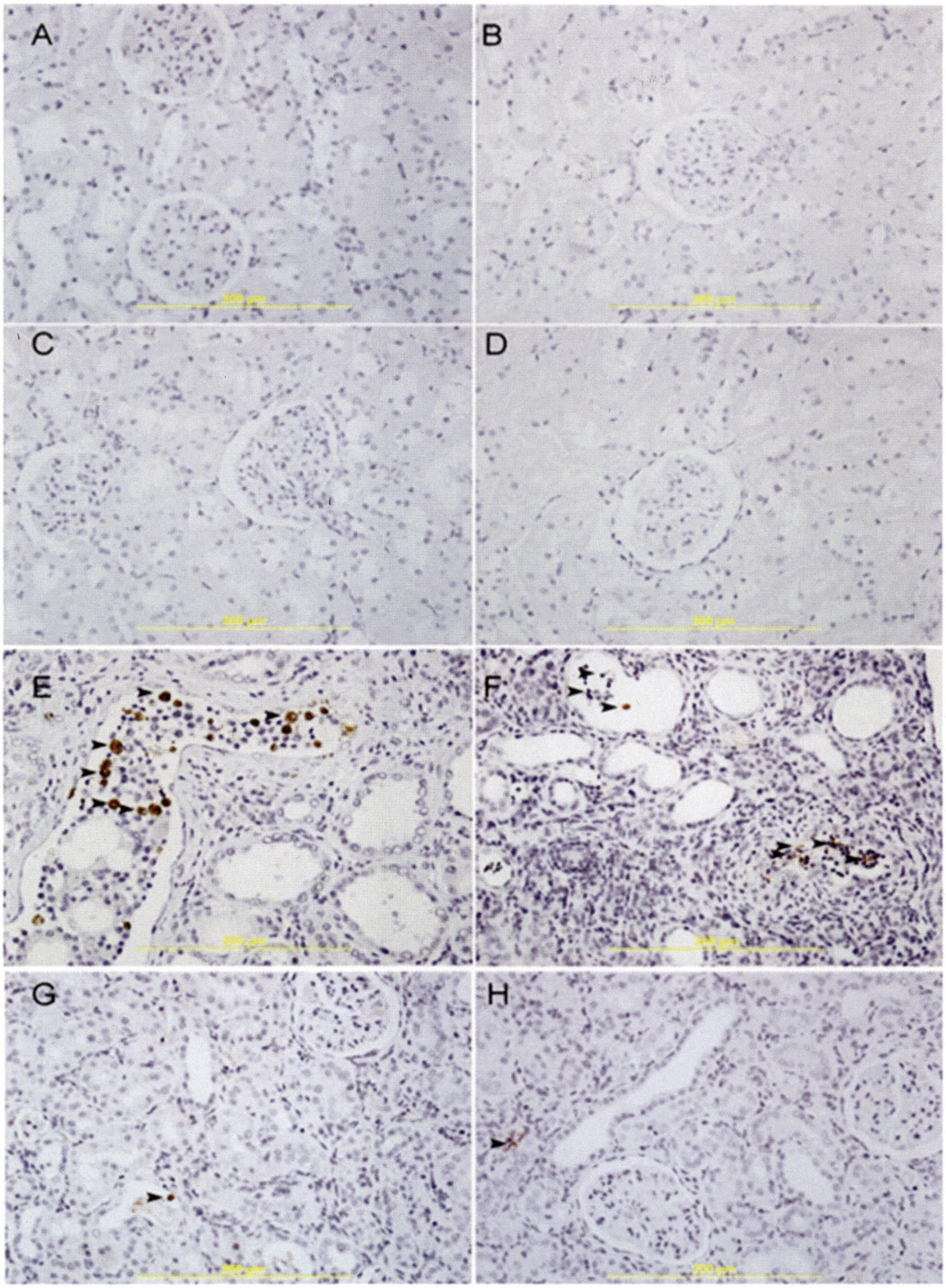

Figure 8. Representative photograph of sections of renal tissue of rats treated with saline (A), saline + swimming exercise, SE (B), gum acacia, GA (C), GA + SE (D), adenine (E), adenine + SE (F), adenine + GA (G) and adenine + GA + SE (H), and analyzed immunohistochemically (anticaspase-3, streptavidin–biotin immunohistochemical method). Sections (**A**), (**B**), (**C**) and (**D**) showed normal kidney architecture and no apoptotic cells. Sections (**E**) and (**F**) both showed acute tubular necrosis with tubular distention and necrotic material and many apoptotic cells showing brown cytoplasmic staining (arrow head). Sections (**G**) and (**H**) both showed a similar degree of improvement in the histological appearance with few focal areas of acute tubular necrosis and very few apoptotic cells showing brown cytoplasmic staining (arrow head).

8-isoprostane, which is a prostaglandin (PG)-F2-like compound that belongs to the F2 isoprostane class. It is produced *in vivo* by the free radical-catalyzed peroxidation of arachidonic acid, and its concentration is increased in conditions and diseases involving oxidative stress [39]. Urinary 8-oxo-2'-deoxyguanosine (8-oxo- dG) concentration is another measure of oxidative DNA stress [28].

Table 3. Evaluation of necrosis and fibrosis in kidneys from rats with chronic kidney disease induced by adenine (A) feeding (0.25% w/w, 5 weeks), and the influence of gum acacia (GA) [15% w/v in drinking water, 5 weeks] with or without swimming exercise (SE) thereon.

Group	% Necrosis	Necrosis Score	% Fibrosis	Fibrosis Score
Saline -treated	0 ± 0^a	0	0 ± 0^a	0
Saline + SE	0 ± 0^a	0	0 ± 0^a	0
A -treated	71.1 ± 2.9^b	3	41.3 ± 2.3^b	2
A –treated + SE	69.8 ± 3.7^b	3	42.1 ± 2.0^b	2
GA	0 ± 0^a	0	0 ± 0^a	0
GA + SE	0 ± 0^a	0	0 ± 0^a	0
A + GA	18.2 ± 0.97^c	1	3.35 ± 0.09^c	1
A + GA + SE	17.8 ± 2.0^c	1	3.42 ± 0.07^c	1

Values in the table are means ± SEM (n = 6 rats).
Values with different superscripts are statistically different (*P* less than 0.05).

Different modes of exercise, including SE, are established to be beneficial in CKD and its cardiovascular and other complications in humans [27,31] and animals [31,28]. The mechanism by which SE ameliorates CKD is not known with certainty, but it has been hypothesized that the basis of the obtained benefits are probably multifactorial [40], and include the beneficial effect of SE on the oxidative status of the tissues. Although there is no unanimity in the literature regarding the influence of exercise on inflammation and oxidative stress, moderate SE is believed to be effective in preventing inflammation and oxidative damage in tissues of rats [32,33], but severe/acute exercise has been shown to produce the opposite effect in humans and rats [34,35]. In our present experiments employing moderate SE, we found that SE did not significantly alter the renal concentration/activity of the measured incidence of oxidative stress (except SOD activity, which was increased), probably reflecting the adequacy of the defensive antioxidant oxidative abilities in these animals. Adenine – induced CKD, as reported before, significantly and markedly decreased the anti-oxidants measured [20,37], an action that was significantly abrogated by either GA or SE given alone, and even more when combined.

In conclusion, we aimed to ascertain experimentally if combining two strategies for mitigating the effects of CKD (viz administration of GA, a nephroprotectant [26] and SE [14] would influence the effects of CKD. Judging by the results of several biochemical and physiological (but not all) parameters measured, there seems to be a significant positive impact in the condition with SE. Therefore, on the whole, these results suggest that the ameliorative action of GA can be enhanced by SE. Previously, it has been reported that significant clinical benefits are obtained from GA treatment in CKD patients who are on a low-protein diet [26]. In future experiments, it would be of interest to see the effect of other modes of exercise with different intensities on the same parameters, and also the possible effect of SE on CKD patients on GA both with and without a low-protein diet.

Author Contributions

Conceived and designed the experiments: BHA. Contributed reagents/materials/analysis tools: BHA MZ MIW SAA JY AN. Contributed to the writing of the manuscript: BHA MZ KAB AN. Conducted the histopathology and immunohistochemistry: SA. Conducted the biochemical experiments: MZ KAB MIW JY AN. Conducted the animal experimentation: AR. Carried out the Western blotting: SAA.

References

1. Harambat J, van Stralen KJ, Kim JJ, Tizard E (2012) Epidemiology of chronic kidney disease in children. Pediatr Nephrol 27: 363–373.
2. Hossain MP, Goyder EC, Rigby JE, El Nahas M (2009) CKD and poverty: a growing global challenge. Am J Kidney Dis 53: 166–174.
3. Briasoulis A, Bakris GL (2013) Chronic kidney disease as a coronary artery disease risk equivalent. Curr Cardiol Rep 15: 340.
4. Clapp EL, Bevington A, Smith AC (2012) Exercise for children with chronic kidney disease and end-stage renal disease. Pediatr Nephrol 27: 165–172.
5. Johansen KL, Painter P (2012) Exercise in individuals with CKD. Am J Kidney Dis 59: 126–134.
6. Bronas UG (2009) Exercise training and reduction of cardiovascular disease risk factors in patients with chronic kidney disease. Adv Chronic Kidney Dis 16: 449–458.
7. Sakr HF (2013) Modulation of metabolic and cardiac dysfunctions by swimming in overweight rats on a high cholesterol and fructose diet: possible role of adiponectin. J Physiol Pharmacol 64: 231–240.
8. Heiwe S, Jacobson SH (2011) Exercise training for adults with chronic kidney disease. Cochrane Database Syst Rev 5: CD003236.
9. Howden EJ, Fassett RG, Isbel NM, Coombes JS (2012) Exercise training in chronic kidney disease patients. Sports Med 42: 473–488.
10. Meredith-Jones K, Waters D, Legge M, Jones L (2011) Upright water-based exercise to improve cardiovascular and metabolic health: a qualitative review. Complement Ther Med 19: 93–103.
11. Tanaka H (2009) Swimming exercise: impact of aquatic exercise on cardiovascular health. Sports Med 39: 377–387.
12. Segura-Orti E, Johansen KL (2010) Exercise in end-stage renal disease. Semi Dial 23: 422–30.
13. Luiz Rda S, Silva KA, Rampaso RR, Antônio EL, Montemor J, et al. (2013) Exercise attenuates renal dysfunction with preservation of myocardial function in chronic kidney disease. PLoS One 8(2): e55363.
14. Peng CC, Chen KC, Hsieh CL, Peng RY (2012) Swimming exercise prevents fibrogenesis in chronic kidney disease by inhibiting the myofibroblast transdifferentiation. PLoS One 7(6): e37388.
15. Kücükköylü S, Rump LC (2013) Cardiovascular morbidity and mortality in renal diseases. Dtsch Med Wochenschr 138: 721–724.
16. Ali BH, Al-Salam S, Al Za'abi M, Waly MI, Ramkumar A, et al. (2013) New model for adenine-induced chronic renal failure in mice, and the effect of gum acacia treatment thereon: Comparison with rats. J Pharmacol Toxicol Methods 68: 384–393.
17. Ali AA, Ali KE, Fadlalla AE, Khalid KE (2008) The effects of gum arabic oral treatment on the metabolic profile of chronic renal failure patients under regular haemodialysis in Central Sudan. Nat Prod Res 22: 12–21.
18. Al Mosawi AJ (2009) Six-year dialysis freedom in end-stage renal disease. Clin Exp Nephrol 13: 494–500.
19. Ali BH, Al-Salam S, Al Husseni I, Kayed RR, Al-Masroori N, et al. (2010) Effects of Gum Arabic in rats with adenine-induced chronic renal failure. Exp Biol Med (Maywood) 235: 373–382.
20. Ali BH, Al-Husseni I, Beegam S, Al-Shukaili A, Nemmar A, et al. (2013) Effect of gum arabic on oxidative stress and inflammation in adenine-induced chronic renal failure in rats. PLoS One 8: e55242.

21. Ali BH, Al Za'abi M, Ramkumar A, Yasin J, Nemmar A (2014) Anemia in adenine-induced chronic renal failure and the influence of treatment with gum acacia thereon. Physiol Res In press.
22. Ali BH, Ziada A, Al Husseni I, Beegam S, Al-Ruqaishi B, et al. (2011) Effect ofAcacia gum on blood pressure in rats with adenine-induced chronic renal failure. Phytomedicine 18: 1176–1180.
23. Neto OB, Abate DT, Júnior MM, Mota GR, Orsatti FL, et al. (2013) Exercise training improves cardiovascular autonomic activity and attenuates renal damage in spontaneously hypertensive rats. J Sports Sci Med 12: 52–59.
24. Gegentonglaga, Yoshizato H, Higuchi Y, Toyota Y, Hanai Y, et al. (2013) Variable alteration of regional tissue oxygen pressure in rat hippocampus by acute swimming exercise. Life Sci 93: 773–777.
25. Al Za'abi M, Ali BH, Al Toubi M (2013) HPLC-fluorescence method for measurement of the uremic toxin indoxyl sulfate in plasma. J Chromatogr Sci 51: 40–43.
26. Ali BH, Ziada A, Blunden G (2009) Biological effects of gum arabic: a review of some recent research. Food Chem Toxicol 47: 1–8.
27. Pechter U, Ots M, Mesikepp S, Zilmer K, Kullissaar T, et al. (2003) Beneficial effects of water-based exercise in patients with chronic kidney disease. Int J Rehabil Res 26: 153–156.
28. Ishikawa Y, Gohda T, Tanimoto M, Omote K, Furukawa M, et al. (2012) Effect of exercise on kidney function, oxidative stress, and inflammation in type 2 diabetic KK-A(y) mice. Exp Diabetes Res 2012: 702948.
29. Babiker R, Merghani TH, Elmusharaf K, Badi RM, Lang F, et al. (2012) Effects of Gum Arabic ingestion on body mass index and body fat percentage in healthy adult females: two-arm randomized, placebo controlled, double-blind trial. Nutr J 11: 111.
30. Koufaki P, Mercer TH, Naish PF (2002) Effects of exercise training on aerobic and functional capacity of end-stage renal disease patients. Clin Physiol Funct Imaging 22: 115–124.
31. Kutner NG (2007) How can exercise be incorporated into the routine care of patients on dialysis? Int Urol Nephrol 39: 1281–1285.
32. Smart N, Steele M (2011) Exercise training in haemodialysis patients: a systematic review and meta-analysis. Nephrology (Carlton) 16: 626–632.
33. Cechella JL, Leite MR, Dobrachinski F, da Rocha JT, Carvalho NR, et al. (2014) Moderate swimming exercise and caffeine supplementation reduce the levels of inflammatory cytokines without causing oxidative stress in tissues of middle-aged rats. Amino Acids In press.
34. Ranadive SM, Kappus RM, Cook MD, Yan H, Lane AD, et al. (2014) Effect of acute moderate exercise on induced inflammation and arterial function in older adults. Exp Physiol In press.
35. Deminice R, Trindade CS, Degiovanni GC, Garlip MR, Portari GV, et al. (2010) Oxidative stress biomarkers response to high intensity interval training and relation to performance in competitive swimmers. J Sports Med Phys Fitness 50: 356–362.
36. Deminice R, Jordao AA (2012) Creatine supplementation reduces oxidative stress biomarkers after acute exercise in rats. Amino Acids 43: 709–715.
37. Diwan V, Mistry A, Gobe G, Brown L (2013) Adenine-induced chronic kidney and cardiovascular damage in rats. J Pharmacol Toxicol Methods 68: 197–207.
38. Fuchs TC, Hewitt P (2011) Biomarkers for drug-induced renal damage and nephrotoxicity-an overview for applied toxicology. AAPS J 3: 615–631.
39. Knight SF, Yuan J, Roy S, Imig JD (2010) Simvastatin and tempol protect against endothelial dysfunction and renal injury in a model of obesity and hypertension. Am J Physiol Renal Physiol 298: F86–94.
40. Heiwe S, Jacobson SH (2011) Exercise training for adults with chronic kidney disease. Cochrane Database Syst Rev 10: CD003236.

15

TRPC6 Single Nucleotide Polymorphisms and Progression of Idiopathic Membranous Nephropathy

Julia M. Hofstra[1], Marieke J. H. Coenen[2], Mascha M. V. A. P. Schijvenaars[2], Jo H. M. Berden[1], Johan van der Vlag[1], Lies H. Hoefsloot[2¤a], Nine V. A. M. Knoers[2¤b], Jack F. M. Wetzels[1], Tom Nijenhuis[1]*

1 Department of Nephrology, Radboud university medical center, Nijmegen, the Netherlands, **2** Department of Human Genetics, Radboud university medical center, Nijmegen, the Netherlands

Abstract

Background: Activating mutations in the Transient Receptor Potential channel C6 (TRPC6) cause autosomal dominant focal segmental glomerular sclerosis (FSGS). TRPC6 expression is upregulated in renal biopsies of patients with idiopathic membranous glomerulopathy (iMN) and animal models thereof. In iMN, disease progression is characterized by glomerulosclerosis. In addition, a context-dependent TRPC6 overexpression was recently suggested in complement-mediated podocyte injury in e.g. iMN. Hence, we hypothesized that genetic variants in TRPC6 might affect susceptibility to development or progression of iMN.

Methods & Results: Genomic DNA was isolated from blood samples of 101 iMN patients and 292 controls. By direct sequencing of the entire TRPC6 gene, 13 single nucleotide polymorphisms (SNPs) were identified in the iMN cohort, two of which were causing an amino acid substitution (rs3802829; Pro15Ser and rs36111323, Ala404Val). No statistically significant differences in genotypes or allele frequencies between patients and controls were observed. Clinical outcome in patients was determined (remission n = 26, renal failure n = 46, persistent proteinuria n = 29, follow-up median 80 months {range 51–166}). The 13 identified SNPs showed no association with remission or renal failure. There were no differences in genotypes or allele frequencies between patients in remission and progressors.

Conclusions: Our data suggest that TRPC6 polymorphisms do not affect susceptibility to iMN, or clinical outcome in iMN.

Editor: Michael Edward Zwick, Emory University School Of Medicine, United States of America

Funding: Financial support was provided by a Dutch Kidney Foundation grant (OW08) for J. M. H and J. F. M. W., a Kolff Career Stimulation Grant from the Dutch Kidney Foundation (KJPB 07.0001), a grant from the Genzyme Renal Innovations Program (GRIP) and a Ruby Diabetes Research Grant from the Dutch Diabetes Fund (2009.80.118) for T. N. http://www.nierstichting.nl http://www.genzyme.com/Responsibility/Grants-and-Giving.aspx http://www.diabetesfonds.nl The funders had no role in study design, data collection and analysis, decision to publish, or preparation of the manuscript.

Competing Interests: The authors have declared that no competing interests exist.

* Email: Tom.Nijenhuis@Radboudumc.nl

¤a Current address: Department of Clinical Genetics, Erasmus Medical Centre, Rotterdam, the Netherlands
¤b Current address: Department of Medical Genetics, Utrecht Medical Centre, Utrecht, the Netherlands

Introduction

Membranous nephropathy (MN) is the leading cause of nephrotic syndrome in the adult Caucasian population and is characterized by immune complex deposition in the subepithelial layer of the glomerular basement membrane. In one third of patients, MN is caused by an underlying disease such as a malignancy, infection or a systemic disease. Until recently, no underlying cause could be identified in two thirds of patients and, therefore, the disease was considered to be idiopathic (iMN) in these patients. [1] In 2009 Beck *et al.* discovered antibodies against the M-type phospholipase A_2 receptor (PLA_2R), a membrane glycoprotein located on the podocyte, in patients with iMN. [2] Further studies showed that antibodies against PLA_2R are present in approximately 70% of Caucasian patients with active disease. [3,4] This finding thus provided evidence that iMN is an autoimmune disease.

A recent genome-wide association study showed that genetic variants in *HLA-DQA1* and *phospholipase A2 receptor* (*PLA2R1*) were most significantly associated with biopsy-proven iMN. [5] Association with *HLA* regions has been identified in many autoimmune diseases, the association with the *PLA2R1* gene supports the key role of the anti-PLA2R antibodies in the pathogenesis of the disease. In an additional study we assessed if rare genetic variants within the coding region of the *PLA2R1* gene could explain antibody formation. Although sequencing of the complete coding sequence of *PLA2R1* in 95 patients with iMN confirmed associations of common single nucleotide polymorphisms (SNPs) with iMN, rare variants were present in only a minority of patients (9%). [6] This data questions why iMN is rare, as these SNPs occur frequently in the general population. It could be hypothesized that a rare combination of (relatively) common events (genetic variants and/or environmental factors) might constitute the pathogenetic trigger. In addition to *HLA* and *PLA2R1*, variants in other genes might be involved.

One of the biggest unresolved issues in patients with iMN is the highly variable disease course. Spontaneous remission occurs in about 40–50% of patients, but another 30–50% of patients progresses to end stage renal disease within 10 years. [7] Although several predictive strategies have been proposed, it remains difficult to identify patients with a high risk of disease progression. [8,9] Progression of disease is accompanied by glomerulsclerosis in renal biopsies. [10]

The Transient Receptor Potential channel C6 (TRPC6) is an ion channel that is expressed in podocytes at the slit diaphragm {Figure 1}. [11] This complex of interconnected proteins provides both physical linkage as well as a signaling platform that regulates podocyte behavior and architecture, and thereby affects glomerular permeability. TRPC6 was recognized as an important slit diaphragm component after *TRPC6* gain-of-function mutations were shown to be responsible for autosomal dominant focal segmental glomerulosclerosis (FSGS), a leading cause of steroid-resistant nephrotic syndrome that can rapidly progress to end-stage renal disease (ESRD). [11–15] Animal studies show that podocyte-specific transgenic TRPC6 overexpression leads to albuminuria and histological findings similar to human FSGS. [14,16] However, glomerular *TRPC6* expression is also increased in acquired human proteinuric diseases. Importantly, this occurs in human MN, as well as in the passive Heymann nephritis animal model for MN. [13,17] Furthermore, angiotensin II (AngII) activates specific TRPC6-mediated intracellular pathways in the podocyte. [17–20] Angiotensin receptor blockers, angiotensin converting enzyme inhibitors and calcineurin inhibitors, all three utilized to treat proteinuria in MN, were shown to inhibit these TRPC6-mediated cascades. [17,19] Thus, TRPC6 is not only primarily involved in the pathogenesis of FSGS, but could also mediate podocyte damage and/or progression to ESRD in other proteinuric diseases like MN. Therefore, we hypothesized that sequence variations in the *TRPC6* gene could affect susceptibility to development and/or progression of iMN.

In the present study, we screened a cohort of 101 biopsy-proven iMN patients for *TRPC6* sequence variations by direct sequencing of all 13 exons of the *TRPC6* gene. Furthermore, we assessed whether genetic variants were associated with disease progression and outcome in patients with iMN.

Subjects and Methods

Patients

The present study included iMN patients referred to our centre between 1995 and 2007. In all patients, the diagnosis of iMN was established by renal biopsy and secondary causes were excluded according to local routine clinical work up. [21] Baseline data on age, sex and ethnicity were present for all patients. To allow subgroup analysis of anti-PLA_2R positive patients, the presence of anti-PLA2R antibodies in the serum was evaluated. Serum samples at diagnosis were available for most patients. The assay for measuring anti-PLA_2R antibodies has been previously described. [22]

iMN patients were evaluated using a standardized protocol as previously described. [23] Patients were prospectively followed, and data on treatment and outcome (e.g. remission and renal survival) are obtained. For the current study we evaluated the occurrence of spontaneous remissions and/or renal failure. Spontaneous remission was defined as proteinuria <2.0 g/day with stable renal function in a patient not treated with immunosuppressive agents. Renal failure/progression was defined as an increase in serum creatinine >25% from baseline with a serum creatinine >135 µmol/l or an increase >50% from baseline.

Ethics statement

The study was approved by the ethics committee of the Radboud university medical center (Commissie Mensgebonden Onderzoek (CMO) Regio Arnhem Nijmegen, nr.9701-0016). All patients gave written informed consent prior to participation in the study.

Sequencing

DNA was purified from blood samples using salt extraction according to a previously described protocol. [24] All exons including splice sites in the *TRPC6* gene were sequenced. Sense and antisense primers were designed using Primer3. [25] PCR primers and conditions are given in Table 1. PCR products were purified using Multiscreen filter plates (Millipore Carrigtwohill, Cork, Ireland). Purified products were used for Sanger sequence analysis (bidirectional) with dye-termination chemistry (BigDye Terminator, version 3) on a 3730 DNA analyzer (Applied Biosystems, Inc., Foster City, CA, USA).

Analysis

TRPC6 sequences were analyzed for the presence of genetic variants in comparison with the published reference sequence for human *TRPC6* (mRNA NM_004621.5). Ethnically matched population allele frequencies of the identified variants were obtained from the 1000 Genomes project (1000 Genomes release 10 - March 2012). [26] Variants were considered to be common (previously reported with allele frequency >1%), rare (previously reported with allele frequency <1%), or novel (not previously reported in the 1000 Genome project nor in dbSNP 136).

SNP genotyping. SNPs that lead to amino acid substitutions, and/or that were rare (previously with allele frequency <1%), completed with SNPs that had a the minor allele frequency in the patient cohort of >10%, were selected for genotyping in 292 healthy individuals from the same geographical region (Table 2). Genotyping was performed using Taqman allelic discrimination assays (Invitrogen, Bleiswijk, The Netherlands) according to the instructions of the manufacturer. The fluorescent signal for allelic discrimination was determined after amplification using an end-point reading on the 7500 Fast Real-time System (Applied Biosystems). Automated allele calling was performed by allelic discrimination plots using SDS 1.4 software (Applied Biosystems). We included 5% duplicate samples in each plate as quality control.

Association analysis. Frequencies of SNPs identified in iMN patients were compared with genotype data of 379 Caucasian controls that were downloaded from the 1000 Genomes project (release 10). In an attempt to increase power, data of 292 healthy controls were added for variants in 5 SNPs, as detected with Taqman assay. Association analyses were performed using the whole genome analysis toolset PLINK (version 1.07). [27] Significance was set a $p<0.05$. SNPs with an allele frequency of 0.1 and higher were used to construct haplotypes. Haplotype analysis was also performed using PLINK. Next, frequencies of SNPs identified in patients with progressive disease (renal failure) were compared with frequencies observed in patients with a spontaneous remission of proteinuria as described above.

Power calculations. In order to be able to estimate the effect size of the genetic variants, we performed a genetic power calculation using the online Harvard Genetic Power Calculator (http://pngu.mgh.harvard.edu/~purcell/gpc/). We calculated the effect size that could be excluded with 80% power and a

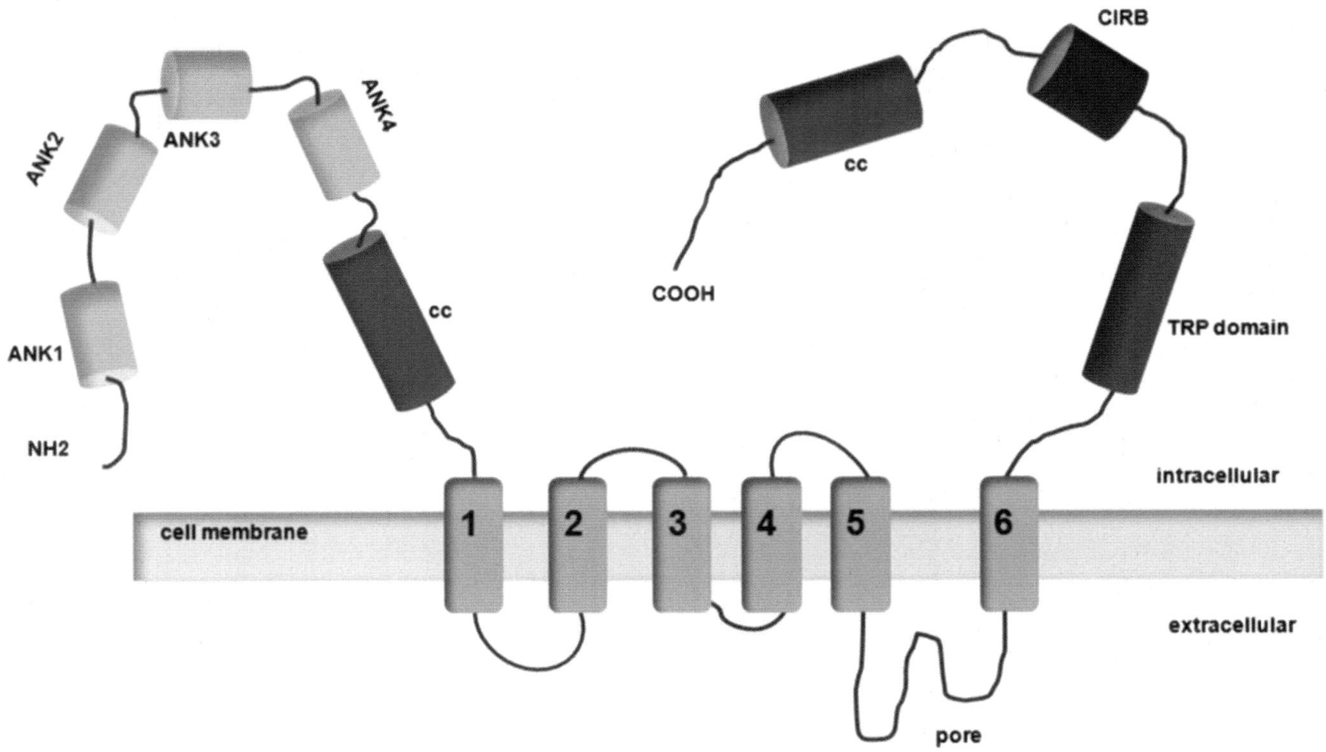

Figure 1. TRPC6 topology. Structure of the TRPC6 monomer. TRPC6 belongs to the large family of TRP channels, which contain six transmembrane domains, one pore-forming region and large intracellular N- and C-tails. Four subunits are required to assemble a functional channel. In the pococyte, TRPC6 is part of the slit diaphragm multiprotein complex. TRP: transient receptor potential, ANK: Ankyrin repeat, cc: coiled–coiled domain, CIRB: CaM/IP3R-binding domain.

two-sided p-value of 0.05, for various frequencies of the high-risk allele (ranging from 0.200 to 0.008).

Results

Patient characteristics

A total of 101 patients with biopsy proven iMN were included in the present study. Patients were mostly male (77%) and mean age at diagnosis was 51±15 years. All patients were of self-reported Caucasian ancestry. Serum samples at onset of disease were available for 92 patients, anti-PLA_2R antibodies were present in 62 samples (67%).

Sequencing

In 101 patients with iMN we identified eight sequence variants in the coding region of the *TRPC6* gene (Table 2). Of the eight coding variants observed, six were common SNPs and two were rare (See Methods for definitions). These rare variants (c.888G>A and c.2142G>T) were both encountered once in two different patients in a heterozygous state, but did not result in amino acid changes (synonymous mutations). Only two of the common SNPs resulted in an amino acid substitution (rs3802829; Pro15Ser and rs36111323, Ala404Val). Four additional common SNPs were observed in the intron regions, as well as one rare variant in the 5′ UTR (c1-10 C>A). The latter was present in 5 patients, all in a heterozygous state.

Association between *TRPC6* variants and occurrence of iMN

Control data were obtained from the 1000 Genomes project as described. To increase power to detect possible genotype frequency differences between our iMN cohort and the general population, 292 healthy Caucasian controls from the same geographical area were included as an additional control group for the frequency of five SNPs. These five SNPs were selected by previously specified criteria. Association analysis showed that there were no significant differences in the allele frequencies of both the coding and non-coding SNPs between the 101 iMN patients and ethnically matched controls (Table 2). Based on our power calculations, the effect sizes that could be excluded for the various frequencies of the high-risk allele were above 1.6 to 4. For the two SNPs leading to amino acid substitutions in exons, these were 1.7 and 1.8, respectively.

When analyzing associations for the subgroup of PLA_2R positive patients (n = 62), the synonymous SNP rs12366144 was more frequently present in patients than in controls (p = 0.02) (Table 2). However, when correcting for the multiple testing of 12 SNPs, (p-value should be less than 0.05/12 = 0.00417), this significant association disappeared. Haplotype analysis was performed including all available SNPs, but no significant associations were determined.

Association between *TRPC6* variants and clinical outcome

After a median follow-up of 80 months (range 15–166) spontaneous remission had occurred in 26 patients, and 46 patients had progressed to renal failure. Of the remaining patients, six had persistent proteinuria >2.0 gram/day with stable renal

Table 1. Primers used to sequence the 13 exons of *TRPC6*.

Exon	F/R primer	Primer sequence 5′—3′
1	F primer	GTCTGCCCAGGTCCAGTTC
1	R primer	GTACACACGCGGGTTCAG
2_01	F primer	GATGAATGGCAAGTCATTTGG
2_01	R primer	AACCTCTTGCCTTCAGCAAA
2_02	F primer	GCCAATGAGCATCTGGAAAT
2_02	R primer	AGCCGTCATGACTGGATCTT
2_03	F primer	GATTGAACGGCCTCATGATT
2_03	R primer	GGTAGCGATCACAACTTTTGC
3	F primer	AACGTGGTATTCTCCATTATTGC
3	R primer	AGCACCAACAAGAACCAAAA
4	F primer	GCCATTTGTTTGTTGCCTGT
4	R primer	TGGAGATAAGATTTTTCCCCACT
5	F primer	GGAGATCATTGGAATGTGCAG
5	R primer	AATGAACCCAAGGCAACTGT
6	F primer	TTGGGACCAAATTTTGAAGG
6	R primer	GAGAATTGTGCAGTAACCGAACT
7	F primer	GGAGACTTCCATTCGAAAACC
7	R primer	CCAAAACATTATCCCATGGAC
8	F primer	TCACTAATTTGCAGACACTAAACAA
8	R primer	CGAAGAGCAGTCCATGCTT
9	F primer	CGATCACTGGGGTCTGAGAG
9	R primer	AAAGGGATGTGGCATAGTGG
10	F primer	AGGGAAGAACCCCGTAAGAA
10	R primer	GCTTCTGAACATCTGTCCCTTT
11	F primer	TTGGCAGCCACAAAGTCTAA
11	R primer	AAGAATCACATAGTTCAAGAACCTAAA
12	F primer	GGCTCACTACAGGGAGGAAG
12	R primer	GCTCTCCAGGCACTCTGC
13	F primer	TTTCCTCCTGTCCCACAGTC
13	R primer	GGCTCCAGATGATAGGATGG

F, forward; R, reverse.

function, 19 patients were censored for outcome analysis because of treatment with immunosuppressive agents, and four patients were lost to follow-up. None of the 13 identified *TRPC6* sequence variations correlated with remission or renal failure (Table 3). An additional analysis comparing those patients in whom spontaneous remission occurred (n = 26) to all others (n = 75) also did not show differences between groups (data not shown).

Discussion

In this study, 13 SNPs in the gene encoding *TRPC6* were identified in our cohort of 101 biopsy-proven iMN patients. None of the identified SNPs was associated with the occurrence of iMN *per se*. In addition, the presence of *TRPC6* SNPs was not associated with clinical outcome in terms of remission rate, persistence of proteinuria or progression to renal failure. Thus, our data do not confirm the hypothesis that *TRPC6* SNPs could confer susceptibility to, or alter the clinical course in iMN.

Pathogenesis of iMN has been an unsolved mystery for decades. The histological features of MN were first described in 1957. [28] The characteristic finding in kidney biopsies of subepithelial deposits that consisted of IgG and complement pointed to an immunological disease ontology. In a rat model of MN, Heymann's nephritis, the disease is caused by IgG antibodies targeting megalin, a protein expressed by both rat tubular cells and podocytes. [29] Since megalin is not present on human podocytes, other pathophysiological mechanisms and other antigenic targets have been considered. A major breakthrough came with the discovery by Beck *et al.* of circulating auto-antibodies against the M-type Phospholipase A_2 receptor (PLA2R), a protein expressed by human podocytes, in the majority of patients with iMN. [2] Anti-PLA2R antibodies in iMN are mainly of the IgG4 subclass, both in serum and in biopsies. IgG4 is considered not to activate complement, but immune deposits in iMN contain large amount of complement C3. It has been suggested that anti-PLA2R antibodies might activate the lectin pathway of the complement cascade by binding to Mannose Binding Lectin. [30] However, the mechanism by which the antibodies finally lead to the membranous phenotype with severe podocyte damage is still unknown. Furthermore, the trigger for autoantibody formation remains unclear. A rare combination of (relatively) common events (genetic variants and/or environmental factors) might serve as a pathogenetic trigger in a multi-hit setting.

Next to these remaining questions on pathogenetic issues, the substantial interindividual variability in the course and prognosis of the iMN is also unexplained as yet. Why is the disease benign with a single episode and spontaneous remission in some patients, and do other patients progress to ESRD after several treatment resistant episodes? The genetic profile of the patient may be one of the aspects contributing to this interindividual variability. In another glomerulopathy, IgA nephropathy, common polymorphisms in several genes (*MYH*, *TLR9*) were associated with disease progression and development of ESRD. [31,32] Since *TRPC6* gain-of-function mutations cause podocyte injury leading to hereditary FSGS, glomerular TRPC6 expression is increased in MN, and glomerulosclerosis occurs in progressive MN, we hypothesized that polymorphisms in *TRPC6*, contribute to the susceptibility to develop iMN and/or progress to end-stage renal disease. Of note, Chen *et al.* previously showed that three *TRPC6* SNPs, which they selected on reasons that were not clearly defined, did not correlate with the occurrence of MN. [33] In our study, all exons were sequenced including splice sites in the *TRPC6* gene to identify polymorphisms in the coding regions of *TRPC6* in an unbiased manner. While we identified *TRPC6* SNPs in iMN patients, we found no association of these SNPs with disease occurrence or progression, although based on the number of patients in our cohort a limited effect size could have been missed. This means that the alleles we identified could still have functional effects on TRPC6 channel activity, of which the resulting clinical effect would fall under the effect size we can rule out. However, the majority of the identified SNPs [11] were either intronic or synonomous, minimizing the chance of any functional relevance. The two SNPs causing predicted amino acid substitutions, although of interest, clearly did not contribute to the development of MN in all patients.

In the PLA2R positive patients, one SNP showed an association, but the statistical significance of this association was lost after correction for multiple testing. In terms of genetic association studies, our cohort is quite small and we, therefore, cannot exclude that our study is underpowered to find existing associations, especially with regard to haplotypes. As only the coding regions of the *TRPC6* gene were sequenced, information on intronic polymorphisms and/or SNPs in the promoter region of the gene that might influence expression of the TRPC6 protein, is lacking.

Table 2. *TRPC6* variants in patients with iMN (n = 101).

Chr	position	name	ref	All	CEU AF	AF patients	p-value	AF PLA2R	p-value*	ref cDNA	cDNA	prot. level	effect	exon	observations
11	101454244	rs191383391	G	G/T	0.017**	0.025	0.44	0.024	0.56	C	c.-10C>A		5′-ÚTR	1	
11	101454192	rs3802829	G	G/A	0.093**	0.089	0.85	0.113	0.48	C	c.43C>T	p.Pro15Ser	missense	1	NH2-terminal region
11	101453995	rs17096918	C	C/T	0.083	0.069	0.52	0.081	0.93	G	c.170+70G>A		intron		
11	101375549	rs10501986	T	T/C	0.480	0.495	0.71	0.492	0.81	A	c.171-20A>G		intron		
11	101374812	rs144891994	C	C/T	0 ^	0.005	NA	0.008	NA	G	c.888G>A	p.Thr296Thr	synonymous	2	CCD
11	101374626	rs4542378	G	G/A	0.480	0.490	0.80	0.492	0.81	C	c.945+129C>T		intron		
11	101359750	rs36111323	G	G/A	0.135**	0.165	0.24	0.156	0.52	C	c.1211C>T	p.Ala404Val	missense	4	linker region between CCD & TMD1
11	101347093	rs12366144	A	A/G	0.250**	0.292	0.20	0.347	0.02	T	c.1683T>C	p.Asn561Asn	synonymous	6	linker region between TMD3 & TMD4
11	101342958	rs61743044	G	G/A	0.020	0.020	1.00	0.024	0.75	C	c.2115C>T	p.Tyr705Tyr	synonymous	8	linker region between TMD5 & TMD6
11	101342931	rs144891994	C	C/A	0.008	0.005	0.66	0	0.32	G	c.2142G>T	p.Thr714Thr	synonymous	8	TMD 6
11	101325970	rs7105083	G	G/A	0.263	0.238	0.47	0.266	0.93	C	c.2485-138C>T		intron		
11	101325788	rs72984209	G	G/A	0.077	0.054	0.28	0.081	0.87	C	c.2529C>T	p.Phe843Phe	synonymous	11	
11	101323770	rs12805398	C	C/T	0.140**	0.158	0.49	0.153	0.69	G	c.2712G>A	p.Gln904Gln	synonymous	13	

Chr = chromosome; position = basepair position based on UCSC genome browser version Human Feb. 2009 (GRCh37/hg19) assembly; name = rs identifier; ref = genomic reference allele; all = alleles; CEU AF = allele frequencies variant allele in control population. Control population consists of Caucasian population from 1000 Genomes project (release 10 - March 2012), complemented with data form 292 geographically matched controls for variants marked with **; ^ = not reported in 1000 Genomes project; AF patient = patient minor allele frequencies; p-value = comparison allele frequencies controls and patients; AF PLA2R = minor allele frequencies in PLA2R positive patients (n = 62); p-value* = comparison allele frequencies controls and PLA2R positive patients; genomic level = NC_000002.11; ref cDNA = reference allele cDNA (given that TRPC6 is on the negative strand); cDNA = NM_004621.5; prot. level = NP_004612.2; CCD = coiled-coiled domain; TMD = transmembrane domain.

Table 3. Genotypes in iMN patients with clinical remission versus patients with renal failure.

	Genotype	Remission n = 26 (%)		Renal Failure n = 46 (%)		p-value*
rs191383391	CC	25	(96.2)	43	(93.5)	0.64
	CA	1	(3.8)	3	(6.5)	
rs3802829	CC	22	(84.6)	37	(80.4)	0.68
	CT	4	(15.4)	9	(19.6)	
rs17096918	GG	23	(88.5)	37	(80.4)	0.40
	GA	3	(11.5)	9	(19.6)	
rs10501986	AA	9	(34.6)	10	(21.7)	0.09
	AG	15	(57.7)	25	(54.3)	
	GG	2	(7.7)	11	(23.9)	
rs144891994	GG	26	(100)	46	(100)	1.00
rs4542378	CC	9	(34.6)	9	(19.6)	0.09
	CT	15	(57.7)	27	(58.7)	
	TT	2	(7.7)	10	(21.7)	
rs36111323*	GG	19	(73.1)	31	(67.4)	0.74
	GA	7	(26.9)	14	(30.4)	
rs61743044	CC	26	(100)	43	(93.5)	1.00
	CT	0	(0)	3	(6.5)	
rs12366144	TT	16	(61.5)	20	(43.5)	0.18
	TC	9	(34.6)	23	(50.0)	
	CC	1	(3.8)	3	(6.5)	
rs145077205	GG	25	(96.2)	46	(100)	0.18
	GT	1	(3.8)	0	(0)	
rs7105083	CC	15	(57.7)	26	(56.5)	0.91
	CT	10	(38.5)	18	(39.1)	
	TT	1	(3.8)	2	(4.3)	
rs72984209	CC	23	(88.5)	41	(89.1)	0.93
	CT	3	(11.5)	5	(10.9)	
rs12805398	GG	18	(69.2)	32	(69.6)	0.88
	GA	8	(30.8)	14	(30.4)	

*N = 45 for renal failure.
*P-value for minor allele frequencies-comparison (Mann-Whitney U).

Since it is *TRPC6* gain-of-function that is associated with podocyte injury, transcriptionally-mediated increased or diminished *TRPC6* expression as a result of genetic variants in *TRPC6* regulatory regions, might influence susceptibility and prognosis.

However, assuming that *TRPC6* SNPs do not affect occurrence and progression in iMN, the question still remains why TRPC6 is overexpressed in iMN. Since TRPC6 is overexpressed in several human glomerular diseases and animal models of podocyte injury and glomerular disease, it could be a common effector in the resulting podocyte injury.[13,17] We have previously shown that AngII-mediated activation of the deleterious calcineurin/NFAT pathway, which includes Ca^{2+} influx through TRPC6 itself, leads to enhanced transcriptional expression of TRPC6 in the podocyte. [17] In addition, antiproteinuric agents like angiotensin receptor blockers, angiotensin converting enzyme inhibitors, calcineurin inhibitors and vitamin D normalize TRPC6 expression in podocyte injury and experimental glomerular disease. [17,34] Alternatively, an interesting hypothesis could be that e.g. anti-PLA2R antibodies actually activate PLA2R on the surface of the podocyte. In cell types other than podocytes, Ca^{2+} influx was demonstrated to be coupled to PLA2R activation. [35] Hypothetically, binding of anti-PLA2R antibodies to PLA2R on the podocyte could activate Ca^{2+} influx through TRPC6 and/or increase TRPC6 expression. A recent study from Kistler et al.,suggests that increasing TRPC6 expression might at first actually serve to protect the podocyte from complement-mediated injury, which seems crucial in MN. [36] Eventually, prolonged TRPC6 overexpression might then become deleterious. While *TRPC6* SNPs do not appear to alter susceptibility to iMN occurrence and progression, this new hypothesis suggests that TRPC6 indeed plays a pathophysiological role in iMN.

Author Contributions

Conceived and designed the experiments: JMH MJHC JFMW TN. Performed the experiments: JMH MJHC MMVAPS. Analyzed the data: JMH MJHC TN. Contributed reagents/materials/analysis tools: MJHC LHH NVAMK. Contributed to the writing of the manuscript: JMH MJHC TN JB JvdV JFMW TN.

References

1. Glassock RJ (1992) Secondary membranous glomerulonephritis. Nephrol Dial Transplant 7 Suppl 1: 64–71
2. Beck LH Jr, Bonegio RG, Lambeau G, Beck DM, Powell DW, Cummins TD, et al. (2009) M-type phospholipase A2 receptor as target antigen in idiopathic membranous nephropathy. N Engl J Med 361: 11–21
3. Ronco P, Debiec H (2012) Pathogenesis of membranous nephropathy: recent advances and future challenges. Nat Rev Nephrol 8: 203–213
4. Hofstra JM, Wetzels JF (2012) Anti-PLA(2)R antibodies in membranous nephropathy: ready for routine clinical practice? Neth J Med 70: 109–113
5. Stanescu HC, Arcos-Burgos M, Medlar A, Bockenhauer D, Kottgen A, Dragomirescu L, et al. (2011) Risk HLA-DQA1 and PLA(2)R1 alleles in idiopathic membranous nephropathy. The New England journal of medicine. 364: 616–626
6. Coenen MJ, Hofstra JM, Debiec H, Stanescu HC, Medlar AJ, Stengel B, et al. (2013) Phospholipase A2 Receptor (PLA2R1) Sequence Variants in Idiopathic Membranous Nephropathy. J Am Soc Nephrol. 24: 677–683
7. van den Brand JA, Hofstra JM, Wetzels JF (2011) Low-molecular-weight proteins as prognostic markers in idiopathic membranous nephropathy. Clin J Am Soc Nephrol 6: 2846–2853
8. Hofstra JM, Fervenza FC, Wetzels JF (2013) Treatment of idiopathic membranous nephropathy. Nature reviews Nephrology 9: 443–458
9. van den Brand JA, Hofstra JM, Wetzels JF (2012) Prognostic value of risk score and urinary markers in idiopathic membranous nephropathy. Clin J Am Soc Nephrol 7: 1242–1248
10. Heeringa SF, Branten AJ, Deegens JK, Steenbergen E, Wetzels JF (2007) Focal segmental glomerulosclerosis is not a sufficient predictor of renal outcome in patients with membranous nephropathy. Nephrol Dial Transplant 22: 2201–2207
11. Reiser J, Polu KR, Moller CC, Kenlan P, Altintas MM, Wei C, et al. (2005) TRPC6 is a glomerular slit diaphragm-associated channel required for normal renal function. Nat Genet 37: 739–744
12. Winn MP, Conlon PJ, Lynn KL, Farrington MK, Creazzo T, Hawkins AF, et al. (2005) A mutation in the TRPC6 cation channel causes familial focal segmental glomerulosclerosis. Science 308: 1801–1804
13. Moller CC, Wei C, Altintas MM, Li J, Greka A, Ohse T, et al. (2007) Induction of TRPC6 channel in acquired forms of proteinuric kidney disease. J Am Soc Nephrol 18: 29–36
14. Krall P, Canales CP, Kairath P, Carmona-Mora P, Molina J, Carpio JD, et al. (2010) Podocyte-specific overexpression of wild type or mutant trpc6 in mice is sufficient to cause glomerular disease. PLoS One 5: e12859.
15. Hofstra JM, Lainez S, van Kuijk WH, Schoots J, Baltissen MP, Hoefsloot LH, et al. (2013) New TRPC6 gain-of-function mutation in a non-consanguineous Dutch family with late-onset focal segmental glomerulosclerosis. Nephrol Dial Transplant 28: 1830–1838
16. Goel M, Sinkins WG, Zuo CD, Estacion M, Schilling WP (2006) Identification and localization of TRPC channels in the rat kidney. Am J Physiol Renal Physiol. 290(5):F1241–F52.
17. Nijenhuis T, Sloan AJ, Hoenderop JG, Flesche J, van GH, Kistler AD, et al. (2011) Angiotensin II contributes to podocyte injury by increasing TRPC6 expression via an NFAT-mediated positive feedback signaling pathway. Am J Pathol 179: 1719–1732
18. Zhang H, Ding J, Fan Q, Liu S (2009) TRPC6 up-regulation in Ang II-induced podocyte apoptosis might result from ERK activation and NF-kappaB translocation. Exp Biol Med 234: 1029–1036
19. Schlondorff J, Del CD, Carrasquillo R, Lacey V, Pollak MR (2009) TRPC6 mutations associated with focal segmental glomerulosclerosis cause constitutive activation of NFAT-dependent transcription. Am J Physiol Cell Physiol 296: C558–C569
20. Eckel J, Lavin PJ, Finch EA, Mukerji N, Burch J, Gbadegesin R, et al. (2011) TRPC6 enhances angiotensin II-induced albuminuria. J Am Soc Nephrol 22: 526–535
21. Hofstra JM, Wetzels JF (2012) Management of patients with membranous nephropathy. Nephrol Dial Transplant 27: 6–9
22. Debiec H, Ronco P (2011) PLA2R autoantibodies and PLA2R glomerular deposits in membranous nephropathy. N Engl J Med 364: 689–690
23. Branten AJ, du Buf-Vereijken PW, Klasen IS, Bosch FH, Feith GW, Hollander DA, et al. (2005) Urinary excretion of beta2-microglobulin and IgG predict prognosis in idiopathic membranous nephropathy: a validation study. J Am Soc Nephrol 16: 169–174
24. Miller SA, Dykes DD, Polesky HF (1988) A simple salting out procedure for extracting DNA from human nucleated cells. Nucleic Acids Res 16:1215
25. Rozen S, Skaletsky H (2000) Primer3 on the WWW for general users and for biologist programmers. Methods Mol Biol 132: 365–386
26. GenomesProject (2010) A map of human genome variation from population-scale sequencing. Nature 467: 1061–1073
27. Purcell S, Neale B, Todd-Brown K, Thomas L, Ferreira MA, Bender D, et al. (2007) PLINK: a tool set for whole-genome association and population-based linkage analyses. Am J Hum Genet 81: 559–575
28. Jones DB (1957) Nephrotic glomerulonephritis. Am J Pathol 33: 313–329
29. Kerjaschki D, Farquhar MG (1982) The pathogenic antigen of Heymann nephritis is a membrane glycoprotein of the renal proximal tubule brush border. Proc Natl Acad Sci USA 79: 5557–5561
30. Ma H, Sandor DG, Beck LH (2013) The role of complement in membranous nephropathy. Semin Nephrol 33: 531–542
31. Suzuki H, Suzuki Y, Narita I, Aizawa M, Kihara M, Yamanaka T, et al. (2008) Toll-like receptor 9 affects severity of IgA nephropathy. J Am Soc Nephrol 19: 2384–2395
32. Cheng W, Zhou X, Zhu L, Shi S, Lv J, Liu L, et al. (2011) Polymorphisms in the nonmuscle myosin heavy chain 9 gene (MYH9) are associated with the progression of IgA nephropathy in Chinese. Nephrol Dial Transplant 26: 2544–2549
33. Chen WC, Chen SY, Chen CH, Chen HY, Lin YW, Ho TJ, et al. (2010) Lack of association between transient receptor potential cation channel 6 polymorphisms and primary membranous glomerulonephritis. Renal failure 32: 666–672
34. Sonneveld R, Ferre S, Hoenderop JG, Dijkman HB, Berden JH, Bindels RJ, et al. (2013) Vitamin D down-regulates TRPC6 expression in podocyte injury and proteinuric glomerular disease. Am J Pathol 182: 1196–1204
35. Brooks RC, McCarthy KD, Lapetina EG, Morell P (1989) Receptor-stimulated phospholipase A2 activation is coupled to influx of external calcium and not to mobilization of intracellular calcium in C62B glioma cells. J Biol Chem 264: 20147–20153
36. Kistler AD, Singh G, Altintas MM, Yu H, Fernandez IC, Gu C, et al. (2013) Transient Receptor Potential Channel 6 (TRPC6) Protects Podocytes during Complement-mediated Glomerular Disease. J Biol Chem 288: 36598–36609

16

Laboratory Test Surveillance following Acute Kidney Injury

Michael E. Matheny[1,2,3,4*], Josh F. Peterson[2,3], Svetlana K. Eden[4], Adriana M. Hung[1,5], Theodore Speroff[1,3,4], Khaled Abdel-Kader[5], Sharidan K. Parr[5], T. Alp Ikizler[5], Edward D. Siew[5]

1 Geriatrics Research Education & Clinical Center (GRECC), Tennessee Valley Healthcare System (TVHS), Veteran's Health Administration, Nashville, TN, United States of America, **2** Department of Biomedical Informatics, Vanderbilt University School of Medicine, Nashville, TN, United States of America, **3** Division of General Internal Medicine, Department of Medicine, Vanderbilt University School of Medicine, Nashville, TN, United States of America, **4** Department of Biostatistics, Vanderbilt University School of Medicine, Nashville, TN, United States of America, **5** Division of Nephrology, Department of Medicine, Vanderbilt University School of Medicine, Nashville, TN, United States of America

Abstract

Background: Patients with hospitalized acute kidney injury (AKI) are at increased risk for accelerated loss of kidney function, morbidity, and mortality. We sought to inform efforts at improving post-AKI outcomes by describing the receipt of renal-specific laboratory test surveillance among a large high-risk cohort.

Methods: We acquired clinical data from the Electronic health record (EHR) of 5 Veterans Affairs (VA) hospitals to identify patients hospitalized with AKI from January 1st, 2002 to December 31st, 2009, and followed these patients for 1 year or until death, enrollment in palliative care, or improvement in renal function to estimated GFR (eGFR) $\geq$60 L/min/1.73 m^2. Using demographic data, administrative codes, and laboratory test data, we evaluated the receipt and timing of outpatient testing for serum concentrations of creatinine and any as well as quantitative proteinuria recommended for CKD risk stratification. Additionally, we reported the rate of phosphorus and parathyroid hormone (PTH) monitoring recommended for chronic kidney disease (CKD) patients.

Results: A total of 10,955 patients admitted with AKI were discharged with an eGFR$<$60 mL/min/1.73 m^2. During outpatient follow-up at 90 and 365 days, respectively, creatinine was measured on 69% and 85% of patients, quantitative proteinuria was measured on 6% and 12% of patients, PTH or phosphorus was measured on 10% and 15% of patients.

Conclusions: Measurement of creatinine was common among all patients following AKI. However, patients with AKI were infrequently monitored with assessments of quantitative proteinuria or mineral metabolism disorder, even for patients with baseline kidney disease.

Editor: Cordula M. Stover, University of Leicester, United Kingdom

Funding: This work was partially funded through a number of research grants. MEM was supported by Veterans Administration HSR&D Career Development Award CDA-08-020 and Veterans Administration HSR&D Investigator Initiated Research IIR-11-292, which also includes TS as co-investigator. EDS was supported by National Institutes of Health Grant 5K23 DK088964-02. AH was supported by Veterans Administration CSR&D Career Development Award 2-031-09S. JFP was supported by National Library of Medicine R01 LM009965-01. TAI was supported by U01DK82192 from the National Institute of Diabetes, Digestive and Kidney Diseases, and Clinical Translational Science Award 1UL-1RR024975 from the National Center for Research Resources. The views presented in this work are solely those of the authors and do not necessarily represent the position or the policy of the U.S. Department of Veterans Affairs or the National Institutes of Health. The funders had no role in study design, data collection and analysis, decision to publish, or preparation of the manuscript.

Competing Interests: The authors have declared that no competing interests exist.

* Email: michael@matheny.info

Introduction

Patients surviving AKI are at increased risk for long-term loss of kidney function and mortality [1,2,3,4,5,6]. As AKI identifies both patients at risk for developing incident CKD along as well as acceleration of disease among those with prevalent chronic kidney disease (CKD) [7,8], characterizing the patterns of care following AKI is an important first step to developing strategies that can potentially improve outcomes among AKI survivors. Kidney function and proteinuria may also predict recurrent AKI [9], a potentially important mechanism for potential disease progression following AKI [10].

Recently published guidelines by the Kidney Disease Improving Global Outcomes (KDIGO) panel recommend that patients who have experienced AKI be evaluated with a follow-up serum creatinine by 3 months to assess for resolution, new onset, or worsening of pre-existing CKD and to consider patients without CKD to be at 'increased' risk [11]. Current clinical practice guidelines for patients with CKD recommend they be appropriately monitored for disease progression (i.e. serum creatinine), the development of risk factors that associate with disease progression (i.e. proteinuria), and complications of kidney disease that may contribute to morbidity and mortality (e.g. disorders of mineral metabolism) [12]. The CKD guidelines state that dipstick screening for proteinuria among the general population is acceptable but advocate more quantitative and specific measurements including albumin-to-creatinine ratio (ACR) or protein-to-creatinine ratio (PCR) in patients deemed to be at 'increased' risk for progressive disease [13]. A summary of these recommendations is presented in Table 1 among patients with acute kidney injury, chronic kidney disease, and diabetes.

We sought to determine the frequency of laboratory surveillance among survivors of AKI with evidence of impaired kidney function at the time of discharge. We hypothesized that AKI survivors would be infrequently assessed for kidney function recovery and proteinuria, and that patients with persistent impairment of kidney function would not be assessed for disorders of mineral metabolism (an early complication of chronic renal dysfunction) [14,15]. We evaluated these hypotheses by examining the frequency and timing of measurement of serum creatinine, proteinuria, and serum phosphorous or intact parathyroid hormone (PTH) among AKI survivors within a regional Veterans Affairs (VA) Integrated Service Network (VISN 9) Health Care system.

Materials and Methods

Study Setting and Design

The study cohort pooled data from five Veterans Administration (VA) medical centers located in Nashville, TN, Murfreesboro, TN, Lexington, KY, Louisville, KY, and Huntington, WV. The VA is an integrated care network that includes acute inpatient hospitals, outpatient primary care and sub-specialty clinics, outpatient pharmacies, rehabilitation facilities, and long-term care facilities and domiciliaries. All VA clinical providers and allied health personnel are required to use the same electronic health record (EHR) for documentation and execution of all clinical care.

A retrospective cohort was collected of all adult (≥18 years) patients with a hospital admission complicated by AKI from January 1st, 2002 to December 31st, 2009. The Tennessee Valley Health System (TVHS) Veteran's Health Administration Institutional Review Board (IRB) and Research & Development Committees approved this study. This study was executed under expedited review with a waiver of HIPAA and informed consent approved by the IRB, written informed consent was not required. Because accurate date/time stamps were required for much of the work, full de-identification was not possible for the data, but removal of all patient names, social security numbers, and other identifiers except for dates of birth and death were performed in the initial data preparation step prior to analysis.

Data Collection

All data were collected from the regional data warehouse, which included demographic information (e.g., age, gender, race, admitting service, and location), inpatient and outpatient procedure and diagnosis codes using CPT and ICD9 coding, chemistry and hematology laboratory data, fee basis records (non-VA care ordered by a VA provider), and inpatient and outpatient computerized provider order entry records.

Data are available through VA Informatics and Computing Infrastructure, which provides access to the VA electronic health record data for research purposes (http://www.hsrd.research.va.gov/for_researchers/vinci/). We are willing to share the SQL database extraction, transformation, and load scripts used to prepare the data and the R statistical code used in the analysis upon request to the corresponding author.

Data Definitions

Acute kidney injury was defined as a 0.3 mg/dl or 50% increase in serum creatinine from the baseline serum creatinine to the peak inpatient serum creatinine, based on the Stage I definition of the Acute Kidney Injury Network (AKIN) creatinine criteria [16]. Based on our prior validation work, the baseline creatinine was defined as the mean observed outpatient serum creatinine value between 7–365 days prior to admission [17]. Estimated Glomerular Filtration Rate (eGFR) for all serum creatinine measures was calculated using the abbreviated Modification of Diet and Renal Disease (MDRD) equation as these were the values clinicians were provided [18], and CKD was defined as a baseline eGFR< 60 mL/min/1.73 m^2 [13].

Other chronic comorbidities (diabetes mellitus, hypertension, coronary artery disease, congestive heart failure, and peripheral arterial disease) were defined using administrative CPT and ICD-9 diagnostic codes collected from data prior to hospital admission,

Table 1. Summary of KDIGO and American Diabetes Association (ADA) recommendations regarding surveillance among acute kidney injury, chronic kidney disease, and diabetic patient cohorts.

Clinical Setting	Laboratory Test(s)	Monitoring Recommendation
Acute Kidney Injury [47]	Serum Creatinine	3 months following AKI to assess for CKD:
		If CKD, use CKD monitoring recommendations
		If not CKD, consider as increased CKD risk
After Acute Kidney Injury without Chronic Kidney Disease [47]	Serum Creatinine, Any Urine Protein	Recommend undergoing testing to estimate renal function and markers of chronic kidney disease but do not specify an interval
Chronic Kidney Disease [15]	Serum Creatinine, Any Urine Protein, Urine Quantitative Protein	Every 12 months or every 4–6 months with GFR<30 or moderately increased proteinuria. Quantitative assessment preferred over dipstick urine protein.
Chronic Kidney Disease [15,48]	Serum PTH, Serum Phosphate	Measurement at least once to establish baseline, with subsequent frequency of testing determined on an individual basis, with reasonable monitoring intervals every 12 months or every 3–6 months for GFR<30
Diabetes [49]	Urine Quantitative Protein	Every 12 months

and detailed in Appendix S1. Extensive ICD-9 validation work has been performed previously in the Veterans Affairs [19] and in general populations [20]. Additional related ICD-9 codes used were aimed at increasing sensitivity to these validated codes.

Cohort Inclusion/Exclusion Criteria

Patients were included if they had at least one outpatient serum creatinine measurement between 7 and 365 days prior to admission, at least one inpatient creatinine, and were hospitalized for greater than 24 hours [21]. For patients with multiple eligible AKI admissions, only the first qualifying admission was chosen. In order to select patients with continuity of care in the VA system beyond an isolated inpatient admission, patients were required to have encounters with the VA on two different dates within a year prior to the admission. An encounter was defined as any inpatient or outpatient diagnostic code, outpatient pharmacy fill record, laboratory test measurement, radiology test evaluation, pathology test measurement, or outpatient clinic visit within the VA or through VA fee basis care. Patients were excluded if they had end stage renal disease (ESRD) defined as receiving chronic dialysis therapy through ICD9 or CPT codes, a recorded dialysis procedure within 48 hours before admission, or had a baseline eGFR≤15 mL/min/1.73 m^2. Patients with a history of renal transplant were also excluded. Patients still receiving dialysis therapy within 48 hours of discharge or receiving hospice/palliative care prior to discharge were excluded. Patient hospitalizations >30 days were also excluded because of systematic differences and complications in patients requiring care for long inpatient stays. Finally patients who died or experienced an improvement of renal function to ≥60 mL/min/1.73 m^2 prior to discharge were excluded.

Outcome Definitions

The primary outcomes were time from discharge to follow-up of serum creatinine, any proteinuria, quantitative proteinuria, and PTH or phosphorus as separate assessments. For any proteinuria, quantitative proteinuria, PTH, and phosphorus measurements, the times to improvement in kidney function, mortality, and hospice enrollment were included in the model as competing outcomes due to the lack of rationale for performing ongoing monitoring in those situations. Only mortality and hospice enrollment were modeled as competing risks for serum creatinine follow-up.

The definition of serum creatinine was all blood, serum, or plasma creatinine measurements performed. Urinary protein evaluation was separated into any proteinuria measurement and quantitative measurements restricted to spot microalbumin or albumin tests, protein to creatinine ratio tests, and timed urine collections for albumin and protein. The composite outcome of measurements of PTH or phosphorus included all such measurements in blood, serum, or plasma. Death was ascertained through an aggregate of administrative codes, the national death index, patient family reports, personnel direct family contact, and federal third party notifications.

Statistical Analysis

Pre-admission patient demographics and chronic clinical conditions were summarized as medians and interquartile ranges (IQRs) for continuous variables and frequencies (%) for categorical variables. We used cumulative incidence functions (CIF) to estimate cumulative probabilities for occurrence of laboratory testing, improvement to eGFR≥60 mL/min/1.73 m^2, and death or hospice care (treating these events as competing risks) [22,23]. Because the occurrence of death, hospice or improvement of clinical condition preclude the need for monitoring of kidney injury, these outcomes are competing events effecting the proper estimation of incidence of surveillance using CIF whereas Kaplan-Meier function analysis would overestimate the probability of laboratory test surveillance. A competing risk analysis accounts for patient outcomes, as noted above, whose occurrence results in patients no longer being recommended to receive laboratory surveillance for proteinuria and mineral bone disease (MBD). Furthermore, reporting the cumulative probabilities of competing events that potentially explain non-receipt of care as well as the proportion of patients who "remain at risk" who have not yet received care may help provide some clinical context to facilitate interpretation of the true "gap" in care.

The following set of models measure the cumulative incidence at 3 months and 12 months for 1) laboratory testing surveillance occurring prior to renal function improvement, death, or hospice care, 2) renal function improvement without prior laboratory testing surveillance and prior to death or hospice care, and 3) death or hospice care without prior renal function improvement or surveillance testing. The models provide charting of surveillance incidence relative to the incidence of the competing factors and provide estimates of the proportion of surveillance testing and those remaining at risk at 3 months and 12 months post discharge. Patients who didn't have laboratory test evaluation, improvement to eGFR≥60 mL/min/1.73 m^2, death or hospice care at the 12th month of the surveillance period were censored. Aalen's variance estimator was used to estimate confidence intervals of cumulative probabilities [24] and confidence intervals for the proportion remaining at risk were calculated using the Greenwood method. In addition to the overall cohort analysis, stratified analyses of patients with a baseline eGFR≥60 mL/min/1.73 m^2 versus <60 mL/min/1.73 m^2, diabetes, or hypertension, were all separately performed. All analyses were performed using the R software for statistical computing, version 2.12.1 (http://www.r-project.org/).

Results

Subject Characteristics

After applying inclusion and exclusion criteria (Figure 1), the study cohort included 10,955 patients with AKI during hospitalization who survived to discharge without hospice referral, dialysis-dependence, or an eGFR>60 mL/min/1.73 m^2. Baseline cohort patient demographics and comorbidities prior to the index admission for the overall cohort and sub-cohorts with diabetes and hypertension are shown in Table 2. The median age of patients was 70 years (IQR: 60–78) with rates of chronic disease including diabetes mellitus of 57%, hypertension 88%, coronary artery disease 58%, congestive heart failure 34%, and peripheral vascular disease 21%. Of note, 5136 (47%) of patients had evidence of preadmission CKD defined by an outpatient baseline eGFR<60 mL/min/1.73 m^2. The distribution of AKI severity during the index hospitalization using AKIN criteria included 8790 (80%) patients with AKIN stage I, 1063 (10%) with AKIN stage II, and 1099 (10%) with AKIN stage III injury.

Serum Creatinine Measurement

The cumulative incidence of serum creatinine testing adjusted for competitive risks within the full cohort was 68.7% (95% CI: 67.8–69.6) at 3 months and 85.3% (95% CI: 84.7–86.0) at 12 months. Only 4.9% of surviving patients did not have a creatinine measurement by the end of the follow-up period.

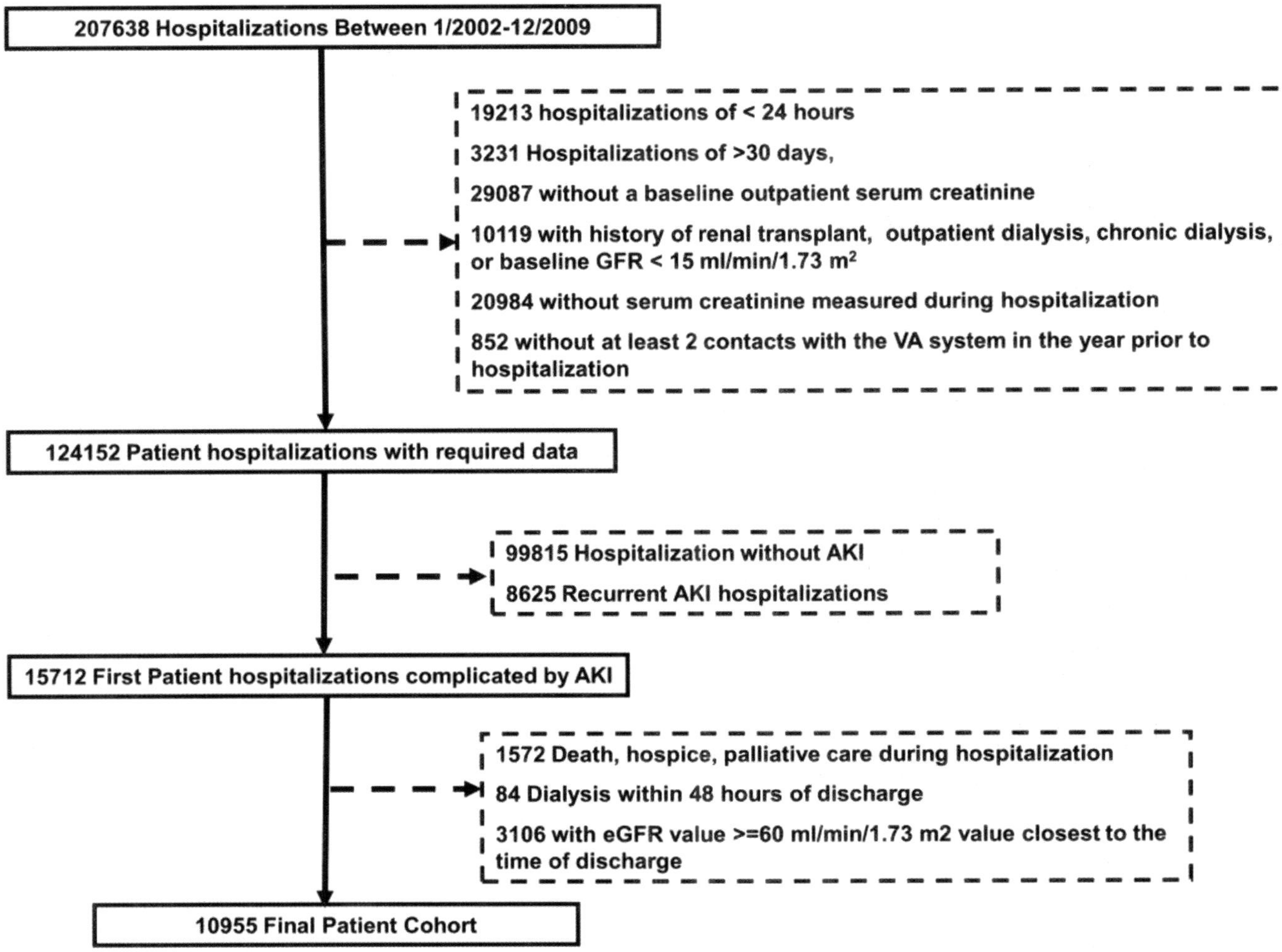

Figure 1. Study population flowchart. In each exclusion block, patients can appear in more than one exclusion criteria.

Table 2. Demographics and Baseline Characteristics.

Variable	Full Cohort	Hypertension Sub-Cohort	Diabetes Sub-Cohort
Sample		9593	6196
Age	70 (60–78)	71 (61–79)	71 (61–79)
Men, n(%)	10667 (97%)	9375 (98%)	6066 (98%)
White, n(%)	9615 (88%)	8409 (88%)	5477 (88%)
Diabetes mellitus, n(%)	6196 (57%)	5806 (61%)	6196 (100%)
Hypertension, n(%)	9593 (88%)	9593 (100%)	5806 (94%)
Coronary artery disease, n(%)	6385 (58%)	5993 (62%)	4164 (67%)
Congestive heart failure, n(%)	3711 (34%)	3505 (37%)	2580 (42%)
Peripheral vascular disease, n(%)	2351 (21%)	2241 (23%)	1670 (27%)
Chronic Kidney Disease, n(%)			
CKD IIIa (eGFR 45–59 mL/min/1.73 m^2)	2703 (25%)	2511 (26%)	1657 (27%)
CKD IIIb (eGFR 30–44 mL/min/1.73 m^2)	1772 (16%)	1672 (17%)	1204 (19%)
CKD IV (eGFR 15–29 mL/min/1.73 m^2)	661 (6%)	627 (7%)	449 (7%)
Median [IQR] Baseline Creatinine (mg/dl)	1.25 (1.02–1.58)	1.30 (1.05–1.60)	1.30 (1.07–1.66)
Median baseline estimated GFR, [IQR] mL/min/1.73 m^2	62 (47–79)	60 (46–76)	58 (44–75)
Median Length of Stay, [IQR], Days	4.9 (2.8–8.6)	4.9 (2.8–8.3)	4.9 (2.8–8.6)

Continuous variables presented as median (interquartile range). GFR = glomerular filtration rate.

Urinary Protein Measurement

We measured the cumulative incidences of any dipstick or quantitative urinalysis measurement (Table 3, Figures 2b and 3b). Among the entire cohort, 33.7% underwent proteinuria testing measurement by 12 months prior to experiencing improvement of kidney function or death/hospice. A total of 10.2% of patients did not receive any proteinuria assessment at the end of follow-up. This number was 14.2% among patients with a baseline eGFR <60 ml/min/1.73 m^2.

We also measured the cumulative incidence of quantitative proteinuria (Table 3, Figures 2c, 3c). We found that 12.3% of the study cohort had quantitative proteinuria measurement prior to improving kidney function or experiencing death/hospice. Among survivors with persistently decreased eGFR<60 ml/min/1.73 m^2, 21.2% of patients did not receive quantitative proteinuria assessment by the end of follow-up. This rate increased to 33.7% among survivors with a baseline eGFR<60 ml/min/1.73 m^2.

PTH or Phosphorus Measurement

Lastly, we found that 15.3% of patients had PTH or phosphorus measured by 12 months prior to improving kidney function (52.6%) or dying/receiving hospice care (12.1%) (Table 4, Figures 2d, 3d). Patients with baseline CKD had a higher likelihood of receiving PTH or phosphorus testing compared to those with normal pre-admission renal function (26.3% versus 5.6%). Among patients with pre-existing CKD, nearly one-third (31.3%) had neither a PTH nor phosphorus measured within 12 months.

Summary of Results

Figure 4 is a summary of results summarizing the proportions of AKI patients who did not have any surveillance testing by 12 months adjusted for competing events.

Sensitivity Analyses

In order to evaluate potential systematic differences for those patients with moderate to severe injury, we repeated our analysis defining AKI as only KDIGO Stage II–III injury (i.e. a minimum doubling of baseline serum creatinine or dialysis), and made them available in Appendix S2. The rates of improvement to eGFR ≥60 mL/min/1.73 m^2 were lower across all groups and strata at 30 days but were relatively similar at 365 days. Overall patterns of creatinine, any proteinuria, and quantitative proteinuria measurement were very similar, but PTH or phosphorus measurement increased from 15% to 24% in this population.

Because we found that a portion of those patients with baseline eGFR<60 mL/min/1.73 m^2 experienced an eGFR≥60 mL/min/1.73 m^2 at least once in the surveillance period following hospitalized AKI, we evaluated the eGFR values for patients with a baseline eGFR of <60 and 45–59 mL/min/1.73 m^2, respectively, at the time of admission. We found that approximately 10% and 17% of these patients had an eGFR above 60 mL/min/1.73 m^2 in the 180 days prior to admission, and approximately 12% and 20% of these patients experienced an eGFR above 60 mL/min/1.73 m^2 in the year following the hospitalization with AKI.

Discussion

In this study, we aimed to describe the rates of measurement of serum creatinine, proteinuria, and PTH and phosphorus among patients who survive AKI, an event associated with high risk for future loss of kidney function [8]. We found that serum creatinine

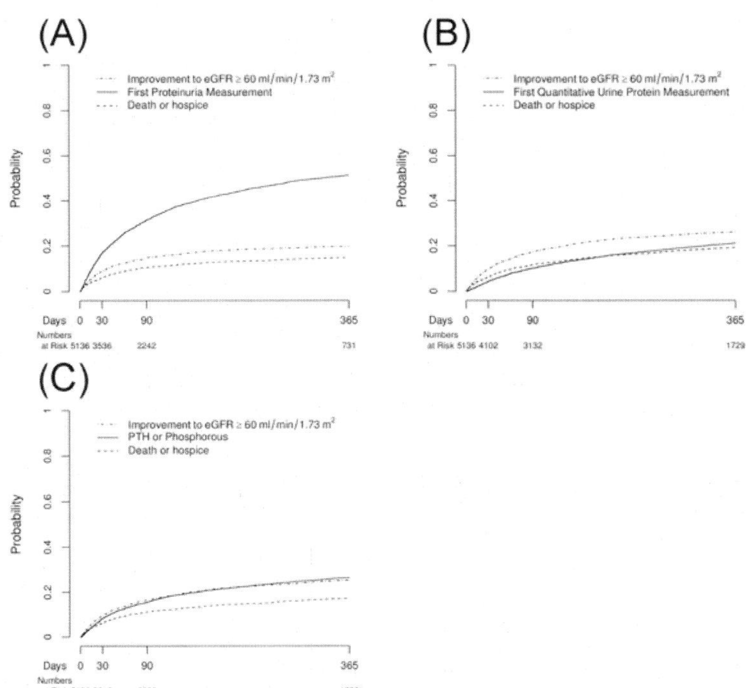

Figure 2. Cumulative Incidences of (A) Any Proteinuria Measurement, (B) Quantitative Proteinuria Measurement, and (C) PTH or Phosphorus Measurement Each Analyzed with Improvement in Kidney Function, and Death or Hospice as Competing Risks for one year following hospital discharge among Patients with Baseline eGFR<60 mL/min/1.73 m^2.

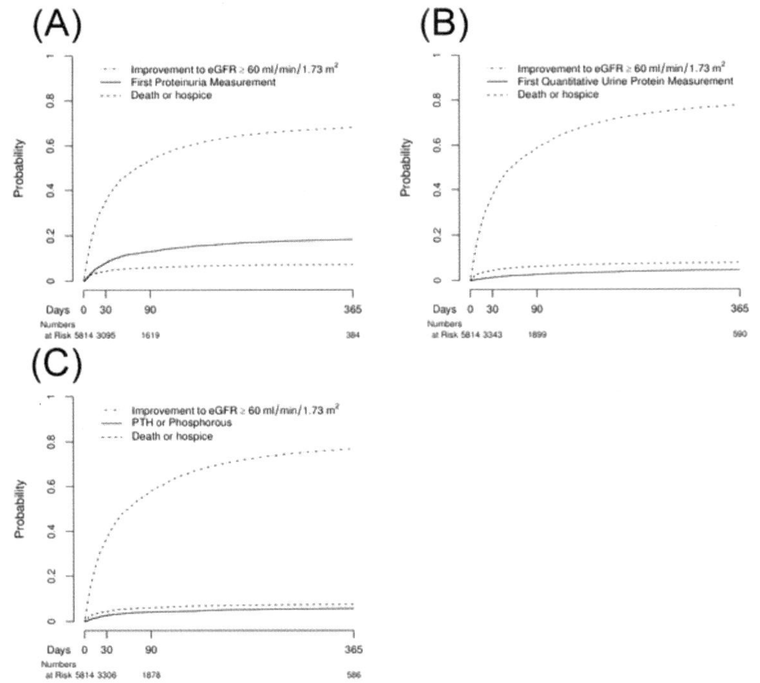

Figure 3. Cumulative Incidences of (A) Any Proteinuria Measurement, (B) Quantitative Proteinuria Measurement, and (C) PTH or Phosphorus Measurement Each Analyzed with Improvement in Kidney Function, and Death or Hospice as Competing Risks for one year following hospital discharge among Patients with Baseline eGFR ≥ 60 mL/min/1.73 m².

and any proteinuria measurements were common following AKI. However, measurement of quantitative proteinuria and mineral metabolism among AKI survivors with persistent decreases in kidney function post-hospitalization were infrequently measured.

The most striking finding from this study are the paradoxically low rates of quantitative proteinuria assessments, especially among patients with pre-existing CKD. For example, among patients with baseline CKD who survived to 12 months, only 39% underwent quantitative proteinuria testing at 1 year. Sub-analyses among patients with diabetes and among patients with hypertension confirm the consistent pattern of low rates of assessment among each of those sub-groups with co-existing CKD. There was a small increase in surveillance among those patients with both diabetes and pre-existing CKD, but approximately a third of the patient population did not receive surveillance by one year. To emphasize the importance of this finding, both the CKD guidelines and the diabetes guidelines strongly recommend quantitative protein annually at a minimum.

In addition to being a key risk factor for CKD progression [25,26], the presence of proteinuria is an important risk factor for AKI [7,9,27]. Accumulating data suggest that loss of kidney function in this population can often be non-linear and punctuated by recurrent episodes of AKI. [28,29,30] Consequently, monitoring for the development or worsening of proteinuria following an AKI event may be an important component of developing future risk reduction strategies. Because the longer term risks of AKI superimposed on CKD have only recently garnered increased attention, we suspect providers were unlikely to alter their established norms of care for CKD patients in our cohort.

While disorders of mineral metabolism have been observed during AKI [31], the extent to which AKI influences downstream derangements in mineral metabolism is unknown. KDOQI recommends initial laboratory assessment of PTH, calcium, phosphorus for all CKD patients followed by periodic surveillance depending on the severity and progression of CKD [30]. Although guidelines regarding management of mineral and bone disease are in need of higher quality evidence, we do not believe this justifies a nihilistic approach. Although changes in MBD markers are more prevalent in CKD Stage IV, approximately 10% of stable CKD stage 3 patients will develop hyperphosphatemia while 20–40% of stable CKD 3a–3b patients will develop secondary hyperparathyroidism [15]. Whether clinicians recommend dietary or pharmacologic interventions or watchful waiting while assessing for clinical manifestations, providers will require occasional lab testing to thoughtfully inform these decisions. Only about one quarter of patients with pre-existing CKD had PTH or phosphorous measured and over one-third were still eligible for surveillance by the end of the follow-up period. This is consistent with prior CKD literature, which has shown infrequent testing of phosphorus (26% to 68%) and PTH (3% to 38%), depending on the cohort and CKD severity [32,33,34]. The latter is particularly relevant given that patients with CKD who experience AKI are among those at the highest risk of experiencing accelerated decline to ESRD [35].

Early nephrology referral among both veteran and general populations with CKD has been shown to improve outcomes [36,37,38,39,40], but the rates of referral are low in both general outpatient settings and among those with recent hospitalized AKI [36,41]. However, with recent data indicating continued rises in disease incidence [5], it is unlikely that the nephrology workforce will have the capacity to care for most of these patients. Consequently, the ability of primary caregivers to identify those at highest risk will be of increasing relevance to both streamline appropriate referral and targeting those for future interventions. Recent publications suggest that common lab values including serum phosphate and albuminuria can be used in predictive models to identify CKD patients at increased risk for end-stage renal disease [42] [43]. Similar work is needed in patients with

Table 3. (A) Urinary Proteinuria and (B) Quantitative Proteinuria each in Competing Incidence Functions with Improvement in Kidney Function (eGFR≥60 mL/min/1.73 m^2) and Death or Hospice Care.

Event	Cohort	Baseline eGFR	3 months	12 months
(A) Any Proteinuria Measurement				
Any Proteinuria Measurement	All	≥60	13.0% (12.1–13.8)	18.2% (17.2–19.2)
	HTN	≥60	13.6% (12.6–14.5)	19.2% (18.1–20.3)
	DM	≥60	14.6% (13.3–15.9)	20.4% (19.0–21.9)
	All	<60	31.4% (30.2–32.7)	51.3% (49.9–52.6)
	HTN	<60	31.8% (30.5–33.1)	51.8% (50.3–53.2)
	DM	<60	33.8% (32.2–35.4)	55.0% (53.3–56.7)
Improvement to eGFR≥60 mL/min/1.73 m^2	All	≥60	53.5% (52.2–54.8)	68.0% (66.8–69.2)
	HTN	≥60	53.3% (51.8–54.7)	67.8% (66.5–69.1)
	DM	≥60	54.2% (52.4–56.0)	67.7% (66.0–69.4)
	All	<60	14.7% (13.7–15.7)	19.7% (18.6–20.8)
	HTN	<60	14.6% (13.6–15.6)	19.7% (18.6–20.9)
	DM	<60	14.0% (12.8–15.2)	18.3% (17.0–19.7)
Death or Hospice Care	All	≥60	5.9% (5.4–6.6)	7.2% (6.5–7.9)
	HTN	≥60	5.7% (5.1–6.4)	7.0% (6.3–7.8)
	DM	≥60	5.6% (4.8–6.5)	7.0% (6.1–8.0)
	All	<60	10.5% (9.7–11.4)	14.8% (13.9–15.8)
	HTN	<60	10.0% (9.2–10.8)	14.3% (13.3–15.3)
	DM	<60	9.7% (8.7–10.7)	13.8% (12.6–15.0)
Proportion Remaining at Risk	All	≥60	27.8% (26.7–29.0)	6.6% (6.0–7.2)
	HTN	≥60	27.7% (26.5–39.0)	6.0% (5.3–6.7)
	DM	≥60	25.7% (24.1–27.3)	4.9% (4.1–5.6)
	All	<60	43.7% (42.3–45.0)	14.2% (13.3–15.2)
	HTN	<60	44.0% (42.5–45.4)	14.2% (13.3–15.2)
	DM	<60	42.8% (41.1–44.5)	12.9% (11.8–14.1)
(B) Quantitative Proteinuria Measurement				
Quantitative Proteinuria Measurement	All	≥60	2.7% (2.3–3.2)	4.5% (3.9–5.0)
	HTN	≥60	3.1% (2.6–3.6)	5.0% (4.4–5.7)
	DM	≥60	4.6% (3.9–5.4)	7.5% (6.6–8.5)
	All	<60	10.2% (9.4–11.0)	21.1% (20.0–22.3)
	HTN	<60	10.4% (9.6–11.3)	21.6% (20.5–22.8)
	DM	<60	12.6% (11.5–13.7)	26.7% (25.2–28.2)
Improvement to eGFR≥60 ml/min/1.73 m^2	All	≥60	58.7% (57.4–59.9)	77.6% (76.6–78.7)
	HTN	≥60	58.4% (57.0–59.8)	77.8% (76.6–79.0)
	DM	≥60	59.3% (57.5–61.1)	77.1% (75.5–78.6)
	All	<60	17.3% (16.3–18.4)	26.1% (24.9–27.3)
	HTN	<60	17.2% (16.2–18.3)	25.9% (24.7–27.2)
	DM	<60	16.5% (15.3–17.8)	24.2% (22.8–25.7)
Death or Hospice Care	All	≥60	6.2% (5.6–6.8)	7.8% (7.1–8.5)
	HTN	≥60	5.9% (5.3–6.6)	7.6% (6.8–8.3)
	DM	≥60	5.9% (5.0–6.8)	7.7% (6.8–8.7)
	All	<60	11.7% (10.9–12.6)	19.2% (18.1–20.3)
	HTN	<60	11.2% 910.3–12.1)	18.7% (17.6–19.8)
	DM	<60	10.7% (9.6–11.7)	17.9% (16.6–19.2)
Proportion Remaining at Risk	All	≥60	32.7% (31.5–33.9)	10.1% (9.4–10.9)
	HTN	≥60	32.9% (31.5–34.2)	9.6% (8.8–10.5)
	DM	≥60	30.4% (28.7–32.1)	7.8% (6.8–8.7)
	All	<60	61.0% (59.6–62.3)	33.7% (32.4–35.0)
	HTN	<60	61.4% (60.0–62.8)	33.8% (32.5–35.2)

Table 3. Cont.

Event	Cohort	Baseline eGFR	3 months	12 months
	DM	<60	60.6% (58.9–62.2)	31.2% (29.6–32.8)

The CIF was calculated in the entire cohort, among those with baseline eGFR≥60 mL/min/1.73 m^2, and among those with baseline eGFR<60 mL/min/1.73 m^2. Indicates the cumulative incidence probabilities and 95% confidence limits for each event and time interval during the surveillance period. HTN = Hypertension Sub-Cohort. DM = Diabetic Sub-Cohort.

AKI superimposed on CKD. As assessment for proteinuria and disorders of mineral metabolism are the precursors to effective management and potentially risk assessments, these results highlight the need to disseminate the components of nephrologist specialty care to primary care.

This study has a number of strengths. It is a multi-site study of a population of Veterans that leverages detailed laboratory and electronic health record data to establish rates of test measurement among a cohort with a high prevalence of CKD, diabetes, and hypertension. The study adds to the literature by providing estimates of surveillance among both the general high risk cohort of AKI survivors as well as the sub-group with pre-existing CKD. This study also included sensitivity analyses and evaluation for more severe degrees of injury. Stratification by baseline eGFR did show some threshold effects, particularly when the baseline was close to 60 mL/min/1.73 m^2. However this reflects a clinically significant threshold for care, so we included analyses for the whole population and stratified by baseline eGFR to improved interpretation flexibility. In addition, severity of injury was noted to impact the rapidity but not the final rate of recovery and receipt of PTH and phosphorus measurement.

We recognize several study limitations. The veteran patient population may limit generalizability to other care settings. Excluding patients with lengths of stay greater than 30 days may potentially bias the population towards a healthier one, but this represents a very different sub-population within the VA, largely among patients extended rehabilitation, placement or psychosocial barriers to discharge, and for these reasons we excluded them. As

Table 4. Cumulative Incidences for Receipt of PTH or Phosphorus, Improvement in Kidney Function (eGFR≥60 mL/min/1.73 m^2), and Death or Hospice Care in the entire cohort, among those with baseline eGFR≥60 mL/min/1.73 m^2, and among those with baseline eGFR<60 mL/min/1.73 m^2.

Event		Baseline eGFR	3 months	12 months
PTH or Phosphorus Measurement	All	≥60	4.1% (3.6–4.6)	5.6% (5.1–6.2)
	HTN	≥60	4.0% (3.5–4.6)	5.5% (4.9–6.2)
	DM	≥60	3.9% (3.2–4.6)	5.5% (4.7–6.4)
	All	<60	15.5% (14.5–16.5)	26.3% (25.1–27.5)
	HTN	<60	16.0% (15.0–17.0)	27.0% (25.7–28.2)
	DM	<60	16.7% (15.4–18.0)	28.3% (26.8–30.0)
Improvement to eGFR≥60 mL/min/1.73 m^2	All	≥60	57.8% (56.5–59.1)	76.8% (75.7–77.8)
	HTN	≥60	57.9% (56.5–59.3)	77.5% (76.3–78.6)
	DM	≥60	59.7% (57.9–61.4)	78.6% (77.1–80.1)
	All	<60	16.6% (15.6–17.7)	25.2% (24.0–26.4)
	HTN	<60	16.5% (15.5–17.6)	25.1% (23.8–26.3)
	DM	<60	15.9% (14.7–17.2)	24.0% (22.5–25.4)
Death or Hospice Care	All	≥60	6.0% (5.5–6.7)	7.5% (6.9–8.2)
	HTN	≥60	5.8% (5.2–6.5)	7.3% (6.6–8.1)
	DM	≥60	5.8% (5.0–6.7)	7.5% (6.6–8.5)
	All	<60	11.2% (10.4–12.1)	17.3% (16.2–18.3)
	HTN	<60	10.7% (9.8–11.6)	16.7% (15.6–17.7)
	DM	<60	10.2% (9.2–11.3)	16.2% (14.9–17.4)
Proportion Remaining at Risk	All	≥60	32.3% (31.1–33.5)	10.1% (9.3–10.9)
	HTN	≥60	32.6% (31.3–33.9)	9.7% (8.8–10.5)
	DM	≥60	30.8% (29.2–32.5)	8.4% (7.4–9.4)
	All	<60	56.9% (55.5–58.2)	31.3% (30.0–32.6)
	HTN	<60	57.1% (55.7–58.5)	31.4% (30.0–32.7)
	DM	<60	57.6% (55.9–59.2)	31.6% (30.0–33.2)

Indicates the cumulative incidence probabilities and 95% confidence limits for each event and time interval during the surveillance period.

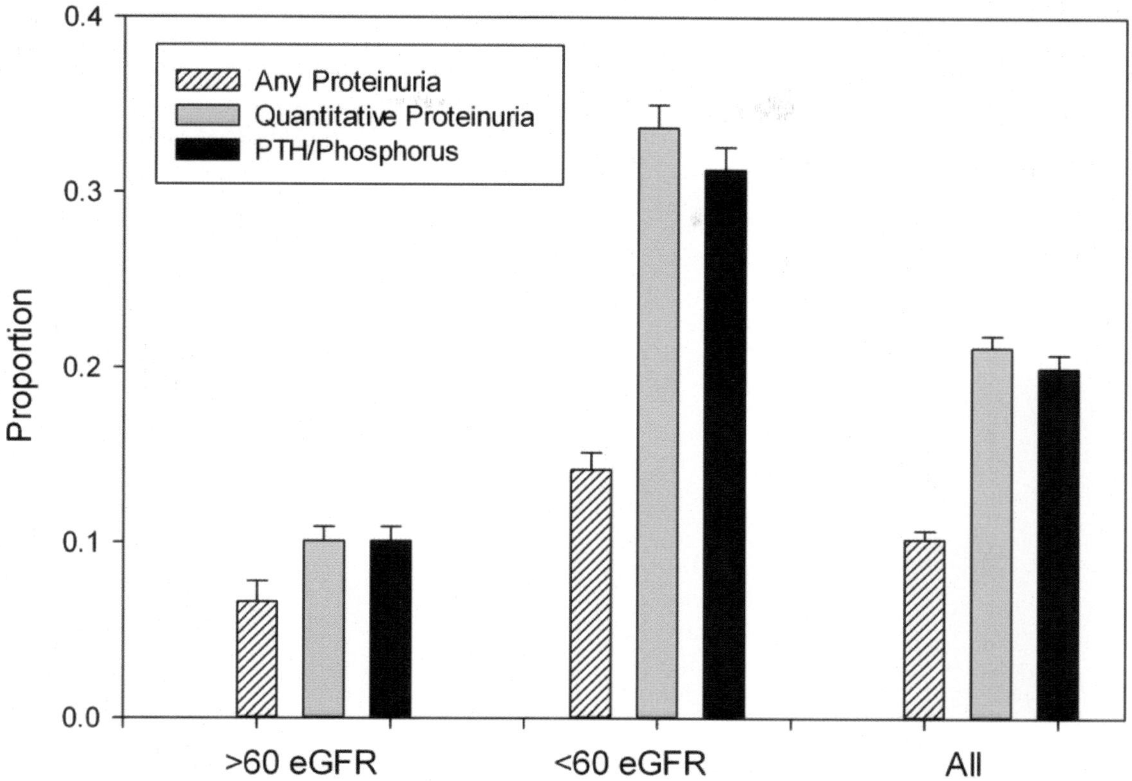

Figure 4. Proportion of patients Remaining at Risk (Still Eligible without Receipt) for Measurement of Any Proteinuria, Quantitative Proteinuria, or PTH or Phosphorus at one year post-discharge in the entire cohort, among those with baseline eGFR≥60 mL/min/1.73 m^2, and among those with baseline eGFR<60 mL/min/1.73 m^2. Indicates the cumulative incidence probabilities with competing risks from Improvement in Kidney Function (eGFR≥60 mL/min/1.73 m^2) and Death or Hospice Care, and 95% confidence limits included.

noted above, we also did not evaluate the test result values in the follow-up period to determine whether they were abnormal or if clinical care changed in response to test ascertainment, and so a portion of those tested may not have received the recommended care following surveillance. While providers may have appropriately used ACEi or ARBs and optimally controlled BP without quantifying proteinuria, the literature on quality of CKD care suggests this is unlikely [44,45,46]. In addition, it is possible that some patients obtaining care at an outside healthcare facility were not captured. However, restriction of the cohort to those patients with frequent contacts with the VA likely limited this bias towards not receiving the recommended care, and rates of serum creatinine measurement were quite high, indicating that laboratory surveillance was conducted on the majority of these patients within the VA. Lastly, as optimal post-AKI management remains to be defined, it is yet unknown the extent that modifying risk factors such as proteinuria improve outcomes in this patient population and will likely require formal testing in future trials. However, we employed conservative criteria for appropriate laboratory surveillance, and in many patients, optimal surveillance is likely to consist of closer monitoring.

In summary, patients received high rates of serum creatinine surveillance following hospitalization complicated by acute kidney injury, but rates of monitoring for quantitative proteinuria, PTH, and phosphorus measurement were low among the patients, regardless of AKI severity. Clinicians delivering outpatient care to these patients following hospitalization, particularly among those patients with additional risk factors for worsening kidney disease, such as pre-existing CKD and diabetes, should ensure that patients receive the recommended laboratory test follow-up. These findings highlight opportunities to improve clinical care among AKI survivors receiving a majority of care outside of nephrology specialist care [41]. Opportunities that exist for improving proteinuria and CKD-MBD management include increasing the frequency of nephrology management for high risk patients and providing educational as well as clinical decision support tools to assist primary care providers.

Author Contributions

Conceived and designed the experiments: MEM JFP TS TAI EDS. Performed the experiments: MEM EDS. Analyzed the data: MEM SKE. Contributed reagents/materials/analysis tools: MEM JFP AMH TS KA EDS SKP. Wrote the paper: MEM JFP SKE AMH TS KA TAI EDS SKP.

References

1. Coca SG, Yusuf B, Shlipak MG, Garg AX, Parikh CR (2009) Long-term risk of mortality and other adverse outcomes after acute kidney injury: a systematic review and meta-analysis. Am J Kidney Dis 53: 961–973.
2. Waikar SS, Curhan GC, Wald R, McCarthy EP, Chertow GM (2006) Declining mortality in patients with acute renal failure, 1988 to 2002. J Am Soc Nephrol 17: 1143–1150.
3. Uchino S, Kellum JA, Bellomo R, Doig GS, Morimatsu H, et al. (2005) Acute renal failure in critically ill patients: a multinational, multicenter study. Jama 294: 813–818.
4. Chertow GM, Burdick E, Honour M, Bonventre JV, Bates DW (2005) Acute kidney injury, mortality, length of stay, and costs in hospitalized patients. J Am Soc Nephrol 16: 3365–3370.
5. Hsu RK, McCulloch CE, Dudley RA, Lo LJ, Hsu CY (2013) Temporal changes in incidence of dialysis-requiring AKI. J Am Soc Nephrol 24: 37–42.
6. Hsu CY, Chertow GM, McCulloch CE, Fan D, Ordonez JD, et al. (2009) Nonrecovery of kidney function and death after acute on chronic renal failure. Clin J Am Soc Nephrol 4: 891–898.
7. Hsu CY, Ordonez JD, Chertow GM, Fan D, McCulloch CE, et al. (2008) The risk of acute renal failure in patients with chronic kidney disease. Kidney Int 74: 101–107.
8. Coca SG, Singanamala S, Parikh CR (2011) Chronic kidney disease after acute kidney injury: a systematic review and meta-analysis. Kidney Int.
9. Grams ME, Astor BC, Bash LD, Matsushita K, Wang Y, et al. (2010) Albuminuria and estimated glomerular filtration rate independently associate with acute kidney injury. J Am Soc Nephrol 21: 1757–1764.
10. Thakar CV, Christianson A, Himmelfarb J, Leonard AC (2011) Acute kidney injury episodes and chronic kidney disease risk in diabetes mellitus. Clin J Am Soc Nephrol 6: 2567–2572.
11. Kellum JA, Lameire N (2013) Diagnosis, evaluation, and management of acute kidney injury: a KDIGO summary (Part 1). Crit Care 17: 204.
12. (2002) K/DOQI clinical practice guidelines for chronic kidney disease: evaluation, classification, and stratification. Am J Kidney Dis 39: S1–266.
13. (2013) Summary of Recommendation Statements. Kidney inter Suppl 3: 5–14.
14. (2003) K/DOQI clinical practice guidelines for bone metabolism and disease in chronic kidney disease. Am J Kidney Dis 42: S1–201.
15. Group KDIGOKCW (2013) KDIGO 2012 Clinical Practice Guideline for the Evaluation and Management of Chronic Kidney Disease. Kidney International 3 Suppl.: 1–150.
16. Mehta RL, Kellum JA, Shah SV, Molitoris BA, Ronco C, et al. (2007) Acute Kidney Injury Network: report of an initiative to improve outcomes in acute kidney injury. Crit Care 11: R31.
17. Siew ED, Ikizler TA, Matheny ME, Shi Y, Schildcrout JS, et al. (2012) Estimating baseline kidney function in hospitalized patients with impaired kidney function. Clin J Am Soc Nephrol 7: 712–719.
18. Levey A, Greene T, Kusek JW, Beck GJ (2000) A simplified equation to predict glomerular filtration rate from serum creatinine [Abstract]. J Am Soc Nephrol 11.
19. Singh JA (2009) Accuracy of Veterans Affairs databases for diagnoses of chronic diseases. Preventing chronic disease 6: A126.
20. Grams ME, Plantinga LC, Hedgeman E, Saran R, Myers GL, et al. (2011) Validation of CKD and related conditions in existing data sets: A systematic review. American journal of kidney diseases: the official journal of the National Kidney Foundation 57: 44–54.
21. Siew ED, Matheny ME, Ikizler TA, Lewis JB, Miller RA, et al. (2010) Commonly used surrogates for baseline renal function affect the classification and prognosis of acute kidney injury. Kidney Int 77: 536–542.
22. Kalbfleish J, Prentice RL (1980) The Statistical Analysis of Failure Time Data. New York: John Wiley & Sons, Inc.
23. Gray RJ (1988) A Class of K-sample Tests for Comparing the Cumulative Incidence of a Competing Risk. Annals of Statistics 16: 1141–1154.
24. Aalen O (1978) Nonparametric Estimation of Partial Transition Probabilities in Multiple Decrement Models. Annals of Statistics 6: 534–545.
25. Ruggenenti P, Perna A, Remuzzi G (2001) ACE inhibitors to prevent end-stage renal disease: when to start and why possibly never to stop: a post hoc analysis of the REIN trial results. Ramipril Efficacy in Nephropathy. J Am Soc Nephrol 12: 2832–2837.
26. Jafar TH, Stark PC, Schmid CH, Landa M, Maschio G, et al. (2001) Proteinuria as a modifiable risk factor for the progression of non-diabetic renal disease. Kidney Int 60: 1131–1140.
27. Uhlig K, Berns JS, Kestenbaum B, Kumar R, Leonard MB, et al. (2010) KDOQI US commentary on the 2009 KDIGO Clinical Practice Guideline for the Diagnosis, Evaluation, and Treatment of CKD-Mineral and Bone Disorder (CKD-MBD). Am J Kidney Dis 55: 773–799.
28. Li L, Astor BC, Lewis J, Hu B, Appel LJ, et al. (2012) Longitudinal progression trajectory of GFR among patients with CKD. Am J Kidney Dis 59: 504–512.
29. O'Hare AM, Batten A, Burrows NR, Pavkov ME, Taylor L, et al. (2012) Trajectories of kidney function decline in the 2 years before initiation of long-term dialysis. Am J Kidney Dis 59: 513–522.
30. Moe S, Drueke T, Cunningham J, Goodman W, Martin K, et al. (2006) Definition, evaluation, and classification of renal osteodystrophy: a position statement from Kidney Disease: Improving Global Outcomes (KDIGO). Kidney Int 69: 1945–1953.
31. Zhang M, Hsu R, Hsu CY, Kordesch K, Nicasio E, et al. (2011) FGF-23 and PTH levels in patients with acute kidney injury: A cross-sectional case series study. Ann Intensive Care 1: 21.
32. Hoy T, Fisher M, Barber B, Borker R, Stolshek B, et al. (2007) Adherence to K/DOQI practice guidelines for bone metabolism and disease. The American journal of managed care 13: 620–625.
33. Kausz AT, Guo H, Pereira BJ, Collins AJ, Gilbertson DT (2005) General medical care among patients with chronic kidney disease: opportunities for improving outcomes. J Am Soc Nephrol 16: 3092–3101.
34. Winkelmayer WC, Levin R, Avorn J (2003) The nephrologist's role in the management of calcium-phosphorus metabolism in patients with chronic kidney disease. Kidney Int 63: 1836–1842.
35. Ishani A, Xue JL, Himmelfarb J, Eggers PW, Kimmel PL, et al. (2009) Acute kidney injury increases risk of ESRD among elderly. J Am Soc Nephrol 20: 223–228.
36. Tseng CL, Kern EF, Miller DR, Tiwari A, Maney M, et al. (2008) Survival benefit of nephrologic care in patients with diabetes mellitus and chronic kidney disease. Arch Intern Med 168: 55–62.
37. Chan MR, Dall AT, Fletcher KE, Lu N, Trivedi H (2007) Outcomes in patients with chronic kidney disease referred late to nephrologists: a meta-analysis. Am J Med 120: 1063–1070.
38. Chow KM, Szeto CC, Law MC, Kwan BC, Leung CB, et al. (2008) Impact of early nephrology referral on mortality and hospitalization in peritoneal dialysis patients. Perit Dial Int 28: 371–376.
39. Winkelmayer WC, Owen WF Jr, Levin R, Avorn J (2003) A propensity analysis of late versus early nephrologist referral and mortality on dialysis. J Am Soc Nephrol 14: 486–492.
40. Khan SS, Xue JL, Kazmi WH, Gilbertson DT, Obrador GT, et al. (2005) Does predialysis nephrology care influence patient survival after initiation of dialysis? Kidney Int 67: 1038–1046.
41. Siew ED, Peterson JF, Eden SK, Hung AM, Speroff T, et al. (2012) Outpatient nephrology referral rates after acute kidney injury. J Am Soc Nephrol 23: 305–312.
42. Tangri N, Inker LA, Tighiouart H, Sorensen E, Menon V, et al. (2012) Filtration markers may have prognostic value independent of glomerular filtration rate. J Am Soc Nephrol 23: 351–359.
43. Drawz PE, Goswami P, Azem R, Babineau DC, Rahman M (2013) A simple tool to predict end-stage renal disease within 1 year in elderly adults with advanced chronic kidney disease. J Am Geriatr Soc 61: 762–768.
44. Philipneri MD, Rocca Rey LA, Schnitzler MA, Abbott KC, Brennan DC, et al. (2008) Delivery patterns of recommended chronic kidney disease care in clinical practice: administrative claims-based analysis and systematic literature review. Clin Exp Nephrol 12: 41–52.
45. Tuot DS, Plantinga LC, Hsu CY, Powe NR (2012) Is awareness of chronic kidney disease associated with evidence-based guideline-concordant outcomes? Am J Nephrol 35: 191–197.
46. Plantinga LC, Miller ER 3rd, Stevens LA, Saran R, Messer K, et al. (2009) Blood pressure control among persons without and with chronic kidney disease: US trends and risk factors 1999–2006. Hypertension 54: 47–56.
47. Group KDIGOKAKIW (2012) KDIGO Clinical Practice Guideline for Acute Kidney Injury. Kidney inter Suppl 2: 1–138.
48. (2009) KDIGO clinical practice guideline for the diagnosis, evaluation, prevention, and treatment of Chronic Kidney Disease-Mineral and Bone Disorder (CKD-MBD). Kidney International - Supplement: S1–130.
49. (2004) Nephropathy in Diabetes. Diabetes Care 27: s79–s83.

17

Role of Far Infra-Red Therapy in Dialysis Arterio-Venous Fistula Maturation and Survival: Systematic Review and Meta-Analysis

Khalid Bashar[1]*, Donagh Healy[1], Leonard D. Browne[2], Elrasheid A. H. Kheirelseid[1], Michael T. Walsh[2], Mary Clarke - Moloney[1], Paul E. Burke[1], Eamon G. Kavanagh[1], Stewart Redmond Walsh[3]

1 Department of vascular surgery, University Hospital Limerick, Limerick, Ireland, **2** Centre for Applied Biomedical Engineering Research (CABER), Department of Mechanical, Aeronautical & Biomedical Engineering, Materials and Surface Science Institute, University of Limerick, Limerick, Ireland, **3** Department of surgery, National University of Ireland, Galway, Ireland

Abstract

Introduction: A well-functioning arteriovenous fistula (AVF) is the best modality for vascular access in patients with end-stage renal disease (ESRD) requiring haemodialysis (HD). However, AVFs' main disadvantage is the high rate of maturation failure, with approximately one third (20%–50%) not maturing into useful access. This review examine the use of Far-Infra Red therapy in an attempt to enhance both primary (unassisted) and secondary (assisted) patency rates for AVF in dialysis and pre-dialysis patients.

Method: We performed an online search for observational studies and randomised controlled trials (RCTs) that evaluated FIR in patients with AVF. Eligible studies compared FIR with control treatment and reported at least one outcome measure relating to access survival. Primary patency and secondary patency rates were the main outcomes of interest.

Results: Four RCTs (666 patients) were included. Unassisted patency assessed in 610 patients, and was significantly better among those who received FIR (228/311) compared to (185/299) controls (pooled risk ratio of 1.23 [1.12–1.35], p = 0.00001). In addition, the two studies which reported secondary patency rates showed significant difference in favour of FIR therapy-160/168 patients - compared to 140/163 controls (pooled risk ratio of 1.11 [1.04–1.19], p = 0.003).

Conclusion: FIR therapy may positively influence the complex process of AVF maturation improving both primary and secondary patency rates. However blinded RCTs performed by investigators with no commercial ties to FIR therapy technologies are needed.

Editor: Daniel Schneditz, Medical University of Graz, Austria

Funding: The authors have no support or funding to report.

Competing Interests: The authors have declared that no competing interests exist.

* Email: khalidbashar@rcsi.ie

Introduction

The number of patients with end stage renal disease (ESRD) requiring haemodialysis (HD) is steadily rising, a trend that is expected to continue [1]. Vascular access is a critical component in successful HD. A well-functioning arteriovenous fistula (AVF) is the best modality for HD vascular access [2–6]. AVF maturation is a complex process of remodelling. The newly formed fistula has to form a low resistance circuit capable of dilation to accommodate the increased blood flow required for HD. The AVF also has to be cannulated repeatedly with ease. The need for re-intervention to maintain patency should be minimal [2–4,6,7].

AVFs' main disadvantage is the high rate of maturation failure, with approximately one third (20%–50%) not maturing into useful access [8–10]. AVFs have higher primary failure rates to mature compared to grafts [8,11,12]. However they last longer, and with exclusion of fistulas that fail to mature primarily, the cumulative patency from formation to permanent failure is superior to grafts. AVFs also require fewer secondary interventions in the form of angioplasty, stenting or thrombectomy [8,13–16]. AVFs are associated with fewer complications compared to AVG and CVC in terms of infection, death, vascular access salvage procedures and hospitalizations [15,16]. Also, a mature AVF has a lower incidence of thrombosis and stenosis. This translates into prolonged patency rates and lower risk for infection [1,17–20].

Maturation of AVF depends on variable biomechanical forces. Remodelling of the arterial limb is characterised by vessel dilatation and outward hypertrophic remodelling of the intimal layer. Remodelling at the venous end can be accompanied by aggressive intimal thickening resulting in inward hypertrophic remodelling. Intimal hyperplasia (IH) is defined as the abnormal migration and proliferation of vascular smooth muscle cells provoked by injury, inflammation or stretch with associated

Table 1. Results of the study quality assessment.

Included study	Domain	Support for judgement	DH's judgement
Lai 2013 ESVS [37]	Random sequence generation	The method of generating the random sequence was not described.	Unclear
	Allocation concealment	No description of methods for maintaining allocation concealment.	Unclear
	Blinding of participants and personnel	Participants and personnel were not blinded. Dysfunctional access signs and other referral criteria could have a subjective component.	High risk of bias
	Blinding of outcome assessment	Outcome assessors were not blinded. Dysfunctional access signs and other referral criteria could have a subjective component.	High risk of bias
	Incomplete outcome data	Loss to follow up was minimal. Analysis was not by intention to treat. 9/59 control group patients crossed over to the intervention group potentially leading to bias in favour of the intervention	Unclear
	Selective reporting	No link to the protocol was given	Unclear
	Other sources of bias	None	Not available
Lin 2007 J Am Soc Neph [35]	Random sequence generation	A computerised minimisation algorithm was used	Low risk of bias
	Allocation concealment	Allocation sequence was kept by a study nurse who would not disclose allocations until time of intervention. Diagnosing malfunction in a fistula could have had a subjective element.	Unclear
	Blinding of participants and personnel	Participants and personnel were not blinded.	High risk of bias
	Blinding of outcome assessment	Outcome assessors were not blinded. Diagnosing malfunction in a fistula could have had a subjective element.	High risk of bias
	Incomplete outcome data	Loss to follow up was minimal and was similar between groups and was unlikely to influence results	Low risk of bias
	Selective reporting	Protocol was not available.	Unclear
	Other sources of bias	None	Not available
Lin 2013 AJKD [38]	Random sequence generation	A computer generated sequence was used	Low risk of bias
	Allocation concealment	Sealed opaque envelope were used to conceal allocation. There was no information in the manuscript or protocol on who had access to the envelopes and whether they were opened sequentially	Unclear
	Blinding of participants and personnel	No blinding. Diagnosing malfunction in a fistula could have had a subjective element.	High risk of bias
	Blinding of outcome assessment	Ultrasonographers were blinded however patients were not blinded. Diagnosing malfunction in a fistula could have had a subjective element.	High risk of bias
	Incomplete outcome data	Loss to follow up was similar between groups and unlikely to influence results	Low risk of bias
	Selective reporting	Link to protocol was provided (NCT01138254). Trial was not prospectively registered and there were several changes made including changes to outcomes.	High risk of bias
	Other sources of bias	None	Not available
Lin 2013 Neph Dial Transplant [36]	Random sequence generation	A computer generated sequence was used	Low risk of bias

Table 1. Cont.

Included study	Domain	Support for judgement	DH's judgement
	Allocation concealment	Sealed opaque envelope were used to conceal allocation. Two study nurses had access to the envelopes and there was no information in the manuscript or protocol on whether they were opened sequentially	Unclear
	Blinding of participants and personnel	No blinding. Diagnosing malfunction in a fistula could have had a subjective element.	High risk of bias
	Blinding of outcome assessment	No blinding. Diagnosing malfunction in a fistula could have had a subjective element.	High risk of bias
	Incomplete outcome data	Loss to follow up was similar between groups and unlikely to influence results	Low risk of bias.
	Selective reporting	All outcomes that were mentioned in the protocol were reported. The subgrouping based on polymorphisms of heme oxygenase-1 was not prespecified	Low risk of bias
	Other sources of bias	None	Not available

deposition of extracellular matrix in the intimal layer of the vein [21–23].

Far infra-red FIR therapy, which is a form of heat therapy, has been implicated in improvement of endothelial function and haemodynamics in coronary arteries, probably through up-regulating endothelial nitric oxide synthase (eNOS) expression in arterial endothelium leading to improved cardiac function in patients with chronic heart diseases [24]. Repeated leg hyperthermia using FIR has been shown to reduce oxidative stress in bed ridden type II diabetics [25].

FIR has also been reported to show encouraging results in phantom limb pain control [26], stimulation of the secretion of TGF-beta1 and activation of fibroblasts which may promote better wound healing independent of skin blood flow and skin temperature [27,28], reduction of both stress and fatigue levels of patients with end stage renal disease (ESRD) and stimulates the autonomic nervous system in those who are receiving regular haemodialysis (HD) [29].

This review was designed to examine the effect of FIR on AVF maturation using primary and secondary patency rates as the main outcomes of interest.

Methods

This systematic review and meta-analysis were conducted according to the Preferred Reporting Items for Systematic Review and Meta-Analysis (PRISMA) guidelines [30].

Eligibility Criteria

We included observational studies or randomised controlled trials (RCTs) that examined FIR therapy in patients with AVFs and ESRD. Eligible studies reported on AVF patency rates in FIR and non-FIR groups at one year or more following initiation of FIR therapy. Cases series and case reports were excluded. There was no restriction with regard to publication status or language.

Search strategy

A search of the literature for relevant studies was conducted in March 2014. We searched Medline without date restriction using the free text "far infra-red". Additionally we used the strategy (["far infra-red" OR "far infrared" OR "post conditioning"] AND ["arteriovenous fistula" "dialysis" OR "end stage renal disease" OR "dialysis access" OR "access survival" OR "primary patency" OR "secondary patency" OR "fistula maturation]") to search CINAHL, EMBASE, the Cochrane library and Google Scholar. Bibliographies of included studies were searched for additional studies.

Abstracts of the relevant titles were subsequently obtained and evaluated for eligibility (KB, DH). Any remaining uncertainty was resolved by examination of the full article (KB, DH). Discussion with a third author (SRW) resolved discrepancies in cases of disagreement regarding eligibility.

The relevant outcomes for this review were primary patency – defined as unassisted AVF patency rates after at least 12 months of follow up - and secondary patency – defined as assisted patency rates after at least 12 months of follow up. The incidence of salvage procedures (endoluminal procedures or surgical procedures) for dysfunctional fistulas during follow up was a secondary outcome.

Data Collection

Data were extracted and checked for accuracy by two reviewers (KB, DH) independently and recorded on a Microsoft Excel spreadsheet. Any disagreements in extracting data were discussed between two reviewers (KB, DH), and if not settled this was resolved by consulting with a third reviewer (SRW). The following information regarding participant characteristics were recorded: age, sex, presence of co-morbidities, start of HD, primary and secondary patency rates, AVF salvage procedures, underlying cause of ESRD, definition of first AVF malfunction and overall access survival. The trials' inclusion and exclusion criteria were also recorded.

Quality assessment for risk of bias

The risk of bias for each study was assessed according to the criteria outlined in the in the Cochrane Handbook for Systematic Reviews of Interventions [31]. For each included study; the method used to perform random sequence generation, allocation concealment and blinding was described. The study was then

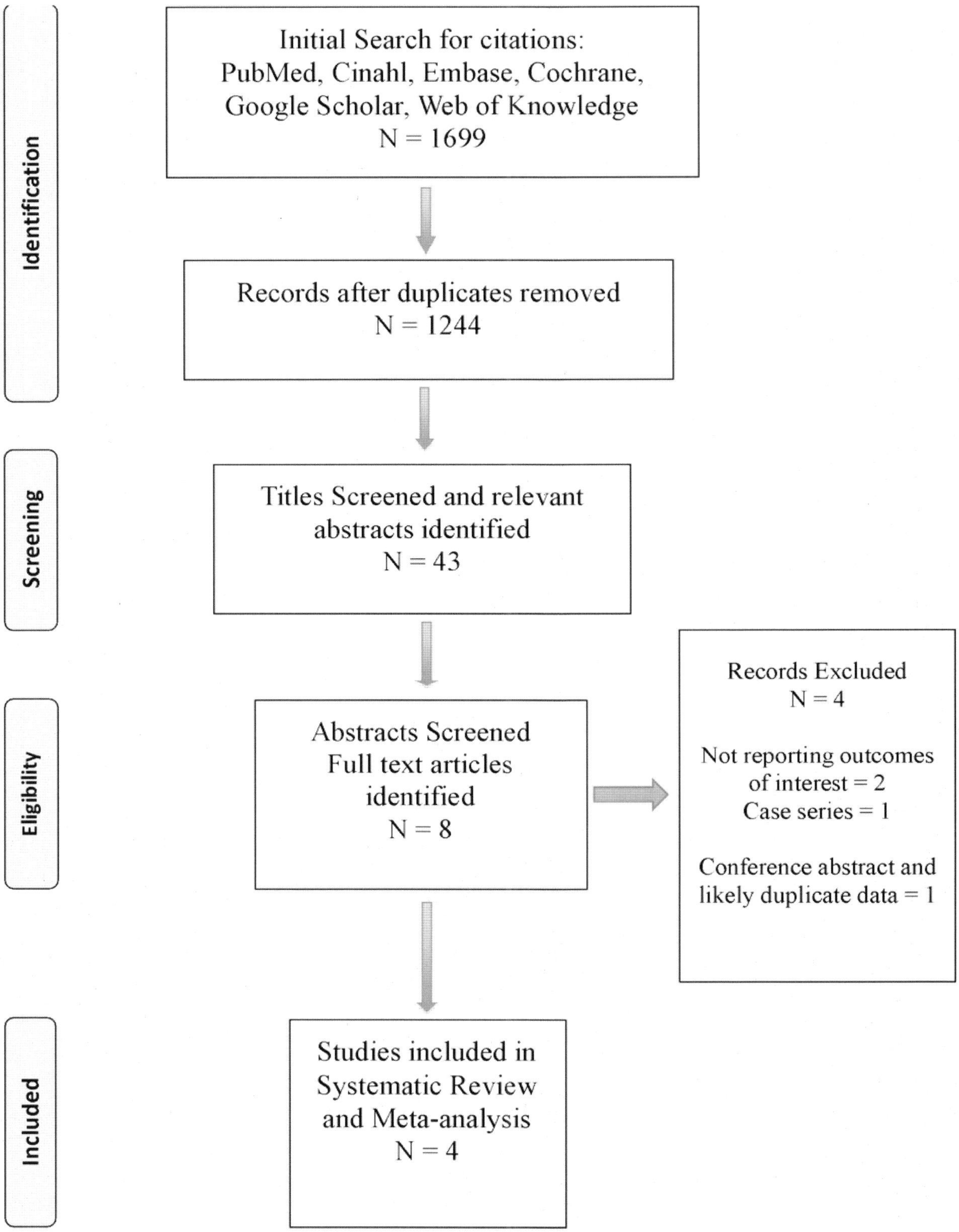

Figure 1. PRISMA 2009 Flow Diagram.

scrutinised for incomplete data outcomes, selective reporting and other potential sources of bias. Where possible, study protocols were obtained from trial registries to ascertain whether there was selective reporting within studies [Table 1].

Data analysis

Statistical analyses were performed using Review Manager version 5.2.8 [32]. Pooled risk ratios were calculated using the random effects model of DerSimonian and Laird [33]. For

Table 2. Inclusion & exclusion criteria and definition of AVF malfunction for included studies.

Study	Inclusion criteria	Exclusion criteria	Definition of AVF malfunction
Lin 2007 [35]	(1) Receiving 4 h of maintenance HD therapy three times weekly for at least 6 months at Taipei Veterans General Hospital, (2) Using a native AVF as the current vascular access for more than 6 months, without interventions within the last 3 months, and (3) Creation of AVF by cardiovascular surgeons in our hospital with the standardized surgical procedures of venous end-to-arterial side anastomosis in the upper extremity.	During the 1-yr follow-up, patients would be excluded from the study because of the following censoring criterion: (1) Renal transplantation, (2) Death with a functioning access, (3) Shifting to peritoneal dialysis, and (4) Loss of follow-up.	The need for any interventional procedure (surgery or angioplasty) to correct an occlusive or malfunctioning AVF that cannot sustain an extracorporeal blood flow >200 ml/min during HD after exclusion of the following stenosis-unrelated events: Infectious complication, progressive aneurysmal formation, or steal syndrome.
Lin 2013_AJKD [38]	(1) Aged 18–80 years, (2) Had CKD with estimated glomerular filtration rate (eGFR) of 5–20 mL/min/1.73 m^2, (3) Were not anticipated to receive dialysis or kidney transplantation within the next 3 months, and (4) Were undergoing AVF creation with venous end-to-arterial side anastomosis in the upper extremity.	(1) Those receiving an arteriovenous graft or cuffed tunnelled double-lumen catheter as the type of permanent vascular access, (2) Heart failure of New York Heart Association functional class III or IV, and (3) Episode of cardio- or cerebrovascular event or receiving intervention therapy within 3 months prior to screening.	The need for any interventional procedure (surgery or angioplasty) to correct an occlusive or malfunctioning fistula which could not sustain an extracorporeal blood flow >200 mL/min during HD after excluding the following stenosis-unrelated events, such as infectious complication, progressive aneurysmal formation or steal syndrome.
Lai_2013 [37]	(1) Received two or more PTA on the target lesions at upper extremities, with the last PTA successfully performed within the week before patient enrolment, and (2) After successful completion of at least 1 week of HD treatment, the patients with AVF or AVG were consecutively enrolled and randomly assigned to either a post-PTA FIR radiation group or a control group receiving the usual form radiation therapy at a 1:1 ratio.	(1) Received HD treatments other than three times a week, (2) Had previously received FIR radiation Therapy, (3) Received implantation of an endovascular stent, (4) Had multiple lesions that a single radiation field did not cover or the central lesion was considered too deep to be irradiated, (5) Missed FIR radiation treatments exceeding 10%, (6) Underwent renal transplantation, (7) Switched to peritoneal dialysis treatments, and (8) Had any severe disease with an estimated life expectancy of less than 1 year.	A significant lesion was defined as a lumen loss of 50% or more compared with adjacent normal vessel on angiography following dysfunctional diagnosis based on clinical signs suggestive of stenosis.
Lin_2013_NDT [36]	(1) Receiving 4 h of maintenance HD therapy three times weekly for at least 6 months at Taipei Veterans General Hospital, (2) Using a native AVF as the present vascular access for >6 months, without interventions within the last 3 months, and (3) Creation of AVF by cardiovascular surgeons in our hospital with the standardized surgical procedures of venous end-to-arterial side anastomosis in the upper extremity.	Received an AV graft as the first vascular access.	The need for any interventional procedure (surgery or angioplasty) to correct an occlusive or malfunctioning fistula which could not sustain an extracorporeal blood flow >200 mL/min during HD after excluding the following stenosis-unrelated events, such as infectious complication, progressive aneurysmal formation or steal syndrome.

continuous outcome variables the weighted mean difference (WMD) was calculated. The presence of statistical heterogeneity between studies was evaluated using the Cochran's Q statistic. P-values less than 5% were considered as statistically significant. Publication bias was assessed visually using a funnel plot, and additionally by comparing fixed and random effects modelling in a sensitivity analysis – this is a recognised method that can detect the influence of small-study effects [34].

Results

Study Selection

The results of the study selection process are summarized in the PRISMA flow diagram (Figure 1). The initial search yielded a total of 1669 citations, with 1244 citations remaining following removal of duplicates. The titles of these citations were screened with a total of 43 titles deemed potentially relevant. The abstracts of those titles were examined and eight full text articles were subsequently retrieved and examined. After assessing for eligibility

Table 3. Patients' Characteristics across included studies.

Study	Patients		Age		Gender M:F		Diabetes		Hypertension		Hx of AVF failure		Time on HD		Withdrawals
	FIR	Control	FIR	Control	FIR	Control	FIR	Control	FIR	Control	FIR	Control	FIR	Control	
Lin 2007 [35]	63/72	64/73	61.9±14.4	59.2±19.0	37:35	38:35	25	24	40	39	33	34	85.2±41.1	79.2±42.2	Creation of another vascular access because of the poor response to angioplasty: 1 patient receiving FIR therapy and four patients in control group. Patients were censored in case of: Renal transplantation ($n = 3$), death with a functioning access ($n = 5$), shifting to peritoneal dialysis ($n = 4$) or loss of follow-up ($n = 1$).
Lin 2013_AJKD [38]	60	62	63.2±18.5	63.0±14.4	32:28	35:27	28	23	18	20	-	-	Pre-dialysis	Pre-dialysis	Lost to F/U: FIR = 1; Control = 1. Shifting to PD: FIR = 1; Control = 1. Death e AVF: FIR = 2; Control = 3. Renal transplantation: FIR = 1. New AVF (Infection): Control = 1. D/C intervention: FIR = 2; Control = 1.
Lin 2013_NDT [36]	119/139	120/141	61.3±14.1	62.8±15.9	79:60	71:70	45	47	80	90	47	45	66.0±59.1	75.9±58.0	Underwent creation of another vascular access due to non-stenotic lesions: 3 patients receiving FIR therapy and 2 patients in the control group. Patients were censored in case of: Renal transplantation (n = 5), death with a functioning access (n = 15), shift to peritoneal dialysis (n = 5) or loss of follow-up (n = 9).
Lai 2013 [37]	69	50	62.7±10.9	63.1±12.5	32:37	24/26	42	28	48	38	All	All	50.4±42.0	58.8±56.4	Crossover patients: 9 from Control to FIR.

Study or Subgroup	FIR Events	FIR Total	Control Events	Control Total	Weight	Risk Ratio M-H, Random, 95% CI	Year
Lin 2007	55	64	46	68	23.2%	1.27 [1.05, 1.54]	2007
Lai 2013	17	69	9	50	1.6%	1.37 [0.67, 2.82]	2013
Lin 2013_AJKD	52	59	43	61	24.3%	1.25 [1.04, 1.51]	2013
Lin 2013_NDT	104	119	87	120	50.9%	1.21 [1.06, 1.37]	2013
Total (95% CI)		**311**		**299**	**100.0%**	**1.23 [1.12, 1.35]**	
Total events	228		185				

Heterogeneity: $Tau^2 = 0.00$; $Chi^2 = 0.33$, $df = 3$ ($P = 0.96$); $I^2 = 0\%$

Test for overall effect: $Z = 4.45$ ($P < 0.00001$)

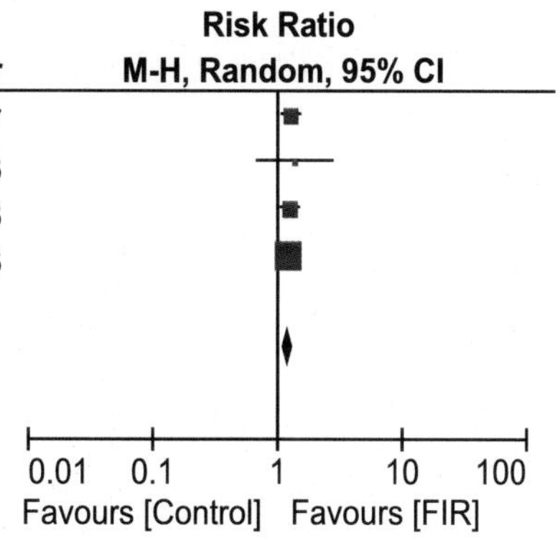

Figure 2. Forest Plot showing Primary AVFs patency at 12 months.

criteria, four RCT's were included in the review [35–38]. Three of those studies reported on patients with history of previous AVF who had been on HD prior to FIR therapy [35–37], while one study reported on patients with newly formed AVF not on HD [38]. We were not able to include another study by Lin et al [39] with a follow up of 3 months for primary patency rates as it was a conference abstract only, also we had concerns that the data in this study was used in another study by the same author [36] that has already been included in this review. Three studies were excluded from the final analysis after going through the full articles. Shipley et al followed their patients for six months in a case series of 20 patients – no control group - and reported maturation in 10 of those patients [40]. Two studies did not report on the outcomes of interest to the author of this systematic review [29,41].

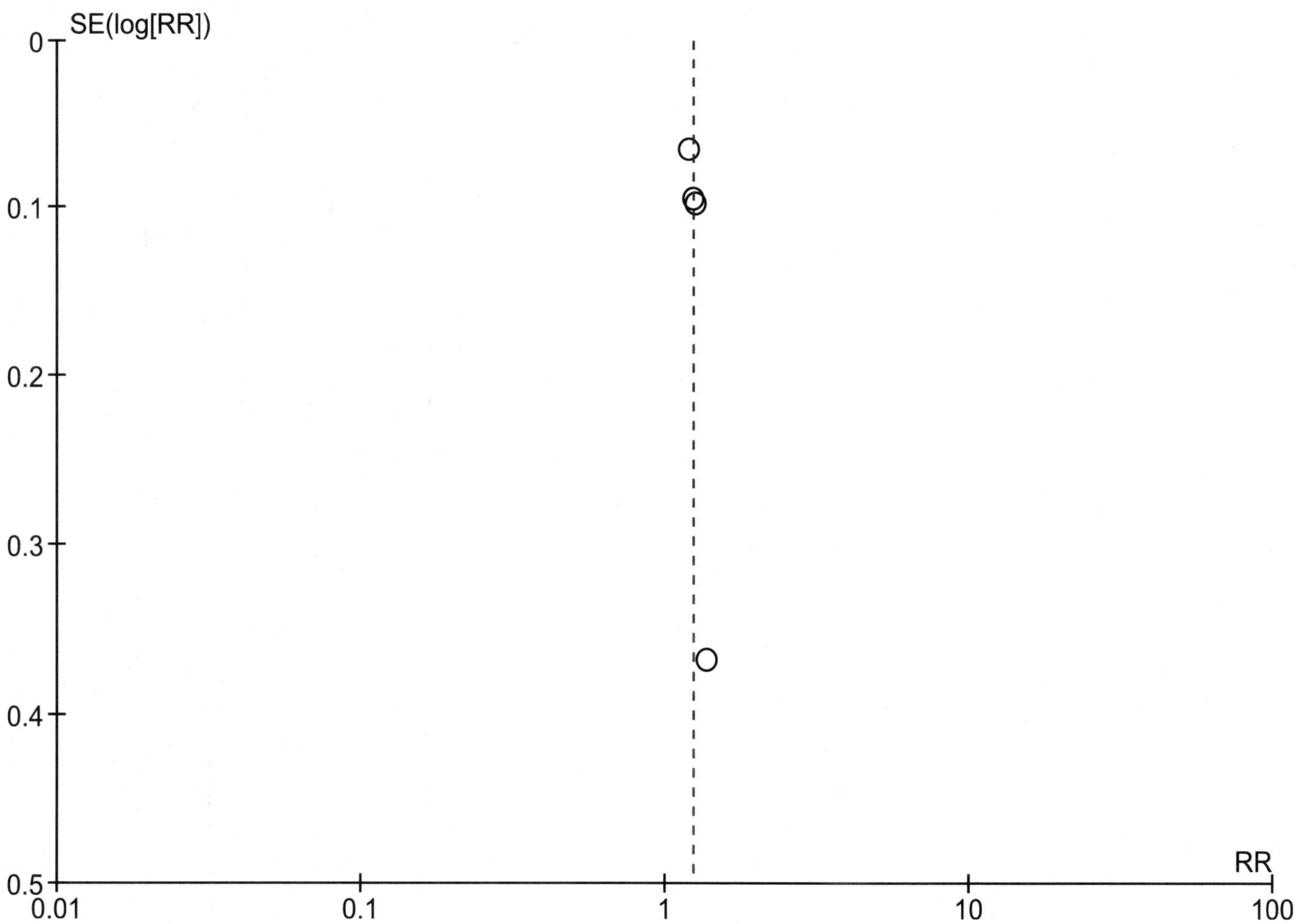

Figure 3. Funnel plot for Primary AVFs patency at 12 months.

Study or Subgroup	FIR Events	FIR Total	Control Events	Control Total	Weight	Risk Ratio M-H, Random, 95% CI	Year
Lin 2007	55	64	46	68	30.6%	1.27 [1.05, 1.54]	2007
Lin 2013_NDT	104	119	87	120	67.2%	1.21 [1.06, 1.37]	2013
Lai 2013	17	69	9	50	2.2%	1.37 [0.67, 2.82]	2013
Total (95% CI)		**252**		**238**	**100.0%**	**1.23 [1.10, 1.37]**	
Total events	176		142				

Heterogeneity: Tau² = 0.00; Chi² = 0.31, df = 2 (P = 0.86); I² = 0%
Test for overall effect: Z = 3.79 (P = 0.0001)

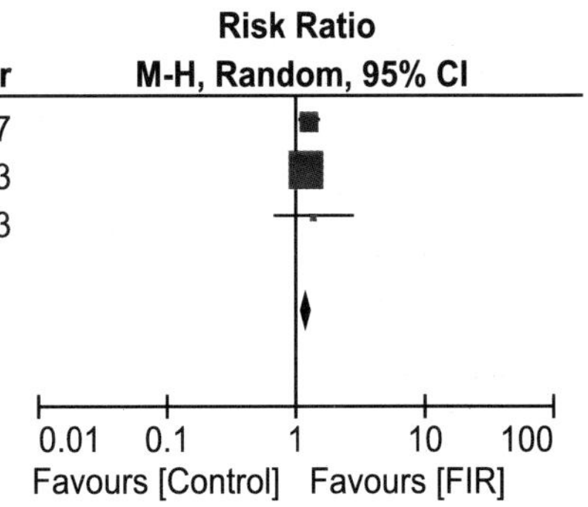

Figure 4. Forest Plot showing Primary AVFs patency at 12 months, Lin et al RCT on new AVFs excluded.

Characteristics of included studies

Far Infrared (FIR) technique. All studies included used the same technique for delivering of FIR therapy. WS TY101 FIR emitter (WS Far Infrared Medical Technology Co., Ltd., Taipei, Taiwan) was used in all studies which generates electromagnetic waves with wavelengths in the range between 5 and 25 (peak at 5–8.2 μm). The top radiator was set at a height of 20–30 cm above the surface of the AVF with the treatment time set at 40 min during HD three times per week.

Participants

The four studies included 666 patients, with 340 patients randomised to receive FIR therapy – median age 62.3±14.5 SD, while 326 were randomised to the control group – median age 62.0±14.5 SD. 348 patients were males–180 in FIR group and 168 in the control group, while females were 318, of those 160 received FIR therapy and 158 were controls.

Inclusion and exclusion criteria of studies are outlined in [Table 2], along with the definition of AVF malfunction for each of the included studies.

Apart from Lin et al who evaluated the effects of FIR in pre-dialysis patients with newly formed AVFs [38], the remaining RCTs included patients who already started HD. Mean time on HD in months for Lin et al [35] was 85.2±41.1 for FIR group and 79.2±42.2 for the control group, for Lai et al [37] FIR = 50.4±42 and control = 58.8±56.4 and for Lin et al in 2013 [36] FIR = 66.0±59.1 and control = 75.9±58.0. All patients in included trials received FIR therapy for 40 minutes per session three times a week for the duration of the study.

Lai et al studied patients with history of dysfunctional AVFs and repeated angioplasty. The mean life of the AVFs for their patients was 21.8±23.0 months for FIR group and 23.5±22.6 months for the controls [37]. 33 patients from 72 had history of AVF malfunction and 14 patients required surgical intervention, while 20 patients had a total of 49 angioplasty procedures in the FIR group compared to 34 patients from 73 with history of AVF malfunction, 13 of those required surgical intervention and 20 patients with total of 46 angioplasty procedures in the control group, in the RCT by Lin et al in 2007 [35]. Similarly, 47 patients had history of AVF malfunction with 12 patients requiring surgery from 139 and 35 patients underwent 79 angioplasty procedures in the FIR group, compared to 45 patients with history of malfunction, 13 patients of those required surgery and 32 patients underwent angioplasty as a salvage procedure in the control group in the study by Lin et al in 2013 [36]. All patients in both FIR and control groups had angioplasty procedures prior to recruitment in the study by Lai et al [37], while none of the patients included by Lin et al had a history of either surgical or angioplasty salvage procedures since they were all first time AVFs [38]. Lai et al had 9 of their patients who were initially randomised to the control group crossing over to the FIR group based on their request [37]. Clinical maturation was reported in 49 (81.7%) patients of 60 who received FIR therapy by Lin et all, compared to 37 (59.7%) from the 62 control subjects [38]. Sub -group analysis by age, gender and diagnosis of hypertension was not possible as this was not included in studies, and we did not have access to the raw data used by the authors. Other patients' characteristics are detailed in [Table 3].

Primary - unassisted - patency rates at 1 year

All of the 4 included studies (610 patients) reported on unassisted – primary – patency rate after 12 months of follow-up on the FIR therapy. 228/311 patients in FIR group had primarily patent AVFs at 12 months compared to 185/299 patients in the

Study or Subgroup	FIR Events	FIR Total	Control Events	Control Total	Weight	Risk Ratio M-H, Random, 95% CI
Lin 2013_AJKD	58	59	52	61	41.2%	1.15 [1.03, 1.29]
Lin 2013_NDT	102	109	88	102	58.8%	1.08 [0.99, 1.19]
Total (95% CI)		**168**		**163**	**100.0%**	**1.11 [1.04, 1.19]**
Total events	160		140			

Heterogeneity: Tau² = 0.00; Chi² = 0.71, df = 1 (P = 0.40); I² = 0%
Test for overall effect: Z = 2.97 (P = 0.003)

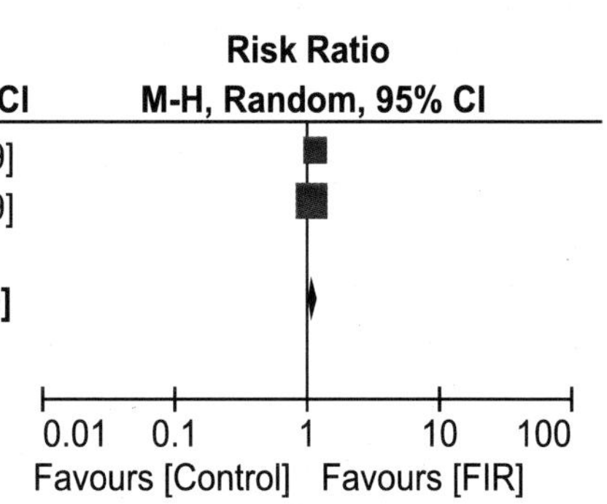

Figure 5. Forest plot showing assisted patency rates at 12 months.

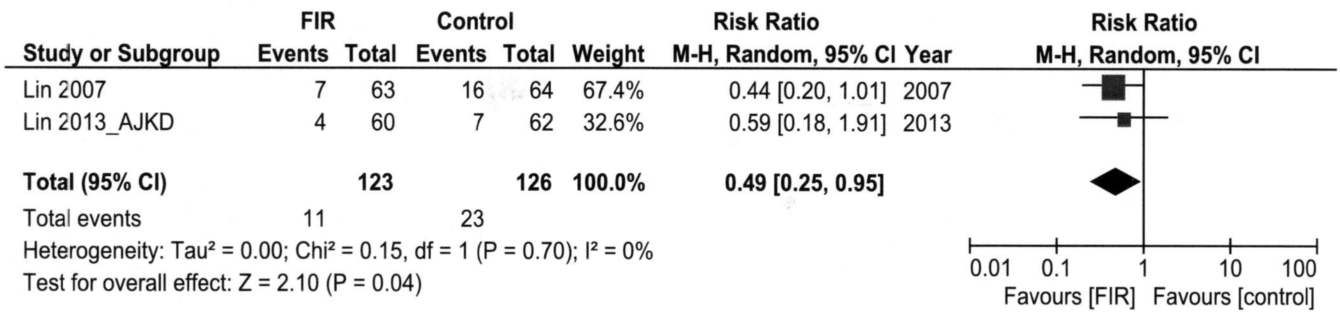

Figure 6. Forest plot showing surgical intervention for AVF malfunction.

control group. Pooled results showed significant difference between the two groups, with those who received FIR showing better primary patency rates compared to control (Pooled risk ratio = 1.23 [1.12, 1.35], 95% CI, p = 0.00001) [Figure 2]. There was no evidence of statistical heterogeneity (Cochran's Q = 0.33; degree of freedom (DF) = 3; p = 0.96; $I^2 = 0\%$). The funnel plot did not suggest bias [Figure 3], and the result was unchanged when fixed effects modelling was used (pooled risk ratio1.24 [1.13–1.37], 95% CI, p<0.0001).

Excluding the RCT by Lin et al on newly formed AVFs in pre-dialysis patients [38] from the analysis for primary patency after 12 months, the remaining studies (490 patients) showed better results in the FIR group with 176/252 AVFs being patent at 12 months compared to 142/238 in the control group [35–37]. This was statistically significant (Pooled risk ratio = 1.23 [1.10, 1.37], 95% CI, p = 0.0001) [Figure 4]. There was no evidence of statistical heterogeneity (Cochran's Q = 0.31; degree of freedom (DF) = 2; p = 0.86; $I^2 = 0\%$).

Secondary - assisted - patency rates

Data could be retrieved from 2 studies (331 patients) for analysis of assisted – secondary – patency rates at 12 months following salvage procedures [36,38]. 160/168 patients in the FIR group had patent AVFs following intervention for dysfunctional fistulas, compared to 140/163 patients in the control arm. Pooled results showed statistically significant difference favouring FIR therapy (Pooled risk ratio = 1.11 [1.04–1.19]; 95% CI, p = 0.003) [Figure 5]. There was no evidence of statistical heterogeneity (Cochran's Q = 0.71; degree of freedom (DF) = 1; p = 0.40; $I^2 = 0\%$).

Intervention

Two studies [35,38] (249 patients) reported the need for intervention to salvage a dysfunctional AVF. Patients who received FIR therapy required less interventions, 11/123 patients compared to 23/126 patients in the control group. The difference was significant (Pooled risk ratio = 0.49 [0.25–0.985; 95% CI; p = 0.04) [Figure 6]. There was no evidence of statistical heterogeneity (Cochran's Q = 0.15; degree of freedom (DF) = 1; p = 0.70; $I^2 = 0\%$).

Discussion

This review identified four studies (666 patients) which evaluated the use of FIR therapy to improve primary and secondary patency rates for AVFs in patients with ESRD. They all reported significant improvement in the outcome measures assessed in this review in favour of FIR therapy. Three of those studies (490 patients) were carried out on patients already started HD sessions, and one study (122 patients) focused on pre-dialysis first time AVF maturation. All four trials following some form of randomisation, and the demographics of patients in included studies did not differ significantly. Pooled analysis showed that primary - unassisted - patency was significantly better in the FIR group (pooled risk ratio of 1.23 [1.12–1.35], p value of 0.0001). Secondary – assisted – patency was reported in two studies (279 patients) and was found to be significantly better in those who received FIR therapy (pooled risk ratio of 1.19 [1.07–1.31], p value of 0.0008).

Post-conditioning using Far Infra-Red therapy has been shown to increase the level of heme oxygenase-1 (HO-1) expression which protects against Ischaemia/reperfusion injury in study by Tu et al [42]. HO-1 is a known vasodilator and at the same time inhibits proliferation of vascular smooth muscle cells, platelet aggregation, and vasospasm leading to favourable conditions for maturation of AVFs. Also, Ikeda et al repeated thermal therapy was shown to up-regulate endothelial nitric oxide synthase expression in Syrian hamsters [24], a finding that was validated by Akasaki et al, who also reported increased angiogenesis via (eNOS) following repeated thermal therapy in mice with hindlimb ischemia. [43]. Kipshidze et al irradiated cultures of rabbit endothelial cells and smooth muscle cells with different doses of non-ablative infrared. They found that non-ablative infrared laser inhibited neointimal hyperplasia after coronary arteries angioplasty in cholesterol-fed rabbits for up to 60 days [44]. FIR therapy is still considered a novel treatment for AVF although the technique has been described since 2007 by Lin et al [35]. This review demonstrated a beneficial use of FIR therapy that improved both primary and secondary patency rates across all studies included. This statistically significant difference was consistent even when one excluded study for having only 3 months of follow-up was added to the sensitivity analysis [39]. Also, excluding the only RCT found by the authors on newly formed AVF did not alter the outcome of the pooled analysis in terms of significance.

FIR therapy was also shown to improve access flow (Qa). The study by Lin et al – which was one of the RCTs included in the review - showed that 40 min of FIR therapy in a single HD session could increase access flow of AVF by about 50 mL/min with a 1-year effect of improving Qa by up to 150 mL/min and increasing unassisted patency of AVF by about 18% in comparison with controls [35].

A serious limiting factor of this systematic review is that the four RCTs came from the same institution (Yang-Ming University in Taiwan), and three of the four were authored by the same two authors (Lin-cc and Yang-wc) [35,36,38]. Dr Lin-cc reported that he was receiving lecture fees from WS Far Infrared Medical Technology, the company that makes the infrared machines used in the studies raising the potential of bias.

Also, all the RCTs were performed in an unblinded fashion, which can impact outcomes as demonstrated by the fact that in one study nine patients opted to join the FIR group despite initially being allocated as controls. Blinding in clinical trials involving FIR therapy would involve additional costs in making machines that resemble the ones used to deliver FIR therapy. Those machines should be convincing to both staff and patients if effective double blinding is to be considered. However, blinding can be attempted by placing a screen between the FIR device and the patient. Also, double-blinding can be achieved by placing a box over the device and then creating simple mock devices that also appear as boxes. This review provides a thorough examination of published evidence supporting the use of FIR therapy to promote AVF access maturation in patients with ESRD in HD, and also for those who are likely to require dialysis in the near future. The meta-analysis showed overwhelming support for regular use of FIR therapy, however there were limitations that need to be considered. Finally, this review may serve to guide future advances in using repeated thermal therapy in postconditioning of AVFs.

Conclusion

Results from four RCTs suggest that regular use of FIR therapy in haemodialysis and pre-haemodialysis patients, in particular those with AVFs, can positively influence AVF function. However, more blinded randomised controlled, multicentre and international clinical trials are required. We also hope to see sub-group analysis in those studies, particularly by age (e.g. using 65 as cut-off), gender and diagnosis of hypertension.

Author Contributions

Conceived and designed the experiments: KB DH EK SRW MCM PB EK MW LB. Performed the experiments: KB DH EK SRW MCM PB EK MW LB. Analyzed the data: KB DH EK SRW MCM PB EK MW. Contributed reagents/materials/analysis tools: KB DH. Contributed to the writing of the manuscript: KB DH EK SRW MCM PB EK MW LB.

References

1. Frankel A (2006) Temporary access and central venous catheters. Eur J Vasc Endovasc Surg 31: 417–422.
2. NKF-KDOQI (2006) 2006 Updates Clinical Practice Guidelines and Recommendations.
3. Hoggard J, Saad T, Schon D, Vesely TM, Royer T (2008) Guidelines for venous access in patients with chronic kidney disease. A Position Statement from the American Society of Diagnostic and Interventional Nephrology, Clinical Practice Committee and the Association for Vascular Access. Semin Dial 21: 186–191.
4. Polkinghorne KR, Chin GK, Macginley RJ, Owen AR, Russell C, et al. (2013) KHA-CARI guideline: Vascular access - central venous catheters, arteriovenous fistulae and arteriovenous grafts. Nephrology (Carlton).
5. Stolic R (2013) Most important chronic complications of arteriovenous fistulas for hemodialysis. Med Princ Pract 22: 220–228.
6. McCann M, Einarsdottir H, Van Waeleghem JP, Murphy F, Sedgewick J (2008) Vascular access management 1: an overview. J Ren Care 34: 77–84.
7. Dixon BS (2006) Why don't fistulas mature? Kidney Int 70: 1413–1422.
8. Allon M, Robbin ML (2002) Increasing arteriovenous fistulas in hemodialysis patients: problems and solutions. Kidney Int 62: 1109–1124.
9. Rayner HC, Pisoni RL, Gillespie BW, Goodkin DA, Akiba T, et al. (2003) Creation, cannulation and survival of arteriovenous fistulae: data from the Dialysis Outcomes and Practice Patterns Study. Kidney Int 63: 323–330.
10. Lok CE, Oliver MJ, Su J, Bhola C, Hannigan N, et al. (2005) Arteriovenous fistula outcomes in the era of the elderly dialysis population. Kidney Int 67: 2462–2469.
11. Allon M, Lockhart ME, Lilly RZ, Gallichio MH, Young CJ, et al. (2001) Effect of preoperative sonographic mapping on vascular access outcomes in hemodialysis patients. Kidney Int 60: 2013–2020.
12. Oliver MJ, McCann RL, Indridason OS, Butterly DW, Schwab SJ (2001) Comparison of transposed brachiobasilic fistulas to upper arm grafts and brachiocephalic fistulas. Kidney Int 60: 1532–1539.
13. Allon M (2007) Current management of vascular access. Clin J Am Soc Nephrol 2: 786–800.
14. Dixon BS, Novak L, Fangman J (2002) Hemodialysis vascular access survival: upper-arm native arteriovenous fistula. Am J Kidney Dis 39: 92–101.
15. Ocak G, Rotmans JI, Vossen CY, Rosendaal FR, Krediet RT, et al. (2013) Type of arteriovenous vascular access and association with patency and mortality. BMC Nephrol 14: 79.
16. Polkinghorne KR, McDonald SP, Atkins RC, Kerr PG (2004) Vascular access and all-cause mortality: a propensity score analysis. J Am Soc Nephrol 15: 477–486.
17. Spergel LM, Ravani P, Roy-Chaudhury P, Asif A, Besarab A (2007) Surgical salvage of the autogenous arteriovenous fistula (AVF). J Nephrol 20: 388–398.
18. Brunori G, Bandera A, Valente F, Laudon A (2008) [Vascular access for dialysis in elderly: AVF versus permanent CVC]. G Ital Nefrol 25: 614–618.
19. McCann M, Einarsdottir H, Van Waeleghem JP, Murphy F, Sedgewick J (2010) Vascular access management III: central venous catheters. J Ren Care 36: 25–33.
20. Ma A, Shroff R, Hothi D, Lopez MM, Veligratli F, et al. (2013) A comparison of arteriovenous fistulas and central venous lines for long-term chronic haemodialysis. Pediatr Nephrol 28: 321–326.
21. Cox JL, Chiasson DA, Gotlieb AI (1991) Stranger in a strange land: the pathogenesis of saphenous vein graft stenosis with emphasis on structural and functional differences between veins and arteries. Prog Cardiovasc Dis 34: 45–68.
22. Davies MG, Hagen PO (1994) Pathobiology of intimal hyperplasia. Br J Surg 81: 1254–1269.
23. Newby AC, Zaltsman AB (2000) Molecular mechanisms in intimal hyperplasia. J Pathol 190: 300–309.
24. Ikeda Y, Biro S, Kamogawa Y, Yoshifuku S, Eto H, et al. (2001) Repeated thermal therapy upregulates arterial endothelial nitric oxide synthase expression in Syrian golden hamsters. Jpn Circ J 65: 434–438.
25. Kawaura A, Tanida N, Kamitani M, Akiyama J, Mizutani M, et al. (2010) The effect of leg hyperthermia using far infrared rays in bedridden subjects with type 2 diabetes mellitus. Acta Med Okayama 64: 143–147.
26. Huang CY, Yang RS, Kuo TS, Hsu KH (2009) Phantom limb pain treated by far infrared ray. Conf Proc IEEE Eng Med Biol Soc 2009: 1589–1591.
27. Toyokawa H, Matsui Y, Uhara J, Tsuchiya H, Teshima S, et al. (2003) Promotive effects of far-infrared ray on full-thickness skin wound healing in rats. Exp Biol Med (Maywood) 228: 724–729.
28. Capon A, Mordon S (2003) Can thermal lasers promote skin wound healing? Am J Clin Dermatol 4: 1–12.
29. Su LH, Wu KD, Lee LS, Wang H, Liu CF (2009) Effects of far infrared acupoint stimulation on autonomic activity and quality of life in hemodialysis patients. Am J Chin Med 37: 215–226.
30. Liberati A, Altman DG, Tetzlaff J, Mulrow C, Gotzsche PC, et al. (2009) The PRISMA statement for reporting systematic reviews and meta-analyses of studies that evaluate health care interventions: explanation and elaboration. PLoS Med 6: e1000100.
31. Higgins JP, Altman DG, Gotzsche PC, Juni P, Moher D, et al. (2011) The Cochrane Collaboration's tool for assessing risk of bias in randomised trials. BMJ 343: d5928.
32. The Nordic Cochrane Centre TCc (2012) Review Manager (RevMan) [Computer Program]. Version 5.2.
33. DerSimonian R, Laird NM (1983) Evaluating the Effect of Coaching on SAT Scores: A Meta-Analysis. Harvard Educational Review 53: 1–15.
34. Sterne JAC EM, Moher D (2011) Chapter 10: Addressing reporting biases. Higgins JPT, Green S (editors) Cochrane Handbook for Systematic Reviews of Intervention Version 5.1.0.
35. Lin CC, Chang CF, Lai MY, Chen TW, Lee PC, et al. (2007) Far-infrared therapy: a novel treatment to improve access blood flow and unassisted patency of arteriovenous fistula in hemodialysis patients. J Am Soc Nephrol 18: 985–992.
36. Lin CC, Chung MY, Yang WC, Lin SJ, Lee PC (2013) Length polymorphisms of heme oxygenase-1 determine the effect of far-infrared therapy on the function of arteriovenous fistula in hemodialysis patients: a novel physicogenomic study. Nephrol Dial Transplant 28: 1284–1293.
37. Lai CC, Fang HC, Mar GY, Liou JC, Tseng CJ, et al. (2013) Post-angioplasty far infrared radiation therapy improves 1-year angioplasty-free hemodialysis access patency of recurrent obstructive lesions. Eur J Vasc Endovasc Surg 46: 726–732.
38. Lin CC, Yang WC, Chen MC, Liu WS, Yang CY, et al. (2013) Effect of Far Infrared Therapy on Arteriovenous Fistula Maturation: An Open-Label Randomized Controlled Trial. Am J Kidney Dis.
39. W.-C LC-CY (2012) Far infrared therapy improves arteriovenous fistula maturation. Nephrology Dialysis Transplantation Conference: 50th ERA-EDTA Congress Istanbul Turkey Conference Start: 20120524 Conference End: 20120527.

40. Shipley T, Adam J, Sweeney D, Fenwick S, Mansy H, et al. (2012) Does far infrared therapy aid av fistula maturation and maintenance?. Nephrology Dialysis Transplantation Conference: 49th ERA-EDTA Congress Paris France Conference Start: 20120524 Conference End: 20120527 Conference Publication: (varpagings) 27 (ii261).
41. Lin CH, Lee LS, Su LH, Huang TC, Liu CF (2011) Thermal therapy in dialysis patients - a randomized trial. Am J Chin Med 39: 839–851.
42. Tu YP, Chen SC, Liu YH, Chen CF, Hour TC (2013) Postconditioning with far-infrared irradiation increases heme oxygenase-1 expression and protects against ischemia/reperfusion injury in rat testis. Life Sci 92: 35–41.
43. Akasaki Y, Miyata M, Eto H, Shirasawa T, Hamada N, et al. (2006) Repeated thermal therapy up-regulates endothelial nitric oxide synthase and augments angiogenesis in a mouse model of hindlimb ischemia. Circ J 70: 463–470.
44. Kipshidze N, Nikolaychik V, Muckerheidi M, Keelan MH, Chekanov V, et al. (2001) Effect of short pulsed nonablative infrared laser irradiation on vascular cells in vitro and neointimal hyperplasia in a rabbit balloon injury model. Circulation 104: 1850–1855.

18

Innate-Like and Conventional T Cell Populations from Hemodialyzed and Kidney Transplanted Patients Are Equally Compromised

Marine Baron[1], Renata Belo[1], Dominique Cathelin[2,3], Lucia Moreira-Teixeira[1], Claire Cartery[4], Eric Rondeau[2,3], Laurent Mesnard[2,3]*❡, Maria Leite-de-Moraes[1]*❡

1 INEM (Institut Necker Enfants Malades), CNRS UMR 8253, INSERM UMR 1151, Université Paris Descartes, Sorbonne Paris Cité, France, Hôpital Necker Enfants Malades, Paris, France, **2** INSERM UMR S 702, Université Pierre et Marie Curie, Assistance Publique-Hôpitaux de Paris, Hôpital Tenon, Paris, France, **3** AP-HP, Hôpital Tenon, Urgences Néphrologiques & Transplantation Rénale, Universite Pierre et Marie Curie, Paris, France, **4** Nephrology and Dialysis, Tenon Hospital, Assistance Publique-Hôpitaux de Paris, Hôpital Tenon, Paris, France

Abstract

Clinicians are well aware of existing pharmacologically-induced immune deficient status in kidney-transplanted patients that will favor their susceptibility to bacterial or viral infections. Previous studies indicated that advanced Stage 4–5 Chronic Kidney Disease might also be regarded as an immune deficiency-like status as well, even though the mechanisms are not fully understood. Here, we analyzed the *ex vivo* frequency and the functional properties of both conventional and innate-like T (ILT) lymphocyte subsets in the peripheral blood of 35 patients on hemodialysis, 29 kidney transplanted patients and 38 healthy donors. We found that peripheral blood cell count of ILT cells, as iNKT (invariant Natural Killer T) and MAIT (mucosal-associated invariant T), were significantly decreased in hemodialyzed patients compared to healthy controls. This deficiency was also observed regarding conventional T cells, including the IL-17-producing $CD4^+$ Th17 cells. Pertaining to regulatory T cells, we also noticed major modifications in the global frequency of $CD4^+CD25^+Foxp3^+$ T lymphocytes, including the resting suppressive $CD45RA^+Foxp3^{lo}$ and activated suppressive $CD45RA^-Foxp3^{hi}$ T cell subpopulations. We found no significant differences between the immune status of hemodialyzed and kidney-transplanted subjects. In conclusion, we demonstrated that both ILT and conventional T cell numbers are equally impaired in hemodialyzed and kidney-transplanted patients.

Editor: Johan K. Sandberg, Karolinska Institutet, Sweden

Funding: This work was supported by research grants from CNRS (Centre National de la Recherche Scientifique), René Descartes University, INSERM (Institut National de la Santé et de la Recherche Médicale), FRM (Fondation pour la Recherche Medicale), Day Solvay Foundation and FCT (Fundaçao para a Ciência e a Tecnologia). The funders had no role in study design, data collection and analysis, decision to publish, or preparation of the manuscript.

* Email: maria.leite-de-moraes@parisdescartes.fr (MLM); laurent.mesnard@tnn.aphp.fr (LM)

❡ These authors contributed equally to this work.

Introduction

Chronic kidney disease (CKD) is a common disease characterized by the progressive loss of the renal function that may lead to the initiation of treatment by replacement therapy such as hemodialysis or kidney transplantation (KT). Besides classical complication of chronic renal failure such as hypertension, fluid overload, hypocalcemia or even anemia, complications as a result of infections, especially caused by bacteria, are also an important source of morbidity and mortality in these patients, particularly at the terminal stage (CKD-5) [1]. A possible explanation for this susceptibility to infections is their frequent hospitalization, overuse of antibiotics and other confounding factors like diabetes or auto-immune related disease that are commonly associated with their kidney disease. Therefore, compromised immune responses may also explain this susceptibility to infectious agents [2]. Indeed, immunological abnormalities reported so far for CKD-5 patients include reduced phagocytic functions, defective antigen presentation and impaired B and T cell responses [3–8]. The mechanisms responsible for these deficiencies are not fully elucidated.

T lymphocytes are currently considered as major players to coordinate adaptive immune responses against infections. Recently, several studies highlighted the participation of a new group of T cells, called innate-like T (ILT) cells, which are on the frontier between innate and adaptive immune responses. Here, we focused our attention on two ILT populations, namely invariant Natural Killer T (iNKT) and mucosal-associated invariant T (MAIT) cells that display conserved significant homologies between mouse and human [9,10,11]. These lymphocytes produce a broad range of cytokines few minutes after stimulation allowing them to modulate both innate and acquired immunity in a large spectrum of inflammatory diseases [9,10,11,12]. They express a highly restricted T cell receptor (TCR) repertoire composed in humans of a single invariant Vα24Jα18 and Vα7.2Jα33 for iNKT and MAIT cells, respectively. In contrast to conventional T cells that recognize peptides, iNKT cells recognize glycolipids presented by CD1d while MAIT cells are activated by vitamin B metabolites

Table 1. Patient demographic characteristics.

Characteristic	Value
Non-transplanted patient	
N	35
Age (yr; mean ± SEM)	40.4±1.74
Gender (female/male)	13/22
Cause of ESRD:	
Vascular nephropathy (hypertensive sclerosis, thrombotic microangiopathy)	8
Autoimmune related nephropathy (systemic lupus erythematosus, Wegener granulomatosis, rheumatoid purpura, idiopathic GEM)	8
Primary glomerulonephritis (focal segmental glomerulosclerosis, IgA nephropathy, Alport syndrome)	7
Secondary glomerulonephritis (diabetes mellitus, type 1 diabetes, sickle cell disease)	5
Tubulointerstitial nephritis (reflux nephropathy, myeloma)	4
Congenital/hereditary nephropathy (polycystic kidney)	4
Unknown	1
Blood lymphocyte counts per mm^3 (mean ± SEM)	1335±187
Transplanted patient	
N	29
Age (yr; mean ± SEM)	40.1±1.83
Gender (female/male)	10/19
Years post-transplantation (mean ± SEM)	3.34±0.59
Cause of ESRD:	
Primary glomerulonephritis (Alport syndrome, IgA nephropathy, focal segmental glomerulosclerosis)	7
Congenital/hereditary nephropathy (polycystic kidney, Fabry disease, tuberous sclerosis, Bor syndrome)	6
Unknown	6
Tubulointerstitial nephritis (reflux nephropathy)	5
Vascular nephropathy (hypertensive sclerosis, atypical hemolytic uremic syndrome)	4
Autoimmune related nephropathy (systemic lupus erythematosus)	1
Blood lymphocyte counts per mm^3 (mean ± SEM)	1316±147
MDRD (mL/min; mean ± SEM)	61.9±4.03
Healthy donors	
N	38
Age (yr; mean ± SEM)	30.7±2.2
Gender (female/male)	15/23
Blood lymphocyte counts per mm^3 (mean ± SEM)	1794±213

Two hemodialysed patients had glomerulonephritis and vascular nephropathy at the same time.

presented by the MHC-related protein 1 (MR1) molecules [13,14]. Both iNKT and MAIT cells are generally regarded as protective against infections and we reported that iNKT cells also attenuated the development of anti-glomerular basement membrane glomerulonephritis in a murine model [15,16,17,18]. Herein, we analyzed the frequency of these innate-like T lymphocytes, namely iNKT and MAIT cells, and of conventional T cells in the peripheral blood of CKD-5/Hemodialyzed (HD) and kidney transplanted patients.

Materials and Methods

Patients

Patient demographic characteristics and most relevant clinical data are shown in Table 1. All patients entered in this study after providing their informed consent. The study was conducted according to the procedures of the Declaration of Helsinki and to local ethic committee rules (Commission de Protection des Personnes, Ile de France). Patient's anonymity was protected. Thirty-seven HD patients, 31 kidney transplanted patients and 38 healthy volunteer's donors, considered here as controls, (Table 1) (obtained after signed informed consent managed by the French Blood Department) participated in the study.

Cell preparation

Blood samples were obtained from CKD or kidney transplanted patients (End Stage Renal Disease) from Tenon Hospital (Kidney Emergencies and Renal Transplantation and nephrology and hemodialysis units), Paris, France. All analyses were performed on freshly isolated peripheral blood mononuclear cells (PBMC) from 10 to 20 mL of blood by density-gradient centrifugation (Ficoll-Paque PLUS; GE Healthcare). Cell-surface staining was performed in PBS buffer containing 2% FCS and 0.01% NaN_3 on ice, as previously described [12,19]. Cells were first stained with PBS57-loaded or empty-CD1d-tetramers (National Institutes of Health Tetramer Core Facility), then with the following directly

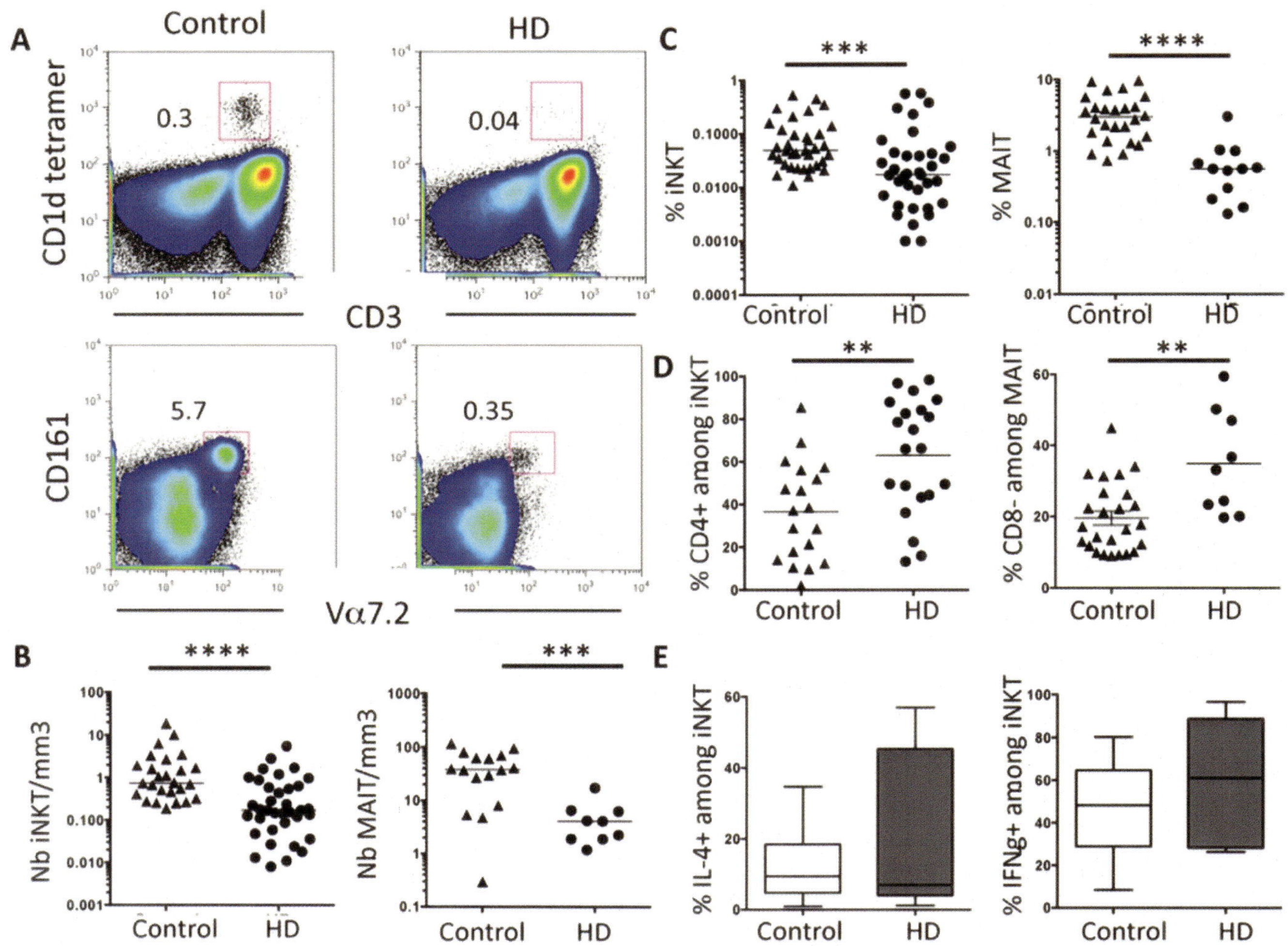

Figure 1. iNKT cell deficit in HD patients. (A) iNKT cells were double stained by anti-CD3 and the PBS57-loaded CD1d-tetramer. Representative FACS profile showing the percentage of iNKT and MAIT cells in control versus HD patients. (B and C) HD patients had significant low numbers (B) and percentage (C) of peripheral blood iNKT and MAIT cells when compared to healthy donors. Bars represent the median. (D) The frequency of $CD4^+$ and $CD8^-$ subsets respectively among gated iNKT and MAIT cells in control versus HD patients is represented. (E) The percentage of IL-4^+ or $IFN\gamma^+$ cells among gated iNKT lymphocytes was assessed after 5 h stimulation with PMA and ionomycin. Box-and-whisker plots are used to represent the distributions. The bottom and the top of a box represent the 5th and 95th percentiles, and the bar in the box shows the median. **, $P<0.001$; ***, $P<0.0005$; ****, $P<0.0001$ versus controls.

conjugated monoclonal antibodies (eBioscience): anti-CD3, anti-CD4, anti-CD8, anti-CD25, anti-CD45RA, anti-CD161, anti-TCRV**α**7.2 and/or anti-Foxp3. Intra-cellular analysis of Foxp3 was performed after fixation and permeabilization using Foxp3 staining buffers (eBioscience). Data were acquired on a FACS-Canto II flow cytometer (BD Biosciences) with the use of FACSDiva Version 6.1.3 software (BD Biosciences) and were analyzed with the FlowJo Version 8.5.3 software (TreeStar). Lymphocyte subpopulations were analyzed within the lymphocyte gate on forward and side-scatter plots. Results were expressed in absolute numbers per mm^3 of peripheral blood.

Intracellular cytokine staining

For intracellular cytokine staining, PBMC were incubated for five hours with PMA (25 ng/mL), Ionomycin (1 µg/mL) and Brefeldin A (10 µg/mL, all from Sigma-Aldrich). Cells were stained with CD1d-tetramer, washed and fixed with 4% paraformaldehyde and permeabilized with 0.5% saponin (Sigma-Aldrich) before further incubated with anti-CD3, anti-CD4, anti-CD8, anti-IL-4, anti-IFN**γ** anti-IL-17 antibodies. Isotype-matched antibodies were used to define marker settings for cytokines antibodies.

Statistical Analysis

Statistical analyses were performed using GraphPad Prism (version 6.0 for Mac OS X, San Diego, California USA). Groups were compared using the nonparametric Mann-Whitney U test for non-normally distributed variables. All p values were two-tailed, and the statistical significance level was defined as a $p<0.05$.

Results and Discussion

Clinical data are presented at Table 1. In sum, of the 35 HD patients, 13 were female and 22 male, with an age of 40.4 ± 1.6 (range 19-59) years at the time of blood collection. The gender and age of healthy donors were 15 females/23 males, 30.7 ± 2.2 years old (range 20–64). The cause of ESRD (End Stage Renal Disease) for these HD patients was vascular nephropathy (8 patients), autoimmune related nephropathy (8 patients), primary glomeru-

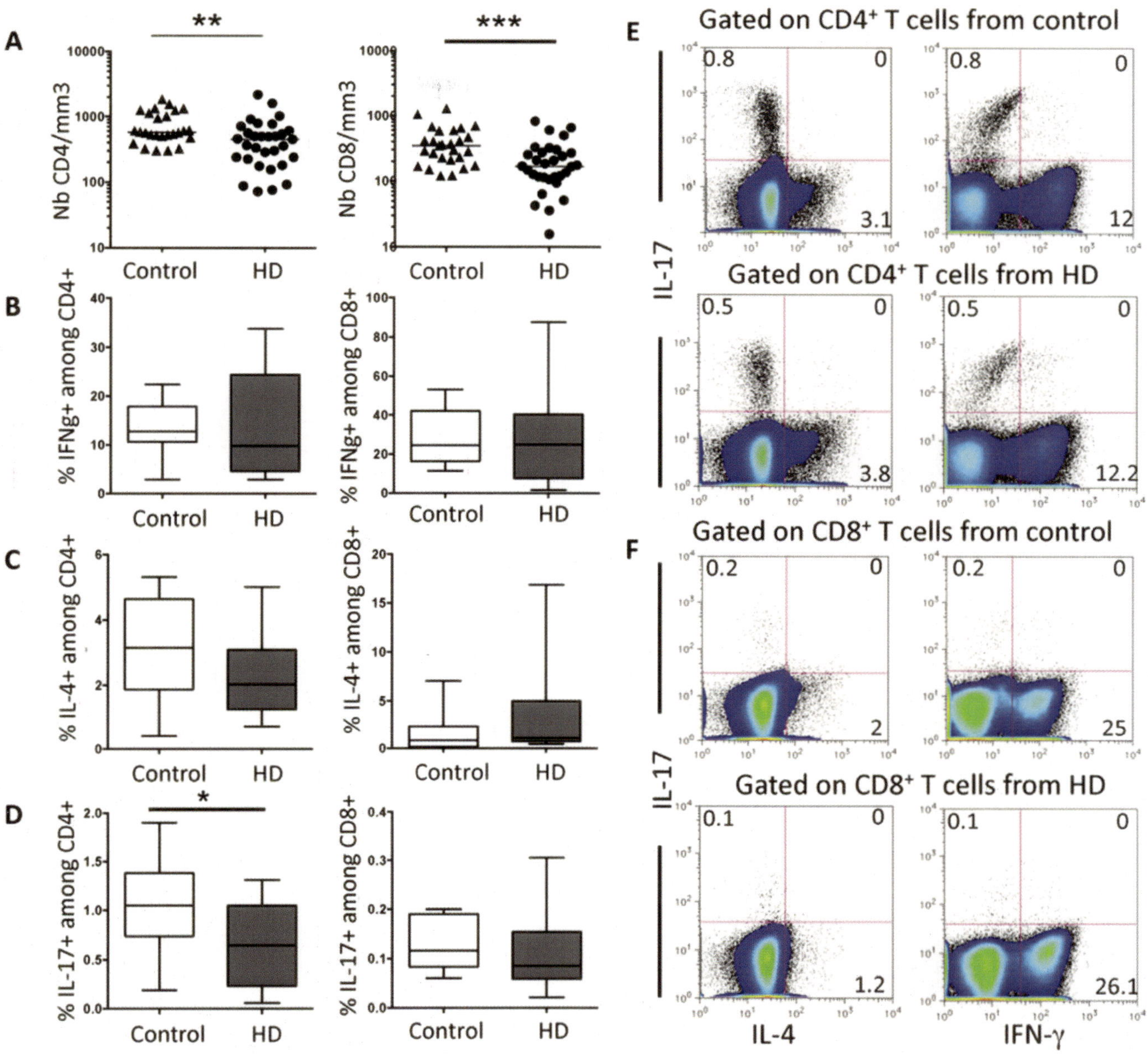

Figure 2. CD4$^+$ and CD8$^+$ T cell numbers are reduced in HD patients. (A) CD4$^+$ and CD8$^+$T cell numbers are significant decreased in the peripheral blood of HD patients compared to healthy donors. Bars represent the median. (B) The percentage of IFNγ$^+$ cells among gated CD8$^+$ or CD4$^+$ T lymphocytes or (C) the percentage of IL-4$^+$ and IL-17$^+$ cells among gated CD4$^+$ T lymphocytes was assessed after 6 h stimulation with PMA and ionomycin. Box-and-whisker plots are used to represent the distributions. The bottom and the top of a box represent the 5th and 95th percentiles, and the bar in the box shows the median. *, $P<0.01$; **, $P<0.001$; ***, $P<0.0005$ versus controls. Representative FACS analysis of IL-4, IL-17 and IFNγ production by gated CD4$^+$ (E) or CD8$^+$ (F) T cells from health donor controls (top) or HD patients (bottom) are represented.

lonephritis (7 patients), secondary glomerulonephritis (5 patients), tubulointerstitial nephritis (4 patients), congenital/hereditary nephropathy (4 patients) or unknown (1 patient). Two HD patients had both glomerulonephritis and vascular nephropathy. Eleven HD patients received corticoids associated or not with immunossuppressive drugs (calcineurin inhibitors or selective inhibitors of inosine monophosphate dehydrogenase or antimetabolite-drug). All analysis performed in our study were made including or not these patients. Statistic differences reported below were obtained whatever immunosuppressed patients were excluded or not (data not shown). For this reason, they were maintained in the study.

Among the 31 kidney-transplanted patients, 11 were female and 20 male, with an age of 39.7±1.7 (range 20–59) years at the time of blood collection. Patients were analyzed about 3.34±0.59 years post-transplantation. The cause of ESRD for these KD patients was primary glomerulonephritis (7 patients), congenital/hereditary nephropathy (6 patients), unknown (6 patient), tubulointerstitial nephritis (5 patients), vascular nephropathy (4 patients), autoimmune related nephropathy (2 patients) or secondary glomerulonephritis (1 patient). Their MDRD was 62.1±3.78 mL/min.

Herein, we analyzed the frequency of iNKT and MAIT cells in the peripheral blood of CKD-5/Hemodialyzed (HD) patients. iNKT cells were identified by CD1d/PBS57 tetramers and MAIT

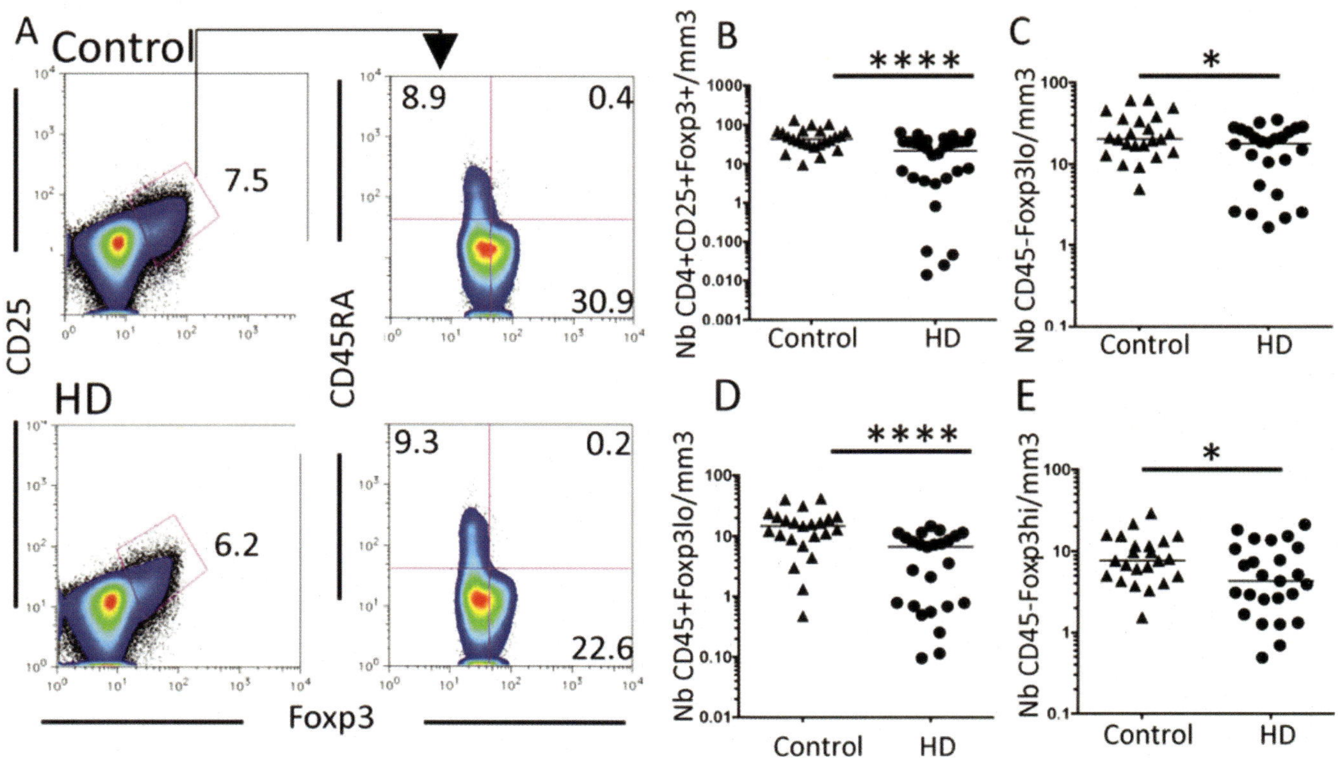

Figure 3. Global Foxp3$^+$ T cell numbers are reduced in HD patients. (A) Representative FACS analysis of CD4$^+$CD25$^+$Foxp3$^+$T cells and their distinct subsets on PBMC from control (top) and HD patients (bottom). (B) CD4$^+$CD25$^+$Foxp3$^+$T cell numbers are reduced in HD patients. (C to E) Among these gated cells, cytokine-secreting CD45RA$^-$Foxp3^{lo} nonsuppressive (C), resting suppressive CD45RA$^+$Foxp3^{lo} (D) and activated suppressive CD45RA$^-$Foxp3^{hi} (E) cells, all these subsets are reduced in HD patients compared to controls. Bars represent the median. *, P<0.01; ****, P<0.0001.

cells by the expression of CD3, CD161 and TCR Vα7.2 chain (Figure 1A). We found that the absolute number of iNKT and MAIT cells was drastically reduced in HD patients compared to control healthy donors (Figure 1B). We confirmed previous reports showing that the number of total CD3$^+$ T cells was diminished in these patients (808.2±130/mm^3 in HD patients versus 1296±156/mm^3 in health donors) [20]. iNKT and MAIT cell deficiency was also observed in terms of percentage among gated CD3$^+$ T cells (Figure 1C), thus confirming their pronounced deficiency in HD patients. In addition, the subset distribution of these particular T cell populations was also committed since we found that the percentage of CD4$^+$ and CD8$^-$ subsets were enhanced among gated iNKT and MAIT cells, respectively (Figure 1D) compared to controls. The reduced number of these distinct iNKT or MAIT subsets limited a more accurate analysis of their specific cytokine profile. However, *ex vivo* analysis of cytokine-producing capacities did not outline significant differences in the percentage of IL-4$^+$ or IFNγ^+ among gated iNKT cells

Table 2. Numbers of distinct T cell populations in the peripheral blood of kidney-transplanted versus healthy donors.

T cell populations	Number per mm3 in		p
	transplanted patients	healthy donors	
iNKT	0.76±0.15	2.31±0.78	0.0360
MAIT	3.78±1.28	44.76±8.50	0.0107
CD4	501.4±70.4	765.7±85.1	0.0098
CD8	365.3±51.7	407.0±53.9	0.4875
CD4+Foxp3+CD25+	22.46±4.87	51.81±6.43	0.0005
CD45RA-Foxp3lo	16.26±3.45	25.94±3.31	0.0394
CD45RA+Foxp3lo	7.12±1.65	15.78±2.27	0.0036
CD45RA-Foxp3hi	4.20±0.90	9.71±1.36	0.0017

Results are expressed as mean ± SEM of cell counts in the peripheral blood of kidney-transplanted versus healthy donors. Mann Whitney test was used to compare the sample.
p<0.05 are considered as significant.

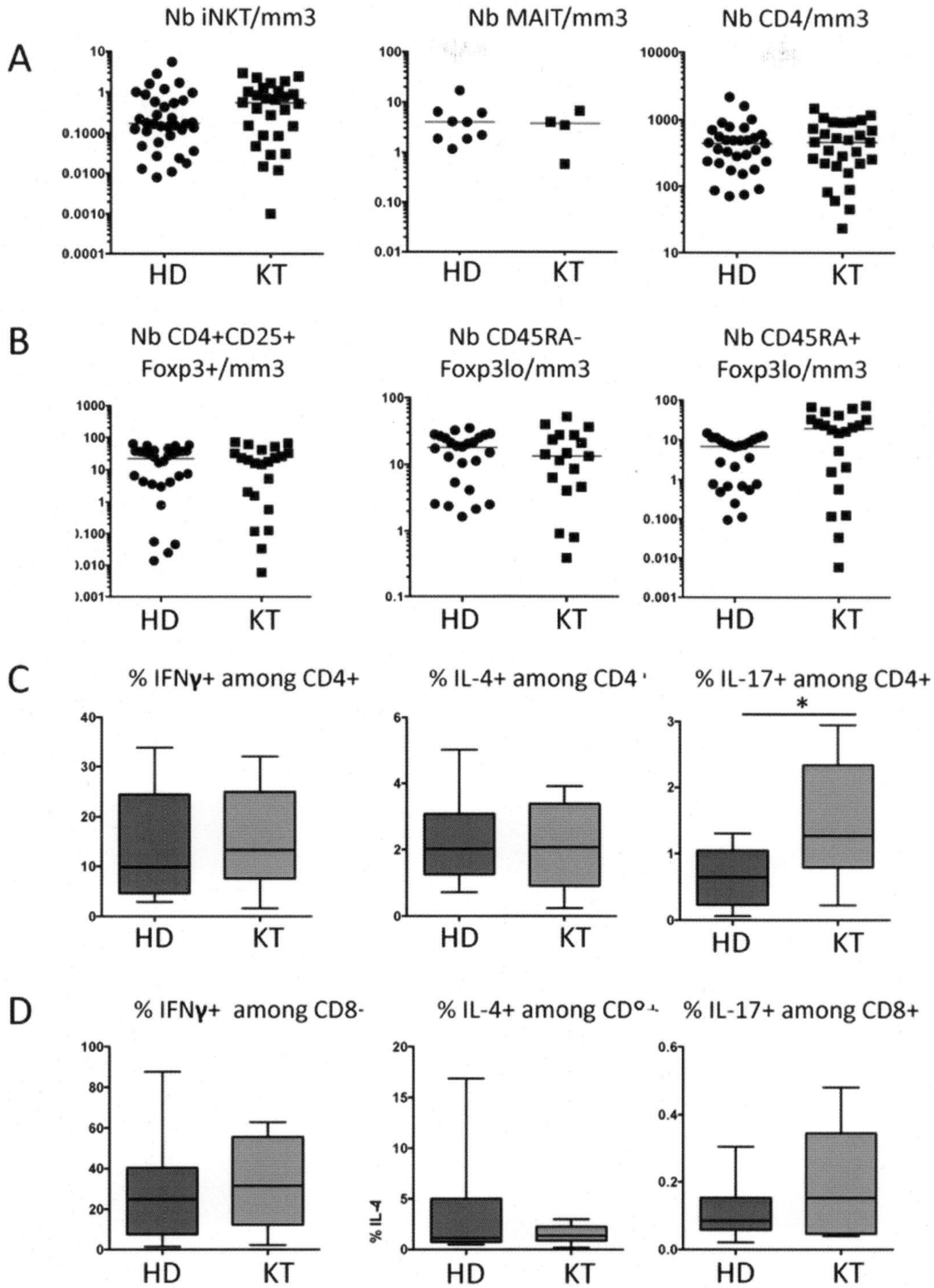

Figure 4. Both ILT and conventional T cells are equally deficient in HD and KD patients. (A) HD patients had no significant differences in their number of iNKT, MAIT, $CD4^+$ and $CD8^+$ T cells when compared to kidney transplanted (KT) patients. Bars represent the median. (B) $CD4^+CD25^+Foxp3^+$T cell numbers are similarly reduced in HD as in KD patients. Among these gated cells, cytokine-secreting $CD45RA^-Foxp3^{lo}$ nonsuppressive, resting suppressive $CD45RA^+Foxp3^{lo}$ and activated suppressive $CD45RA^-Foxp3^{hi}$ cell levels, are also similar in HD and KD patients. (C and D) The percentage of $IFN\gamma^+$, $IL\text{-}4^+$ or $IL\text{-}17^+$ cells among gated $CD4^+$ (C) or $CD8^+$ (D) T lymphocytes was assessed after 6 h stimulation with PMA and ionomycin. Box-and-whisker plots are used to represent the distributions. The bottom and the top of a box represent the 5th and 95th percentiles, and the bar in the box shows the median. (A and B) Bars represent the median. *, $P<0.01$.

between patients and healthy controls (Figure 1E) indicating that these cells are functional, but yet in very few numbers in HD patients.

Deficiency in peripheral blood cell count and percentage was also observed in HD patients concerning CD4$^+$ and CD8$^+$ T cells (Figure 2A). Using a short, 6 hours, polyclonal stimulation, we found no significant difference in the ability of *ex vivo* CD4$^+$ T cells to secrete IFNγ (Figure 2B and 2E). Similarly, the percentage of IFNγ-producing CD8$^+$ T cells was unchanged in HD patients compared to controls (Figure 2B and 2F). This was also true regarding IL-4-producing CD4$^+$ (Figure 2C and 2E) or CD8$^+$ T cells (Figure 2C and 2F). Conversely, the frequency of IL-17A (or IL-17)-producing CD4$^+$ T cells was significantly reduced in HD patients (Figure 2D and 2E). No significant difference was observed concerning the ability of CD8+ T cells from HD patients to secrete IL-17 (Figure 2D and 2F). IL-17-producing Th17 CD4$^+$ T cells are usually considered as playing an important role against infections including fungal infections [21]. Polymorphisms within the IL-17E and IL-17RA genes are associated with end stage renal disease [22], suggesting that IL-17 family or its receptors could influence the severity of the kidney inflammatory response. Together, our findings reveal that CD4$^+$ T cells in HD patients are impaired in number with a pronounced deficiency in their IL-17-producing subset, namely CD4$^+$ Th17 cells.

In addition to the analysis of *ex vivo* cytokine-producing capacities, we also focused our attention on regulatory Foxp3$^+$CD4$^+$ T (Treg) cells that play a key role in the regulation of inflammatory responses. Treg cells are usually designed as CD25^{high}Foxp3$^+$ cells. We found that HD patients presented a global deficiency in the CD4$^+$Foxp3$^+$CD25$^+$ T cells count (Figure 3A and 3B). Previous reports have highlighted that TCR activated human T cells can express Foxp3 and CD25 but these cells are not suppressive [23,24]. To address this issue, new combinations of markers are now used to distinguish suppressive from nonsuppressive Foxp3$^+$ T cells. A pertinent example is the analysis of CD45RA expression associated with distinct levels of Foxp3 [25] (Figure 3A). This approach revealed that the peripheral number of cytokine-secreting CD45RA$^-$Foxp3^{lo} nonsuppressive (Figure 3C), resting suppressive CD45RA$^+$Foxp3^{lo} (Figure 3D) and activated suppressive CD45RA$^-$Foxp3^{hi} (Figure 3E) T cell subpopulation were significantly reduced in HD patients compared to controls. Globally these findings endorse the above results showing that the immune system of HD patients is dysregulated not only at the level of non conventional ILT iNKT and MAIT cells but also of conventional effector and regulatory T cells. This global immune dysregulation might favor the susceptibility of these patients to infections.

These results aimed us to ask a key question: are these immune deficits observed in HD patients similar to those reported in kidney-transplanted persons? Kidney transplantation is a common treatment for HD patients. We confirmed an immune deficit in kidney-transplanted patients in terms of T cell counts when compared to healthy donors (Table 2). Interestingly, the analysis of kidney-transplanted patients clearly shows that their immune system is equally impaired as those from ERDS patients since we found no significant difference between the distinct ILT and conventional T cell populations tested (Figure 4). Indeed, the number of peripheral blood iNKT, MAIT, CD4$^+$, CD8$^+$ and CD4$^+$CD25$^+$Foxp3$^+$ T cell populations, including CD45RA$^-$Foxp3^{lo} nonsuppressive, resting suppressive CD45RA$^+$Foxp3^{lo} T cell and activated suppressive CD45RA$^-$Foxp3^{hi} T cell subpopulations were similar in kidney transplanted and HD patients (Figure 4A and 4B). Concerning their cytokine profile, the frequency of CD4- or CD8-producing IFNγ or IL-4 was similar between HD and KT patients (Figure 4C and 4D). IL-17-producing T cells was slightly different since the percentage of IL-17$^+$ among gated CD4^s T cells was enhanced in KT compared to HD patients (Figure 4C). However, this was not confirmed in terms of total cell counts of IL-17-producing CD4$^+$ T cells (5.9 ± 2.6 versus $4.3 \pm 1.2 \times 10^3$/ml for HD versus KT patients, respectively).

Overall, our findings clearly show that HD patients presented similar immune dysfunctions as transplanted patients. This information is of high clinical value, because clinicians are well aware of the poor immunological status of transplanted patients but underestimate the immunological status of HD patient *per se*. Furthermore, our findings concerning ILT cells, namely MAIT and iNKT cells, are the first evidence that these lymphocytes are reduced in the peripheral blood of HD and kidney-transplanted patients. Their deficiency likely favors the susceptibility of these patients to infections. T cell counts were also reduced in terms of conventional T cell subsets namely CD8$^+$, CD4$^+$, Th17, CD4$^+$CD25$^+$Foxp3$^+$ and their subsets: nonsuppressive CD45RA$^-$Foxp3^{lo}, resting suppressive CD45RA$^+$Foxp3^{lo} T cell and activated suppressive CD45RA$^-$Foxp3^{hi} T cell subpopulations. The low number of resting suppressive CD45RA$^+$Foxp3^{lo} and activated suppressive CD45RA$^-$Foxp3^{hi} T cell subsets, could contribute to the global dysregulation of the immune systems observed so far in CKD and transplanted patients.

In conclusion, kidney failure results in a global T cells immune dysfunction that can contribute to enhance the risk of complications due to infections in particular. Our, data reinforce the underestimated immune dysfunction found in HD patients, which appears similar to kidney-transplanted patients. Overall our findings emphasize the importance of tight clinical fellow-up of hemodialyzed patients, especially in an infectious context.

Acknowledgments

We are especially indebted to NIH Tetramer facilities for providing CD1d/PBS57 tetramers. This work was supported by research grants from CNRS (Centre National de la Recherche Scientifique), René Descartes University, INSERM (Institut National de la Santé et de la Recherche Médicale), FRM (Fondation pour la Recherche Medicale), Day Solvay Foundation and FCT (Fundaçao para a Ciência e a Tecnologia).

Author Contributions

Conceived and designed the experiments: MB LM MLM. Performed the experiments: MB RB DC LMT. Analyzed the data: MB LM MLM. Contributed reagents/materials/analysis tools: CC ER. Wrote the paper: MB LM MLM.

References

1. Sarnak MJ, Jaber BL (2000) Mortality caused by sepsis in patients with end-stage renal disease compared with the general population. Kidney Int 58: 1758–1764.
2. Jaber BL (2005) Bacterial infections in hemodialysis patients: pathogenesis and prevention. Kidney Int 67: 2508–2519.
3. Lewis SL, Van Epps DE (1987) Neutrophil and monocyte alterations in chronic dialysis patients. Am J Kidney Dis 9: 381–395.
4. Jaber BL, Cendoroglo M, Balakrishnan VS, Perianayagam MC, King AJ, et al. (2001) Apoptosis of leukocytes: basic concepts and implications in uremia. Kidney Int Suppl 78: S197–205.
5. Vanholder R, Ringoir S (1993) Infectious morbidity and defects of phagocytic function in end-stage renal disease: a review. J Am Soc Nephrol 3: 1541–1554.

6. Verkade MA, van Druningen CJ, Vaessen LM, Hesselink DA, Weimar W, et al. (2007) Functional impairment of monocyte-derived dendritic cells in patients with severe chronic kidney disease. Nephrol Dial Transplant 22: 128–138.
7. Raska K Jr, Raskova J, Shea SM, Frankel RM, Wood RH, et al. (1983) T cell subsets and cellular immunity in end-stage renal disease. Am J Med 75: 734–740.
8. Peraldi MN, Berrou J, Metivier F, Toubert A (2013) Natural killer cell dysfunction in uremia: the role of oxidative stress and the effects of dialysis. Blood Purif, 35 Suppl 2:14–19.
9. Bendelac A, Savage PB, Teyton L (2007) The biology of NKT cells. Annu Rev Immunol 25: 297–336.
10. Kronenberg M (2005) Toward an understanding of NKT cell biology: progress and paradoxes. Annu Rev Immunol 23: 877–900.
11. Le Bourhis L, Guerri L, Dusseaux M, Martin E, Soudais C, et al. (2011) Mucosal-associated invariant T cells: unconventional development and function. Trends Immunol 32: 212–218.
12. Moreira-Teixeira L, Resende M, Coffre M, Devergne O, Herbeuval JP, et al. (2011) Proinflammatory environment dictates the IL-17-producing capacity of human invariant NKT cells. J Immunol 186: 5758–5765.
13. Kawano T, Cui J, Koezuka Y, Toura I, Kaneko Y, et al. (1997) CD1d-restricted and TCR-mediated activation of valpha14 NKT cells by glycosylceramides. Science 278: 1626–1629.
14. Kjer-Nielsen L, Patel O, Corbett AJ, Le Nours J, Meehan B, et al. (2012) MR1 presents microbial vitamin B metabolites to MAIT cells. Nature 491: 717–723.
15. Berzins SP, Smyth MJ, Baxter AG (2011) Presumed guilty: natural killer T cell defects and human disease. Nat Rev Immunol 11: 131–142.
16. Paget C, Trottein F (2013) Role of type 1 natural killer T cells in pulmonary immunity. Mucosal Immunol 6: 1054–1067.
17. Le Bourhis L, Guerri L, Dusseaux M, Martin E, Soudais C, et al. (2011) Mucosal-associated invariant T cells: unconventional development and function. Trends Immunol 32: 212–218.
18. Mesnard L, Keller AC, Michel ML, Vandermeersch S, Rafat C, et al. (2009) Invariant natural killer T cells and TGF-beta attenuate anti-GBM glomerulonephritis. J Am Soc Nephrol 20: 1282–1292.
19. Moreira-Teixeira L, Resende M, Devergne O, Herbeuval JP, Hermine O, et al. (2012) Rapamycin combined with TGF-beta converts human invariant NKT cells into suppressive Foxp3+ regulatory cells. J Immunol 188: 624–631.
20. Deenitchina SS, Ando T, Okuda S, Kinukawa N, Hirakata H, et al. (1995) Cellular immunity in hemodialysis patients: a quantitative analysis of immune cell subsets by flow cytometry. Am J Nephrol 15: 57–65.
21. Cypowyj S, Picard C, Marodi L, Casanova JL, Puel A (2012) Immunity to infection in IL-17-deficient mice and humans. Eur J Immunol 42: 2246–2254.
22. Kim YG, Kim EY, Ihm CG, Lee TW, Lee SH, et al. (2012) Gene polymorphisms of interleukin-17 and interleukin-17 receptor are associated with end-stage kidney disease. Am J Nephrol 36: 472–477.
23. Ziegler SF (2006) FOXP3: of mice and men. Annu Rev Immunol 24: 209–226.
24. Gavin MA, Rasmussen JP, Fontenot JD, Vasta V, Manganiello VC, et al. (2007) Foxp3-dependent programme of regulatory T-cell differentiation. Nature 445: 771–775.
25. Miyara M, Yoshioka Y, Kitoh A, Shima T, Wing K, et al. (2009) Functional delineation and differentiation dynamics of human CD4+ T cells expressing the FoxP3 transcription factor. Immunity 30: 899–911.

Hypertension and Hyperglycemia Synergize to Cause Incipient Renal Tubular Alterations Resulting in Increased NGAL Urinary Excretion in Rats

Ana M. Blázquez-Medela[2,3], Omar García-Sánchez[2,3], Víctor Blanco-Gozalo[1,2,4], Yaremi Quiros[2,4], María J. Montero[2], Carlos Martínez-Salgado[1,2,3], José M. López-Novoa[2,3], Francisco J. López-Hernández[1,2,3]*

1 Instituto de Estudios de Ciencias de la Salud de Castilla y León-Instituto de Investigación Biomédica de Salamanca (IECSCYL-IBSAL), Unidad de Investigación, Hospital Universitario de Salamanca, Salamanca, Spain, **2** Departamento de Fisiología y Farmacología, Universidad de Salamanca, Salamanca, Spain, **3** Instituto Reina Sofía de Investigación Nefrológica, Fundación Iñigo Álvarez de Toledo, Madrid, Spain, **4** Bio-inRen, S.L., Salamanca, Spain

Abstract

Background: Hypertension and diabetes are the two leading causes of chronic kidney disease (CKD) eventually leading to end stage renal disease (ESRD) and the need of renal replacement therapy. Mortality among CKD and ESRD patients is high, mostly due to cardiovascular events. New early markers of risk are necessary to better anticipate the course of the disease, to detect the renal affection of additive risk factors, and to appropriately handle patients in a pre-emptive and personalized manner.

Methods: Renal function and NGAL urinary excretion was monitored in rats with spontaneous (SHR) or L-NAME induced hypertension rendered hyperglycemic (or not as controls).

Results: Combination of hypertension and hyperglycemia (but not each of these factors independently) causes an increased urinary excretion of neutrophil gelatinase-associated lipocalin (NGAL) in the rat, in the absence of signs of renal damage. Increased NGAL excretion is observed in diabetic animals with two independent models of hypertension. Elevated urinary NGAL results from a specific alteration in its tubular handling, rather than from an increase in its renal expression. In fact, when kidneys of hyperglycaemic-hypertensive rats are perfused *in situ* with Krebs-dextran solution containing exogenous NGAL, they excrete more NGAL in the urine than hypertensive rats. We also show that albuminuria is not capable of detecting the additive effect posed by the coexistence of these two risk factors.

Conclusions: Our results suggest that accumulation of hypertension and hyperglycemia induces an incipient and quite specific alteration in the tubular handling of NGAL resulting in its increased urinary excretion.

Editor: Nick Ashton, The University of Manchester, United Kingdom

Funding: This work was supported by grants from the Junta de Castilla y León (Consejería de Educación, HUS02B06; Consejería de Sanidad, GRS80/A/06; and Excellence Group, GR-100), Spain; Instituto de Salud Carlos III (FIS, PI081900, PI11/02278, PS0901067; and RETIC 06/0016, RedinRen), Madrid, Spain; and Fundación Renal Íñigo Álvarez de Toledo, Madrid, Spain. AMB-M and OG-S were recipients of a fellowship from the Instituto de Salud Carlos III, Madrid, Spain. The funders had no role in study design, data collection and analysis, decision to publish, or preparation of the manuscript.

Competing Interests: JMLN and FJLH are minority share-holders of Bio-inRen, S.L., a biotechnology company in the field of diagnostic of renal diseases.

* Email: flopezher@usal.es

Introduction

Hypertension and diabetes are known to eventually damage target organs including the heart, blood vessels and the kidneys. Hypertension and diabetes often lead to a progressive and irreversible loss of kidney function known as chronic kidney disease (CKD). Hypertensive and diabetic CKD take place during months or years, finally leading to end-stage renal disease (ESRD) [1,2], characterized by renal failure and the absolute need of renal replacement therapy (RRT), in the form of renal transplant or dialysis [1,3]. Diabetes and hypertension are the world leading causes of ESRD [4]. The presence of an increasing number of comorbid conditions increases in turn the risk of cardiovascular episodes or of inception and progression of chronic diseases. However, the additive effect of comorbidities on risk statement is hitherto bereft of quantitative markers, which might be useful for stratifying patients pre-emptively according to their individual risk.

Controlling hypertension and hyperglycemia is the most effective strategy to minimize hypertensive and diabetic nephropathies. However, effective treatments are missing for halting CKD progression and reversing the accumulated injury. The most effective drugs available (most prominently, inhibitors of the renin-angiotensin system) are only capable of slowing down renal disease progression [5,6]. Still, they are useful for preventing the need of RRT during the patient's lifetime, in some cases; or for postponing RRT installation and thus reducing the time during which it is applied. This has an enormous health and socioeconomic repercussion, because of the impairment in life quality and the high and disproportionate cost derived from dialysis, which consumes about 2% of the total health expenditure, whereas it is applied to 0.1% of the population [7–10]. Consequently, a critical aspect of CKD handling, both from the sanitary and the economic points of view, is the effective and early diagnosis. Traditionally, CKD diagnosis has been mostly performed through the detection of signs of renal dysfunction, most prominently of glomerular filtration estimated from the plasma creatinine concentration. However, the equivalent of over 60% of the renal mass is voided by the time renal dysfunction symptoms appear. For this reason, the discovery of earlier markers poses an urgent challenge in order to enhance therapeutic efficacy. The most developed of these new markers is the urinary excretion of albumin. Over excretion of small amounts of albumin (30–300 mg/day; termed microalbuminuria) is detected early in the course of diabetic and hypertensive nephropathy before other markers are evident [11]. Microalbuminuria is the result of subtle alterations in the sieving properties of the glomerular filtration barrier, in tubular reabsorption, or both. Accumulated clinical information has demonstrated that early microalbuminuria is a factor of progression and bad prognosis [11]. The level of circulating tumor necrosis factor (TNF) receptors has also been shown to predict renal function decline [12,13] and ESRD [13–15] in diabetic patients.

Another promising marker under development is urinary neutrophil gelatinase-associated lipocalin (NGAL). NGAL is normally found in the blood. However, its serum and urinary levels increase during inflammation, renal and cardiovascular diseases, certain types of cancer and other conditions [16]. Because of this, this molecule has gained attention in the last decade as a potential biomarker [17]. Indeed, urinary NGAL (uNGAL) has been developed most intensively as an early and sensitive marker of acute kidney injury [18]. It anticipates the course of disease earlier than conventional markers, such as serum creatinine, and has an enhanced prognostic value [19]. Urinary NGAL also correlates with the renal damage inflicted by cisplatin [20,21], cyclosporine [22] and with outcome after kidney allograft transplantation [23]; and it has been suggested as a potential marker of the transition from AKI to CKD [24]. Moreover, serum and urinary NGAL have been shown to correlate with different chronic renal diseases of glomerular and tubular origin [16,25,26], including diabetic nephropathy in mice [27] and humans [28], and hypertensive nephropathy [29]. In this study, we attempted to study the utility of the evolution of uNGAL to detect and monitor potential additive effects of the comorbid factors hypertension and diabetes in the rat.

Methods

All reagents were purchased from Sigma (Madrid, Spain), except where otherwise indicated.

Animals and experimental protocol

Male Wistar (Animal Experimentation Service of the University of Salamanca, Salamanca, Spain) and SHR rats (Charles River, Barcelona, Spain) weighing 200–250 g were used. Rats were treated in accordance with the Declaration of Helsinki Principles on the Advice on Care and Use of Animals referred to in: law 14\/2 007 (3 July) on Biomedical Research, Conseil de l'Europe (published in Official Daily N. L358/1-358/6, 18-12-1986), Government Spanish (Royal Decree 223/1 988, (14 March) and Order of 13-10-1989, and Official Bulletin of the State b. 256, pp. 31349–31362, 28-10-1990). The procedure was approved by the Bioethics Committee of the University of Salamanca. Animals were treated with care through the experiments. Except when allocated in metabolic cages for short periods of time (2–3 days), rats were housed 6 per cage under controlled environmental conditions with regulated light/darkness cycles in the University of Salamanca Experimental Animal Service. Rats were fed ad libitum with regular chow and they had free access to water. All surgical procedures were performed under inhalational anaesthesia with 3% isoflurane (2-chloro-2-(difluoromethoxy)-1,1,1-trifluoro-ethane; Schering Plough, Madrid), in 1 L/min oxygen flow. A single dose of buprenorphine (0.01 mg/kg) was administered before awakening to minimize post-surgical pain. Humane policy was implemented, although it was rarely necessary in our experiments. Rats showing evident behavioural signs of illness, pain or distress at any time, including reduced movement, abnormal resting postures, voluntary starvation, ruffled hair, etc. were immediately euthanized with CO_2.

Rats were rendered diabetic (or not, as controls) with a single injection of streptozotocin (60 mg/kg body weight), and monitored during 3 months. A subset of control and diabetic Wistar rats was treated with L-nitro-arginine methyl ester (L-NAME; 40 mg/kg/day in the drinking water for 7 weeks), starting one week after streptozotocin injection, as a second model of hypertension (combined or not with diabetes). Blood pressure was monitored in conscious animals by the tail cuff method (Cibertec, Madrid, Spain). For glycemic control, diabetic rats were injected daily with the necessary dose of insulin to keep glycemia at about 400 mg/dL. Glycemia was measured weekly with commercial reactive strips (Bayer, Leverkusen, Germany) in a drop of blood from the tail. At different time points, rats were allocated in individual metabolic cages for 24-hour urine sample collection. Urine was cleared by centrifugation, and it was stored at −80°C until use. At different time points after streptozotocin injection, rats were anaesthetized, and the kidneys were perfused by the aorta with heparinised saline solution (0.9% NaCl) and immediately dissected. Animals were killed by exsanguination under anaesthesia. One kidney was frozen in liquid nitrogen and subsequently kept at −80°C for Western blot studies. The other one was fixed in buffered 3.7% p-formaldehyde for histological studies. Blood samples were also obtained in heparinized capillaries at different time points by a small incision in the tail tip. Blood was centrifuged and serum was kept at −80°C until use.

Histological studies

Paraffin blocks were made with fixed kidneys and 5-μm tissue sections were stained with Masson's trichrome for the evaluation of fibrosis. Photographs were taken under an Olympus BX51 microscope connected to an Olympus DP70 colour, digital camera (Olympus, Tokyo, Japan).

Biochemical measurements

Serum and urinary creatinine (Cr_s and Cr_u respectively) and blood urea concentration were measured by means of the automated analyzer Reflotron (Roche Diagnostics, Barcelona, Spain; lower detection limit of 0.5 mg/dL). Urine protein concentration was measured by the Bradford method [30]. Urine NAG content was determined by a colorimetric method with a commercial kit (Roche Diagnostics, Barcelona, Spain) based on the conversion of 3-cresolsulfonphthaleinyl-N-acetyl-β-D-glucosaminide into the purple 3-cresol-cresolsulfonphthaleinyl. Albuminuria was measured with a commercial ELISA following the manufacturer's instructions (Bethyl Laboratories, Montgomery, TX, USA).

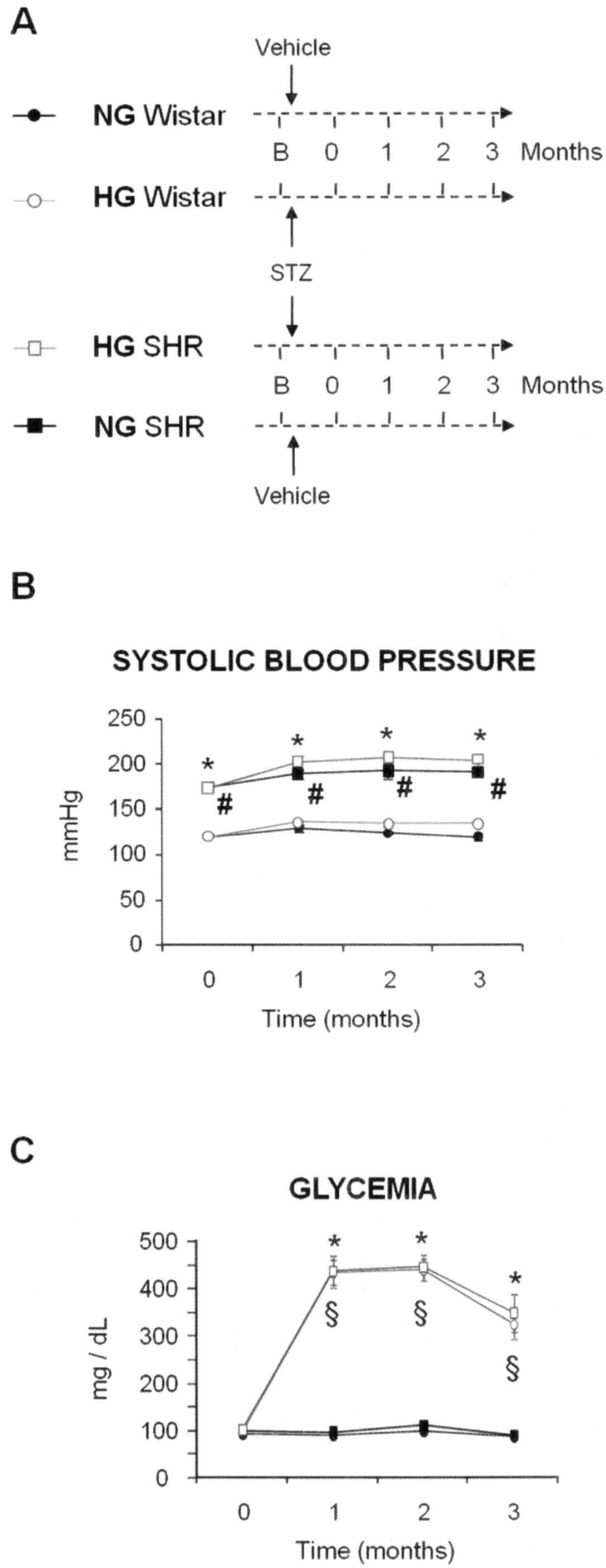
A
Vehicle
NG Wistar
B 0 1 2 3 Months
HG Wistar
STZ
HG SHR
B 0 1 2 3 Months
NG SHR
Vehicle
B
SYSTOLIC BLOOD PRESSURE
250
200
150
100
50
0
mmHg
0 1 2 3
Time (months)
C
GLYCEMIA
500
400
300
200
100
0
mg / dL
0 1 2 3
Time (months)

Figure 1. Experimental model, blood pressure and glycemia. Evolution of systolic blood pressure (B; n = 10–12 per group), glycemia (C; n = 10–12 per group), during 3 months in normoglycemic (NG) and hyperglycemic (HG) Wistar and SHR rats. Panel A shows a schematic representation of the experimental model. Data represent the mean ± standard error. *p<0.01 vs. NG Wistar. #p<0.01 vs. HG Wistar. §p<0.01 vs. NG SHR.

Western blot

Western blots were run with (i) urine samples (a volume of urine from each animal corresponding to the same excretion fraction, up to 24 µL of urine; or 21 µL per sample in kidney perfusion experiments), (ii) tissue extracts (100 µg total protein per sample) prepared by homogenizing the kidneys with a tissue mixer (Ultra-Turrax T8, IKA-Werwe) at 4°C in homogenization buffer (140 mM NaCl, 20 mM Tris-HCl pH = 7.5, 0.5 M ethylenediaminetetraacetic acid -EDTA-, 10% glycerol, 1% Igepal CA-630, 1 µg/mL aprotinin, 1 µg/mL leupeptin, 1 µg/mL pepstatin A, 1 mM phenylmethylsulphonyl fluoride -PMSF-), or (iii) albumin-free blood serum. Albumin was removed from serum with a column-based, commercial kit based on the immunological retention of rat albumin (Qproteome Murine Albumin Depletion Kit, Quiagen). Samples were separated by electrophoresis in 10–15% acrylamide gels (Mini Protean II system, BioRad, Madrid, Spain). Immediately, proteins were electrically transferred to an Immobilon-P membrane (Millipore, Madrid, Spain). Membranes were probed with antibodies against NGAL (MBL, Woburn, MA, USA) and albumin (Abcam, Cambridge, UK). An anti-GM2AP polyclonal antibody was produced and used as described [31]. A control peptide for NGAL (MBL, Woburn, MA, USA) was also used in some experiments to ascertain the specificity of the NGAL signal, according to the manufacturer's instructions.

Gene expression analysis. RT-PCR-amplification of NGAL and GAPDH was performed on mRNA samples obtained from kidney tissue with the next primers: for rat NGAL, 5′-TCTGGGCCTAAGGATAACAAC-3′ and 5′-AGACAGGTGGGACCTGAACCA-3′; for rat GAPDH, 5′-TGAAGGTCGGTGTGAACGGATTTGGC-3′ and 5′-CATGTAGGCCATGAGGTCCACCAC-3′. PCR conditions were: 1×(95°C×5 min); n×(95°C×1 min+T_m×1 min+72°C×1 min); 1×(72°C×5 min); where n was 35 for NGAL and 30 for GAPDH, and T_m was 64°C for NGAL, and 55.9°C for GAPDH.

Excretion studies with *in situ* perfused kidneys. At the end of the treatment, some hyperglycaemic SHR rats were anesthetized and an extracorporeal circuit for kidney perfusion was set up, as described elsewhere [32], with some modifications. Briefly, the renal artery, vein and ureter of the right kidney were ligated. The renal artery and vein of the left kidney and the urinary bladder were cannulated. Oxygenated and warm (37°C) Krebs-dextran [40 g/L of dextran (molecular weight 64 K–76 K) in Krebs solution (118.3 mM NaCl, 4.7 mM KCl, 1.8 mM $CaCl_2$, 1.2 mM $MgSO_4$, 1.2 mM KH_2PO_4, 25 mM $NaHCO_3$, 0.026 mM EDTA, 11.1 glucose, pH = 7.4)] was perfused through the renal artery at 3 mL/min, and was discarded through the renal vein. Urine fractions were collected from a catheter placed in the urinary bladder, starting before the perfusion with Krebs (when blood was still passing through the kidney), and during 2 hours after perfusion with Krebs started. In addition, similar experiments were carried out in hyperglycaemic and normoglycemic SHR, in which an excess of rat NGAL (42 ng/mL; Adipogen, San Diego, CA, USA) was added to the Krebs-dextran solution. As a control of these perfusion experiments, in order to discard a potential artefact derived from surgery or other experimental manoeuvres that would impede NGAL urinary excretion, kidneys were also perfused *in situ* with blood from the carotid artery. For this purpose, the artery, vein and ureter of the left kidney were ligated as above. A catheter was placed in the right carotid artery and connected directly to the renal artery. Urine was collected as above.

In a separate set of experiments, kidney perfusion experiments were carried in normoglycemic Wistar rats. Urine samples were collected from the urinary bladder before and after a bolus injection of sodium maleate (400 mg/kg) or saline (as control) was administered through a catheter placed into the right jugular vein. Sodium maleate was used to block megalin-mediated proximal tubule reabsorption [33,34]. All urine samples were kept at −80°C until further assayed.

Statistical analysis

Data are represented as the mean ± standard error of n experiments performed, as indicated in each case. Statistical comparisons were assessed by the one-way ANOVA analysis followed by the post hoc Tukey's test for multi-group comparisons, and the Student's t test for comparison between two groups. A $p<0.05$ was considered statistically significant.

Results

Evolution of blood pressure, glycemia and renal function in SHR and Wistar, normo and hyperglycemic rats

Blood pressure was significantly higher in SHR than in Wistar through the study. However, no differences in BP were seen between normoglycemic and hyperglycemic rats, either from the SHR or the Wistar strain (figure 1-B). Hyperglycemia was induced in a subset of SHR and Wistar by an injection of streptozotocin (STZ). Glycemia was higher in STZ-treated rats than in controls of either strain, and hyperglycemia was very similar in SHR and Wistar rats (figure 1-C). No renal dysfunction was observed in any of the experimental groups through the study, as evidenced by similar values of plasma creatinine, plasma urea, proteinuria (table 1). Microalbuminuria (figure 2) and N-acetylglucosaminidase (NAG) excretion (figure 2) were higher in hyperglycemic SHR and Wistar rats, compared with their corresponding normoglycemic controls. Microalbuminuria and NAG excretion partly correlated with the profile of urinary output (figure 2), which suggests that a part of their excretion might be due to a wash-out effect rather than to renal injury, as described for other proteins [35]. In any case, no further tubular alteration (if any) was induced by the concomitant presence of hypertension and hyperglycemia. Furthermore, microalbuminuria, NAG and sodium excretion did not correlate with the coexistence of these two risk factors, but merely (if at all) with direct or indirect tubular alterations, adaptations or effects caused exclusively by hyperglycemia. No renal tissue injury was evident on the histological study of renal tissue sections (figure 3). Masson's trichrome staining reveals no signs of fibrosis in any of the experimental conditions, compared to the normal kidney (i.e. in the control group). Furthermore, no gross structural alterations are induced by hyperglycemia, hypertension or the combination of both at this experimental time. Renal corpuscles and tubuli show normal appearance.

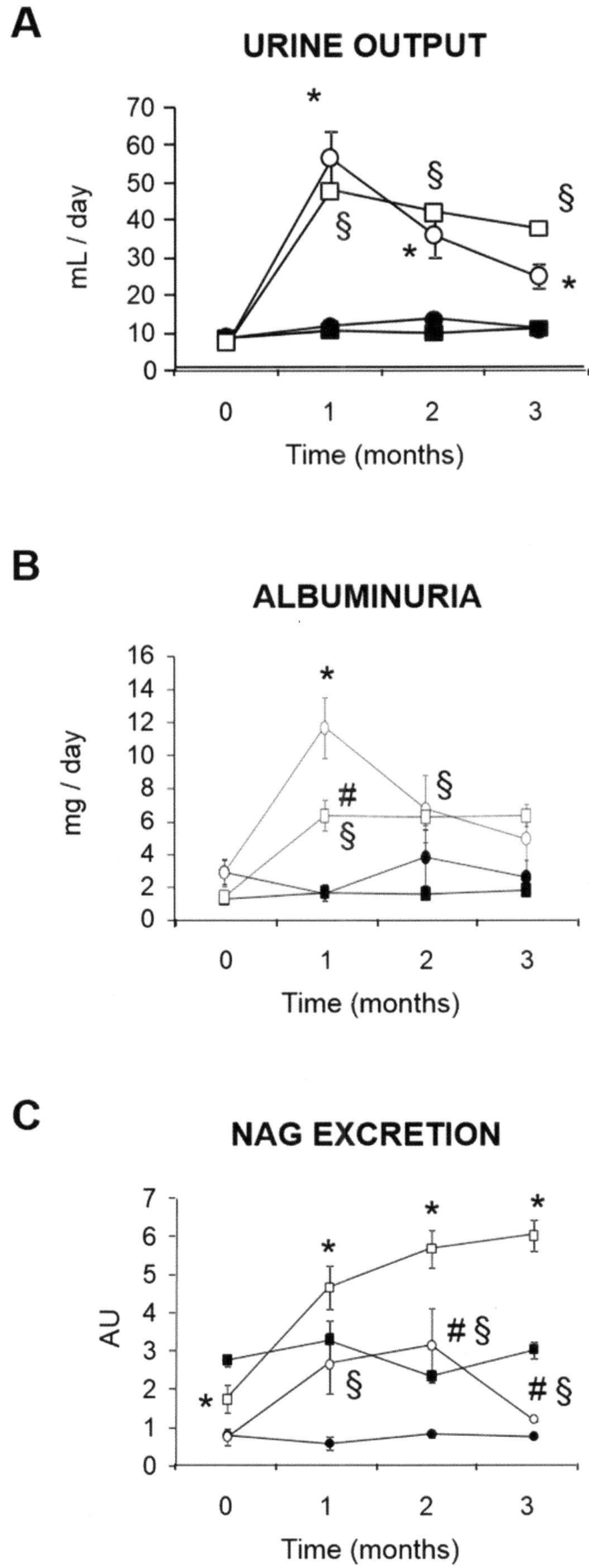
A
URINE OUTPUT
mL / day
70
60
50
40
30
20
10
0
0
1
2
3
Time (months)
*
§
B
ALBUMINURIA
mg / day
16
14
12
10
8
6
4
2
0
Time (months)
#
C
NAG EXCRETION
AU
7
6
5
4
Time (months)

Figure 2. Urinary biochemistry of renal function. Urine output (A; n = 10–12 per group), albuminuria (B; n = 4–6 per group), and NAG excretion (C; n = 4–5 per group) during 3 months in normoglycemic (NG) and hyperglycemic (HG) Wistar and SHR rats. Data represent the mean ± standard error. *p<0.01 vs. NG Wistar. #p<0.01 vs. HG Wistar. §p<0.01 vs. NG SHR.

NGAL urinary excretion is increased in spontaneously hypertensive-diabetic rats

Urinary NGAL excretion, a marker associated to a number of pathological circumstances including early diabetic nephropathy, was not modified by either hypertension or hyperglycemia alone in our experimental setting. However, it increased significantly in rats suffering concomitantly of hypertension (SHR rats) and hyperglycemia (figure 4). Urinary NGAL excretion increased from the first month of hyperglycemia in SHR, and stayed high during the rest of the study.

NGAL urinary excretion is also increased L-NAME-induced hypertensive-diabetic rats

In order to verify that the increased urinary excretion of NGAL was the consequence of the combined effect of hypertension and hyperglycemia, and not of a particular characteristic of the SHR strain when rendered hyperglycaemic, we also studied the effect of hyperglycemia on the excretion of this marker in a model of induced hypertension. For this purpose, we induced hypertension in Wistar rats by chronic treatment with the NO synthase inhibitor L-NAME. As shown in figure 5-D, L-NAME-treated rats became rapidly hypertensive. Hyperglycemia was also induced in a subset of animals, which was maintained at values of blood glucose concentration similar to those in SHR (figure 5-E). Renal function was not impaired in L-NAME-hypertensive and L-NAME-hypertensive-hyperglycemic rats, as indicated by the evolution of plasma creatinine concentration and proteinuria (figure 5-C and 5-G, respectively). Urine output increased in hyperglycemic rats (figure 5-F), probably as a consequence of hyperglycemia. In this setting, NGAL was not increased in the urine in the L-NAME-induced hypertension model. However, when L-NAME treated rats were also rendered hyperglycemic, NGAL appeared in the urine after 7 weeks of hypertension (figure 5-B). This indicates that chronic coexistence of both factors is necessary to induce a synergistic increase in NGAL urinary excretion.

Increased urinary NGAL results from its altered tubular handling

We also aimed at unraveling the origin of the increased urinary NGAL. Figure 6-A shows that the renal tissue NGAL level is not increased in NGAL-excreting rats, that is, in hypertensive-hyperglycemic rats. The reactive band appears a little lower than the typical 25 kDa band found in the urine by us and other authors [36], as shown in the positive control (C+). This could mean that the observed band might not correspond to NGAL. In any case, no

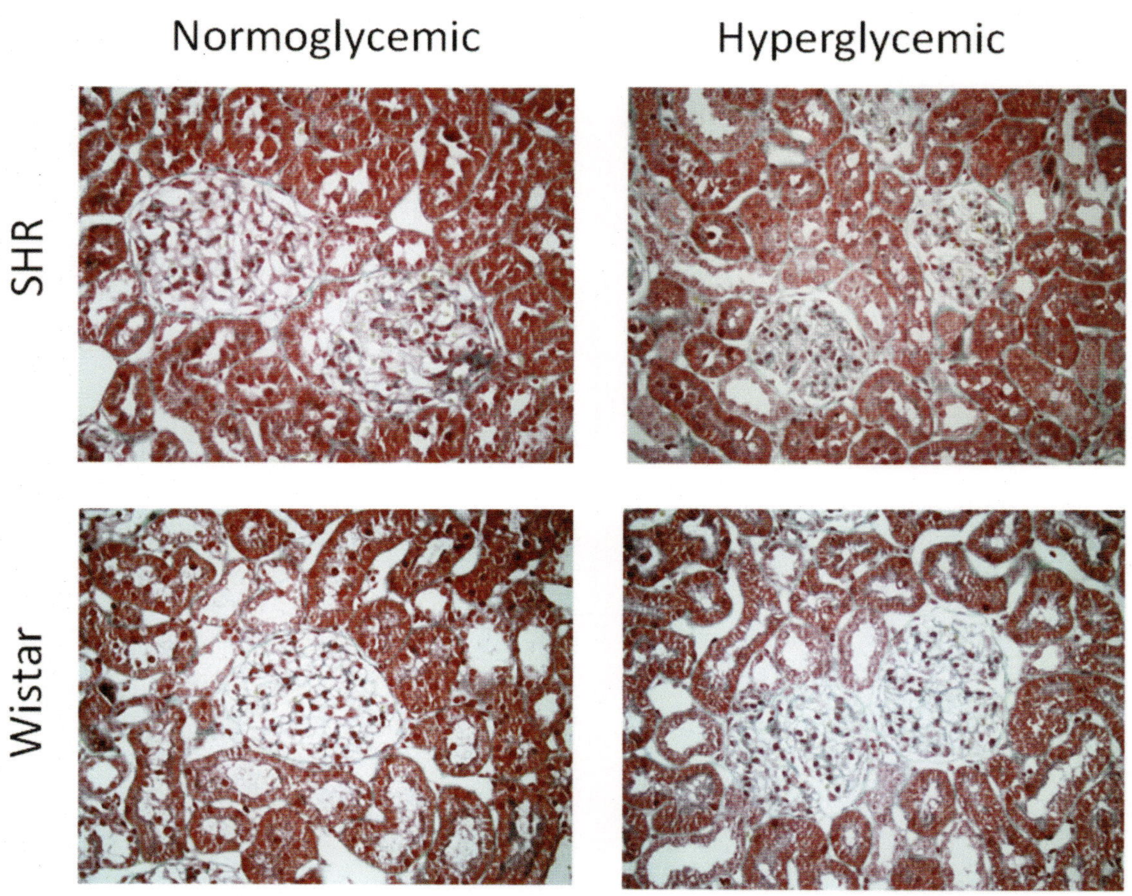

Figure 3. Histological study. Representative images of renal tissue sections stained with Masson's trichrome 3 months after the inception of hyperglycemia (or not, as control) in Wistar and SHR rats. n = 4 animals per group.

Table 1. Evolution of plasma creatinine and urea concentration, and urinary protein excretion during 3 months in normoglycemic (NG) and hyperglycemic (HG) Wistar and SHR rats.

Group	Time (months)	Plasma Creatinine (mg/dL)	Plasma Urea (mg/dL)	Urinary Protein Excretion (mg/day)
NG Wistar	0	<0.5	N.D.	10.4±2.9
	1	<0.5	N.D.	12.9±2.4
	2	<0.5	N.D.	20.1±1.8
	3	<0.5	N.D.	17.9±2.8
HG Wistar	0	<0.5	N.D.	9.5±1.7
	1	<0.5	N.D.	28.2±3.5
	2	<0.5	N.D.	31.2±4.0
	3	<0.5	N.D.	26.5±4.5
NG SHR	0	<0.5	42.8±3.9	25.1±2.1
	1	<0.5	45.4±2.5	20.3±2.6
	2	<0.5	40.4±2.0	15.6±1.9
	3	<0.5	41.1±2.2	14.7±1.5
HG SHR	0	<0.5	37.4±3.5	25.0±1.4
	1	<0.5	62.8±5.5	17.9±4.3
	2	<0.5	54.9±7.2	38.7±3.0
	3	<0.5	49.9±3.2	35.9±4.9

Data represent the mean ± standard error of n = 6 animals per condition. N.D., not determined.

increased expression of NGAL in the renal tissue seems to be able to explain the increased urinary excretion. Moreover, gene expression analysis by RT-PCR showed that neither hypertension or diabetes, nor the combination of both modified the expression of NGAL in renal tissue (figure 6-B). As such, the only other possible source of the urinary NGAL is the blood irrigating the kidneys, which is partially filtered through the glomerular filtration barrier. In fact, when the kidney of hypertensive-hyperglycemic rats is perfused with Krebs

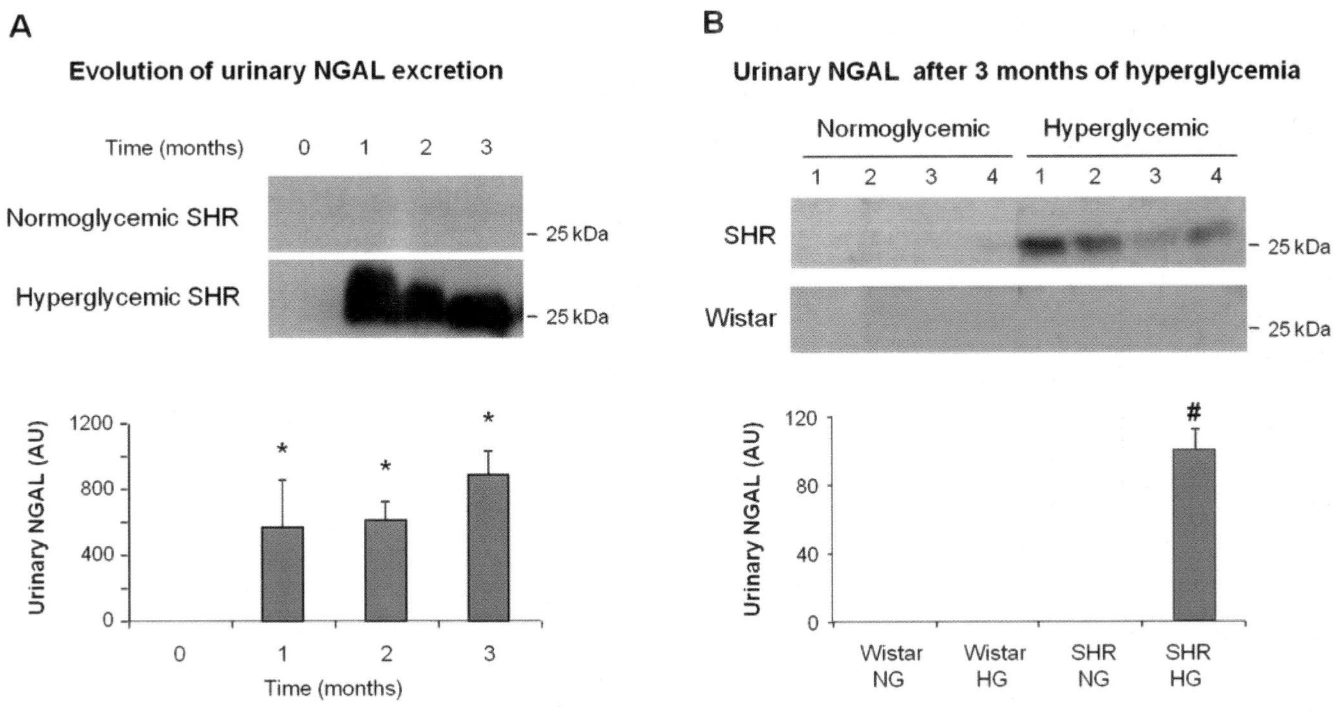

Figure 4. Effect of hyperglycemia and genetic hypertension on NGAL urinary levels. Evolution of NGAL urinary excretion during 3 months (A; n = 3 per group), and level of urinary NGAL after 3 months in different animals per group (B; n = 4 per group), determined by western blot in the urine of normoglycemic (NG) and hyperglycemic (HG) Wistar and SHR rats. Data represent the mean ± standard error. *p<0.01 vs. time 0. #p<0.01 vs. NG Wistar, HG Wistar and NG SHR.

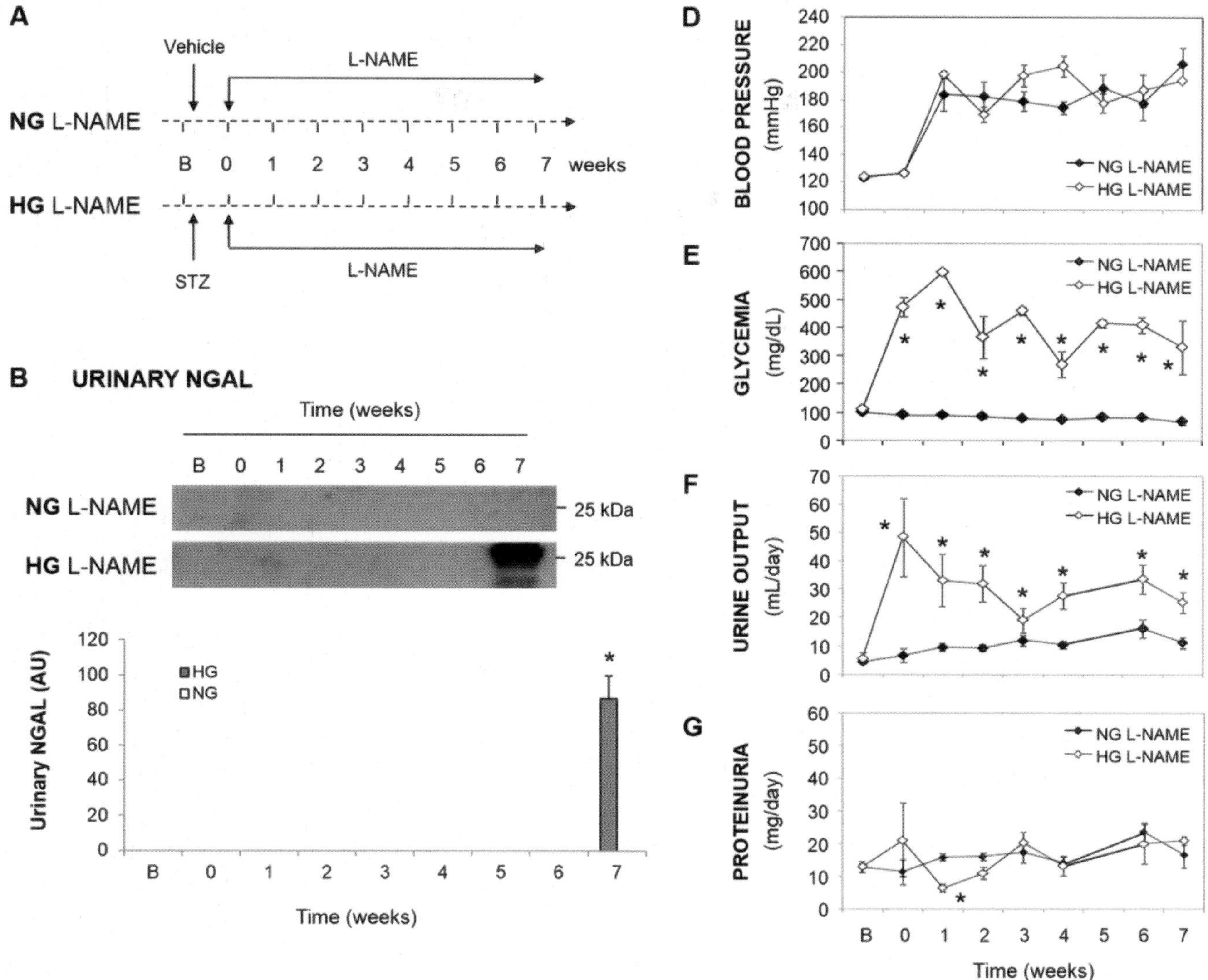

C **PLASMA CREATININE (mg/dL)**

	Time (weeks)			
	B	2	4	7
NG L-NAME	≤ 0.5	≤ 0.5	≤ 0.5	≤ 0.5
HG L-NAME	≤ 0.5	≤ 0.5	≤ 0.5	≤ 0.5

Figure 5. Effect of hyperglycemia and L-NAME-induced hypertension on NGAL urinary levels. Evolution of NGAL urinary excretion and its corresponding densitometric quantification (B; n = 4 per group), plasma creatinine concentration (C; n = 4–6 per group), systolic blood pressure (D; n = 8 per group), glycemia (E; n = 8 per group), urine output (F; n = 8 per group) and proteinuria (G; n = 8 per group) during 7 weeks in Wistar rats rendered hypertensive with L-NAME, in which hyperglycemia was induced in parallel (or not, as control). Panel A shows a schematic representation of the experimental model. Data represent the mean ± standard error. *p<0.001 vs. NG L-NAME. B, basal time point. HG, hyperglycemic. NG, normoglycemic.

solution (which does not contain proteins, but a high molecular weight dextran to compensate for the oncotic pressure of the blood), NGAL is not excreted with the urine any more (figure 7-A). This supports the idea that the NGAL observed in the urine of these rats comes from the blood and not from the renal tissue. Moreover, when exogenous rat NGAL was added to the Krebs solution perfusing the kidney, hypertensive-hyperglycemic rats excreted more NGAL in the urine than hypertensive (normoglycemic) rats (figure 7-B). This further indicates that the renal handling of NGAL is intrinsically altered in hypertensive-hyperglycemic rats. As a control of the perfusion experiments, in order to discard an experimental artifact due to the surgical procedure, when the kidneys of hypertensive-hyperglycemic rats were perfused with their own blood through a catheter connecting the carotid artery with the renal artery, NGAL still appeared in the urine (figure 7-C); whereas no NGAL was detected in these circumstances in the urine of hypertensive

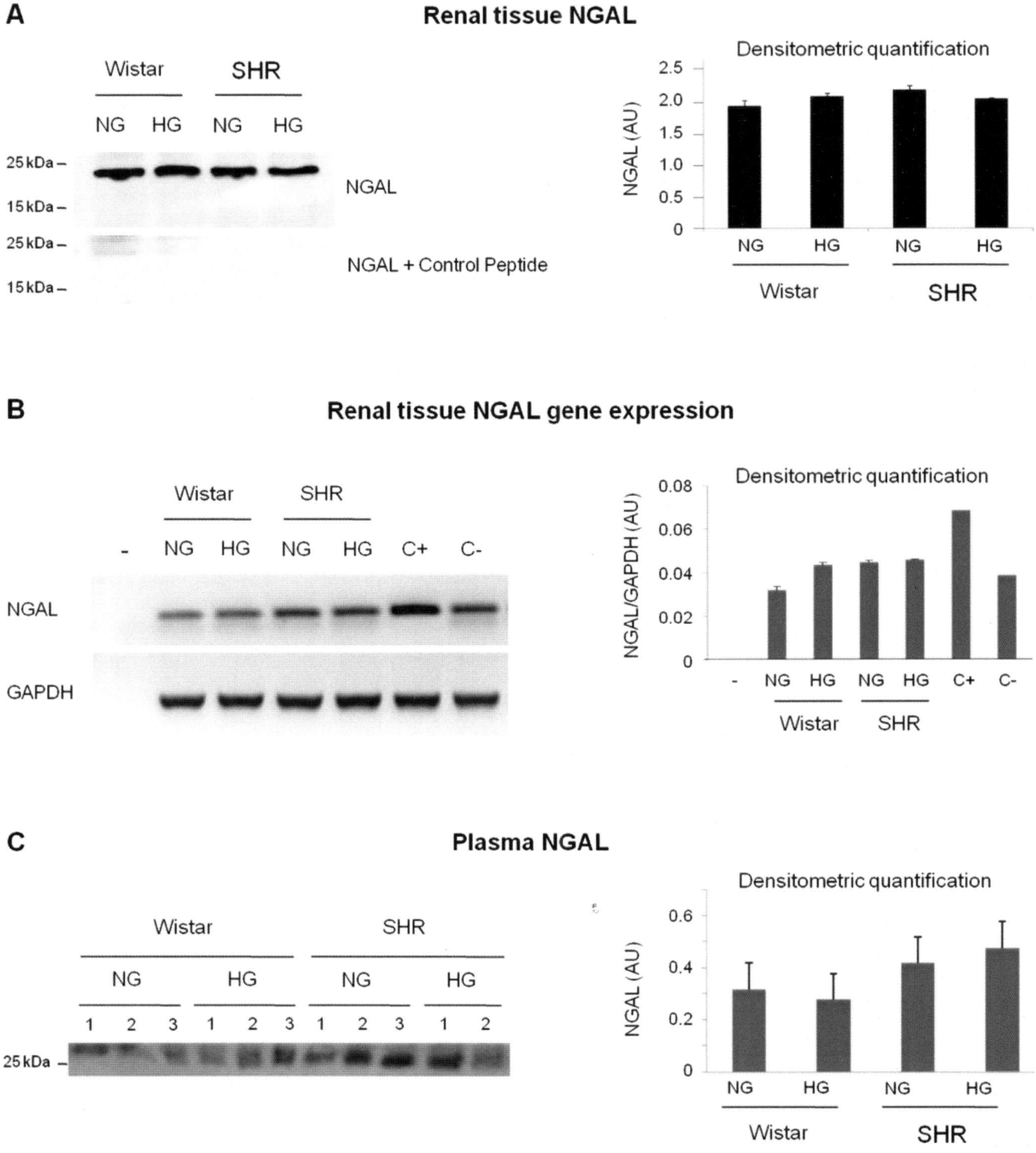

Figure 6. Renal and plasma NGAL are not modified by hyperglycemia and hypertension. Renal tissue NGAL protein levels (A; n = 4–5 per group), renal NGAL gene expression analysis (B; n = 3) and NGAL plasma level (C; n = 2–3 per group), in normoglycemic (NG) and hyperglycemic (HG) Wistar and SHR rats after 3 months of hyperglycemia. In each panel, representative images of Western blot are shown (left) along with the corresponding densitometric quantification (right). In panel B, the next symbols were used: −, H_2O was added in lieu of template DNA (as a PCR control); C+, a renal tissue sample from a ischemia/reperfusion-injured Wistar rat kidney (as a positive control of increased NAGL expression); C−, a renal tissue sample from a sham-operated Wistar rat (as a control for C+).

(normoglycemic) rats. Of note, this latter difference in NGAL excretion when kidneys are perfused in situ with Krebs-dextran containing NGAL is almost identical to the difference in NGAL excretion between hypertensive-hyperglycemic and hypertensive rats when blood perfuses the kidneys.

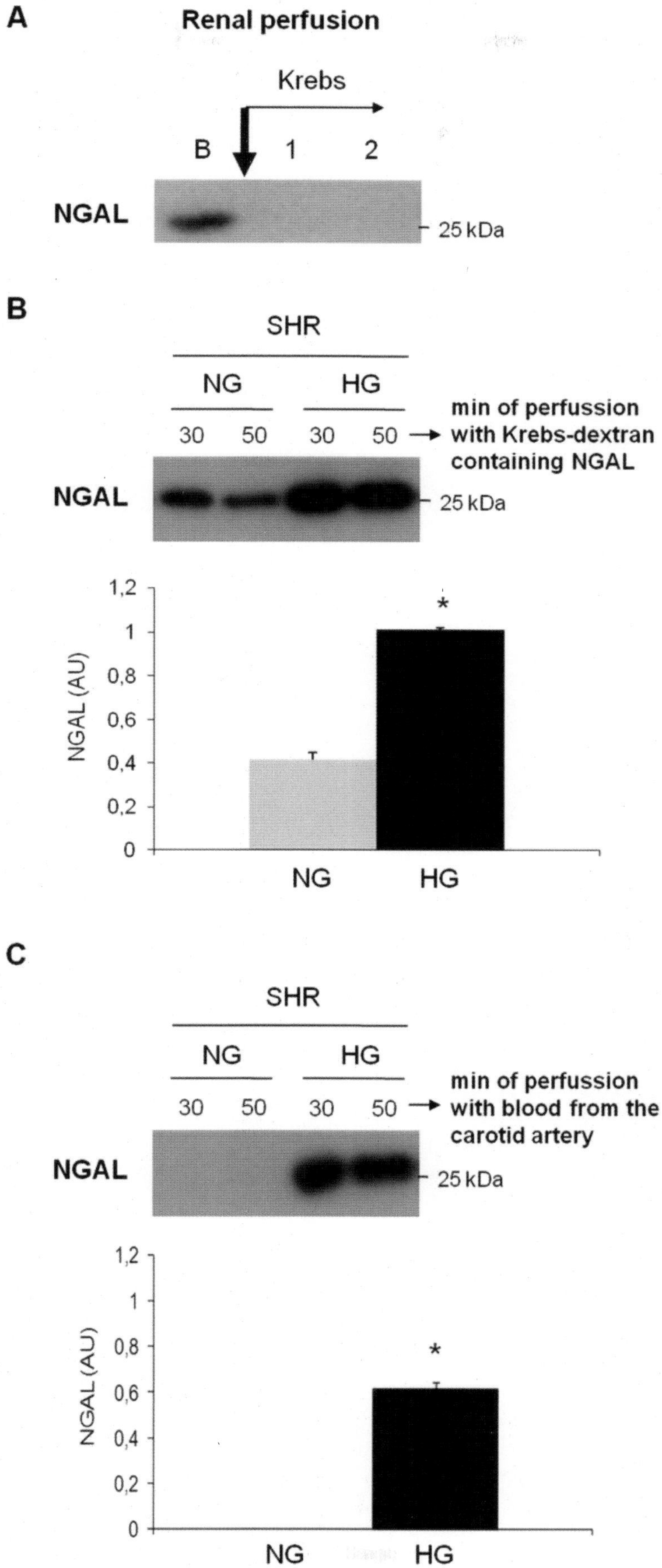
A
Renal perfusion
Krebs
B
1
2
NGAL
25 kDa
B
SHR
NG
HG
30
50
30
50
min of perfussion with Krebs-dextran containing NGAL
NGAL
25 kDa
NGAL (AU)
1,2
1
0,8
0,6
0,4
0,2
0
*
NG
HG
C
SHR
NG
HG
30
50
30
50
min of perfussion with blood from the carotid artery
NGAL
25 kDa
NGAL (AU)
1,2
1
0,8
0,6
0,4
0,2
0
*
NG
HG

Figure 7. Increased NGAL urinary excretion is due to a tubular handling alteration. A) Representative image of Western blot showing the effect of in situ perfusion of the renal vasculature with Krebs-dextran solution on NGAL urinary excretion in 3-month hyperglycemic SHR rats. B represents a basal urine sample before perfusing Krebs solution, when blood still perfuses the kidney. B) Representative image of Western blot showing the effect of adding an excess of NGAL to the Krebs-dextran solution on NGAL urinary excretion in 3-month normoglycemic (NG) and hyperglycemic SHR; and band quantification (lower graphic). C) Representative image of Western blot showing the effect of renal perfusion with the animal's own blood from the carotid artery on NGAL urinary excretion in 3-month normoglycemic (NG) and hyperglycemic SHR; and band quantification (lower graphic). Data represent the average ± standard error of n = 5 per group. *p<0.001 vs. normoglycemic (NG) SHR. AU, arbitrary units.

A potential cause of increased urinary excretion of NGAL would be its increased concentration in the blood, which we examined by western blot. We found no increment in NGAL plasma concentration in hyperglycemic SHR that could explain its increased urinary excretion (figure 6-C). Because low molecular weight proteins (such as NGAL) freely filtrate through the glomerular filtration barrier, the enhanced urinary excretion must be the consequence of altered tubular handling (i.e. reabsorption). *In vivo* inhibition of proximal tubule, megalin/cubilin-driven endocytosis with maleate produced only a brief and transient increase in urinary NGAL, while causing a more sustained excretion of albumin and ganglioside M2 activator protein (figure 8). This indicates that although the megalin/cubilin complex reabsorbs NGAL, other re-uptake mechanisms exist that redundantly participate in NGAL reabsorption.

Discussion

Diabetes and hypertension frequently coexist, and their combination provides additive risk of chronic nephropathy, cardiovascular events and death [37–39]. As an example, diabetes is responsible for 36.8% of diagnosed cases of chronic kidney disease (CKD) in the USA [40]. It is thought that up to 15–30% of type 1 diabetic patients and 20–40% of type 2 will develop renal problems in the evolutionary course of diabetes [1]. Diabetes is the leading cause of ESRD; near 50% of ESRD patients are diabetic. Hypertension is the second leading cause of ESRD. About 51–63% of all patients with CKD are hypertensive. This number grows to 90% in patients over 65 years. In the corresponding general population the incidence of hypertension is 11–13% and 50%, respectively [1]. In this article, we propose uNGAL as a prospective marker of the additive risk of CKD posed by the combination of hypertension and diabetes.

NGAL is a 25 kDa protein of the lipocalin superfamily. This superfamily comprises proteins formed by 8 β-strands composing a β-barrel and enclosing a calyx, which binds and transports low-molecular-weight molecules [41]. In turn, NGAL binds and is transported by cell membrane transporters, such as the megalin-cubilin complex and 24p3 receptor [42]. It is expressed by different epithelia (including renal tubuli) in physiological and pathological circumstances [16,43]. A relation has been proposed between inflammation and NGAL expression in neutrophils and epithelial cells [44]. In agreement, NGAL has been shown to be involved in the repair of ischemic renal tubular epithelium [36]. Indeed, treatment with exogenous NGAL ameliorates the kidney injury caused by ischemia-reperfusion [45]. This effect is thought to be mediated, at least in part, by favouring epithelial cell dedifferentiation, proliferation and, thus, repair. Strikingly though, NGAL-deficient mice are significantly protected against the chronic renal damage induced by 75% nephrectomy [46]. Interestingly, NGAL over-expression in these mice was mediated by hypoxia-inducible factor 1α (HIF-1α). It can be hypothesized that NGAL is expressed as a mediator of an inflammatory response, initially unleashed as a repair response. In such case, NGAL might act as a repair mediator. However, a persistent inflammatory response has been shown to be detrimental for the acute and chronic kidney repair (reviewed in 1 and 2). In those circumstances, NGAL might turn prejudicial overall. Moreover, NGAL has been proposed as a real-time indicator of the progression of chronic renal damage. NGAL also plays a role in the pathogenesis and clinical manifestations of atherosclerosis, acute myocardial infarction and heart failure. It has also been proposed as a potential link between the kidney and the cardiovascular system. In fact, cardiac, vascular and serum levels increase in a number of cardiovascular diseases [47], including those resulting from CKD.

Increasing serum and urinary NGAL correlate with decreasing glomerular filtration and with increasing renal parenchymal degeneration [26,48]. Under these circumstances, the accumulation of NGAL in the blood is related to the reduced filtration; and its increase in the urine is thought to be the consequence of its increased expression by damaged renal compartments, mostly the tubuli. However, the origin of increased uNGAL in our model is not the renal parenchyma, which is not damaged by the time NGAL is detected in the urine, nor increased gene expression or protein levels are detected in renal tissue homogenates from hypertensive and hyperglycaemic animals (figure 6). When the blood is substituted by a protein-free isotonic solution (Krebs), no NGAL is detected in the urine of these animals. Furthermore, when NGAL is added to the Krebs solution in *in situ* perfusion experiments, hypertensive-hyperglycemic kidneys excrete more NGAL in the urine than those in hypertensive rats. This indicates that uNGAL comes from the blood and that there is an intrinsic alteration in the tubular handling of this protein in hypertensive-hyperglycemic rats, most probably a defect in its tubular re-uptake.

Because of its small size, NGAL filters freely through the glomerular barrier. Under normal conditions, filtered NGAL is reabsorbed in the tubules with the concourse of the proximal tubule endocytic complex formed by megalin and cubilin [49]. In this sense, our experiments show that, although the megalin/cubilin complex participates in NGAL reabsorption, there are other redundant mechanisms capable of achieving full NGAL reuptake shortly after megalin/cubilin voidance, as demonstrated in figure 7. As such, the key alterations caused by sustained hypertension and hyperglycemia leading to NGAL urinary over-excretion must be looked for in tubular handling systems different from that of megalin/cubilin. This differs from the mechanism of microalbuminuria in early diabetic nephropathy, which is mainly due to reduced reabsorption through the megalin system. Indeed, both reduced megalin expression [50], and disruption of megalin-dependent reuptake [51] are thought to mediate microalbuminuria, although the precise mechanism is not fully understood. On the contrary, the mechanism underlying hypertensive microalbuminuria is mostly unknown.

Our results point at a potentially new and different utility of NGAL as a diagnostic (or even prognostic) marker in the course of CKD. NGAL appears in the urine upon the chronically synergistic action of hypertension and hyperglycemia, even in the absence of overt nephropathy. In our experimental model, this capability is not achieved by albuminuria, which more closely correlates with

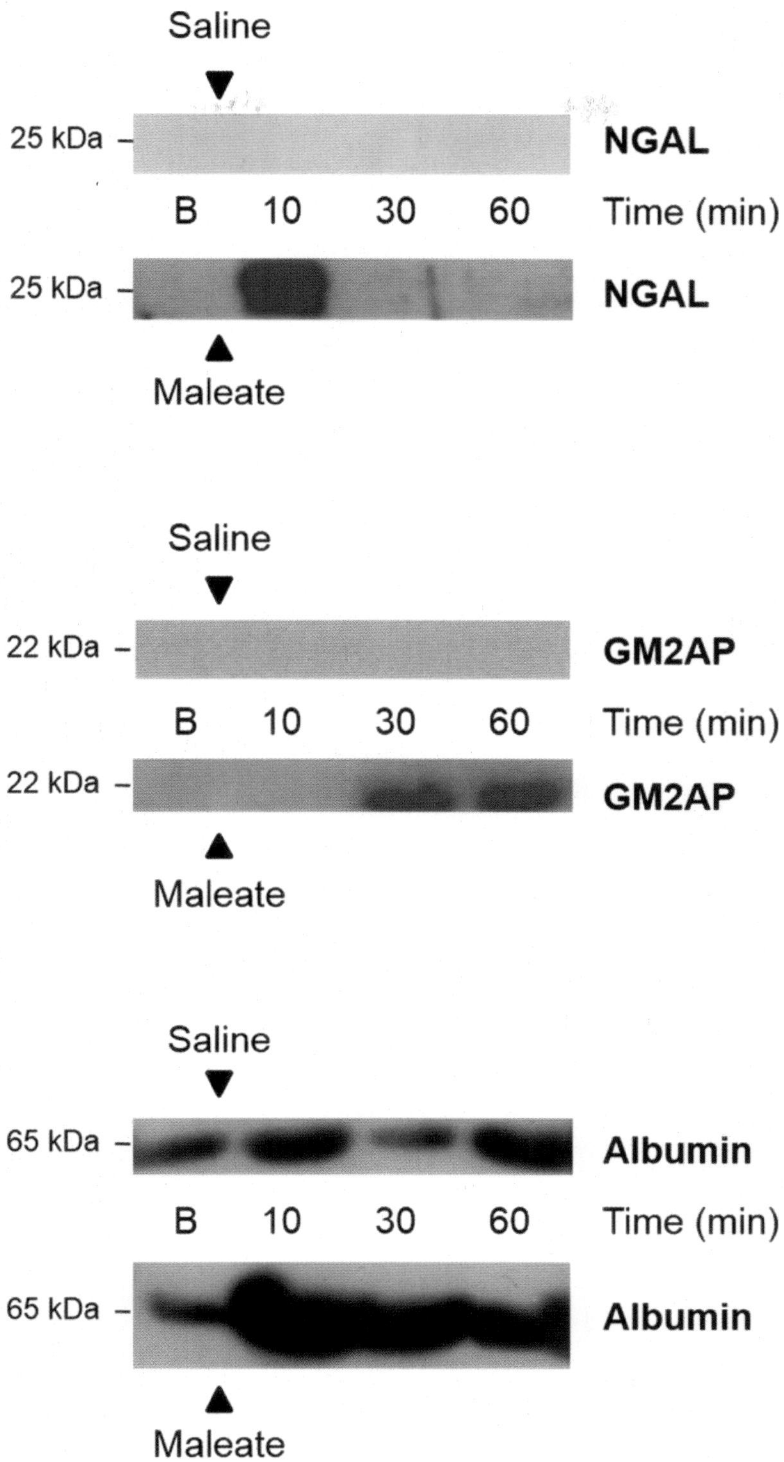

Figure 8. Effect of a single intravenous bolus of maleate (or saline as control) in the urinary excretion of NGAL, GM2AP and albumin during the following hour in normotensive-normoglycemic (Wistar) rats (n = 3 per group).

hyperglycemia and increased urine output than with the additive presence of both risk factors (namely hypertension and hyperglycemia). Both NGAL and albumin are increasingly excreted with the urine as a result of incipient and subtle alterations in their renal handling. However, NGAL might incorporate a new capacity to early detect and quantify the increased risk posed by the synergistic action of hypertension and diabetes; and, prospectively, also to monitor the evolution and prognosis of CKD patients.

Clinical studies are necessary to ascertain the capacity of uNGAL to stratify patients according to their prognosis and their individual risk of progression through CKD, in early stages where no other signs different from microalbuminuria are evident. In perspective, this pre-emptive and personalized stratification would enable us to transform qualitative risk factors (same status for all hypertensive-diabetic patients) into quantitative parameters that score how hypertension and diabetes affect patients in an individual basis with respect to their specific prognosis on CKD progression.

Author Contributions

Conceived and designed the experiments: CMS JMLN FJLH. Performed the experiments: AMBM OGS VBG YQ MJM CMS JMLN FJLH. Analyzed the data: AMBM OGS VBG YQ MJM CMS JMLN FJLH. Contributed to the writing of the manuscript: CMS JMLN FJLH.

References

1. Lopez-Novoa JM, Martinez-Salgado C, Rodriguez-Peña AB, López-Hernández FJ (2010) Common pathophysiological mechanisms of chronic kidney disease: therapeutic perspectives. Pharmacol Ther 128: 61–81.
2. Lopez-Novoa JM, Rodriguez-Peña AB, Ortiz A, Martinez-Salgado C, López Hernández FJ (2011) Etiopathology of chronic tubular, glomerular and renovascular nephropathies: Clinical implications. J Transl Med 9: 13.
3. De Zeeuw D, Hillege HL, de Jong PE (2005) The kidney, a cardiovascular risk marker, and a new target for therapy. Kidney Int Suppl (Suppl 98): S25–S29.
4. Atkins RC (2005) The epidemiology of chronic kidney disease. Kidney Int Suppl (94): S14–S18.
5. Remuzzi G, Benigni A, Remuzzi A (2006) Mechanisms of progression and regression of renal lesions of chronic nephropathies and diabetes. J Clin Invest 116: 288–296.
6. Carrero JJ, Stenvinkel P (2011) Predialysis chronic kidney disease in 2010: Novel targets for slowing CKD progression. Nat Rev Nephrol 7: 65–66.
7. Xue JL, Ma JZ, Louis TA, Collins AJ (2001) Forecast of the number of patients with end-stage renal disease in the United States to the year 2010. J Am Soc Nephrol 12: 2753−2758.
8. Winkelmayer WC, Weinstein MC, Mittleman MA, Glynn RJ, Pliskin JS (2002) Health economic evaluations: The special case of end stage renal disease treatment. Med Decis Mak 22: 417−430.
9. Szczech LA, Lazar IL (2004) Projecting the United States ESRD population: Issues regarding treatment of patients with ESRD. Kidney Int Suppl (90): S3−S7.
10. U.S. Renal Data System, USRDS (2009) 2009 Annual Data Report: Atlas of end-stage renal disease in the United States. Bethesda, MD: National Institutes of Health, National Institute of Diabetes and Digestive and Kidney Diseases http://www.usrds.org/2009/slides/indiv/INDEX_CKD.HTML.
11. Basi S, Fesler P, Mimran A, Lewis JB (2008) Microalbuminuria in type 2 diabetes and hypertension: a marker, treatment target, or innocent bystander? Diabetes Care (Suppl 2): S194–S201.
12. Gohda T, Niewczas MA, Ficociello LH, Walker WH, Skupien J, et al. (2012) Circulating TNF receptors 1 and 2 predict stage 3 CKD in type 1 diabetes. J Am Soc Nephrol 23: 516–524.
13. Gohda T, Tomino Y (2013) Novel biomarkers for the progression of diabetic nephropathy: soluble TNF receptors. Curr Diab Rep 13: 560–566.
14. Niewczas MA, Gohda T, Skupien J, Smiles AM, Walker WH, et al. (2012) Circulating TNF receptors 1 and 2 predict ESRD in type 2 diabetes. J Am Soc Nephrol 23: 507–515.
15. Izumi Y, Yabe D, Taniguchi A, Fukushima M, Nakai Y, et al. (2013) Circulating TNF receptor 2 is associated with the development of chronic kidney disease in non-obese Japanese patients with type 2 diabetes. Diabetes Res Clin Pract 99: 145–150.
16. Soni SS, Cruz D, Bobek I, Chionh CY, Nalesso F, et al. (2010) NGAL: a biomarker of acute kidney injury and other systemic conditions. Int Urol Nephrol 42: 141–150.
17. Vaidya VS, Ferguson MA, Bonventre JV (2008) Biomarkers of acute kidney injury. Annu Rev Pharmacol Toxicol 48: 463–493.
18. Devarajan P (2010) Neutrophil gelatinase-associated lipocalin: a promising biomarker for human acute kidney injury. Biomark Med 4: 265–280.
19. Devarajan P (2008) Neutrophil gelatinase-associated lipocalin (NGAL): a new marker of kidney disease. Scand J Clin Lab Invest Suppl 241: 89–94.
20. Mishra J, Mori K, Ma Q, Kelly C, Barasch J, et al. (2004) Neutrophil gelatinase-associated lipocalin: a novel early urinary biomarker for cisplatin nephrotoxicity. Am J Nephrol 24: 307–315.
21. Gaspari F, Cravedi P, Mandalà M, Perico N, de Leon FR, et al. (2010) Predicting Cisplatin-Induced Acute Kidney Injury by Urinary Neutrophil Gelatinase-Associated Lipocalin Excretion: A Pilot Prospective Case-Control Study. Nephron Clin Pract 115: c154–c160.
22. Wasilewska A, Zoch-Zwierz W, Taranta-Janusz K, Michaluk-Skutnik J (2010) Neutrophil gelatinase-associated lipocalin (NGAL): a new marker of cyclosporine nephrotoxicity? Pediatr Nephrol 25: 889–897.
23. Lebkowska U, Malyszko J, Lebkowska A, Koc-Zorawska E, Lebkowski W, et al. (2009) Neutrophil gelatinase-associated lipocalin and cystatin C could predict renal outcome in patients undergoing kidney allograft transplantation: a prospective study. Transplant Proc 41: 154–157.
24. Ko GJ, Grigoryev DN, Linfert D, Jang HR, Watkins T, et al. (2010) Transcriptional analysis of kidneys during repair from AKI reveals possible roles for NGAL and KIM-1 as biomarkers of AKI to CKD transition. Am J Physiol Renal Physiol 298: F1472–F1483.
25. Malyszko J, Bachorzewska-Gajewska H, Sitniewska E, Malyszko JS, Poniatowski B, et al. (2008) Serum neutrophil gelatinase-associated lipocalin as a marker of renal function in non-diabetic patients with stage 2–4 chronic kidney disease. Ren Fail 30: 625–628.
26. Chaudhary K, Phadke G, Nistala R, Weidmeyer CE, McFarlane SI, et al. (2010) The emerging role of biomarkers in diabetic and hypertensive chronic kidney disease. Curr Diab Rep 10: 37–42.
27. Kuwabara T, Mori K, Mukoyama M, Kasahara M, Yokoi H, et al. (2009) Urinary neutrophil gelatinase-associated lipocalin levels reflect damage to glomeruli, proximal tubules, and distal nephrons. Kidney Int 75: 285–294.
28. Bolignano D, Lacquaniti A, Coppolino G, Donato V, Fazio MR, et al. (2009) Neutrophil gelatinase-associated lipocalin as an early biomarker of nephropathy in diabetic patients. Kidney Blood Press Res 32: 91–98.
29. Malyszko J, Bachorzewska-Gajewska H, Malyszko JS, Pawlak K, Dobrzycki S (2008) Serum neutrophil gelatinase-associated lipocalin as a marker of renal function in hypertensive and normotensive patients with coronary artery disease. Nephrology (Carlton) 13: 153–156.
30. Bradford MM (1976) A rapid and sensitive method for the quantitation of microgram quantities of protein utilizing the principle of protein-dye binding. Anal Biochem 72: 248–254.
31. Quiros Y, Ferreira L, Sancho-Martínez SM, González-Buitrago JM, López-Novoa JM, et al. (2010) Sub-nephrotoxic doses of gentamicin predispose animals to developing acute kidney injury and to excrete ganglioside M2 activator protein. Kidney Int 78: 1006–1015.
32. López-Novoa JM, Santos JC, Villamediana LM, Garrote FJ, Thim L, et al. (1986) Renal catabolism of 125I-glicentin. Am J Physiol 250: E545–E550.
33. Bergeron M, Mayers P, Brown D (1996) Specific effect of maleate on an apical membrane glycoprotein (gp330) in proximal tubule of rat kidneys. Am J Physiol Renal Fluid Electrolyte Physiol 271: F908–F916.
34. Nagai J, Tanaka H, Nakanishi N, Murakami T, Takano M (2001) Role of megalin in renal handling of aminoglycosides. Am J Physiol Renal Physiol 281: F337–F344.
35. Martínez Seeber A, Vila SB, Catanzaro OL (1982) The mechanism of urinary kallikrein excretion in the rat. Clin Sci (Lond) 63: 217–218.
36. Mishra J, Ma Q, Prada A, Mitsnefes M, Zahedi K, et al. (2003) Identification of neutrophil gelatinase-associated lipocalin as a novel early urinary biomarker for ischemic renal injury. J Am Soc Nephrol 14: 2534–2543.
37. Mancia G (2005) The association of hypertension and diabetes: prevalence, cardiovascular risk and protection by blood pressure reduction. Acta Diabetol (Suppl 1): S17–S25.
38. Grossman E, Messerli FH (2008) Hypertension and diabetes. Adv Cardiol 45: 82–106.
39. Sahakyan K, Klein BE, Myers CE, Tsai MY, Klein R (2010) Novel risk factors in long-term hypertension incidence in type 1 diabetes mellitus. Am Heart J 159: 1074–1080.
40. U.S. Renal Data System, USRDS 2007 Annual Data Report. Atlas of Chronic Kidney Disease and End-Stage Renal Disease in the United States, National Institutes of Health, National Institute of Diabetes and Digestive and Kidney Diseases. http://www.usrds.org/adr_2007.htm.
41. Flower DR, North AC, Sansom CE (2000) The lipocalin protein family: structural and sequence overview. Biochim Biophys Acta 1482: 9–24.
42. Devireddy LR, Gazin C, Zhu X, Green MR (2005) A cell-surface receptor for lipocalin 24p3 selectively mediates apoptosis and iron uptake. Cell 123: 1293–1305.
43. Cowland JB, Borregaard N (1997) Molecular characterization and pattern of tissue expression of the gene for neutrophil gelatinase-associated lipocalin from humans. Genomics 45: 17–23.
44. Carlson M, Raab Y, Sevéus L, Xu S, Hällgren R, et al. (2002) Human neutrophil lipocalin is a unique marker of neutrophil inflammation in ulcerative colitis and proctitis. Gut 50: 501–506.
45. Mori K, Lee HT, Rapoport D, Drexler IR, Foster K, et al. (2005) Endocytic delivery of lipocalin-siderophore-iron complex rescues the kidney from ischemia-reperfusion injury. J Clin Invest 115: 610–621.
46. Viau A, El Karoui K, Laouari D, Drexler IR, Foster K, et al. (2010) Lipocalin 2 is essential for chronic kidney disease progression in mice and humans. J Clin Invest 120: 4065–4076.
47. Bolignano D, Coppolino G, Lacquaniti A, Buemi M (2010) From kidney to cardiovascular diseases: NGAL as a biomarker beyond the confines of nephrology. Eur J Clin Invest 40: 273–276.
48. Mori K, Nakao K (2007) Neutrophil gelatinase-associated lipocalin as the real-time indicator of active kidney damage. Kidney Int 71: 967–970.

49. Hvidberg V, Jacobsen C, Strong RK, Cowland JB, Moestrup SK, et al. (2005) The endocytic receptor megalin binds the iron transporting neutrophil-gelatinase-associated lipocalin with high affinity and mediates its cellular uptake. FEBS Lett 579: 773–777.

50. Tojo A, Onozato ML, Ha H, Kurihara H, Sakai T, et al. (2001) Reduced albumin reabsorption in the proximal tubule of early-stage diabetic rats. Histochem Cell Biol 116: 269–276.

51. Hryciw DH, Lee EM, Pollock CA, Poronnik P (2004) Molecular changes in proximal tubule function in diabetes mellitus. Clin Exp Pharmacol Physiol 31: 372–379.

20

Urinary CD133$^+$ Extracellular Vesicles Are Decreased in Kidney Transplanted Patients with Slow Graft Function and Vascular Damage

Veronica Dimuccio[1], Andrea Ranghino[2], Loredana Praticò Barbato[3], Fabrizio Fop[4], Luigi Biancone[2], Giovanni Camussi[2], Benedetta Bussolati[1]*

1 Department of Molecular Biotechnology and Health Sciences, University of Torino, Torino, Italy, **2** Department of Medical Sciences, University of Torino, Torino, Italy, **3** Immunogenetics and Transplant Biology Service, Città della Salute e della Scienza Hospital, Torino, Italy, **4** Division of Nephrology, Dialysis and Transplantation, Città della Salute e della Scienza Hospital, Torino, Italy

Abstract

Extracellular vesicles (EVs) present in the urine are mainly released from cells of the nephron and can therefore provide information on kidney function. We here evaluated the presence of vesicles expressing the progenitor marker CD133 in the urine of normal subjects and of patients undergoing renal transplant. We found that EV expressing CD133 were present in the urine of normal subjects, but not of patients with end stage renal disease. The first day after transplant, urinary CD133$^+$ EVs were present at low levels, to increase thereafter (at day 7). Urinary CD133$^+$ EVs significantly increased in patients with slow graft function in respect to those with early graft function. In patients with a severe pre-transplant vascular damage of the graft, CD133$^+$ EVs did not increase at day 7. At variance, the levels of EVs expressing the renal exosomal marker CD24 did not vary in the urine of patients with end stage renal disease or in transplanted patients in respect to controls. Sorted CD133$^+$ EVs were found to express glomerular and proximal tubular markers. These data indicate that urinary CD133$^+$ EVs are continuously released during the homeostatic turnover of the nephron and may provide information on its function or regenerative potential.

Editor: Ines Armando, Universtiy of Maryland Schoool of Medicine, United States of America

Funding: This work was supported by Regione Piemonte, PISTEM project. Dr. Dimuccio was recipient of a long term Fellowship from the ERA-EDTA. The funders had no role in study design, data collection and analysis, decision to publish, or preparation of the manuscript.

* Email: benedetta.bussolati@unito.it

Introduction

Extracellular vesicles (EVs) are circular fragments of membrane released from the endosomal compartment or shed from the surface membranes of most cell types [1]. EVs express surface receptors and contain proteins and extracellular RNA shared in great part with the cell of origin and their presence has been identified in all biological fluids [1,2]. In the urine, EVs are considered to mainly derive from cells of the nephron, with a minimal contribution of the lower urinary collecting system cells [3]. Indeed, proteomic analysis of urinary EVs identified membrane and cytosolic proteins, which have characteristics of renal tubule epithelial cells of different nephron segments and of podocytes [3,4]. Urinary EVs can therefore provide quantitative and qualitative information on the state of the kidney [5], thus suggesting their use as biomarkers in renal pathology.

After kidney transplantation from deceased donor, ischemia-reperfusion injury of the graft causes renal tubular epithelial cell necrosis and apoptosis leading to loss of organ function [6,7]. A slow or delayed graft function may affect approximately 25% of transplant recipients, causing a significant increase in early transplant-related morbidity and a long term decrease of graft survival [6]. The current approach to clinical management of episodes of renal dysfunction during the first six months after transplantation is mainly based on the results of a percutaneous allograft biopsy [7]. In addition, advances in non-invasive immune monitoring for rejection, such as measurements of signs of cellular immune response, are currently available [8]. However, non invasive tools for evaluation of renal damage and regeneration would be required to guide effective therapeutic interventions.

Intrinsic mechanisms of tissue repair and regeneration occur in the mammalian kidney to re-acquire functionality after ischemic, toxic or inflammatory insults [9]. Recent evidence indicates that cells with characteristics of progenitors, expressing the stem cell marker CD133 and lacking differentiation markers, are present in different segments of the human nephron, being localized in the Bowman capsule of glomeruli, in proximal tubules as well as in inner medullary papilla region including Henle's loop and S3 limb segment [10–12]. In addition, CD133$^+$ cells in the cortex increase in number after acute renal damage, suggesting their role in renal repair after injury [13]. In particular, the number of CD133$^+$ cells was reported to increase in tubules of transplanted patients undergoing delayed graft function as a result of acute renal injury

[13], as well as of patients with proteinuric glomerular diseases [14,15].

Somatic stem and precursor cells of nervous and hematopoietic origin have been shown to release CD133-carrying EVs [16,17] and their level in the spinocerebral fluids associated to pathological conditions [18,19]. We therefore reasoned that $CD133^+$ cells along the nephron could similarly release CD133-carrying EVs and that the presence of these EVs in the urine may provide information on the physiopathological state of the kidney or on its regenerative ability. Indeed, CD133-carrying EVs were previously reported in the urine of normal subjects [20]. In the present study, we aimed to better characterize the urinary $CD133^+$ EVs and to assess their levels in normal subjects and in patients with chronic and acute renal dysfunction. In particular, $CD133^+$ EVs were evaluated in patients with end stage renal disease and in kidney transplanted patients with early or slow graft function, at different days after transplantation.

Materials and Methods

Ethical statement

i) Urine samples: the study was conducted using urine samples from normal human volunteers and transplanted patients. Approval from the San Giovanni Battista Hospital Review Board was obtained, and written informed consent was given by each participant. ii) HLA typing sera from multiparous women: HLA typing sera were obtained from multiparous women by the HLA typing laboratory of our hospital following approval of the San Giovanni Battista Hospital Review Board and stored in an anonymous fashion. All participants gave written consent for their samples to be used in research. iii) kidneys from deceased donors: the evaluation of vascular lesions was performed on protocol biopsies of kidneys from deceased donors prior to transplantation. All organ donor next of kin gave written consent for use of the donor samples in research (as part of the overall protocol and consent for organ donation), as approved by the Regional Transplant Institutional Board.

Patients

Urine samples were obtained from normal human volunteers and transplanted patients. Levels of $CD133^+$ EVs were compared in transplanted patients ($n = 25$), in age-matched controls ($n = 20$) and in end stage renal disease (ESRD) patients with residual diuresis ($n = 5$). All patient information is presented in Table 1. In addition, in selected experiments, urinary EVs were obtained from urine pooled from normal subjects ($n = 10$, age: 28 ± 3, M/F: 4/6).

Evs isolation and count

Urinary EVs from transplanted patients were collected from 80 ml of urine drained by a vescical catheter, from a 6-hours collection, at the first (D1) and the seventh (D7) day after the transplant. In selected patients ($n = 6$), urine was also collected after 30 days. Urine from controls (control normal subjects) and ESRD patients was obtained from 80 ml of the second morning urine or of a 6-hours collection. In addition urine was collected from normal subjects after an oral water load. After voiding, a water load of 20 ml/kg was given orally for 30 minutes. Urine was collected for 6 hours [21].

Urine was centrifuged at 2500 rpm for 15 minutes to pellet cells and Tamm-Horsfall protein. The supernatant was supplemented with protease inhibitor (Sigma) and NaN_3 10 mM (Fluka), filtered through a 0.8 µM filter (Millipore) and then ultracentrifuged at 100.000 g for 1 hour at 4°C. The pellet was resuspended in RPMI (Sigma) and 1% DMSO (Sigma) was added to allow freezing storage in −80°C until use.

EV quantification. For cytofluorimetric and Western Blot analysis, samples were quantified through a proteic Bradford assay. Urinary EVs were also analysed by nanoparticle tracking analysis (NTA), using the NanoSight LM10 system (NanoSight Ltd, Amesbury, UK), configured with a 405 nm laser and a high sensitivity digital camera system (OrcaFlash2.8, Hamamatsu C11440, NanoSight Ltd) as previously described [22]. Briefly, EVs coming from 80 ml of urine were resuspended in 100 µl of vesicle-free physiologic solution (Fresenius Kabi, Runcorn, UK). Each sample was then diluted 1:1000 in the same solution. For this analysis, a monochromatic laser beam at 405 nm was applied to the diluted suspension of EVs. For each sample, three videos of 30 seconds duration were recorded and number of particles/ml and mean size was averaged. NTA post-acquisition settings were optimized and kept constant between samples, and each video was then analysed to give the mean, mode, and median vesicle size together with an estimation of the concentration.

Sorting of $CD133^+$ fraction

Sorting of $CD133^+$ EVs was performed on urine pools obtained from the second morning urine of normal subjects. $CD133^+$ EVs were isolated by magnetic cell sorting, using the CD133 MicroBead Kit applied to the MACS system (Miltenyi Biotec, Auburn, CA). Briefly, urinary EVs were collected from a total volume of 200 ml of urine. The relative pellet, obtained after the 100.000 g ultracentrifugation, was resuspended in 100 µl of ultracentrifuged vesicle-free MACS Buffer, then 100 µl of FcR Blocking Reagent and 100 µl of CD133 MicroBeads were added. This mix was incubated for 30 minutes at 4°C. Hereafter 250 µl of vesicle-free MACS buffer was added to stop the coupling reaction of the antibody to the EVs. The final sample volume of 550 µl was totally applied onto the LS-column for the EVs separation as recommended by the manufacturer's instructions. $CD133^-$ EVs, finally present in a buffer suspension of 9 ml, and the $CD133^+$ EVs, present in a buffer suspension of 5 ml, were then collected through a further 100.000 g centrifuge. Both $CD133^+$ and $CD133^-$ EVs pellets were analyzed using Western blot analysis. For nanoparticle tracking analysis, $CD133^+$ EVs were sorted using an indirect labelling that allows removal magnetic beads with the APC multisorting kit (Miltenyi). Briefly, pelleted EVs were stained with the APC conjugated CD133 mAb (1:20 dilution, 10 minutes at 4°C), ultracentrifuged, and then sorted with the APC-multi-sorting kit following the manufacture's instructions.

Cytofluorimetric analysis

Flow cytometry analysis was performed with a FACSCalibur machine using CellQuest software (Becton Dickinson Bioscience Pharmingen, Franklyn Lake, NJ, USA). As EVs are too small for FACScan analysis, we bound EVs to surfactant-free white aldehyde/sulfate latex beads 4% w/v, 4 µm diameter (Molecular Probes, Invitrogen) [23]. We incubated 5 µl beads with 15 µg EVs for 10–15 minutes at RT and then overnight at 4°C in a final volume of 1 ml PBS-BSA 0.5%. Then the adsorbed EVs were divided in different vials and incubated with antibodies diluted 1:50, for 15 minutes at 4°C. The adsorbed EVs were then washed and analyzed with a FACSCalibur and CellQuest software. Flow cytometry was performed using anti-human monoclonal antibodies (MAbs): APC-conjugated CD133 (AC133; Miltenyi, Auburn, CA, USA); FITC conjugated CD24, PE-conjugated CD9, PE-conjugated CD81 (Becton Dickinson) and anti-Rab5 (Santa Cruz Biotechnology, Santa Cruz, CA, USA). Comparison of urinary EVs among groups was performed by evaluating the relative

Table 1. Characteristics of the transplanted patients, ESRD patients and normal subjects in the study.

	Early graf function (n = 13)	Slow graft function (n = 12)	
RECIPIENTS			
Age, years	53.8±14.1	56.1±12.1	ns
Sex, (M/F)	6/7	11/2	
Cause of chronic kidney disease	Unknown, 3; Chronic pyelonephritis, 2; APKD, 2; Gn, 5; nephroangiosclerosis, 1.	Unknown, 1; Chronic pyelonephritis, 3; Gn, 5; nephroangiosclerosis, 1; diabetic nephropathy, 2; hemolytic-uremic syndrome, 1.	
Prior treatment			
Hemodialysis, No (%)	11 (84)	10 (77)	ns
Peritoneal dialysis, No (%)	2 (15.3)	3 (23)	ns
Time on dialysis (months)	51.1±48.9	71.5±126	ns
Retransplant, No (%)	3 (23)	3 (23)	ns
Panel reactive Antibody >20%, No (%)	2 (15.3)	1(7.7)	ns
≥4 HLA mismatches, No (%)	12 (100%)	11 (84%)	ns
LD/DD	0/13	1/12	ns
Cold ischemia time, h	14.5±5	14.1±5.5	ns
Induction ID, No. (%)			
Basiliximab	13 (100)	11 (84)	ns
Rituximab	0	1 (7)	ns
No induction	0	1 (7)	ns
Maintenance ID, No. (%)			
Tacrolimus	13 (100)	12 (92)	ns
Mycophenolate mofetil	11 (84)	12 (92)	ns
Steroid	13 (100)	13 (100)	ns
Urine 24-h volume (ml)			
Before transplantation	577±701	700±730	ns
day 1 post-transplant	2875±2799	1110±989	p = 0.02
day 7 post-transplant	3706±1098	3881±2025	ns
GFR			ns
day 1 post-transplant	14.2±6.5	12.8±4.3	ns
day 7 post-transplant	45.2±23	14.3±5.4	p = 0.0001
DONORS			
Age, years	60.9±20.5	67.3±11	ns
ECD, No (%)	11 (84%)	11 (84%)	ns
GFR (ml/min)	98.8±49	84.3±17	ns
Hypertension, No (%)	8 (61.5)	9 (69.2)	ns
Diabetes, No (%)	3 (23)	1 (7.7)	
Histological score			
Glomerular sclerosis	1.2±0.4	0.9±0.3	p = 0.04
Tubular atrophy	0.2±0.4	0.1±0.3	ns
Interstitial fibrosis	0.5±0.5	0.3±0.5	ns
Arterial and arteriolar narrowing	1.2±0.4	0.9±0.5	ns
Final score	3±1	2.2±0.9	p = 0.04
ESRD patients (n = 5)			
Age, yrs	54.4±17,6		
Sex, (M/F)	1/4		

Table 1. Cont.

	Early graf function (n = 13)	Slow graft function (n = 12)
Cause of chronic kidney disease	APKD, 2; Unknown, 1; nephroangiosclerosis, 1; Cisplatin-induced nephropathy, 1	
Urine 24-hours volume (ml)	1780±705	
CONTROL SUBJECTS (n = 20)		
Age, yrs	51.8±17.1	
Sex, (M/F)	11/9	

ECD: expanded criteria donors according to Crystal City Meeting criteria [35]. **GFR:** glomerular filtration rate. **Histological score:** performed on pretransplant biopsies according to a semiquantitative method [25]. **APKD:** adult polycystic kidney disease; **Gn:** glomerulonephritis; **LD:** living donor; **DD:** deceased donor. **ID:** immunosuppressive therapy. **ESRD:** end-stage kidney disease. Continuous variables are express as mean ± SD.

amount of EVs positive for a selected marker in respect to all EVs, in conditions where the same quantity of EVs was tested (15 μg protein, corresponding roughly to 1×10^{12} urinary EVs/μg protein, as evaluated by Bradford protein analysis and NTA, respectively). This protein amount was selected by preliminary experiments using different amounts of EVs (from 1 to 50 μg,) that showed no increase in CD133 level at concentration higher than 15 μg (Figure S1). To assess vesicle binding to latex beads, $CD133^+$ or $CD133^-$ EVs were labelled with Vibrant Dil cell-labeling solution (Molecular Probes by Life Techonologies) and processed for fluorescence analysis. No difference was observed in $CD133^+$ or $CD133^-$ EV fluorescence (Figure S1).

Western Blot

For protein analysis, both the $CD133^+$ and the $CD133^-$ fractions of EVs were lysed at 4°C for 30 minutes in RIPA buffer (20 nM Tris-HCl, 150 nM NaCl, 1% deoxycholate, 0.1% SDS, 1% Triton X-100, pH 7.8) supplemented with protease and phosphatase inhibitors cocktail and PMSF (Sigma). When the protein concentration was lower than 2 mg/ml a protocol was used to precipitate, and then concentrate, 10 μg of proteins [24]. Briefly, the volume corresponding to 10 μg was brought to 250 μl with deionized water, and then 800 μl of Methanol, 200 μl of Chloroform and dH2O were added. The mix was strongly vortexed and centrifuged at 12000 rpm for 2 minutes. The upper phase was removed and 600 μl of MetOH was added. After a centrifuge the upper part was removed and the pellet was left to dry under the hood. The remaining dried pellet was resuspended in a proper volume of Laemmli Buffer and the sample was loaded onto the gel. Aliquots of the cell lysates containing 10 μg proteins, as determined by the Bradford method, were run on 10% acrylamide gel SDS-PAGE under reducing conditions. The transfer of proteins onto a PVDF membrane was performed in a 7 minutes transfer program of the iBlot™ Dry Blotting System (Life Technology). The following primary antibodies were used: CD133/1 (clones AC133 and W6B3C1) (Miltenyi), rabbit polyclonal CD133 (Abcam) both at 1:500 dilution; CD81, CD9 and CD63 (all from Becton Dickinson) at 1:200 dilution; Megalin,

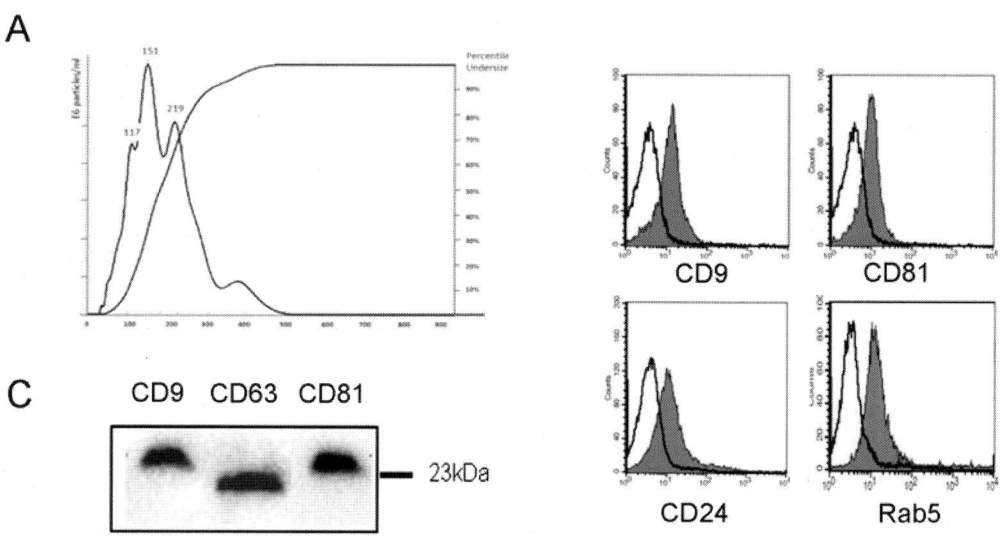

Figure 1. Characterization of normal urinary EVs. Panel A. NanoSight analysis of samples prepared from the urine of normal subjects showing their size distribution profile. A peak at 151 nm was observed. **Panel B and C.** Representative images of the expression of exosome markers by urinary EVs by cytofluorimetric (B) and Western Blot analysis (C). Cytofluorimetric histograms show marker detection (grey area) and isotypic control (dark line). Five different preparations were tested with similar results.

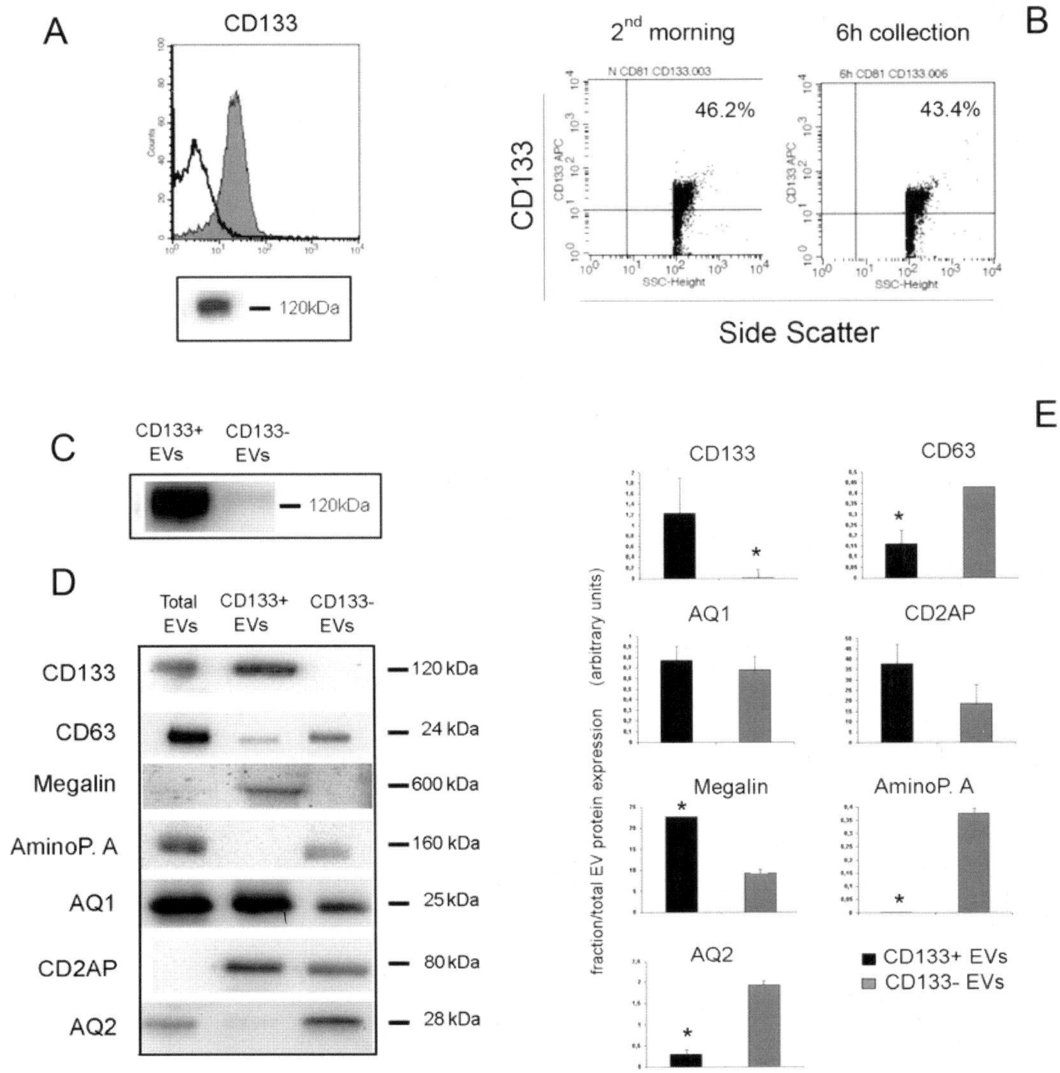

Figure 2. Expression of CD133 by urinary vesicles. Panel A. Representative cytofluorimetric and Western Blot (clone AC133) images of the expression of CD133 by urinary vesicles of normal subjects. The cytofluorimetric histogram shows CD133 detection (grey area) and isotypic control (dark line). **Panel B**. Scatter and fluorescence dot plots showing similar $CD133^{+}$ EV levels in normal urine of a second morning minction or of a 6-hours collection. Plots are representative of three experiments with similar results. **Panel C**. Representative image of CD133 detection in $CD133^{+}$ and $CD133^{-}$ sorted EVs (clone W6B3C1). **Panel D and E**. Representative images and quantification of the expression of different nephron markers by the total urinary EVs and by $CD133^{+}$ and $CD133^{-}$ sorted EVs. Data are mean $\pm$ SD of at least three different experiments and report the marker expression in the sorted fractions normalized on the expression in the Total EVs. AminoP.: Aminopeptidase A, AQ: Aquaporin, CD2AP: CD2 Associated protein. * = $p<0.05$.

Aquaporin-1 (AQ1) and Aquaporin-2 (AQ2) at 1:100 dilution; Aminopeptidase A and CD2 Associated protein (CD2AP) (all from Santa Cruz Biotechnology) at 1:200 dilution.

HLA typing sera. Sera from multiparous women were obtained by the HLA typing laboratory of our hospital. Sera characterized to contain antibodies directed against the HLA class I antigens of the donors were used in order to distinguish the origin of the extracellular vesicles. Typing sera were used at 1:50 dilution in Western Blot experiments. The use of an irrelevant serum gave no signal (data not shown).

Histological evaluation of vascular lesions. Briefly, kidneys from deceased donors underwent a protocol biopsy prior to transplantation in order to quantify the severity of tissue damage according to the histological score proposed by Remuzzi et al [25]. All specimens were evaluated by the same renal pathologist. Specifically, vascular lesions defined as arterial and arteriolar narrowing were scored as follow: 0 absent (n = 7), 1 increased wall thickness but to a degree that is less than the diameter of the lumen (n = 15), 2 wall thickness that is equal or slightly greater to the diameter of the lumen (n = 3), 3 wall thickness that far exceeds the diameter of the lumen with extreme luminal narrowing or occlusion (n = 0).

Statistical methods

Statistical analysis was performed with SPSS (IBM SPSS Statistics, vers. 12.0.0). Continuous variables are presented as median (min–max), according to their distribution. The difference between groups of these variables was analyzed with Mann-Whitney, Wilcoxon or Kruskal-Wallis test.

Categorical variables are presented as fraction and Pearson's or for small samples Fisher's exact test was employed to compare

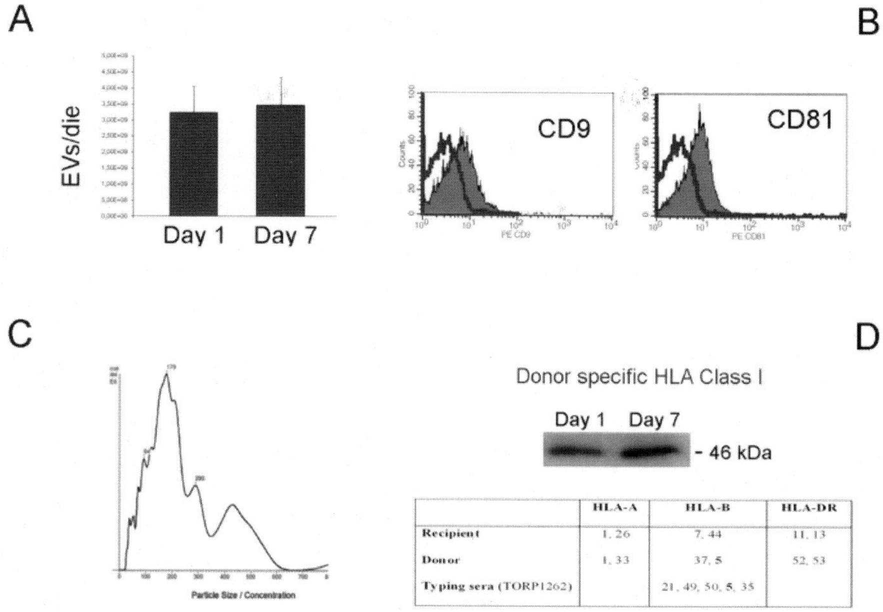

	HLA-A	HLA-B	HLA-DR
Recipient	1, 26	7, 44	11, 13
Donor	1, 33	37, 5	52, 53
Typing sera (TORP1262)		21, 49, 50, 5, 35	

Figure 3. Characterization of urinary EVs in transplanted patients. Urinary EVs were obtained from patients (n = 25) undergoing renal transplant. **Panel A**. Mean number of EVs/day in the urine of transplanted patients were similar at day 1 and 7 after transplant, counted as described in Material and Methods. Data are mean ± SD of all samples. **Panel B and C**. Characterization of EVs showing expression of CD9 and CD81 exosome markers and NanoSight analysis of size distribution profile. Similar results were obtained for samples from all transplanted patients at day 1 and 7. **Panel D**. Representative western blot analysis showing the donor origin of the extracellular vesicle using typing sera containing antibodies directed against HLA class I antigens of the donor not shared by the recipient, at 1 and 7 days after transplant. In the table are reported the HLA typing of the recipient and the donor and the HLA-antigen recognized by the typing serum (TORP1262). HLA-B5 (bold) is present in the donor and not in the recipient. Three patients were tested with similar results.

groups. The odds ratios (OR) were used as a measure of relative risk. Significance level for all tests was set at $p<0.05$.

Results

Detection and characterization of CD133$^+$ urinary EV in normal subjects

EVs were isolated from urine obtained from normal subjects using a two-step differential centrifugation protocol based on a first low-speed centrifugation, followed by filtration trough a 0.8 µm filter to remove cells, cellular debris and apoptotic bodies. The supernatant was subsequently ultracentrifuged at 100,000 g for 1 h to sediment urinary vesicles. Urinary EVs showed a heterogenic size, as evaluated by NanoSight analysis, with a mean peak of 151 nm (Fig. 1A).

Cytofluorimetric analysis of the EVs using latex beads showed presence of typical exosome markers such as CD9, CD81 and Rab5, and of the renal vesicle marker CD24 [26] (Fig. 1B). Figure 1C shows Western Blot analysis of EVs expressing the tetraspanins CD9, CD63 and CD81. We focused our attention on CD133, a stem cell marker expressed in the kidney by progenitors cells [10–12] and previously described in the urinary EVs [20]. We found that CD133$^+$ EVs were detectable at high levels in the urine of normal subjects using cytofluorimetric assay (Fig. 2A). No difference was observed in the levels of CD133$^+$ EV according to the urine collection protocol, as the same results were obtained in the second-morning urine or in a 6 h collection urine of the same subject (Fig. 2B). By Western Blot analysis, CD133 was detected using the stem/progenitor specific antibody against the AC133 isoform, and its molecular weight was compatible with the glycosylated isoform (120 kDa) confirming that EVs expressed the stem/progenitor specific isoform of CD133 [17,20] (Fig. 2A).

To further characterize the possible origin of CD133$^+$ EVs from different nephron segments, we sorted CD133$^+$ EVs and compared the expression of typical nephron markers in the CD133 positive and negative fractions. Sorting CD133$^+$ EVs using magnetic beads provided a specific enrichment of vesicles expressing CD133, that was undetectable in the negative fraction (Fig. 2C). As shown in Fig. 2D and E, the CD133$^+$ fraction expressed CD63 at low levels. The proximal tubular markers AQ1 and Megalin, but not Aminopeptidase A were expressed by CD133$^+$ EVs. In addition, the glomerular marker CD2AP was highly expressed by CD133$^+$ EVs in respect to the negative fraction whereas the collecting duct marker AQ2 was only present in the negative fraction (Fig. 2D and E). These data suggest that CD133$^+$ EVs may have a glomerular and proximal tubular origin. CD133$^+$ and CD133$^-$ EVs did not differ in size, as evaluated by nanoparticle track analysis (Figure S1). Moreover, labelled CD133$^-$ and CD133$^+$ EVs showed similar binding to latex beads, as proved by similar fluorescence intensity (Figure S1).

We next assessed whether the presence of CD133$^+$ EVs within urine might be influenced by parameters such as the urinary flow and urine concentration. After an acute water load, urine (6 h collection) was diluted in respect to a regular water uptake of the same subject (6 h collection); urinary creatinine: 42.3±7.2 g/L vs 119.6±24 mg/dL). The levels of CD133+ EVs did not significantly vary in the same subject according to urine dilution (mean variation 3.8±6.7%, n = 3).

CD133$^+$ urinary Evs are decreased in transplanted patients with SGF

We next evaluated the presence of CD133$^+$ EVs in the urine of transplanted patients at day 1 and 7 after transplant. As soon as 1 day after transplant, EVs were present in the urine and the

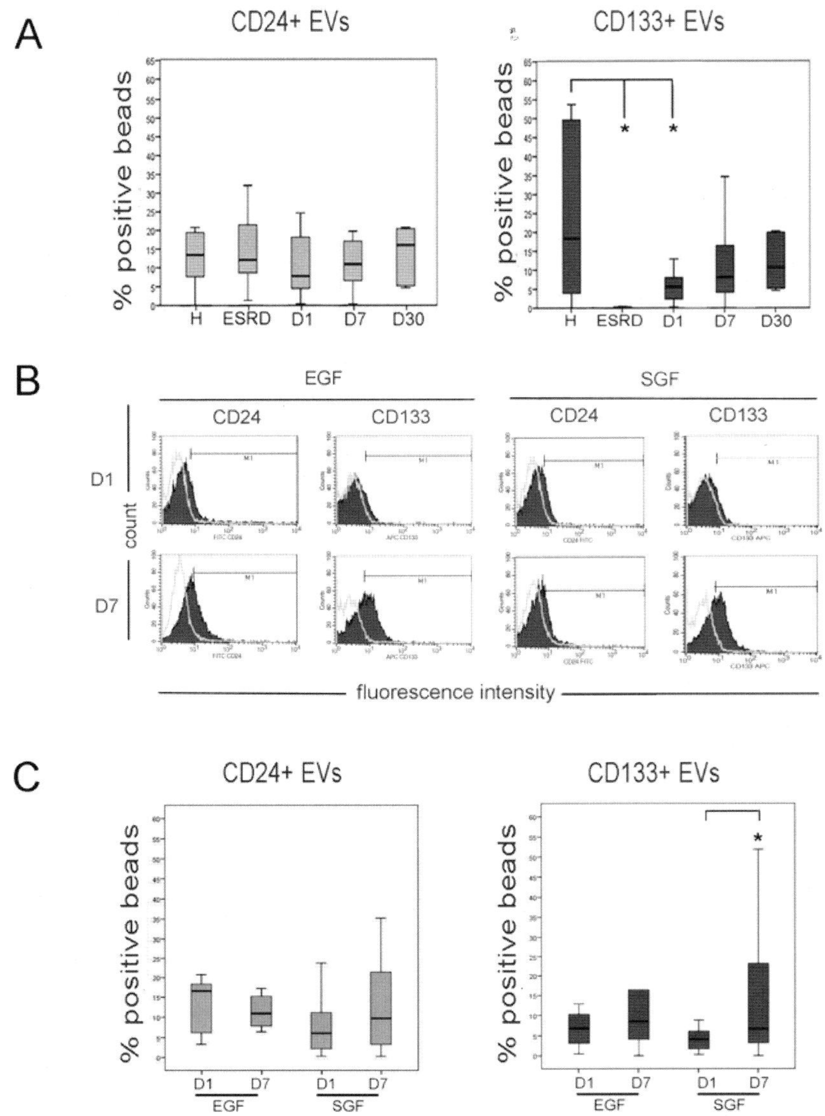

Figure 4. CD24^{+} and CD133^{+} EVs in the urine of normal subjects, ESRD and transplanted patients. Panel A. Levels of urinary CD24^{+} and CD133^{+} EVs in normal subjects (H), ESRD patients with residual diuresis and transplanted patients at day 1, 7 or 30 after transplant (D1, D7 and D30, respectively). A significant reduction of CD133^{+} EVs but not of CD24^{+} EVs was observed in ESRD and transplanted patients at day 1. Data are expressed as % positive beads and are mean ± SD of all samples. **Panel B and C.** Representative cytofluorimetric histograms (B) and median values (C) of CD24^{+} and CD133^{+} EV levels in the urine of patients with EGF (n = 13) and SGF (n = 12) at day 1 and 7 after transplant. Urinary CD133^{+} EVs but not CD24^{+} EVs were lower in EGF patients at day 1, and significantly increased at day 7. Statistical analysis was performed as described in the Materials and methods section. * = $p<0.05$.

production evaluated as EV number/die did not significantly vary within the first 7 days (Fig. 3A). EVs from transplanted patients expressed the exosome markers CD9 and CD81 and a mean size of 179 nm (Fig. 3B and C). To check whether EVs derived from the transplanted kidney rather than from the native kidney or from the lower urinary tract, EVs were stained with anti-HLA Class I Abs recognizing the donor specific antigen isoforms. As shown in Fig. 3D, a band detecting donor specific HLA Class I was present both at 1 and 7 days after transplant.

We evaluated the relative percentage of EVs expressing CD133 using a cytofluorimetric analysis (Fig. 4B). The expression of CD24, a marker of urinary vesicles [26], was used as control. First, to assess whether CD133^{+} EVs specifically derived by a functioning kidney, we analyzed CD133^{+} EVs in ESRD patients with a residual diuresis. No CD133^{+} EVs were detected in the urine of ESRD patients. The level of CD24 was maintained constant in healthy subjects and ESRD patients, indicating a specific loss of CD133^{+} EVs in patients with impairment of the renal function.

CD133^{+} EVs were present in patients undergoing transplant in the first day. However, the CD133^{+} EV levels were significantly lower than those of healthy subjects matched for age and sex with the kidney donors. Levels of CD133^{+} EVs increased 7 days after transplant to levels statistically not different from control subjects (Fig. 4A and Fig. 5). In contrast, no significant difference was observed in the levels of CD24^{+} EVs, suggesting the absence of variation in vesicle production by the kidney. Evaluation of CD133^{+} EV levels at 30 days after transplant in 6 patients did not show significant variation in respect to day 7 (Fig. 4A).

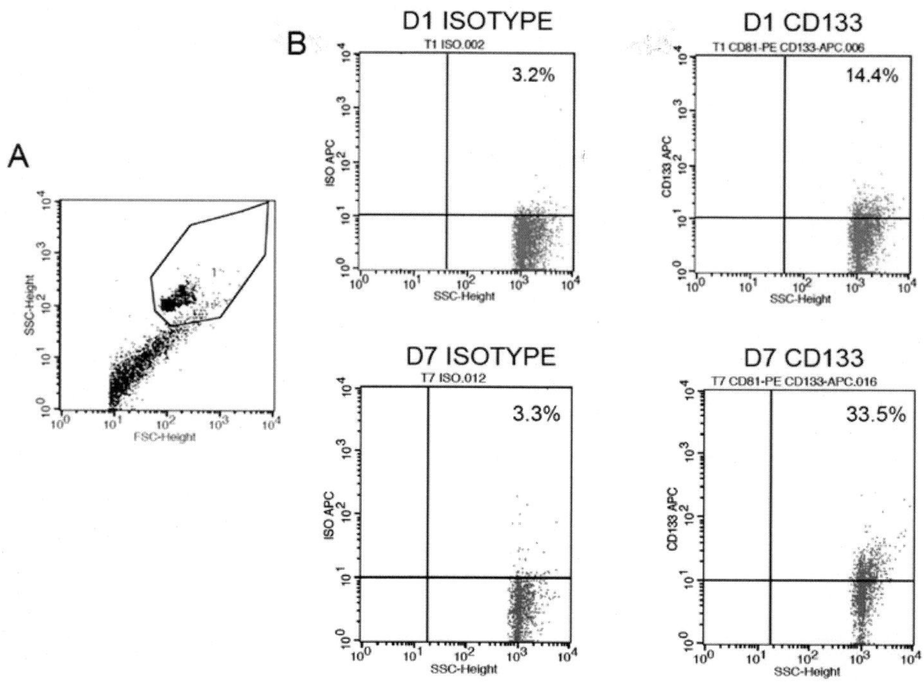

Figure 5. Detection of CD133⁺ EVs in transplanted patients. Panel A and B. Representative dot plots showing the gating strategy of latex bead-conjugated EVs (A) and the fluorescence detection of isotype or CD133 on EVs from a transplanted patients at day 1 or 7.

Transplanted patients were retrospectively divided in respect to kidney function into patients with EGF or SGF, the latter defined as >3 mg/dl creatinine at day 3 [24]. Interestingly, at day 1 the $CD133^+$ EVs were lower in SGF than in EGF patients, although it did not reach a statistical significance (p = 0.08). At day 7, the increase in $CD133^+$ EVs levels was significant only in patients with SGF. Levels of CD24, used as control of the presence of urinary vesicles, did not significantly vary in the different conditions (Fig. 4B and C).

The increase of $CD133^+$ EVs levels from day 1 to day 7 was not related to different urine dilution, as urine concentration did not significantly vary in the first 7 days post-transplant (urinary creatinine concentration: 34±5 mg/dL at day 1vs 29.8±8 mg/dL at day 7), as recently reported [27]. Moreover, the increase was not dependent on a parallel increase in the glomerular filtration, as the glomerular filtration rate increased from day 1 to day 7 only in EGF but not in SGF patients (Table 1).

$CD133^+$ urinary Evs correlate with the severity of the vascular damage in pre-transplanted kidneys

In addition, when patients were divided according to the graft vascular lesions, evaluated as indicated in the material and methods [25], $CD133^+$ EV levels, and not $CD24^+$ EV levels, showed a different increase within time (Fig. 6). In particular, patients with vascular score 2 did not show a recovery of the $CD133^+$ EVs levels at day 7 after transplant. No correlation of $CD133^+$ EVs was found with other parameters such as ischemia time, introduction of calcineurin inhibitors, HLA mismatch or pre-transplant diuresis (Table 2).

Table 2. Correlation of $CD133^+$ EVs and patients' clinical parameters.

		No	$CD133^+$ EVs T1	p*	$CD133^+$ EVs T7	p*
Ischemia (h)	<15	12	4.38 [0.49–11.88]	0.936	8.41[0.00–56.03]	0.503
	>15	13	6.13 [0.28–31.82]		8.00 [0.00–68.68]	
CNI introduction	ab initio	7	5.37 [0.51–11.88]	0.836	11.23 [1.48–62.29]	0.389
	at Crt<2.5	18	5.86 [0.28–31.82]		7.93 [0.00–68.68]	
HLA Mismatches	<4	12	5.48 [0.28–31.82]	0.852	4.24 [0.00–68.68]	0.087
	>4	13	6.13 [0.49–12.88]		8.69 [1.48–62.29]	
Pre-transplant diuresis	>1 L	11	6.65 [0.28–31.82]	0.085	11.77 [0.34–68.68]	0.166
	<1 L	14	2.81 [0.49–12.88]		6.51 [0.00–62.26]	

No correlation was found among $CD133^+$ EVs and ischemia time, introduction of calcineurin inhibitors (CNI), HLA mismatches, and pre-transplant diuresis. Data are expressed are median [min-max], p* = Mann-Withney test.

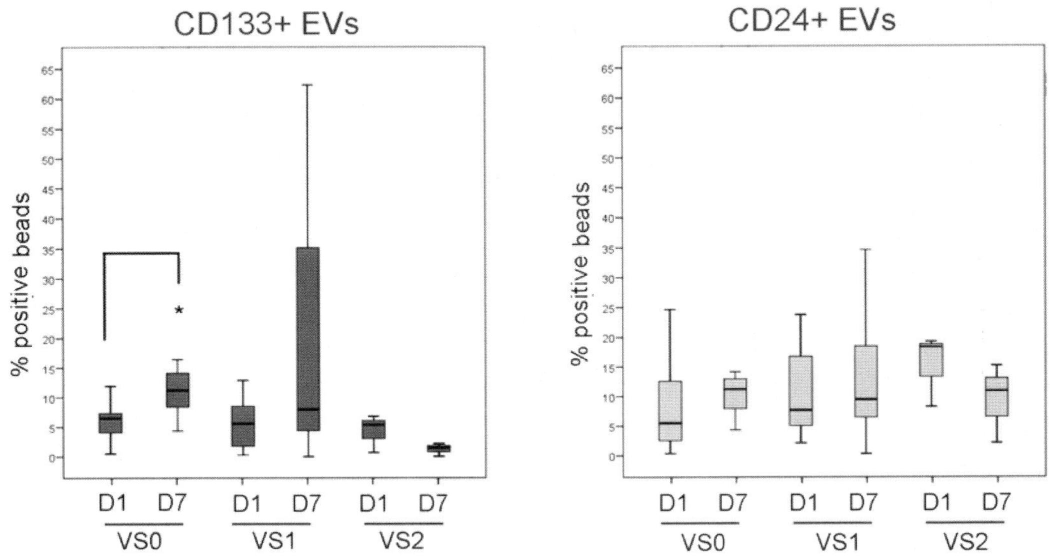

Figure 6. Median values of CD24$^+$ and CD133$^+$ EV levels in the urine of transplanted patients at day 1 and 7 after transplant (D1 and D7), divided according to the graft vascular lesions (VS), as described in Material and methods. No increase in urinary CD133$^+$ EVs was observed in VS2 patients. Statistical analysis was performed as described in the Materials and methods section. * = $p<0.05$.

Discussion

In the present study, we show that CD133$^+$ expressing EVs are present in the urine of normal subjects, but not of patients with ESRD. In the urine of transplanted patients CD133$^+$ EVs were present at low levels the first day after transplant, to increase thereafter (at day 7). In particular, at day 1 the level of CD133$^+$ EVs was lower in patients showing a slow graft function in respect to those with early graft function, then it significantly increased at day 7. Finally, in patients with a severe pre-transplant vascular damage of the graft, CD133$^+$ EVs did not increase at day 7. No significant variation was observed in the presence of CD24$^+$ EVs in patients with ESRD or in transplanted patients.

EVs present in urine could derive both from the cell surface or from intracellular multivescicolar bodies and could be accordingly classified as microvesicles or exosomes, respectively. However, a clear difference based on vesicle markers or dimension is at present of debate [28] and, in the present study, we studied the entire population of EVs present in the urine. The presence of CD133$^+$ EVs in the urine of normal subject and polycystic kidney disease patients was previously reported using Western Blot and immunogold analysis [20,29]. CD133$^+$/CD63$^-$ EVs with a large size (400 nm) were described to be released into body fluids from microvilli of epithelial cells [20]. Other studies reported the biogenesis of CD133$^+$ EVs by multivesicular bodies and their release as CD63$^+$ exosomes [17,30]. The results of our study, showing the presence of CD63 at low levels in CD133$^+$ sorted EVs by Western Blot analysis, suggests that both type of vesicles may be present in urine. The proteomic analysis of urinary EVs previously identified proteins from renal epithelia extending from the glomerular podocytes through the proximal tubules to collecting ducts [3], suggesting that all nephron segments may contribute to their generation. At variance, the origin of CD133$^+$ EVs appeared more restricted to glomeruli and proximal tubules based on the expression of surface markers on CD133$^+$ sorted EVs. Further information in support of the renal origin of CD133$^+$ EVs is provided by their detection immediately after transplantation. Since patients with end stage renal disease did not release CD133$^+$ EVs, the CD133$^+$ EVs found in the urine of transplanted patients the first day after transplant are most likely released by the graft. This is also confirmed by the presence of graft-specific HLA Class I antigens by urinary EVs of transplanted patients. The possible function of the CD133$^+$ EVs in renal physiology still remains to be investigated. It could be however speculated that CD133$^+$ EVs may interact with cells of the nephron, as described for CD133$^+$ EVs released in the urine of polycystic kidney disease patients [29].

In the nervous system, the shedding of CD133$^+$ EVs from the cell surface was regarded as a mechanism of cell differentiation and of neural specification [16]. Similarly, CD133$^+$ EVs are shed by CD133$^+$ hematopoietic stem cells during the process of cell differentiation [17]. Our data show that CD133$^+$ EVs are continuously released by renal cells suggesting the involvement of CD133$^+$ progenitors in the homeostatic turnover of the nephron. The reduction of urinary CD133$^+$ EV levels but not of CD24$^+$ EVs in end stage renal disease indicates that these vesicles are only released by functioning renal tissue, suggesting an exhaustion of the progenitor activity that parallels the loss of kidney function.

It could be therefore speculated that the number of CD133$^+$ EVs may reflect the activity of CD133$^+$ cells in the kidney, as CD133$^+$ EVs were lower in patients with a slow graft function in respect to those with early graft function. In addition, in these latter patients, CD133$^+$ EVs significantly increased after 7 days, possibly underlying that their presence correlates with the graft recovery after tissue damage. Moreover in the same patients the number of CD133$^+$ EVs at day 7 reached levels not significantly different in comparison with normal subjects. Our results parallel the data reported by Loverre et al. [13] showing that CD133$^+$ cells were reduced in renal tissue of pre-transplant delayed graft function patients in respect to early graft function patients. In addition, in delayed graft function patients, an increase of proliferating CD133$^+$ cells was observed 10 days after transplant [13]. These data may further implicate CD133$^+$ cells in the regeneration of renal tissue after injury due to cold ischemia and ischemia-reperfusion, as suggested in several studies [14,15,31]. In addition, in patients with a severe pre-transplant vascular damage, we observed the lack of increase in urinary CD133$^+$ EVs at day 7.

This may imply an inefficient regeneration in the renal tissue of patients with high vascular damage. The lack of variations in $CD24^+$ EVs, used as marker of urinary EVs, indicates that the observed differences in $CD133^+$ EV release do not reflect alteration in EV number but rather in the composition of the vesicle population. Indeed, the relative $CD133^+$ EV levels did not vary in relation to urine concentration or glomerular filtration rate.

Previous studies identified that the amount of membrane particle-associated CD133 was significantly enhanced in patients with glioblastoma and in epileptic patients as compared to healthy adults [18,19]. At variance with these studies, evaluating the amount of CD133 using Western Blot analysis, our study was based on cytofluorimetric evaluation of $CD133^+$ EVs labeled on latex beads. This is a common method to analyze the expression of markers expressed on the EV surface [23]. This method resulted reliable and highly sensitive. In addition, as the results represent a relative expression of positive EVs on the total population, it was not influenced by urine dilution and EV amount in the urine. We are, however, aware that our data do not represent real percentages of $CD133^+$ EVs, as the level of positivity is the result of numerous EVs bound to each bead. These data support the idea that the analysis of urinary $CD133^+$ EVs may represent a possible biomarker for tissue injury or for the repair capacity of the nephron.

The possible use of urinary exosomes as markers of renal damage has already been proposed. For instance, activating transcription factor 3 and Wilms tumor 1 were associated with early tubular and podocyte injury in different experimental models [32]. Moreover, a reduction in the levels of AQ1 in urinary exosomes has been associated with renal ischemia–reperfusion injury in rats [33]. Finally, it has been recently shown that detection of fetuin-A in urinary EVs is a biomarker of renal injury in patients developing acute kidney injury [34]. The evaluation of urinary $CD133^+$ EVs as marker of tubular function and repair may be of interest in acute renal injury, and it could be possibly extended to patients with different levels of chronic renal damage.

Taken together, these results suggest that $CD133^+$ EVs may reflect the activity of $CD133^+$ progenitor cells in renal homeostasis and may provide information on their regenerative potential after acute kidney injury.

Author Contributions

Conceived and designed the experiments: AR BB. Performed the experiments: VD. Analyzed the data: VD FF. Contributed reagents/materials/analysis tools: AR LPB LB. Wrote the paper: GC BB.

References

1. Vlassov AV, Magdaleno S, Setterquist R, Conrad R (2012) Exosomes: current knowledge of their composition, biological functions, and diagnostic and therapeutic potentials. Biochim Biophys Acta 1820: 940–948.
2. van Balkom BW, Pisitkun T, Verhaar MC, Knepper MA (2011) Exosomes and the kidney: prospects for diagnosis and therapy of renal diseases. Kidney Int 80: 1138–1145.
3. Pisitkun T, Shen RF, Knepper MA (2004) Identification and proteomic profiling of exosomes in human urine. Proc Natl Acad Sci U S A 101: 13368–13373.
4. Hogan MC, Johnson KL, Zenka RM, Cristine Charlesworth M, Madden BJ, et al. (2014) Subfractionation, characterization, and in-depth proteomic analysis of glomerular membrane vesicles in human urine. Kidney Int 85: 1225–37.
5. Record M, Subra C, Silvente-Poirot S, Poirot M (2011) Exosomes as intercellular signalosomes and pharmacological effectors. Biochem Pharmacol 81: 1171–1182.
6. Perico N, Cattaneo D, Sayegh MH, Remuzzi G (2004) Delayed graft function in kidney transplantation. Lancet 364: 1814–1827.
7. Marsden PA (2003) Predicting outcomes after renal transplantation–new tools and old tools. N Engl J Med 349: 182–184.
8. Martínez-Flores JA, Serrano M, Morales P, Paz-Artal E, Morales JM, et al. (2014) Comparison of several functional methods to evaluate the immune response on s kidney transplant patients. J Immunol Methods 403: 62–5.
9. Aggarwal S, Moggio A, Bussolati B. (2013) Concise review: stem/progenitor cells for renal tissue repair: current knowledge and perspectives. Stem Cells Transl Med 2: 1011–1019.
10. Sagrinati C, Netti GS, Mazzinghi B, Lazzeri E, Liotta F, et al. (2006) Isolation and characterization of multipotent progenitor cells from the Bowman's capsule of adult human kidneys. J Am Soc Nephrol 17: 2443–2456.
11. Bussolati B, Bruno S, Grange C, Buttiglieri S, Deregibus MC, et al. (2005) Isolation of renal progenitor cells from adult human kidney. Am J Pathol 166: 545–555.
12. Bussolati B, Moggio A, Collino F, Aghemo G, D'Armento G, et al. (2012) Hypoxia modulates the undifferentiated phenotype of human renal inner medullary $CD133^+$ progenitors through Oct4/miR-145 balance. Am J Physiol Renal Physiol 302: F116–F128.
13. Loverre A, Capobianco C, Ditonno P, Battaglia M, Grandaliano G, et al. (2008) Increase of proliferating renal progenitor cells in acute tubular necrosis underlying delayed graft function. Transplantation 85: 1112–1119.
14. Smeets B, Boor P, Dijkman H, Sharma SV, Jirak P, et al. (2013) Proximal tubular cells contain a phenotypically distinct, scattered cell population involved in tubular regeneration. J Pathol 229: 645–659.
15. Kim K, Park BH, Ihm H, Kim KM, Jeong J, et al. (2011) Expression of stem cell marker CD133 in fetal and adult human kidneys and pauci-immune crescentic glomerulonephritis. Histol Histopathol 26: 223–232.
16. Corbeil D, Marzesco AM, Wilsch-Bräuninger M, Huttner WB (2010) The intriguing links between prominin-1 (CD133), cholesterol-based membrane microdomains, remodelling of apical plasma membrane protrusions, extracellular membrane particles, and (neuro)epithelial cell differentiation. FEBS Lett 584: 1659–1664.
17. Bauer N, Wilsch-Bräuninger M, Karbanová J, Fonseca AV, Strauss D, et al. (2011) Haematopoietic stem cell differentiation promotes the release of prominin-1/CD133-containing membrane vesicles–a role of the endocytic-exocytic pathway. EMBO Mol Med 3: 398–409.
18. Huttner HB, Janich P, Köhrmann M, Jászai J, Siebzehnrubl F, et al. (2008) The stem cell marker prominin-1/CD133 on membrane particles in human cerebrospinal fluid offers novel approaches for studying central nervous system disease. Stem Cells 26: 698–705.
19. Huttner HB, Corbeil D, Thirmeyer C, Coras R, Köhrmann M, et al. (2012) Increased membrane shedding–indicated by an elevation of CD133-enriched membrane particles–into the CSF in partial epilepsy. Epilepsy Res 99: 101–106.
20. Marzesco AM, Janich P, Wilsch-Bräuninger M, Dubreuil V, Langenfeld K, et al. (2005) Release of extracellular membrane particles carrying the stem cell marker prominin-1 (CD133) from neural progenitors and other epithelial cells. J Cell Sci 118: 2849–2858.
21. Davis BB, Zenser TV (1993) Evaluation of renal concentrating and diluting ability. Clin Lab Med 13: 131–4.
22. Webber J, Clayton A (2013) How pure are your vesicles? J Extracell Vesicles 2: 18961.
23. Logozzi M, De Milito A, Lugini L, Borghi M, Calabrò L, et al. (2009) High levels of exosomes expressing CD63 and caveolin-1 in plasma of melanoma patients. PLoS One 4: e5219.
24. Wessel D, Flügge UI (1984) A method for the quantitative recovery of protein in dilute solution in the presence of detergents and lipids. Anal Biochem 138: 141–143.
25. Remuzzi G, Grinyò J, Ruggenenti P, Beatini M, Cole EH, et al. (1999) Early experience with dual kidney transplantation in adults using expanded donor criteria. Double Kidney Transplant Group (DKG). J Am Soc Nephrol 10: 2591–2598.
26. Keller S, Rupp C, Stoeck A, Runz S, Fogel M, et al. (2007) CD24 is a marker of exosomes secreted into urine and amniotic fluid. Kidney Int 72: 1095–1102.
27. Jenni F, Riethmüller S, Wüthrich RP (2013) Significance of urine diagnostic tests after renal transplantation. Kidney Blood Press Res 37: 116–23.
28. Raposo G, Stoorvogel W (2013) Extracellular vesicles: exosomes, microvesicles, and friends. J Cell Biol 200: 373–83.
29. Hogan MC, Manganelli L, Woollard JR, Masyuk AI, Masyuk TV, et al. (2009) Characterization of PKD protein-positive exosome-like vesicles. J Am Soc Nephrol 20: 278–288.
30. Marimpietri D, Petretto A, Raffaghello L, Pezzolo A, Gagliani C, et al. (2013) Proteome profiling of neuroblastoma-derived exosomes reveal the expression of proteins potentially involved in tumor progression. PLoS One 8: e75054.
31. Ye Y, Wang B, Jiang X, Hu W, Feng J, et al. (2011) Proliferative capacity of stem/progenitor-like cells in the kidney may associate with the outcome of patients with acute tubular necrosis. Hum Pathol 42: 1132–1141.

32. Zhou H, Cheruvanky A, Hu X, Matsumoto T, Hiramatsu N, et al. (2008) Urinary exosomal transcription factors, a new class of biomarkers for renal disease. Kidney Int 74: 613–621.
33. Sonoda H, Yokota-Ikeda N, Oshikawa S, Kanno Y, Yoshinaga K, et al. (2009) Decreased abundance of urinary exosomal aquaporin-1 in renal ischemia-reperfusion injury. Am J Physiol Renal Physiol 297: F1006–F1016.
34. Zhou H, Pisitkun T, Aponte A, Yuen PS, Hoffert JD, et al. (2006) Exosomal Fetuin-A identified by proteomics: a novel urinary biomarker for detecting acute kidney injury. Kidney Int 70: 1847–1857.
35. Rosengard BR, Feng S, Alfrey EJ, Zaroff JG, Emond JC, et al. (2002) Report of the Crystal City meeting to maximize the use of organs recovered from the cadaver donor. Am J Transplant 2: 701–711.

21

Antihypertensive Medication Classes Used among Medicare Beneficiaries Initiating Treatment in 2007–2010

Shia T. Kent[1]*, Daichi Shimbo[2], Lei Huang[1], Keith M. Diaz[2], Meredith L. Kilgore[3], Suzanne Oparil[4], Paul Muntner[1,4]

1 Department of Epidemiology, University of Alabama at Birmingham, Birmingham, Alabama, United States of America, **2** Center for Behavioral Cardiovascular Health, Department of Medicine, Columbia University Medical Center, New York, New York, United States of America, **3** Department of Health Care Organization and Policy, University of Alabama at Birmingham, Birmingham, Alabama, United States of America, **4** Department of Medicine, Division of Cardiovascular Disease, University of Alabama at Birmingham, Birmingham, Alabama, United States of America

Abstract

Background: After the 2003 publication of the Seventh Report of the Joint National Committee on Prevention, Detection, Evaluation, and Treatment of High Blood Pressure (JNC 7) guidelines, there was a 5–10% increase in patients initiating antihypertensive medication with a thiazide-type diuretic, but most patients still did not initiate treatment with this class. There are few contemporary published data on antihypertensive medication classes filled by patients initiating treatment.

Methods and Findings: We used the 5% random Medicare sample to study the initiation of antihypertensive medication between 2007 and 2010. Initiation was defined by the first antihypertensive medication fill preceded by 365 days with no antihypertensive medication fills. We restricted our analysis to beneficiaries ≥65 years who had two or more outpatient visits with a hypertension diagnosis and full Medicare fee-for-service coverage for the 365 days prior to initiation of antihypertensive medication. Between 2007 and 2010, 32,142 beneficiaries in the 5% Medicare sample initiated antihypertensive medication. Initiation with a thiazide-type diuretic decreased from 19.2% in 2007 to 17.9% in 2010. No other changes in medication classes initiated occurred over this period. Among those initiating antihypertensive medication in 2010, 31.3% filled angiotensin-converting enzyme inhibitors (ACE-Is), 26.9% filled beta blockers, 17.2% filled calcium channel blockers, and 14.4% filled angiotensin receptor blockers (ARBs). Initiation with >1 antihypertensive medication class decreased from 25.6% in 2007 to 24.1% in 2010. Patients initiated >1 antihypertensive medication class most commonly with a thiazide-type diuretic and either an ACE-I or ARB.

Conclusion: These results suggest that JNC 7 had a limited long-term impact on the choice of antihypertensive medication class and provide baseline data prior to the publication of the 2014 Evidence-Based Guideline for the Management of High Blood Pressure in Adults from the Panel Members Appointed to the Eighth Joint National Committee (JNC 8).

Editor: Sadashiva Karnik, Cleveland Clinic Lerner Research Institute, United States of America

Funding: STK was supported by a National Heart, Lung, and Blood Institute (NHLBI) training grant (T32-HL007457-33). DS was supported by an NHLBI program grant (P01-HL047540). KMD was supported by a NHLBI Diversity Supplement (P01-HL047540-19S1). The funders had no role in study design, data collection and analysis, decision to publish, or preparation of the manuscript.

Competing Interests: The authors have declared that no competing interests exist.

* Email: shia@uab.edu

Introduction

In 2002, the Antihypertensive and Lipid-Lowering Treatment to Prevent Heart Attack Trial (ALLHAT) found that in a hypertensive population with at least one additional coronary heart disease (CHD) risk factor, randomization to chlorthalidone (thiazide-type diuretic), amlodpine (calcium channel blocker [CCB]), or lisinopril (angiotensin-converting enzyme inhibitor [ACE-I]) was associated with similar rates of coronary heart disease outcomes [1].Chlorthalidone was associated with a lower risk of heart failure, a secondary outcome. Shortly after the publication of the main results of ALLHAT, the Seventh Report of the Joint National Committee on the Prevention, Detection, Evaluation, and Treatment of High Blood Pressure (JNC 7) published guidelines for the prevention and treatment of hypertension [2].

Based in part on the comparative effectiveness results shown in ALLHAT, and due to their lower cost, JNC 7 supported the use of thiazide-type diuretics as first line therapy for those without a compelling indication for treatment with another antihypertensive drug class. For patients with compelling indications (e.g. chronic kidney disease [CKD]), use of other classes of antihypertensive medication was recommended. Several studies have examined the impact of ALLHAT and JNC 7 on classes of antihypertensive medication being filled by patients initiating treatment [3–5]. These studies reported a 5–10% increase in the initiation of antihypertensive treatment with thiazide-type diuretics after the publication of ALLHAT and JNC 7. However, the majority of patients initiated antihypertensive medication with other drug classes during this period, indicating that JNC 7 guidelines had a limited impact on the choice of drug class. There are few recent data on whether adherence to JNC 7 drug class recommendations has increased or decreased over time. While it is possible that thiazide-type diuretic usage has increased, ACE-Is and CCBs have since decreased in cost [6,7]. Additionally, subsequent trials comparing antihypertensive drug classes on cardiovascular outcomes and a meta-analysis has suggested no substantial differences exist between ACE-Is, angiotensin receptor blockers (ARBs), CCBs, and thiazide-type diuretics [8–12].Also, guidelines and policy statements from various associations and institutions published since JNC 7 have not universally recommended thiazide-type diuretics for patients initiating treatment [13–15]. These factors could influence current trends in choices of first-line therapy among US adults.

The long-term impact of JNC 7 is of relevance to the current and future dissemination of guidelines, such as the recently published 2014 Evidence-Based Guideline for the Management of High Blood Pressure in Adults from the Panel Members Appointed to the Eighth Joint National Committee (JNC 8) [16]. Contemporary data can provide a baseline documentation of whether patients are initiating antihypertensive medication with the classes recommended by JNC 8. Therefore, the goal of the present study was to examine the classes of antihypertensive medication being filled among US Medicare beneficiaries initiating treatment. Additionally, we evaluated the association between patient factors, including demographics and comorbidities, with the initiation of antihypertensive medication classes. To accomplish these goals, we analyzed the 5% random sample of US Medicare beneficiaries initiating antihypertensive medication between 2007 through 2010.

Methods

We conducted a retrospective cohort study of Medicare beneficiaries using the 2006–2010 national 5% random sample from the Centers for Medicare and Medicaid Services (CMS). Medicare is a US federal benefit program that provides health insurance to individuals 65 years of age and older, on disability, or who have end-stage renal disease, through either individual fee-for-service claims or contracts with health care organizations. Specific data used for the current analyses include claims from Medicare fee-for-service Parts A (in-patient), B (out-patient) and D (prescription drug). These data provide Medicare claims data linked by beneficiary across the continuum of care. The CMS and the Institutional Review Board at the University of Alabama at Birmingham approved the study. Beneficiary records were anonymized and de-identified prior to analysis.

The current analysis included Medicare beneficiaries who initiated antihypertensive medication in 2007, 2008, 2009 or 2010. The initial eligibility criterion was defined by filling an antihypertensive medication between January 1, 2007 and December 25, 2010. The date of each beneficiary's first fill for an antihypertensive medication in a calendar year was used as their index fill date. December 25, 2010 rather than December 31, 2010 was chosen for the end of the study period to accommodate a 6 day period to identify additional antihypertensive medication classes filled among patients initiating treatment (see below). To facilitate the identification of prevalent antihypertensive medication users for exclusion from our analyses, beneficiaries were required to have continuous full Medicare coverage (traditional Medicare Parts A and B fee-for-service and Part D coverage) and reside in the 50 United States or Washington DC for the 365 day period preceding the index fill date. This period is referred to as the "look-back" period. To capture medications filled as part of the initial antihypertensive regimen, we required beneficiaries to have full Medicare coverage for 6 days following their index fill date.

To increase the likelihood that the antihypertensive medications were filled to lower blood pressure, we limited the sample to beneficiaries with hypertension, defined by ≥ 2 outpatient physician evaluation and management claims, ≥ 7 days apart, with International Classification of Diseases, 9th Revision (ICD-9) diagnoses of 401.x (malignant, benign or unspecified essential hypertension) during the look-back period. We excluded beneficiaries who were prevalent users of antihypertensive medication defined by any antihypertensive medication fills during the 365 day look-back period. Also, we excluded beneficiaries who were $<$ 65 years of age at the start of the 365 day look-back period or $\geq$ 110 years of age on the date of the index antihypertensive medication fill. To examine possible time trends, we initially created separate yearly cohorts of beneficiaries initiating antihypertensive medication in 2007, 2008, 2009, and 2010. A beneficiary could potentially be counted in multiple years if they had an antihypertensive medication fill more than 365 days prior to the index fill. In subsequent analyses, we pooled the data to create a single cohort that only included each beneficiary's first antihypertensive medication fill in the 2007–2010 time period. A CONSORT diagram showing the inclusion/exclusion of Medicare beneficiaries is provided in Figure S1.

Antihypertensive medication fills

Claims for antihypertensive medications were identified in the Medicare Part D file. Antihypertensive medications filled from the index fill date through the next 6 days were considered to be initiated as part of the same regimen. Antihypertensive medications were grouped into drug classes using classifications from JNC 7, with newer medications identified by review of the study authors (D.S., S.O.). Pills containing two antihypertensive medication classes were considered combination medications and patients were considered to initiate both classes.

Covariates

A priori-selected covariates were used to study the characteristics of Medicare beneficiaries initiating each class of antihypertensive medication. These included age, sex, race/ethnicity, Medicaid buy-in (a measure of poverty) for the entire look-back period, and comorbid conditions that may be considered compelling indications for being prescribed certain antihypertensive medication classes (diabetes, coronary heart disease [CHD], stroke, CKD, and heart failure) [2]. Age, sex, race/ethnicity, and Medicaid buy-in were defined using the Medicare beneficiary enrollment file. Comorbid conditions were defined using claims during the look-back period and previously published algorithms (Appendix S1).

Statistical analyses

Characteristics of Medicare beneficiaries initiating antihypertensive medications were calculated by calendar year of initiation. For each calendar year, the percentages initiating each antihypertensive medication class, initiating >1 class, and initiating antihypertensive treatment with a combination pill were calculated. Among those who initiated therapy with >1 antihypertensive medication class, we examined the pairs of classes that were initiated. P-values for trends across calendar year were calculated in Poisson regression models with calendar year as a continuous variable. Using the pooled 2007–2010 cohort, we calculated the distributions of antihypertensive medication classes initiated for the overall population and in subgroups defined by gender, race/ethnicity (black, white, Hispanic, Asian, or other), the presence or absence of each compelling indication (diabetes, CHD, stroke, CKD, and heart failure), and with any or no compelling indication, separately. We then calculated the risk ratios for initiating each antihypertensive medication class using Poisson regression and sandwich estimators. Initiating each antihypertensive medication class was evaluated in a separate regression model with the comparison group consisting of individuals initiating an antihypertensive medication regimen without that class (e.g., initiating with an ACE-I versus initiating treatment with any other antihypertensive medication classes). Adjusted risk ratios for initiating each antihypertensive medication class were calculated for calendar year of initiation, age, gender, race/ethnicity, Medicaid buy-in, diabetes, CHD, CKD, and heart failure. Adjusted risk ratios for initiating each antihypertensive medication class were also calculated among Medicare beneficiaries without any compelling indications. Lastly, we calculated the percent of beneficiaries in the pooled 2007–2010 cohort who initiated antihypertensive medication with classes recommended by the 2014 JNC 8 guideline. Among beneficiaries without CKD, recommended classes include a thiazide-type diuretic or a CCB for blacks and a thiazide-type diuretic, CCB, ACE-I, or ARB for non-blacks [16]. For beneficiaries with CKD, recommended classes include an ACE-I or an ARB. Analyses were conducted using SAS 9.3 (SAS Institute, Cary, NC).

Results

In 2007, 2008, 2009, and 2010 there were 7,456, 8,769, 8,575, and 8,719 eligible Medicare beneficiaries, respectively, who initiated antihypertensive medication. Characteristics of Medicare beneficiaries in the 5% sample who initiated antihypertensive medications in 2007, 2008, 2009 and 2010 are provided in Table 1. The mean age was 77 years, approximately 80% were white and 37% to 41% were men. Diabetes was the most prevalent comorbid condition, followed by a history of CHD. In each year, approximately 50% of Medicare beneficiaries who initiated antihypertensive medication had a history of diabetes, CHD, stroke, CKD or heart failure. Beneficiaries initiating therapy in later study years were younger and more likely to be male, white, and have diabetes and CKD, and less likely to be black and have had a stroke or heart failure. The presence of any compelling indication (diabetes, CHD, stroke, CKD, and heart failure) for being prescribed certain antihypertensive medication classes was more common in recent study years.

ACE-Is were the most commonly initiated antihypertensive medication class in each year (Table 2). The next most commonly initiated medication classes were beta blockers, thiazide-type diuretics, CCBs, and ARBs. Between 24% and 26% of the cohort initiated antihypertensive medication with >1 class and 11% to 12% initiated treatment with a combination pill. Among those who initiated multiple classes (either with a combination pill or as separate pills), a thiazide-type diuretic with an ACE-I or a thiazide-type diuretic with an ARB were mostly commonly initiated (Table S1). Other antihypertensive medication pairs commonly initiated were an ACE-I with a beta blocker or an ACE-I with a CCB.

Overall, 32,142 Medicare beneficiaries were included in the pooled 2007–2010 cohort. Figure 1 shows antihypertensive medication classes initiated by beneficiary characteristics in this cohort. Compared to females, males were more likely to initiate antihypertensive medication with an ACE-I or beta blocker and less likely to initiate treatment with an ARB or a thiazide-type diuretic. Compared to whites, blacks were more likely to initiate treatment with a thiazide-type diuretic or CCB. Compared to their counterparts without diabetes, beneficiaries with diabetes were more likely to initiate therapy with an ACE-I and less likely to initiate with a thiazide-type or CCB. Those with CHD, stroke, CKD, or heart failure were less likely than those without each respective condition to initiate treatment with an ARB or with a thiazide-type diuretic and more likely to initiate with a loop diuretic or a beta blocker. Those without any compelling indication (diabetes, CHD, stroke, CKD, or heart failure), compared to those with any compelling indication, were less likely to initiate therapy with an ACE-I or beta blocker and more likely to initiate with an ARB or thiazide-type diuretic. Blacks compared with whites, and those with diabetes, a history of stroke, CKD, and heart failure were more likely to initiate treatment with >1 antihypertensive class.

After multivariable adjustment, there was a decline in the initiation of antihypertensive medication with a thiazide-type diuretic over time (Table 3). Specifically, an 8% reduction (risk ratio 0.92; 95% CI 0.86–0.98) in initiation of antihypertensive medication with a thiazide-type diuretic occurred in 2010, compared with 2007. Drug initiation patterns by each compelling indication were similar to those in unadjusted analyses. Older beneficiaries were less likely to initiate treatment with an ACE-I or thiazide-type diuretic and more likely to initiate with a loop diuretic, beta blocker, or CCB. Males were more likely than females to initiate with an ACE-I and were less likely to initiate with an ARB or a thiazide-type or potassium-sparing diuretic. Compared to females, males were more likely to initiate with an ACE-I and less likely to initiate with and ARB, or a thiazide-type or potassium-sparing diuretic. Compared to whites, blacks were less likely to initiate treatment with an ACE-I or loop diuretic and more likely to initiate treatment with a thiazide-type diuretic or CCB. Compared to whites, Hispanics were more likely to initiate antihypertensive medication with an ACE-I or ARB and less likely to initiate with a loop or potassium-sparing diuretic. Asians, compared with whites were more likely to initiate with an ARB or CCB and less likely to initiate treatment with an ACE-I or loop diuretic. Beneficiaries with a Medicaid buy-in were less likely to initiate treatment with an ARB or a thiazide-type or potassium-sparing diuretic, and were more likely to initiate therapy with a loop diuretic.

Drug initiation patterns were similar when limited to beneficiaries without any compelling indications (Table S2). Specifically, in both the overall pooled cohort and among those without any compelling indications, initiation with a thiazide-type diuretic was less common in later study years, and more common in younger, female, and black beneficiaries. One notable difference is that in the overall cohort there was no time trend for initiation with a loop diuretic, but among those without compelling indications loop diuretics were more commonly initiated in later years.

Among beneficiaries in the pooled 2007–2010 cohort, 19,891 (61.9%) initiated antihypertensive treatment with a medication class recommended by JNC 8. Among beneficiaries without CKD, 48.8% of blacks and 66.7% of non-blacks initiated antihypertensive medication with a drug class recommended by JNC 8. Among beneficiaries with CKD, 34.3% initiated antihypertensive medication with an ACE-I or ARB (30.7% of blacks and 34.9% of non-blacks).

Discussion

In the current study of a national sample of older hypertensive US adults we found ACE-Is to be the most commonly initiated class of antihypertensive medication, followed by beta blockers, thiazide-type diuretics, CCBs, and ARBs. Initiation of antihyper-

Table 1. Characteristics of Medicare beneficiaries initiating antihypertensive medication, by calendar year.

	Calendar year				
Characteristic	**2007 (n = 7456)**	**2008 (n = 8769)**	**2009 (n = 8575)**	**2010 (n = 8719)**	**p-value for trend**
Age, years	77.0 (7.6)	77.1 (7.7)	76.8 (7.6)	76.7 (7.6)	<0.001
Male	2753 (36.9%)	3310 (37.7%)	3368 (39.3%)	3540 (40.6%)	<0.001
Race/ethnicity					
White	5933 (79.6%)	7117 (81.2%)	7015 (81.8%)	7189 (82.5%)	<0.001
Black	826 (11.1%)	914 (10.4%)	771 (9.0%)	775 (8.9%)	<0.001
Hispanic	270 (3.6%)	301 (3.4%)	307 (3.6%)	283 (3.2%)	0.27
Asian	220 (3.0%)	220 (2.5%)	274 (3.2%)	252 (2.9%)	0.48
Other	207 (2.8%)	217 (2.5%)	208 (2.4%)	220 (2.5%)	0.32
Medicaid buy-in	2007 (26.9%)	1977 (22.5%)	1916 (22.3%)	1857 (21.3%)	<0.001
Diabetes	1966 (26.4%)	2329 (26.6%)	2346 (27.4%)	2463 (28.2%)	0.003
Coronary heart disease	1310 (17.6%)	1496 (17.1%)	1524 (17.8%)	1516 (17.4%)	0.90
Stroke	583 (7.8%)	661 (7.5%)	583 (6.8%)	600 (6.9%)	0.006
Chronic kidney disease	666 (8.9%)	840 (9.6%)	905 (10.6%)	1041 (11.9%)	<0.001
Heart failure	861 (11.5%)	941 (10.7%)	867 (10.1%)	925 (10.6%)	0.03
Any compelling indication†	3585 (48.1%)	4260 (48.6%)	4207 (49.1%)	4394 (50.4%)	0.002

Numbers in table are mean (standard deviation) for age and number (percent) for other characteristics.
†Others include alpha blockers, central acting agents, direct vasodilators, aldosterone receptor blockers, and renin inhibitors.

tensive medication with a thiazide-type diuretic decreased from 19.2% in 2007 to 17.9% in 2010. No other changes in initiation rates by class occurred between 2007 and 2010. Younger age, female sex, and black race were each associated with a higher likelihood for initiating antihypertensive treatment with a thiazide-type diuretic. However, initiating antihypertensive treatment with a thiazide-type diuretic was uncommon (<30%) in all of the subgroups investigated. Additionally, the percent of beneficiaries initiating antihypertensive treatment with multiple medication classes declined over time from 25.6% in 2007 to 24.1% in 2010.

In 2003, JNC 7 recommended thiazide-type diuretics for patients with uncomplicated hypertension initiating antihypertensive treatment [2]. Several studies have found that initiation of antihypertensive treatment with a thiazide-type diuretic increased after the publication of JNC 7 [3–5]. For example, an analysis of data from a national network of clinics in the US found that the percentage of patients initiating antihypertensive medication with

Table 2. Antihypertensive medication classes initiated among Medicare beneficiaries, by calendar year.

	Calendar year				
Antihypertensive medication class	**2007 (n = 7456)**	**2008 (n = 8769)**	**2009 (n = 8575)**	**2010 (n = 8719)**	**p-value for trend**
Renin angiotensin system blockers	3416 (45.8%)	3919 (44.7%)	3914 (45.6%)	3977 (45.6%)	0.82
ACE-inhibitors	2380 (31.9%)	2662 (30.4%)	2712 (31.6%)	2728 (31.3%)	0.87
Angiotensin receptor blockers	1057 (14.2%)	1280 (14.6%)	1214 (14.2%)	1257 (14.4%)	0.90
All Diuretics	2540 (34.1%)	2999 (34.2%)	2845 (33.2%)	2833 (32.5%)	0.03
Thiazide	1433 (19.2%)	1686 (19.2%)	1616 (18.8%)	1565 (17.9%)	0.03
Loop	929 (12.5%)	1094 (12.5%)	1070 (12.5%)	1090 (12.5%)	0.94
Potassium-sparing	230 (3.1%)	291 (3.3%)	241 (2.8%)	241 (2.8%)	0.06
Beta blockers	2009 (26.9%)	2347 (26.8%)	2290 (26.7%)	2344 (26.9%)	0.93
Calcium channel blockers	1322 (17.7%)	1552 (17.7%)	1442 (16.8%)	1503 (17.2%)	0.21
Others†	417 (5.6%)	481 (5.5%)	489 (5.7%)	527 (6.0%)	0.16
Initiating >1 antihypertensive medication class	1908 (25.6%)	2163 (24.7%)	2090 (24.4%)	2102 (24.1%)	0.03
Initiating a combination pill	899 (12.1%)	993 (11.3%)	963 (11.2%)	966 (11.1%)	0.06

Numbers in table are number (percent).
Numbers of antihypertensive medications initiated are not mutually exclusive; column percentages add to >100%.
Abbreviations: ACE = angiotensin-converting enzyme.
†Others include alpha blockers, central acting agents, direct vasodilators, aldosterone receptor blockers, and renin inhibitors.

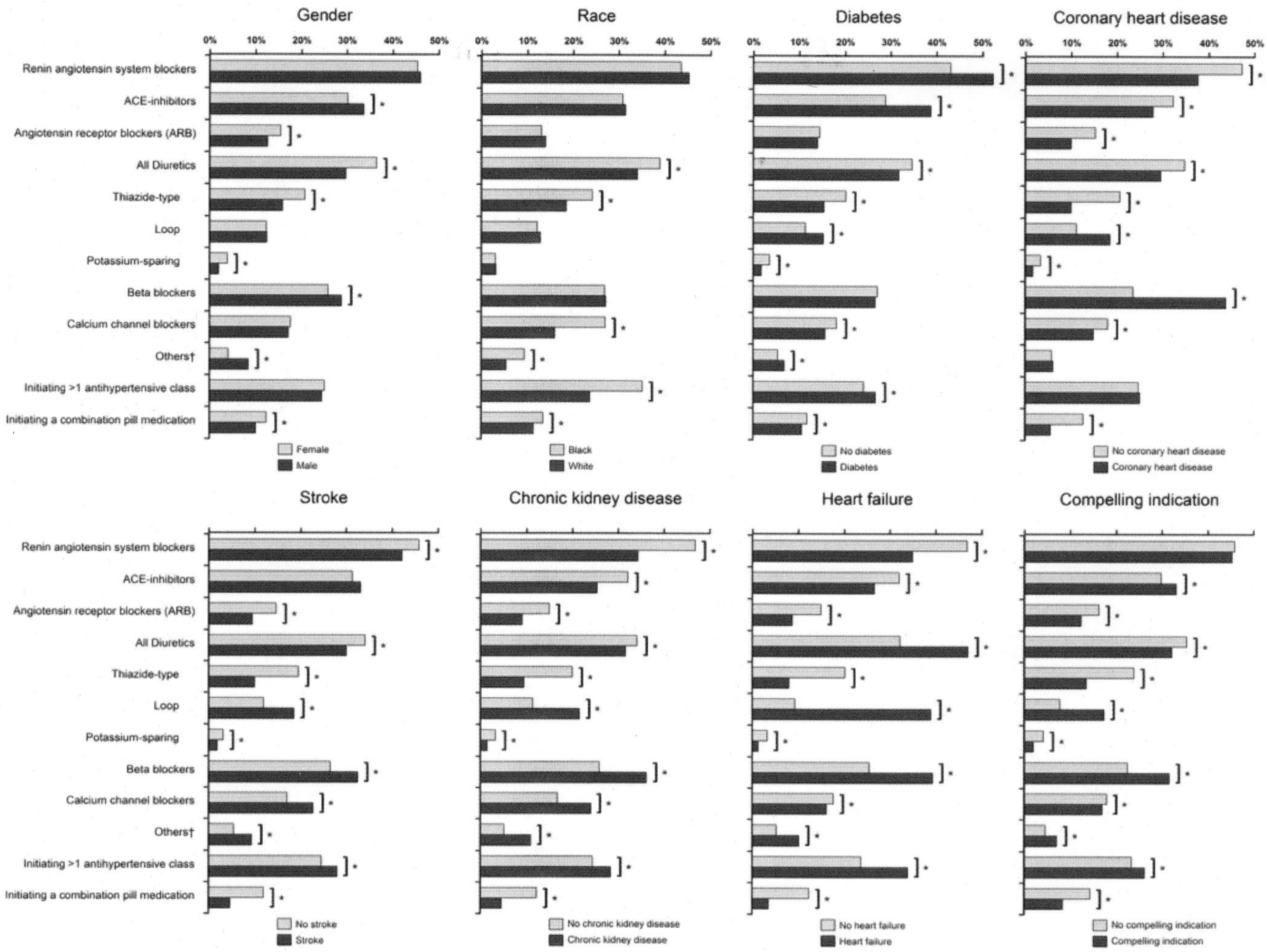

Figure 1. Antihypertensive medication classes initiated among Medicare beneficiaries, by selected covariates. Note: Compelling indication is defined by a beneficiary having diabetes, coronary heart disease, stroke, chronic kidney disease, or heart failure. *$p<0.05$. †Any compelling indication is defined as having diabetes, coronary heart disease, stroke, chronic kidney disease, or heart failure.

a thiazide-type diuretic increased from 29% to 39% after publication of JNC 7 [5]. However, a more recent study in a separate national network of clinics found that only 16% of patients on antihypertensive monotherapy initiated with a thiazide-type diuretic [17]. Results of the current analysis are consistent with the published literature in suggesting that despite the recommendations of the JNC 7 guideline, the majority of US patients do not initiate antihypertensive treatment with a thiazide-type diuretic. Data from the current study also suggest that the proportion of patients initiating antihypertensive medication with a thiazide-type diuretic has decreased modestly in recent years, despite an initial increase following publication of JNC 7. The current study found that the percentages of patients initiating antihypertensive treatment with an ACE-I or CCB were about 31% and 17%, respectively, similar to what has been reported in literature examining initiation rates in the early 2000s [4,5].

Randomized controlled trials following the publication of ALLHAT and JNC 7 that compared cardiovascular risk reduction associated with taking CCBs, ACE-Is, and thiazide-type diuretics have produced mixed results [8–11]. For example, in 2008 a large randomized trial conducted in a high cardiovascular risk hypertensive population reported that combination therapy with an ACE-I and a CCB was superior to the same ACE-I combined with a thiazide-type diuretic in preventing the composite outcome of death from cardiovascular causes, nonfatal myocardial infarction, nonfatal stroke, hospitalization for angina, resuscitation after sudden cardiac arrest, and coronary revascularization (hazard ratio: 0.80; 95% CI: 0.72–0.90) [8]. However, other trials did not find differences in cardiovascular risk associated with ACE-Is [11] or CCBs [10] versus thiazide-type diuretics. In a 2009 pooled analysis of 46 randomized control trials comparing beta blockers, ACE-Is, ARBs, CCBs and thiazide-type diuretics, no drug classes were found to be more effective than others in reducing the incidence of CHD [9]. While CCBs were more effective in preventing stroke compared to other drug classes (relative risk: 0.91; 95% CI: 0.84–0.98), they were less effective in preventing heart failure (relative risk: 1.22; 95% CI: 1.10–1.35). Despite these data, between 2007 and 2010 we found a slight decline in thiazide-type diuretic initiation but did not find a corresponding trend of increasing initiation with an ACE-I or CCB.

Several recent studies have examined prevalent use of antihypertensive medication classes among US adults. The US National Health and Nutrition Examination Survey (NHANES) provide nationally representative data for prevalent antihyperten-

Table 3. Multivariable adjusted risk ratios and 95% confidence intervals for initiating each antihypertensive medication class among Medicare beneficiaries in 2007–2010.

	Antihypertensive medication class initiated							
Characteristic	**ACE-inhibitors (n = 10105)**	**ARBs (n = 4583)**	**Thiazide diuretics (n = 6040)**	**Loop diuretics (n = 3798)**	**Potassium-sparing diuretics (n = 973)**	**Beta blockers (n = 8658)**	**CCBs (n = 593)**	**>1 class (n = 7961)**
Year								
2007	1 (ref)	1 (ref)	ref	1 (ref)	1 (ref)	1 (ref)	1 (ref)	ref
2008	0.95 (0.91–0.99)	1.03 (0.95–1.11)	0.99 (0.93–1.06)	1.03 (0.95–1.11)	1.07 (0.90–1.27)	1.00 (0.95–1.05)	1.00 (0.93–1.07)	0.97 (0.92–1.02)
2009	0.99 (0.95–1.04)	0.99 (0.91–1.06)	0.98 (0.92–1.04)	1.03 (0.95–1.12)	0.93 (0.78–1.11)	1.00 (0.95–1.06)	0.96 (0.90–1.03)	0.97 (0.92–1.03)
2010	0.98 (0.94–1.03)	0.99 (0.92–1.07)	0.92 (0.86–0.98)	1.03 (0.95–1.12)	0.90 (0.75–1.08)	1.01 (0.96–1.06)	0.98 (0.92–1.05)	0.95 (0.90–1.00)
Age								
65–69	1 (ref)	1 (ref)	1 (ref)	1 (ref)	1 (ref)	1 (ref)	1 (ref)	ref
70–74	0.93 (0.89–0.97)	0.95 (0.88–1.03)	0.92 (0.87–0.98)	1.09 (0.98–1.22)	0.99 (0.82–1.18)	1.02 (0.97–1.08)	1.02 (0.94–1.10)	0.90 (0.85–0.95)
75–79	0.85 (0.81–0.90)	0.96 (0.89–1.04)	0.83 (0.77–0.89)	1.41 (1.27–1.56)	0.93 (0.77–1.13)	1.01 (0.96–1.07)	1.16 (1.07–1.25)	0.89 (0.84–0.95)
80–84	0.79 (0.75–0.84)	0.85 (0.78–0.93)	0.78 (0.73–0.84)	1.69 (1.53–1.88)	0.91 (0.74–1.12)	1.09 (1.03–1.15)	1.11 (1.02–1.20)	0.86 (0.81–0.92)
85+	0.73 (0.70–0.78)	0.72 (0.65–0.79)	0.67 (0.62–0.73)	2.23 (2.02 2.46)	0.88 (0.72–1.08)	1.07 (1.01–1.14)	1.20 (1.11–1.30)	0.82 (0.77–0.87)
Male	1.10 (1.06–1.13)	0.84 (0.79–0.88)	0.82 (0.78–0.86)	1.00 (0.95–1.06)	0.55 (0.47–0.64)	1.01 (0.98–1.05)	0.99 (0.94–1.04)	0.95 (0.92–0.99)
Race/ethnicity								
White	1 (ref)	1 (ref)	ref	1 (ref)	1 (ref)	1 (ref)	1 (ref)	1 (ref)
Black	0.95 (0.89–1.00)	1.00 (0.91–1.11)	1.48 (1.38–1.58)	0.80 (0.72–0.88)	1.16 (0.94–1.43)	1.00 (0.95–1.07)	1.68 (1.57–1.80)	1.48 (1.40–1.56)
Hispanic	1.14 (1.05–1.24)	1.28 (1.12–1.48)	1.01 (0.88–1.16)	0.66 (0.55–0.79)	0.61 (0.37–1.02)	0.96 (0.87–1.07)	1.07 (0.93–1.23)	1.03 (0.92–1.15)
Asian	0.73 (0.65–0.82)	1.80 (1.59 2.04)	0.90 (0.77–1.06)	0.48 (0.38–0.61)	0.72 (0.44–1.16)	1.04 (0.93–1.16)	1.51 (1.33–1.71)	1.00 (0.88–1.14)
Other	1.03 (0.93–1.13)	1.22 (1.04–1.43)	0.94 (0.80–1.09)	0.82 (0.67–1.01)	1.19 (0.81–1.74)	0.94 (0.83–1.06)	1.44 (1.26–1.64)	1.20 (1.07–1.35)
Medicaid buy-in	1.01 (0.96–1.05)	0.84 (0.78–0.90)	0.79 (0.74–0.84)	1.33 (1.25–1.42)	0.67 (0.56–0.80)	0.97 (0.93–1.02)	0.95 (0.90–1.01)	0.88 (0.83–0.92)
Diabetes	1.35 (1.30–1.39)	1.01 (0.95–1.08)	0.82 (0.78–0.87)	1.25 (1.18–1.33)	0.58 (0.48–0.69)	0.91 (0.88–0.95)	0.83 (0.78–0.88)	1.06 (1.01–1.10)
Coronary heart disease	0.86 (0.82–0.90)	0.75 (0.69–0.82)	0.60 (0.55–0.65)	1.12 (1.05–1.20)	0.63 (0.51–0.79)	1.74 (1.67–1.81)	0.83 (0.77–0.89)	0.96 (0.91–1.01)
Stroke	1.12 (1.05–1.19)	0.73 (0.64–0.83)	0.60 (0.53–0.68)	1.13 (1.03–1.24)	0.71 (0.52–0.97)	1.12 (1.05–1.19)	1.25 (1.16–1.36)	1.08 (1.01–1.16)
Chronic kidney disease	0.79 (0.74–0.84)	0.73 (0.65–0.81)	0.62 (0.55–0.69)	1.19 (1.10–1.28)	0.64 (0.48–0.86)	1.20 (1.14–1.27)	1.47 (1.37–1.57)	1.06 (1.00–1.13)
Heart failure	0.90 (0.85–0.96)	0.72 (0.65–0.81)	0.54 (0.48–0.61)	3.23 (3.03 3.45)	0.52 (0.38–0.71)	1.25 (1.19–1.32)	0.85 (0.78–0.92)	1.45 (1.37–1.53)

Abbreviations: ACE = angiotensin-converting-enzyme; ARB = Angiotensin receptor blocker; CCB = Calcium channel blocker. The comparison group for each medication class initiated is not initiating that medication class. The comparison group for initiating more than one antihypertensive medication class is initiating only one medication class.

sive medication use. In an analysis of serial NHANES, the overall percentage of individuals with hypertension taking thiazide-type diuretics rose from 22% in 2001–2002 to 28% in 2009–2010 [18]. However, this analysis also found that the percentage of individuals taking ACE-Is, beta blockers, CCBs, or ARBs all rose over the past decade. In addition, antihypertensive polypharmacy has increased over the past decade. Between 2001–2002 and 2009–2010, the percent of US adults with hypertension taking 2 or more classes of antihypertensive medications increased from 37% to 48% [18]. The current study found that the percentage of older US adults initiating antihypertensive treatment with 2 or more classes of medication decreased, albeit modestly, between 2007 and 2010. In the context of the published literature on prevalent antihypertensive medication use, the findings from the current study suggest that patients are increasingly initiating antihypertensive medication with a single class and are subsequently up-titrated to a regimen that includes multiple classes of antihypertensive medication to control blood pressure. This interpretation is supported by a recent study which found that, following publication of JNC 7, patients were initiating antihypertensive medications at a lower systolic and diastolic blood pressure threshold, and thus were less likely to have an indication for multiple classes of medications at the start of therapy [19].

The current study provides data on antihypertensive medication initiation patterns among older US adults in the time period between publication of the JNC 7 and JNC 8 guidelines. Whereas JNC 7 recommended a thiazide-type diuretic as first-line therapy for newly diagnosed patients with hypertension and no other compelling indications, the recently published JNC 8 guideline suggests that in the general nonblack population, including those with diabetes, the initial antihypertensive treatment regimen should include a thiazide-type diuretic, CCB, ACE-I, or ARB. In the general black population, initial antihypertensive treatment should include a thiazide-type diuretic or CCB. Other classes of antihypertensive medication (e.g., beta blockers, alpha blockers) are not recommended for use as first-line antihypertensive therapy in the JNC 8 guideline. Whereas JNC 7 listed several comorbidities that were compelling indications for specific medication classes, JNC 8 only recommended an ACE-I or ARB for those with CKD. We found that 61.9% of Medicare beneficiaries initiated antihypertensive medication in 2007–2010 with an antihypertensive medication class recommended by JNC 8. While this compares favorably to studies that have consistently shown that <40% of patients initiated antihypertensive medication with a thiazide-type diuretic following JNC 7, whether the JNC 8 guideline will affect treatment regimens for patients initiating antihypertensive medication is not yet known and should be investigated in future studies.

Our study has several strengths. We used national data on US adults 65 years of age and older from Medicare. Identifying treatment patterns among older adults is important given their high incidence of hypertension [20] and increased risk for adverse blood pressure-related outcomes including CHD, stroke and end-stage renal disease [21]. Most prior studies have relied on prevalent users of antihypertensive medication. Using Medicare, we were able to assess the initiation of, and secular trends in, antihypertensive medication classes through 2010. This study also has limitations. As with all claims-based analyses, our results depend on the accuracy of claims to identify comorbid conditions and pharmacy fills. While claims-based algorithms for CHD, stroke, diabetes and heart failure have high positive predictive value, algorithms for identifying CKD in Medicare do not [22]. In addition, some beneficiaries may not have submitted claims for reimbursement when initiating antihypertensive medication. However, prior studies suggest that out-of-pocket payments for generic medications among Medicare beneficiaries are not common [23].

Conclusions

Despite the recommendation in JNC 7, in this nationwide study, less than 1 in 5 Medicare beneficiaries initiated antihypertensive medication with a thiazide-type diuretic. The proportion initiating antihypertensive treatment with a thiazide-type diuretic was higher in those without comorbid conditions, but remained below 30% in every subgroup investigated. These data suggest a disconnect between US national guidelines and clinical practice for the treatment of hypertension. Over 30% of Medicare beneficiaries initiated antihypertensive medication with drug classes not recommended as first line therapy in the 2014 JNC 8 guideline. Effective dissemination efforts for the JNC 8 guideline are needed to ensure that patients receive appropriate antihypertensive treatment.

Supporting Information

Figure S1 CONSORT diagram for the analysis Medicare beneficiaries initiating antihypertensive treatment.

Table S1 Most common pairs of antihypertensive medication classes initiated in the pooled 2007–2010 5% Medicare sample who initiated >1 antihypertensive medication, by calendar year.

Table S2 Multivariable adjusted risk ratios for initiating each antihypertensive medication class in the pooled 2007–2010 5% Medicare sample without any compelling indication.

Appendix S1 Compelling indication history claims algorithm definitions.

Author Contributions

Conceived and designed the experiments: STK PM. Analyzed the data: LH. Wrote the paper: STK. Supervised the project: STK PM. Provided medical expertise and input into the study design: SO DS. Contributed to the design of the analyses and provided interpretation of the results: LH. Provided Medicare data expertise and guidance of interpretation of the results: MLK PM. Critical review of the manuscript for content: STK PM DS SO LH MLK KMD.

References

1. Allhat Officers and Coordinators for the Allhat Collaborative Research Group The Antihypertensive Lipid-Lowering Treatment to Prevent Heart Attack Trial (2002) Major outcomes in high-risk hypertensive patients randomized to angiotensin-converting enzyme inhibitor or calcium channel blocker vs diuretic: The Antihypertensive and Lipid-Lowering Treatment to Prevent Heart Attack Trial (ALLHAT). JAMA 288: 2981–2997.
2. Chobanian AV, Bakris GL, Black HR, Cushman WC, Green LA, et al. (2003) The Seventh Report of the Joint National Committee on Prevention, Detection, Evaluation, and Treatment of High Blood Pressure: the JNC 7 report. JAMA 289: 2560–2572. doi: 10.1001/jama.289.19.2560.
3. Xie F, Petitti DB, Chen W (2005) Prescribing patterns for antihypertensive drugs after the Antihypertensive and Lipid-Lowering Treatment to Prevent Heart

Attack Trial: report of experience in a health maintenance organization. Am J Hypertens 18: 464–469. doi: 10.1016/j.amjhyper.2004.11.004.
4. Muntner P, Krousel-Wood M, Hyre AD, Stanley E, Cushman WC, et al. (2009) Antihypertensive prescriptions for newly treated patients before and after the main antihypertensive and lipid-lowering treatment to prevent heart attack trial results and seventh report of the joint national committee on prevention, detection, evaluation, and treatment of high blood pressure guidelines. Hypertension 53: 617–623. doi: 10.1161/HYPERTENSIONAHA.108.120154.
5. Player MS, Gill JM, Fagan HB, Mainous AG, 3rd (2006) Antihypertensive prescribing practices: impact of the antihypertensive and lipid-lowering treatment to prevent heart attack trial. J Clin Hypertens (Greenwich) 8: 860–864.
6. Bian B, Kelton CM, Guo JJ, Wigle PR (2010) ACE Inhibitor and ARB utilization and expenditures in the Medicaid fee-for-service program from 1991 to 2008. J Manag Care Pharm 16: 671–679.
7. Brendt ER, Aitken ML (2011) Brand Loyalty, Generic Entry and Price Competition in Pharmaceuticals in the Quarter Century after the 1984 Waxman-Hatch Legislation. Int J Econ Bus 18: 177–201.
8. Jamerson K, Weber MA, Bakris GL, Dahlof B, Pitt B, et al. (2008) Benazepril plus amlodipine or hydrochlorothiazide for hypertension in high-risk patients. N Engl J Med 359: 2417–2428. doi: 10.1056/NEJMoa0806182.
9. Law MR, Morris JK, Wald NJ (2009) Use of blood pressure lowering drugs in the prevention of cardiovascular disease: meta-analysis of 147 randomised trials in the context of expectations from prospective epidemiological studies. BMJ 338: b1665. doi: 10.1136/bmj.b1665.
10. Black HR, Elliott WJ, Grandits G, Grambsch P, Lucente T, et al. (2003) Principal results of the Controlled Onset Verapamil Investigation of Cardiovascular End Points (CONVINCE) trial. JAMA 289: 2073–2082. doi: 10.1001/jama.289.16.2073.
11. Wing LM, Reid CM, Ryan P, Beilin LJ, Brown MA, et al. (2003) A comparison of outcomes with angiotensin-converting–enzyme inhibitors and diuretics for hypertension in the elderly. N Engl J Med 348: 583–592. doi: 10.1056/NEJMoa021716.
12. Malacco E, Mancia G, Rappelli A, Menotti A, Zuccaro MS, et al. (2003) Treatment of isolated systolic hypertension: the SHELL study results. Blood Press 12: 160–167.
13. Mancia G, De Backer G, Dominiczak A, Cifkova R, Fagard R, et al. (2007) 2007 Guidelines for the Management of Arterial Hypertension: The Task Force for the Management of Arterial Hypertension of the European Society of Hypertension (ESH) and of the European Society of Cardiology (ESC). J Hypertens 25: 1105–1187. doi: 10.1097/HJH.0b013e3281fc975a.
14. Whitworth JA, World Health Organization ISoHWG (2003) 2003 World Health Organization (WHO)/International Society of Hypertension (ISH) statement on management of hypertension. J Hypertens 21: 1983–1992. doi: 10.1097/01.hjh.0000084751.37215.d2.
15. Rosendorff C, Black HR, Cannon CP, Gersh BJ, Gore J, et al. (2007) Treatment of hypertension in the prevention and management of ischemic heart disease: a scientific statement from the American Heart Association Council for High Blood Pressure Research and the Councils on Clinical Cardiology and Epidemiology and Prevention. Circulation 115: 2761–2788. doi: 10.1161/CIRCULATIONAHA.107.183885.
16. James PA, Oparil S, Carter BL, Cushman WC, Dennison-Himmelfarb C, et al. (2013) 2014 Evidence-Based Guideline for the Management of High Blood Pressure in Adults: Report From the Panel Members Appointed to the Eighth Joint National Committee (JNC 8). JAMA. December 18, 2013 ed.
17. Egan BM, Bandyopadhyay D, Shaftman SR, Wagner CS, Zhao Y, et al. (2012) Initial monotherapy and combination therapy and hypertension control the first year. Hypertension 59: 1124–1131. doi: 10.1161/HYPERTENSIONAHA.112.194167.
18. Gu Q, Burt VL, Dillon CF, Yoon S (2012) Trends in antihypertensive medication use and blood pressure control among United States adults with hypertension: the National Health And Nutrition Examination Survey, 2001 to 2010. Circulation 126: 2105–2114. doi: 10.1161/CIRCULATIONAHA.112.096156.
19. Krousel-Wood M, Muntner P, Carson A, Anderson AH, Delaune E, et al. (2012) Hypertension control among newly treated patients before and after publication of the main ALLHAT results and JNC 7 guidelines. J Clin Hypertens (Greenwich) 14: 277–283. doi: 10.1111/j.1751-7176.2012.00609.x.
20. Carson AP, Howard G, Burke GL, Shea S, Levitan EB, et al. (2011) Ethnic differences in hypertension incidence among middle-aged and older adults: the multi-ethnic study of atherosclerosis. Hypertension 57: 1101–1107. doi: 10.1161/HYPERTENSIONAHA.110.168005.
21. Go AS, Mozaffarian D, Roger VL, Benjamin EJ, Berry JD, et al. (2014) Heart disease and stroke statistics–2014 update: a report from the american heart association. Circulation 129: e28–e292. doi: 10.1161/01.cir.0000441139.02102.80.
22. Vlasschaert ME, Bejaimal SA, Hackam DG, Quinn R, Cuerden MS, et al. (2011) Validity of administrative database coding for kidney disease: a systematic review. Am J Kidney Dis 57: 29–43. doi: 10.1053/j.ajkd.2010.08.031.
23. Yun H, Curtis JR, Saag K, Kilgore M, Muntner P, et al. (2013) Generic alendronate use among Medicare beneficiaries: are Part D data complete? Pharmacoepidemiol Drug Saf 22: 55–63. doi: 10.1002/pds.3361.

Lower Blood Glucose and Variability Are Associated with Earlier Recovery from Renal Injury Caused by Episodic Urinary Tract Infection in Advanced Type 2 Diabetic Chronic Kidney Disease

Ping-Fang Chiu[1,2,3], Chia-Lin Wu[3], Ching-Hui Huang[4], Hung-Hsiang Liou[3], Chirn-Bin Chang[3], Horng-Rong Chang[1,2,5]9, Chia-Chu Chang[2,3,6]*9

1 Institute of Medicine, Chung Shan Medical University, Taichung, Taiwan, **2** School of Medicine, Chung Shan Medical University, Taichung, Taiwan, **3** Nephrology Division, Department of Internal Medicine, Changhua Christian Hospital, Changhua, Taiwan, **4** Division of Cardiology, Department of Internal Medicine, Changhua Christian Hospital, Changhua, Taiwan, **5** Division of Nephrology, Department of Internal Medicine, Chung Shan Medical University Hospital, Taichung, Taiwan, **6** Ph.D. Program for Aging, College of Medicine, China Medical University, Taichung, Taiwan

Abstract

Purpose: In our previous study, type 2 diabetic chronic kidney disease (CKD) patients with glomerular filtration rates of <30 mL/min upon hospitalization for urinary tract infection (UTI) were at a risk for acute kidney injury. This study aimed to clarify the effect of glucose and its variability on renal outcomes during admission for the treatment of UTI.

Materials and Methods: Based on the date of renal recovery (RIFLE criteria: acute kidney injury occurred within 1–7 days and was sustained over 1 day), we divided these patients into early- (≤9 days, Group A) and late-recovery (>9 days, Group B) groups. The differences in the continuous and categorical variables of the two groups were assessed separately. The mean glucose levels and their variability (using the standard deviation and the coefficient of standard deviation) were compared at the fasting, midday pre-meal, evening pre-meal, and evening post-meal time points during hospitalization. We have organized the manuscript in a manner compliant with the STROBE (Strengthening the Reporting of Observational Studies in Epidemiology) statement.

Results: Acute kidney injury occurred within the two groups ($p = 0.007$ and $p = 0.001$, respectively). The early-morning blood glucose levels (149.7±44.0 mg/dL) and average blood glucose levels (185.6±52.0 mg/dL) were better in Group A ($p = 0.01$, $p = 0.02$). Group A patients also had lower glucose variability than Group B at the different time points ($p < 0.05$). Group A also had earlier renal recovery. More relevant pathogens were identified from blood in Group B ($p = 0.038$).

Conclusions: Early-morning fasting and mean blood glucose levels and their variability can be good indicators of severe infection and predictors of renal outcome in type 2 diabetic patients with CKD and UTI.

Editor: Francesca D'Addio, San Raffaele Hospital, Italy

Funding: The study was supported by a research grant (97CCHIRP-31) from Changhua Christian Hospital. The funders had no role in study design, data collection and analysis, decision to publish, or preparation of the manuscript.

Competing Interests: The authors have declared that no competing interests exist.

* Email: 27509@cch.org.tw

9 These authors contributed equally to this work.

Introduction

Urinary tract infection (UTI) is a common disease in type 1 and 2 diabetic patients, and diabetic patients are prone to UTI as well [1]. Among diabetic patients, 9–20% of women and 3–11% of men may develop UTI [2], which may result in longer hospitalizations (3- to 5-fold) [3] and higher mortality (7.6% versus 1.6%) [4] in patients with diabetes than in those without diabetes. Additionally, in a previous study, we found that UTI can also lead to acute kidney injury (AKI) in type 2 diabetic chronic kidney disease (CKD) patients who had an estimated glomerular filtration rate (eGFR) of <30 mL/min on admission [5]. Furthermore, AKI episodes can be independent risk factors for renal progression in diabetes CKD patients [6]. The RIFLE criteria for AKI were defined according to the Acute Dialysis Quality Initiative consensus in 2002, and denoted that GFR can abruptly decrease by more than 25% within 1–7 days after admission and may be sustained for longer than 1 day. For almost all type 2 diabetic patients with advanced CKD, renal dysfunction did gradually revert within 6 months after the UTI if they survived and were free from long-term dialysis [5]. The rate of renal recovery was also essential; a shorter recovery period would

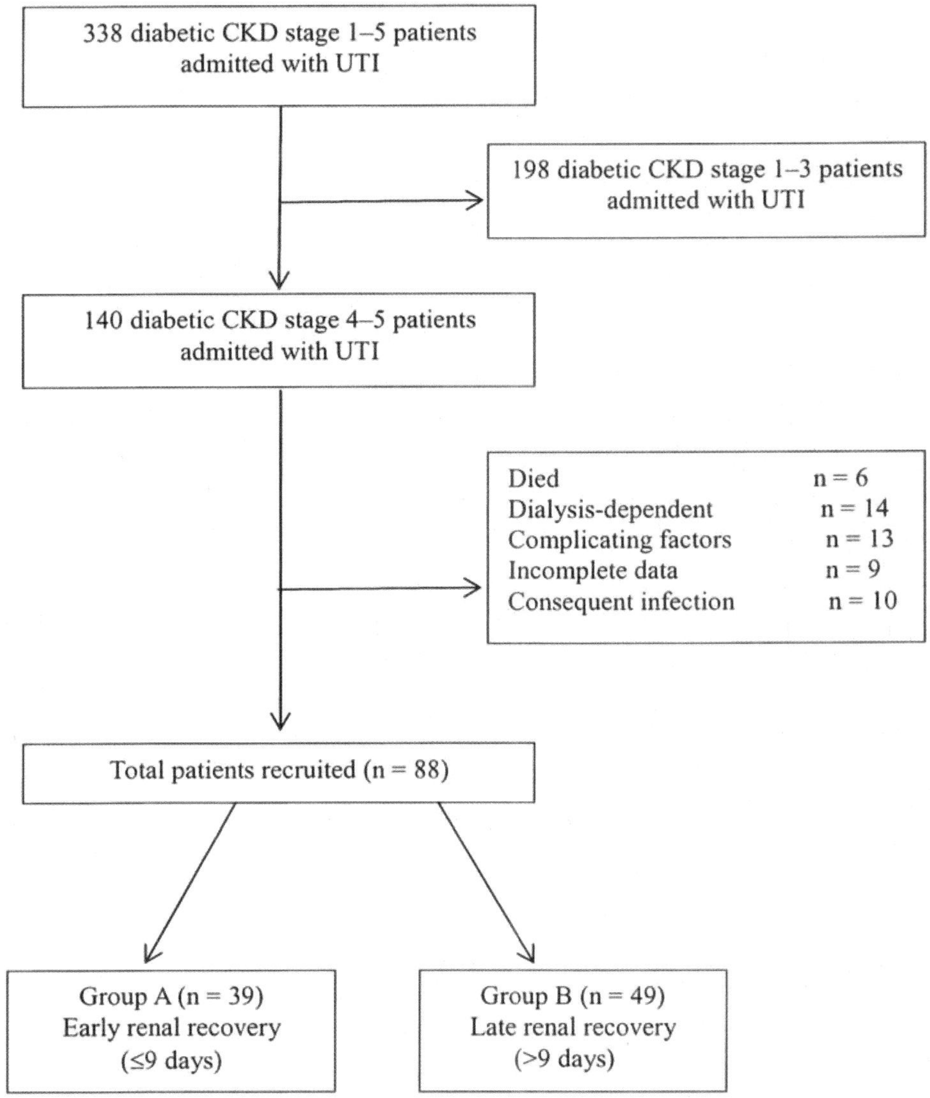

Figure 1. Participant flow diagram depicting the screening/enrollment process.

improve health and reduce the risk of another episode of infection. Possible factors that could affect renal recovery included the baseline GFR, severity or duration of sepsis, and concurrent co-morbidities. Critically ill patients with lower glucose variability have lower short-term or hospital mortality than patients with higher glucose variability [7]. However, the impact of glucose and its fluctuations on renal function during hospitalization from nonfatal infection has not been reported. This study aimed to clarify the association of glucose and its variability during admission and renal outcome in type 2 diabetic patients with CKD and episodic UTI.

Materials and Methods

We enrolled patients that had been managed under CKD care programs, who also had UTI and were admitted to our hospital from 2001 to November 2013. The admission criteria for UTI in our hospital included the presence of a systemic inflammatory response syndrome or a complicated condition involving a major organ. We excluded patients who had untreated obstructive uropathy, those who died, those who were dialysis-dependent after infection, or those who had subsequent hospital-acquired infections. To improve the quality of reporting in observational studies, the manuscript was organized in a manner compliant with the STROBE (Strengthening the Reporting of Observational Studies in Epidemiology) statement [8]. The patient flow chart is shown in Figure 1, which includes the number of patients recruited and excluded from the study. The Modification of the Diet in Renal Disease (MDRD) formula was applied for GFR estimation. The formula used for eGFR was the following:

$$\begin{aligned} \text{GFR (mL/min/1.73 m}^2) = 186 \times \text{serum creatinine}^{-1.154} \\ \times \text{age}^{-0.203} \\ \times 1.212 \text{ (if black)}. \end{aligned}$$

AKI was defined using the RIFLE criteria. When the decrease in eGFR returned to <10% of baseline renal function, the patient was determined to be in renal recovery as defined in previously published manuscripts [9,10]. Based on the date of renal recovery

Table 1. Patient characteristics.

	Group A (n = 39)		Group B (n = 49)		
	Mean	**SD**	**Mean**	**SD**	*p*
Age‡	67.8	8.7	68.4	14.1	0.80
Gender, male†	26.3%		26.5%		0.98
Hypertension†	76.3%		63.3%		0.009*
CVD†	23.7%		24.5%		0.86
Hyperlipidemia†	18.4%		16.3%		0.61
Liver†	15.8%		16.3%		0.89
Stroke†	21.1%		22.5%		0.75
SBP (mmHg)‡	135	26	121	17	0.057
DBP (mmHg)‡	73	17	72	13	0.78
eGFR (ml/min)‡	16.9	7.9	15.4	7.7	0.47
BUN (mg/dL)‡	61.4	41.7	59.6	33.6	0.84
Cr (mg/dL)‡	4.09	2.9	3.99	2.3	0.86
ALT (U/L)‡	23.3	12.3	34.6	29.6	0.03*
HbA1C (%)‡	7.7	2.0	8.2	2.8	0.30
Cholesterol (mg/dL)‡	150.8	62.1	169.6	60	0.79
Triglyceride (mg/dL)‡	170.3	77.9	209.5	80.1	0.51
HDL (mg/dL)‡	37.7	12.8	39.4	17.7	0.90
LDL (mg/dL)‡	89.8	35.6	102.9	44.8	0.76
Uric acid (mg/dL)‡	6.3	1.6	7.9	2.2	0.08
Albumin (g/dL)‡	2.8	0.7	2.7	0.6	0.37
Na (mEq/dL)‡	132.3	6.8	133.0	7.0	0.61
K (mEq/dL)‡	4.6	1.0	4.2	1.1	0.15
WBC ($\times 10^3$)‡	11.3	5.5	13.5	8.3	0.10
Hemoglobin (g/dL)‡	10.4	2.4	10.2	2.5	0.72
Hematocrit (%)‡	30.5	7.7	30.0	7.4	0.77
UPCR (g/g)‡	1.8	2.0	1.1	1.2	0.31
Hospital days§	6.78	3.68	11.5	10.8	0.019*
(median)	6.0		7.5		

Abbreviations: CVD, cardiovascular disease; ALT, alanine aminotransferase; WBC, white blood cell; UPCR, urine protein–creatinine ratio; SBP, systolic blood pressure; DBP, diastolic blood pressure.
†chi-square test.
‡student's t-test.
§Mann–Whitney U test.
*$p<0.05$.

Table 2. Blood glucose levels and renal outcome.

	Group A		Group B		
Glucose (mg/dL)	**mean**	**SD**	**mean**	**SD**	*p*
Fasting	149.7	44.0	181.2	64.5	0.01*
Midday pre-meal	203.7	60.8	228.5	81.9	0.17
Evening pre-meal	209.9	62.5	234.6	74.4	0.11
Evening post-meal	216.0	54.5	228.2	68.8	0.41
mean	185.6	52.0	216.7	69.5	0.02*

Abbreviation: SD, standard deviation.
*$p<0.05$.

Table 3. Glucose variability: standard deviation (SD) and renal outcome.

	Group A		Group B		
Glucose (mg/dL)	**SD mean**	**SD**	**SD mean**	**SD**	***p***
Fasting	46.6	37.9	64.0	32.6	0.03*
Midday pre-meal	64.6	40.1	72.1	40.2	0.46
Evening pre-meal	66.1	37.4	84.6	40.5	0.04*
Evening post-meal	64.0	37.7	83.0	38.3	0.04*

*$p<0.05$.

(GFR decrease within 1–7 days and that was sustained for longer than 1 day) after admission, we divided these patients into early- (≤9 days, Group A) and late-recovery (>9 days, Group B) groups. The basic characteristics of these patients were collected and analyzed in Table 1. The continuous and categorical variable differences, including blood glucose (Table 2–4) and bacteriology (Table 5), of the two groups were assayed separately by the Student's t-test, the Mann–Whitney U test, and the chi-squared test. The mean glucose level and its variability (calculated by the standard deviation and the coefficient of standard deviation: SD/mean) at four fixed time points (fasting, midday pre-meal, evening pre-meal, evening post-meal) during the hospitalization were compared. The patients' survival rates after episodic UTI were analyzed using the Kaplan–Meier method.

Ethics Statement

The CKD care program including ethics and patients' right was guided by the Clinical Care Program Certification and Joint Commission International. This protocol was also approved by the Institutional Review Board of the Changhua Christian Hospital, Taiwan. All subjects gave written informed consent to participate. If patients could not be contacted in any way, the data were categorized as incomplete.

Results

One hundred and forty diabetic CKD patients with eGFR of <30 mL/min who were admitted to the hospital with UTI during the 13 years were evaluated for the study. Fifty-two patients had been excluded because of various causes as reported in Figure 1. Eighty-eight patients (65 females, 23 males) were included. Thirty-nine patients had recovered renal function early (≤9 days, Group A), and 49 patients recovered function late (>9 days, Group B). The baseline characteristics of the patients are listed in Table 1. The age and incidence of comorbidities, such as cardiovascular disease, stroke, and liver disease, were compared between the two groups. The biochemical and hematological data were balanced in both groups, with the exception of alanine aminotransferase (ALT). The estimated GFR series are illustrated in Figure 2. AKI occurred during admission in the two groups ($p=0.007$ and $p=0.001$, respectively), and almost all diabetic patients gradually recovered within 6 months. In contrast, 34 non-diabetic CKD stage 4–5 patients (n = 544; 0.063%, data not shown) were admitted for urosepsis during this period. No significant AKI was observed ($p=0.39$, data not shown).

Microorganisms detected in blood were more notable in Group B (Table 5; $p=0.038$). Urine pathogen culture rates found between both groups were comparable. E. coli was the most commonly isolated pathogen. Moreover, approximately 32% (12 in Group A; 16 in Group B) of patients had cystitis within 3 months before the urosepsis episodes. Two-week antibiotic regimens were prescribed at least for patients with complicated UTI, including first- and second-generation cephalosporins and third-generation cephalosporin/or quinolone (33, 6 in group A; 38, 11 in Group B, respectively). Aminoglycosides were avoided owing to their nephrotoxicity.

The mean early-morning blood glucose levels (149.7±44.0 mg/dL) and average blood glucose levels (185.6±52.0 mg/dL) were better in Group A ($p=0.01$, $p=0.02$; Table 2). Patients in Group A also had lower glucose variability based on the differences in the standard deviation and the coefficient of variation (SD/mean) than patients in Group B at the different time points. There was more relevance in the fasting and the evening post-meal blood glucose levels (Table 3 and 4; $p<0.05$). The trend of glucose variability was also consistently observed at the midday pre-meal and evening pre-meal time points.

The two groups had equivalent long-term patient survival (data not shown). We also adjusted for possible confounding factors that may have contributed to renal recovery using multivariate cox

Table 4. Glucose variability: coefficient of variation (CV) and renal outcome.

	Group A		Group B		
Glucose (mg/dL)	**CV mean**	**SD**	**CV mean**	**SD**	***p***
Fasting	0.29	0.19	0.36	0.14	0.001*
Midday pre-meal	0.30	0.15	0.32	0.16	0.03*
Evening pre-meal	0.32	0.18	0.36	0.15	0.13
Evening post-meal	0.28	0.13	0.35	0.15	0.02*

*$p<0.05$.

Table 5. Bacteriology.

	Group A	Group B	*p*
Blood culture	7	17	0.038*
GNB	5	15	
GPC	2	2	
Urine culture	34	39	0.18
GNB	21	30	
GPC	5	6	
fungus	5	2	
others	3	1	

Abbreviations: GNB, gram-negative bacillus; GPC, gram-positive cocci.
chi-square test.
*$p<0.05$.

proportional hazard regression, including age, severity of infection, and glucose and blood pressure control (Table 6).

Discussion

Diabetes and its complications are the leading cause of end-stage renal disease worldwide. Diabetes patients are vulnerable to UTI. Further, UTI may cause AKI in diabetic CKD patients with an eGFR of <30 mL/min. Furthermore, repeated episodes of AKI are related to rapid progression of renal-failure. The main finding of this study was that better blood glucose control and lower glucose variability during hospitalization in type 2 diabetic patients with CKD could predict earlier renal recovery from UTI.

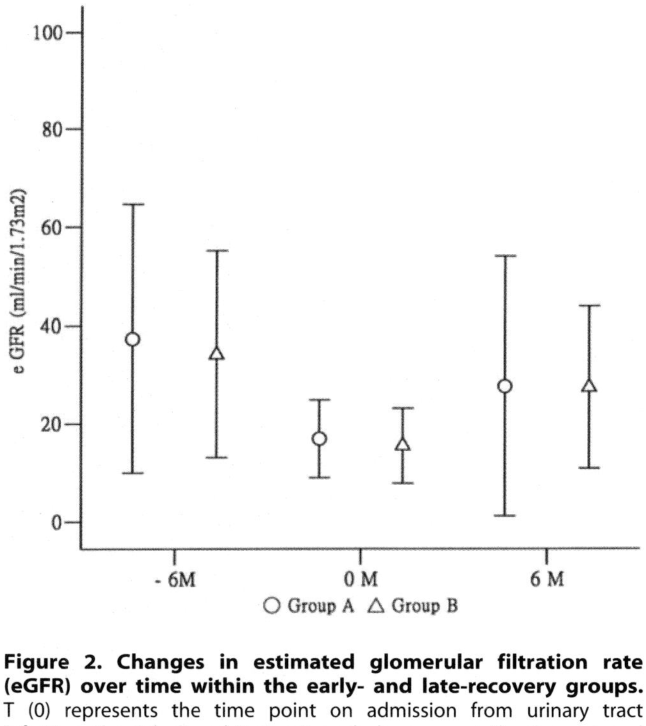

Figure 2. Changes in estimated glomerular filtration rate (eGFR) over time within the early- and late-recovery groups. T (0) represents the time point on admission from urinary tract infection; the "plus" and "minus" symbols represent the time interval after and before admission, respectively. Acute kidney injury occurred in diabetic patients with chronic kidney disease [eGFR at T (0) versus T (−6); $p=0.007$ in Group A; $p=0.001$ in Group B], and eGFR reverted to the trend 6 months later if urinary tract infection was cured.

Because these patients were not critically ill and remained in the ward, glucose measurement at four different time points (fasting, midday pre-meal, evening pre-meal, evening post-meal) was applicable, instead of continued glucose monitoring.

High glycosylated hemoglobin in the diabetic population has been associated with a high incidence of microangiopathy, macroangiopathy, and mortality [11]. Long-term glucose variability has also played a role in the development of microangiopathy and macroangiopathy [12,13]. A study by Monnier et al even suggested that glucose variability may be more deleterious than chronic hyperglycemia in the development of diabetic complications [14]. Acute blood glucose fluctuations during hospitalization for various critical conditions have predicted short-term or in-hospital mortality [15]. The better outcomes were obtained in critical patients with lower glucose variability. This scenario was also found in non-diabetic critically ill patients [16]. Jeon et al demonstrated that pre- and post-operative glucose levels and their variability were associated with the risk of surgical site infection or in-hospital death [17]. Additionally, increased blood glucose variability during hospitalization has been a precursor of sepsis and mortality in burn patients as reported by Alexander et al [18]. Furthermore, a meta-analysis by Haga et al revealed that tight glycemic control might reduce early mortality, the incidence of atrial fibrillation, and the time spent in the intensive care unit after cardiac surgery [19].

In contrast, in data from the reanalysis of the HEART2D study, Siegelaar et al found that a decrease in glucose variability did not reduce cardiovascular events in type 2 diabetic patients after an acute myocardial infarction [20]. The tight blood glucose control in critical patients does not reduce mortality but does increase the risk of hypoglycemia according to meta-analysis studies [21,22]. In the NICE-SUGAR Study, a blood glucose target of 180 mg/dL or less resulted in lower mortality than did a target of 81–108 mg/dL [23]. For non-critically-ill patients treated with insulin, according to the Standards of Medical Care in Diabetes 2013, the pre-meal glucose target should be around 140 mg/dL and post-meal glucose target should be around 180 mg/dL [24]. However, because advanced CKD diabetic patients can be at higher risk of hypoglycemia, sugar control that is less tight seems reasonable. Nevertheless, no current guidelines have been recommended for these patients.

Several possible mechanisms may account for chronic glucose variability. Short-term Type 1 diabetes mellitus (DM) participants with residual β-cell function had lower glucose variability than longer-term Type 1 DM participants (27% versus 42%, respec-

Table 6. Cox proportional hazard regression: hazard ratio of variables and renal injury.

Variable	HR	95% CI	*p*
Glucose (mean)	1.006	1.002–1.010	0.003*
Age	0.979	0.951–1.008	0.150
Hypertension	0.329	0.174–0.619	0.001*
WBC	0.955	0.889–1.025	0.202
HbA1C	0.957	0.844–1.086	0.498

*$p<0.05$.

tively; $p<0.001$) [25]. An autonomic imbalance from increased hypothalamic-pituitary axis activity and cortisol levels can also lead to worsening glucose variability and neuropathy [26,27]. The study by Monnier et al indicated that acute glucose excursion triggered more oxidative stress than chronic sustained hyperglycemia in type 2 diabetic patients. There is a linear correlation between 24-hour urinary excretion rates of 8-Iso Prostaglandin F2 and glycemic variability [28]. The antidiabetic agents, dipeptidyl peptidase IV inhibitors, were found to reduce glucose fluctuations and plasma nitrotyrosine, IL-6, and IL-18 levels ($p<0.05$) in type 2 diabetic patients after 3 months of treatment [29]. Additionally, acute glucose elevation can be highly predictive of infection in critically injured trauma patients, as reported by Bochicchio et al [30]. In our study, it was evident that increased glucose variability in type 2 diabetic patients with CKD and eGFR of <30 mL/min could have delayed the renal recovery from UTI. Additionally, those who had delayed renal recovery also had longer hospital stays.

Another interesting finding was the remarkable pathogen identification rate from blood in Group B. Both C-reactive protein and procalcitonin concentrations can suggest bacterial infection in emergency patients [31,32]. This may imply that hospitalized patients with higher blood glucose and greater variability were in course of more severe inflammation and oxidative stress. Perhaps, infections with concurrent glucose variability may simultaneously influence renal injury and recovery. Elevated liver enzymes were frequently found in septic conditions. Several hepatic biomarkers, including bilirubin, albumin, alkaline phosphatase, aspartate, ALTs, and lactate dehydrogenase, had been evaluated in association with the mortality rate in the intensive care unit by Marshall et al. However, no ideal biomarker has been identified at this time [33].

Several methods were applied for measuring the glucose variability [34]. However, from previous systematic reviews and our study, the magnitude of glycemic variability was highly correlated with the level of the mean glucose value. The degree of correlation of the different measures of glycemic variability was also high [35].

Some limitations in our current study included the following: (1) relative small sample size; (2) single-center evaluation; (3) retrospective analysis; and (4) the use of monitored glucose at fixed time points, instead of continuous glucose monitoring. Whether aggressive control of blood glucose levels during ward hospitalization could improve the recovery of the renal dysfunction would need to be evaluated in a controlled study in the future. However, at least, the glucose levels are a good indicator of severe infection, organ dysfunction, and renal outcome in type 2 diabetic patients with CKD and UTI.

Conclusions

Early-morning fasting and mean blood glucose levels and glucose variability during hospitalization are good indicators of severe infection, and also predictors of renal outcome in type 2 diabetic patients with CKD and UTI.

Author Contributions

Conceived and designed the experiments: PFC CLW CHH CCC HRC. Performed the experiments: PFC CLW CHH CCC HRC. Analyzed the data: PFC CLW HHL CBC. Contributed reagents/materials/analysis tools: CHH CCC. Wrote the paper: PFC CLW CHH CCC.

References

1. Muller LM, Gorter KJ, Hak E, Goudzwaard WL, Schellevis FG, et al. (2005) Increased Risk of Common Infections in Patients with Type 1 and Type 2 Diabetes Mellitus. Clin Infect Dis 41: 281–288.
2. Balachandar MS, Pavković P, Metelko Ž (2002) Kidney infections in diabetes mellitus. Diabetologia Croatica 31: 85–103.
3. Nicolle LE, Friesen D, Harding GK, Roos LL (1996) Hospitalization for acute pyelonephritis in Manitoba, Canada, during the period from 1989 to 1992; impact of diabetes, pregnancy, and aboriginal origin. Clin Infect Dis 22: 1051–1056.
4. Robbins SL, Tucker AW (1944) The cause of death in diabetes. A report of 307 autopsied cases. N Engl J Med 231: 865–868.
5. Chiu PF, Huang CH, Liou HH, Wu CL, Wang SC, et al. (2013) Long-term renal outcomes of episodic urinary tract infection in diabetic patients. J Diabetes Complications 27: 41–43.
6. Thakar CV, Christianson A, Himmelfarb J, Leonard AC (2011) Acute kidney injury episodes and chronic kidney disease risk in diabetes mellitus. Clin J Am Soc Nephrol 6: 2567–2572.
7. Eslami S, Taherzadeh Z, Schultz MJ, Abu-Hanna A (2011) Glucose variability measures and their effect on mortality: a systematic review. Intensive Care Med 37: 583–593.
8. von Elm E, Altman DG, Egger M, Pocock SJ, Gøtzsche PC, et al. (2007) The Strengthening the Reporting of Observational Studies in Epidemiology (STROBE) statement: guidelines for reporting observational studies. BMJ 335: 806–808.
9. Bouman CS, Oudemans-Van Straaten HM, Tijssen JG, Zandstra DF, Kesecioglu J (2002) Effects of early high-volume continuous venovenous hemofiltration on survival and recovery of renal function in intensive care patients with acute renal failure: A prospective, randomized trial. Crit Care Med 30: 2205–2211.
10. Luckraz H, Gravenor MB, George R, Taylor S, Williams A, et al. (2005) Long and short-term outcomes in patients requiring continuous renal replacement therapy post cardiopulmonary bypass. Eur J Cardiothorac Surg 27: 906–909.
11. Zhang Y, Hu G, Yuan Z, Chen L (2012) Glycosylated hemoglobin in relationship to cardiovascular outcomes and death in patients with type 2 diabetes: a systematic review and meta-analysis. PLoS One 7: e42551. doi: 10.1371/journal.pone.0042551.
12. Bragd J, Adamson U, Bäcklund LB, Lins PE, Moberg E, et al. (2008) Can glycaemic variability, as calculated from blood glucose self-monitoring, predict the development of complications in type 1 diabetes over a decade? Diabetes Metab 34: 612–616.
13. Di Flaviani A, Picconi F, Di Stefano P, Giordani I, Malandrucco I, et al. (2011) Impact of glycemic and blood pressure variability on surrogate measures of cardiovascular outcomes in type 2 diabetic patients. Diabetes Care 34: 1605–1609.

14. Monnier L, Colette C, Owens DR 2008) Glycemic variability: the third component of the dysglycemia in diabetes. Is it important? How to measure it? J Diabetes Sci Technol 2: 1094–1100.
15. Eslami S, Taherzadeh Z, Schultz MJ, Abu-Hanna A (2011) Glucose variability measures and their effect on mortality: a systematic review. Intensive Care Med 37: 583–593.
16. Krinsley JS (2008) Glycemic variability: a strong independent predictor of mortality in critically ill patients. Crit Care Med 36: 3008–3013.
17. Jeon CY, Furuya EY, Berman MF, Larson EL (2012) The role of pre-operative and post-operative glucose control in surgical-site infections and mortality. PLoS One 7: e45616. doi: 10.1371/journal.pone.0045616.
18. Pisarchik AN, Pochepen ON, Pisarchyk LA (2012) Increasing blood glucose variability is a precursor of sepsis and mortality in burned patients. PLoS One 7: e46582. doi: 10.1371/journal.pone.0046582
19. Haga KK, McClymont KL, Clarke S, Grounds RS, Ng KY, et al. (2011) The effect of tight glycaemic control, during and after cardiac surgery, on patient mortality and morbidity: A systematic review and meta-analysis. J Cardiothorac Surg 6: 3. Available: http://www.cardiothoracicsurgery.org/content/6/1/3. Accessed 2011 Jan 10.
20. Siegelaar SE, Kerr L, Jacober SJ, Devries JH (2011) A decrease in glucose variability does not reduce cardiovascular event rates in type 2 diabetic patients after acute myocardial infarction. Diabetes Care 34: 855–857.
21. Wiener RS, Wiener DC, Larson RJ (2008) Benefits and risks of tight glucose control in critically ill adults. JAMA 8: 933–944.
22. Griesdale DE, de Souza RJ, van Dam RM, Heyland DK, Cook DJ, et al. (2009) Intensive insulin therapy and mortality among critically ill patients: a meta-analysis including NICE-SUGAR study data. CMAJ 8: 821–827.
23. Finfer S, Chittock DR, Su SY, Blair D, Foster D, et al. (2009) Intensive versus conventional glucose control in critically ill patients. N Engl J Med 360: 1283–1297.
24. American Diabetes Association (2013) Standards of medical care in Diabetes-2013. Diabetes Care 36: S11–S66
25. Sherr J, Tamborlane WV, Xing D, Tsalikian E, Mauras N, et al. (2012) Achievement of target A1C levels with negligible hypoglycemia and low glucose variability in youth with short-term type 1 diabetes and residual β-cell function. Diabetes Care 35: 817–820.
26. Chiodini I, Di Lembo S, Morelli V, Epaminonda P, Coletti F, et al. (2006) Hypothalamic-pituitary-adrenal activity in type 2 diabetes mellitus: role of autonomic imbalance. Metabolism 55: 1135–1140.
27. Tsigos C, Young RJ, White A (1993) Diabetic neuropathy is associated with increased activity of the hypothalamic-pituitary-adrenal axis. J Clin Endocrinol Metab 76: 554–558.
28. Monnier L, Mas E, Ginet C, Michel F, Villon L, et al. (2006) Activation of Oxidative Stress by Acute Glucose Fluctuations Compared With Sustained Chronic Hyperglycemia in Patients With Type 2 Diabetes. JAMA 295:1681–1687
29. Rizzo MR, Barbieri M, Marfella R, Paolisso G (2012) Reduction of oxidative stress and inflammation by blunting daily acute glucose fluctuations in patients with type 2 diabetes: role of dipeptidyl peptidase-IV inhibition. Diabetes Care 35: 2076–2082.
30. Bochicchio GV, Bochicchio KM, Joshi M, Ilahi O, Scalea TM (2010) Acute glucose elevation is highly predictive of infection and outcome in critically injured trauma patients. Ann Surg 252: 597–602.
31. Tudela P, Prat C, Lacoma A, Mòdol Deltell JM, Domínguez J, et al. (2012) Biological markers for predicting bacterial infection, bacteremia, and severity of infection in the emergency department. Emergencias 24: 348–356
32. Riedel S, Melendez JH, An AT, Rosenbaum JE, Zenilman JM (2011) Procalcitonin as a marker for the detection of bacteremia and sepsis in the emergency department. Am J Clin Pathol 135: 182–189
33. Marshall JC, Cook DJ, Christou NV, Bernard GR, Sprung CL, et al. (1995) Multiple organ dysfunction score: a reliable descriptor of a complex clinical outcome. Crit Care Med 23: 1638–1652.
34. Siegelaar SE, Holleman F, Hoekstra JB, DeVries JH (2010) Glucose variability; does it matter? Endocr Rev 31: 171–182.
35. Rodbard D (2012) The challenges of measuring glycemic variability. J Diabetes Sci Technol 6: 712–715.

Survival after Acute Hemodialysis in Pennsylvania, 2005–2007: A Retrospective Cohort Study

Sarah J. Ramer[1]*, Elan D. Cohen[2], Chung-Chou H. Chang[2,3], Mark L. Unruh[4], Amber E. Barnato[2,5,6,7]

1 Rutgers New Jersey Medical School, Newark, New Jersey, United States of America, **2** Division of General Internal Medicine, Department of Medicine, University of Pittsburgh School of Medicine, Pittsburgh, Pennsylvania, United States of America, **3** Department of Biostatistics, University of Pittsburgh Graduate School of Public Health, Pittsburgh, Pennsylvania, United States of America, **4** Division of Nephrology, Department of Internal Medicine, University of New Mexico School of Medicine, Albuquerque, New Mexico, United States of America, **5** Department of Clinical and Translational Science, University of Pittsburgh School of Medicine, Pittsburgh, Pennsylvania, United States of America, **6** Department of Health Policy and Management, University of Pittsburgh Graduate School of Public Health, Pittsburgh, Pennsylvania, United States of America, **7** The CRISMA Laboratory (Clinical Research, Investigation, and Systems Modeling of Acute Illness), Department of Critical Care Medicine, University of Pittsburgh, Pittsburgh, Pennsylvania, United States of America

Abstract

Background: Little is known about acute hemodialysis in the US. Here we describe predictors of receipt of acute hemodialysis in one state and estimate the marginal impact of acute hemodialysis on survival after accounting for confounding due to illness severity.

Materials and Methods: This is a retrospective cohort study of acute-care hospitalizations in Pennsylvania from October 2005 to December 2007 using data from the Pennsylvania Health Care Cost Containment Council. Exposure variable is acute hemodialysis; dependent variable is survival following acute hemodialysis. We used multivariable logistic regression to determine propensity to receive acute hemodialysis and then, for a Cox proportional hazards model, matched acute hemodialysis and non-acute hemodialysis patients 1:5 on this propensity.

Results: In 2,131,248 admissions of adults without end-stage renal disease, there were 6,657 instances of acute hemodialysis. In analyses adjusted for predicted probability of death upon admission plus other covariates and stratified on age, being male, black, and insured were independent predictors of receipt of acute hemodialysis. One-year post-admission mortality was 43% for those receiving acute hemodialysis, compared to 13% among those not receiving acute hemodialysis. After matching on propensity to receive acute hemodialysis and adjusting for predicted probability of death upon admission, patients who received acute hemodialysis had a higher risk of death than patients who did not over at least 1 year of follow-up (hazard ratio 1·82, 95% confidence interval 1·68–1·97).

Conclusions: In a populous US state, receipt of acute hemodialysis varied by age, sex, race, and insurance status even after adjustment for illness severity. In a comparison of patients with similar propensity to receive acute hemodialysis, those who did receive it were less likely to survive than those who did not. These findings raise questions about reasons for lack of benefit.

Editor: Shree Ram Singh, National Cancer Institute, United States of America

Funding: This work was supported by a Doris Duke Clinical Research Fellowship for Medical Students to SR (http://www.ddcf.org/) and by National Institutes of Health grant R01AG035112 to AB (http://www.nih.gov/). The funders had no role in study design, data collection and analysis, decision to publish, or preparation of the manuscript.

Competing Interests: The authors have declared that no competing interests exist.

* Email: sramer@post.harvard.edu

Introduction

Acute hemodialysis (HD), defined as intermittent or continuous, non-peritoneal renal replacement therapy for patients without end-stage renal disease (ESRD), typically in the context of critical illness, is thought to save lives. Overall, however, the prognosis for patients requiring acute HD is poor, with estimates of in-hospital mortality in the literature ranging from 33% [1]-61% [2]. In a large high-quality clinical trial comparing different intensities of renal support for patients with acute kidney injury (AKI), 60-day mortality was nearly 53% [3]; in another such trial, 90-day mortality approached 45% [4]. Moreover, survivors are at high risk for continued renal failure [5–9] and decreased quality of life [10–12], and acute HD adds to the already substantial cost of care for the critically ill in the US [13,14].

Although the US Renal Data System provides detailed information about patients with ESRD undergoing chronic HD, less is known about the epidemiology of acute HD. Several studies, most notably that of Xue and colleagues [1], have reported on the incidence and mortality of AKI among various populations of

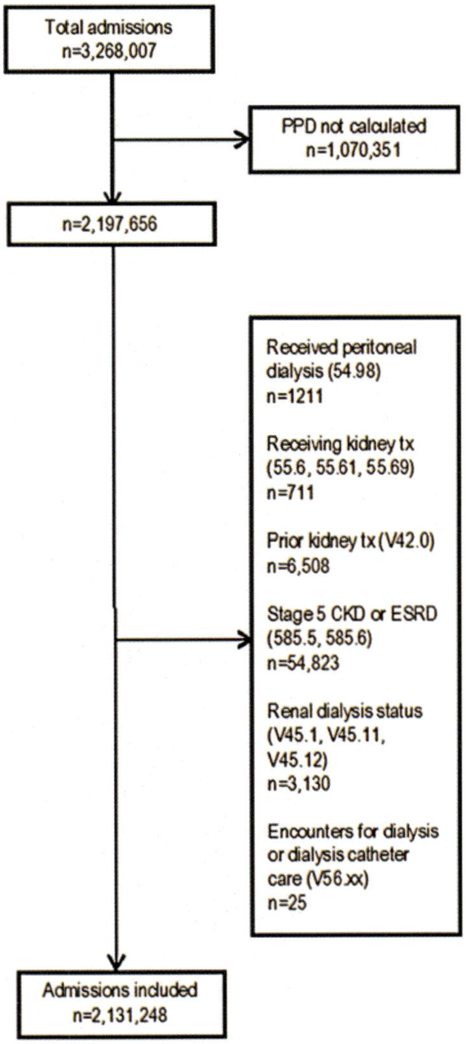

Figure 1. Sample selection process. PPD - predicted probability of death in-hospital, calculated from key clinical findings at admission; tx - transplant; CKD - chronic kidney disease; ESRD - end-stage renal disease.

hospitalized patients in the US [2,6,8]. To our knowledge, however, no study has specifically focused on the predictors of or survival after acute HD.

In the current study, we describe predictors of the receipt of acute HD in a dataset encompassing over 2 million hospital admissions. We then attempt to estimate the marginal impact of acute HD on patient survival after accounting for confounding due to illness severity.

Materials and Methods

Data source

We conducted a retrospective cohort study of adult acute-care hospitalizations in Pennsylvania from October 2005 to December 2007 using data from the Pennsylvania (PA) Health Care Cost Containment Council (PHC4) linked to PA Department of Health death data through December 2008. PHC4 is an independent state agency that collects this data under mandate from the state government. The PHC4 data includes patient demographics, International Classification of Diseases, 9th Revision, Clinical Modification (ICD-9-CM) diagnosis and procedure codes, and the predicted probability of inpatient death at the time of admission for all patients with certain pre-specified diagnosis-related groups (DRGs) and ICD-9-CM codes. (See Text S1. Diagnosis-related groups or International Classification of Diseases, 9th Revision, Clinical Modification principal diagnoses for which the Pennsylvania Health Care Cost Containment Council required predicted probability of inpatient death to be calculated, by year.) The predicted probability of death (PPD) is based upon MediQual mortality models using key clinical findings abstracted from the chart during the first 48 hours of admission. These models significantly out-perform those based upon administrative fields alone, with average c-statistics of 0.86 [15]. It is important to note that the PHC4 data does not include any Current Procedural Terminology (CPT) codes; therefore, it is not possible to distinguish between intermittent HD and all other forms of renal replacement therapy in the PHC4 data.

Exposure variable

Our principal exposure variable was acute HD. We defined acute HD as the receipt of HD (ICD-9-CM procedure code 39.95) by patients without ESRD. We excluded from all analyses admissions with ICD-9-CM diagnosis codes that would indicate current ESRD (585.6, V45.1, V45.11, V45.12, V56.xx), imminent ESRD, i.e., stage 5 chronic kidney disease (CKD) (585.5), or prior ESRD treated with kidney transplant (V42.0). We further excluded admissions with ICD-9-CM procedure codes for kidney transplant (55.6, 55.61, 55.69) or peritoneal dialysis (54.98), as these are procedures that only patients with ESRD undergo. For a flowchart depicting the sample selection process, see Figure 1.

Dependent variable

The primary dependent variable is time to death, in days, from hospital admission. The minimum length of follow-up was one year.

Covariates

Patient-level covariates included demographics, insurance status (commercial and/or Medicare, Medicaid with or without Medicare, and uninsured), principal diagnoses (classified into groups from ICD-9-CM codes using Agency for Healthcare Research and Quality Clinical Classification Software), and illness severity, as measured by the MediQual PPD (available for the 67% of admissions with one of the DRGs or ICD-9-CM codes for which PHC4 required that it be calculated). Hospital-level covariates included number of hospital beds, resident-to-bed ratio (a measure of teaching intensity), percent of patients who are black (a measure of racial concentration, correlated with treatment intensity and risk-adjusted mortality), and a Bayesian shrinkage estimator of the observed-to-expected ratio, i.e., standardized rate, of HD among patients at 95th percentile of PPD upon admission ("end-of-life" HD treatment intensity) [16]. (See Figure S1. Standardized [observed-to-expected] hemodialysis use for patients at high probability of dying upon admission, by hospital, Pennsylvania 2001–2007.)

Statistical analyses

We first descriptively summarized the characteristics of admissions in which patients received acute HD and compared them to admissions in which patients did not receive acute HD by employing chi-squared and t-tests. Using multivariable logistic regression with a random effect for hospital, we calculated a propensity score to receive acute HD based on patient- and hospital-level covariates for every admission, stratified by age (less than 65 years old and 65 years or older). We made the decision to stratify after a graphical analysis showed that the proportion of admissions with acute HD peaked at age 65 and declined thereafter.

On the basis of these propensity scores, we matched admissions with acute HD to those without acute HD in a ratio of 1:5. If a patient had more than one admission, we used only the first admission, even if acute HD was not given in the first admission but was given in a subsequent admission. The rationale for this was to avoid bias, as a patient who underwent acute HD on a 2nd, 3rd, or subsequent admission and then died would seem to have a shorter survival if there was "resetting of the survival clock," so to speak, to the time of that 2nd, 3rd, or subsequent admission. In order to improve the closeness of the matches, we employed matching with replacement, meaning that a non-HD admission could be re-used for matching with an HD admission. To gauge the effectiveness of matching, we used inverse probability treatment weighting to check the covariate balance between the acute HD and non-acute HD groups after propensity score matching. This method allowed us to compare pre- and post-matching samples more accurately since it maintained the original sample size. (See Figure S2. Covariate balance before and after inverse probability treatment weighting by propensity score.)

We plotted Kaplan-Meier survival curves of time to death, up to one year from admission, for admissions with and without acute HD. We then used Cox proportional hazards models to assess the effect of acute HD on survival, with covariate adjustment. Covariates included only patient-level variables, as hospital-level variables were not significantly associated with survival. To reduce indication (severity) bias, we calculated hazards of dying among admissions with and without acute HD, matched for propensity to receive acute HD, with covariate adjustment. We accounted for dependence between patients within a hospital by using the Huber-White sandwich estimator for standard errors. We performed all analyses with Stata version 11 (StataCorp, College Station, TX).

Sensitivity analyses

Along with our main analyses, we performed 3 sensitivity analyses. The first only involved the calculation of propensity scores. Due to the possibility that our sample selection process might have incorrectly classified some HD given to ESRD patients as acute HD, we dropped all patients with Medicare, given that ESRD is a Medicare-qualifying condition, as well as all patients 65 years or older, given that most of them have Medicare, and again ran the multivariable logistic regression models.

The next two sensitivity analyses involved both the calculation of propensity scores and the survival modeling. One used the sample selection process depicted in Figure 1 but then further limited the sample to only admissions that included a stay in the intensive care unit (ICU). We then conducted the same statistical procedures as in the main analysis.

The final sensitivity analysis used the sample selection process depicted in Figure 1 but did not exclude admissions for which the MediQual PPD was not calculated. Instead of using the MediQual PPD as the main risk adjustor, we used the Charlson Comorbidity Index [17,18]. Once again, we then carried out the same statistical procedures as in the main analysis.

Ethics statement

We conducted this research under a data use agreement with PHC4, which acted as an honest broker to merge hospital discharge data with PA Department of Health death records. The University of Pittsburgh Institutional Review Board reviewed and approved the study, which met US federal criteria for exemption from written informed consent because data were not connected to any patient identifiers.

Results

The characteristics of the full sample by acute HD status are detailed in Table 1. Patients who received acute HD differed significantly from those who did not in age, sex, race, and insurance status. Men ($P<0.001$), black patients ($P<0.001$), and insured patients ($P<0.001$) were all more likely to receive acute HD. The most common principal diagnoses among those who received acute HD were acute and unspecified renal failure; septicemia; non-hypertensive congestive heart failure; respiratory failure, insufficiency, or arrest; and diabetes mellitus with complications. As would be expected, acute HD patients were sicker, as reflected in their higher PPD on admission ($P<0.001$) and higher mortality at every time point ($P<0.001$ for all).

As shown in Table 2, in multivariable logistic regression, age, sex, race, and PPD were independently associated with receipt of acute HD. For patients less than 65 years old, increasing age predicted higher odds of receiving acute HD ($P=0.001$); for patients 65 years or older, increasing age predicted lower odds of receiving acute HD ($P<0.001$). In both age groups, male and black patients were more likely to receive acute HD ($P<0.001$ for each). In the under-65 age group, being uninsured was associated with lower odds of receiving acute HD ($P<0.001$). In both age groups, admission to a hospital with a larger bed count ($P<0.001$ in under-65, $P=0.005$ in 65 and older, data not shown) and higher standardized rate of HD among patients at a high probability of dying upon admission were associated with receipt of acute HD ($P<0.001$ for both age groups, data not shown).

The characteristics of the matched sample by acute HD status are displayed in Table 1. Of the 6113 patients who received acute HD in the time period covered by the study, only 3483 did so in their first admission and were therefore eligible for matching. After matching, there was no longer a significant difference between the groups in sex ($P=0.615$). A significant difference persisted for age measured continuously ($P=0.004$), but in the matched sample the patients who received acute HD actually had a lower mean age, as opposed to in the full sample, in which they had a higher mean age. Significant differences also persisted for race ($P<0.001$), insurance status ($P<0.001$), and PPD on admission ($P=0.002$), but as Figure S2 in the supplemental digital content demonstrates, these differences were very much attenuated in the matched sample. Patients who did and did not receive acute HD continued to differ significantly in mortality at every time point ($P<0.001$ for all).

Figure 2 shows Kaplan-Meier curves for patients who did and did not receive acute HD. As would be expected based upon their illness severity, the patients who received acute HD were more likely to die throughout the follow-up period. In the fully adjusted Cox model before propensity score matching, the acute HD patients had a higher risk of death (hazard ratio [HR] 1.78, 95% confidence interval [CI] 1.58–2.00). The survival difference persisted essentially unchanged in the fully adjusted Cox model after propensity score matching (HR 1.82, 95% CI 1.68–1.97; Figure 3).

The sensitivity analysis excluding patients insured by Medicare or 65 years or older produced odds ratios qualitatively unchanged from those obtained from the main analysis. The sensitivity analysis restricted to patients admitted to the ICU differed notably from the main analysis in that, for patients younger than 65, increasing age was not significantly associated with higher odds of

Table 1. Characteristics of full and matched samples by acute hemodialysis status, Pennsylvania 2005–2007.

	Full sample			Matched sample		
	No acute HD	**Acute HD**	**P**	**No acute HD**	**Acute HD**	**P**
Admissions[a] (n)	2,124,591	6,657		17,415	3,483	
Patients (n)	1,283,053	6,113		16,167	3,483	
Female (%)	1,201,352 (57)	3,043 (46)	<0.001	7,856 (45)	1,555 (45)	0.615
Age (yrs)	65.0±17.9	65.5±15.0	0.024	65.2±15.9	64.4±15.5	0.004
Age (%)[b]			<0.001			0.026
21–49	452,764 (21)	1,034 (16)		2,982 (17)	626 (18)	
50–59	321,349 (15)	1,179 (18)		2,883 (17)	625 (18)	
60–69	358,797 (17)	1,439 (22)		3,863 (22)	746 (21)	
70–79	454,958 (21)	1,697 (25)		4,174 (24)	851 (24)	
80+	536,723 (25)	1,308 (20)		3,513 (20)	635 (18)	
Race (%)[b]			<0.001			<0.001
White	1,792,633 (84)	4,899 (74)		13,065 (75)	2,463 (71)	
Black	218,565 (10)	1,393 (21)		3,496 (20)	816 (23)	
Hispanic	38,395 (1.8)	141 (2.1)		292 (1.7)	80 (2.3)	
Asian/Pacific Islander	7,798 (0.37)	27 (0.41)		84 (0.48)	20 (0.57)	
Other/unknown	67,200 (3.2)	197 (3)		478 (2.7)	104 (3)	
Insurance (%)[b]			<0.001			<0.001
Commercial and/or Medicare	1,688,748 (80)	4,642 (70)		12,646 (73)	2,418 (69)	
Medicaid with/without Medicare	404,928 (19)	1,969 (30)		4,601 (26)	1,037 (30)	
Uninsured	30,142 (1.4)	44 (0.66)		168 (0.96)	28 (0.8)	
Primary diagnosis (%)						
Acute and unspecified renal failure	37,021 (1.7)	1,659 (25)	<0.001	4,087 (23)	816 (23)	0.959
Septicemia (except in labor)	55,833 (2.6)	900 (14)	<0.001	2,041 (12)	460 (13)	0.014
Congestive heart failure, non-hypertensive	121,786 (5.7)	547 (8.2)	<0.001	1,204 (6.9)	234 (6.7)	0.678
Respiratory failure, insufficiency, or arrest	33,132 (1.6)	328 (4.9)	<0.001	820 (4.7)	173 (5)	0.513
Diabetes mellitus with complications	40,435 (1.9)	323 (4.9)	<0.001	912 (5.2)	176 (5.1)	0.656
Predicted probability of death upon admission[c]	0.031±0.084	0.14±0.2	<0.001	0.11±0.21	0.13±0.19	0.002
Mortality (%)						
During admission	50,478 (2.4)	1,258 (19)	<0.001	1,480 (8.5)	589 (17)	<0.001
By 90 d post-admit date	194,257 (9.1)	2,309 (35)	<0.001	3,047 (17)	1,059 (30)	<0.001
By 1 yr post-admit date	271,519 (13)	2,837 (43)	<0.001	3,793 (22)	1,315 (38)	<0.001
By 90 d post-admit date, conditional on surviving to discharge	143,873 (6.9)	1,061 (20)	<0.001	1,571 (9.9)	474 (16)	<0.001
By 1 yr post-admit date, conditional on surviving to discharge	221,041 (11)	1,579 (29)	<0.001	2,313 (15)	726 (25)	<0.001

Continuous variables expressed as mean ± standard deviation; categorical variables expressed as n (%).
T-tests used for continuous variables; chi-squared tests used for categorical variables.
[a]All means and proportions are based on admissions, not individual patients.
[b]Due to rounding, percentages may not add up to 100.
[c]Based upon proprietary MediQual mortality model using key clinical findings abstracted from the chart during the first 48 hours of admission.

receiving acute HD (odds ratio 1.00, 95% CI 1.00–1.01, P = 0.85). In the fully adjusted Cox model after propensity score matching, however, the acute HD patients still had a higher risk of death (HR 1.77, 95% CI 1.64–1.92). In the sensitivity analysis that used the Charlson Comorbidity Index rather than the MediQual PPD as the means of risk adjustment, the sample size increased by almost 50% (2,131,248 to 3,174,283) since the admissions for which PPD was not calculated were included. In this larger sample, the hazard ratio for death after acute HD in the fully adjusted Cox model after propensity score matching increased (HR 2.60, 95% CI 2.41–2.80).

Discussion

This work represents one of the first descriptions of the epidemiology of acute HD not limited to Medicare beneficiaries in a large US population. Receipt of acute HD varied by age, sex, race, and insurance status, even after adjustment for patients' underlying illness severity. Furthermore, in a comparison of patients with similar propensity to receive acute HD and adjusted for predicted probability of death upon admission, those who did receive acute HD had a higher risk of death for at least one year compared to those who did not.

Table 2. Independent predictors of receipt of acute hemodialysis, Pennsylvania 2005–2007.[a]

	Age<65		Age≥65	
	Adjusted odds ratio	**95% confidence interval**	**Adjusted odds ratio**	**95% confidence interval**
Age (per year)	1.01	1.00–1.01	0.95	0.94–0.95
Female	0.79	0.73–0.86	0.85	0.79–0.91
Black	1.37	1.24–1.52	1.54	1.37–1.73
Uninsured (vs. Medicare/commercial)	0.49	0.35–0.68	0.58	0.27–1.25
Uninsured (vs. Medicaid ± Medicare)	0.35	0.25–0.48	0.58	0.27–1.27
Primary diagnoses (top 5 by prevalence over all ages)				
Acute and unspecified renal failure	57.9	51.4–65.2	31.3	28.2–34.6
Septicemia (except in labor)	10.8	9.35–12.6	5.57	4.89–6.36
Congestive heart failure, non-hypertensive	6.30	5.31–7.49	3.80	3.34–4.33
Respiratory failure, insufficiency, or arrest	5.55	4.54–6.77	3.12	2.63–3.71
Diabetes mellitus with complications	7.19	6.06–8.54	8.22	6.85–9.86
Predicted probability of inpatient death (per 1% increase)	49.6	40.0–61.4	39.0	32.9–46.3

[a]Based on the full sample.

Our findings that being male or black are independent predictors of receipt of acute HD are consistent with previous findings that these groups are more likely to receive other intensive interventions such as mechanical ventilation [19–21], pulmonary artery catheters [19,20], and cardiopulmonary resuscitation [22]. Other authors have also previously reported a higher rate of renal replacement therapy among critically ill men [19]. Similarly, our finding that the uninsured are much less likely than those with any type of insurance to receive acute HD is in line with a recent report by Lyon and colleagues, who, also working with the PHC4 data, noted that uninsured patients less than 65 years old had a significantly lower probability of receiving acute HD, tracheostomies, and central venous catheters [23]. It should be noted, however, that Lyon's strategy for differentiating acute from chronic HD relied on older ICD-9-CM codes that didn't allow for separation of CKD and ESRD [24]. As such, their strategy may have unnecessarily eliminated from acute HD analyses some CKD patients whose HD was in fact acute. At first glance, after seeing this kind of disparity between the insured and uninsured, one might attribute it to healthcare providers' reluctance to offer expensive therapies to patients who are unlikely to ever be able to pay for them. As Lyon pointed out, though, the disparity could

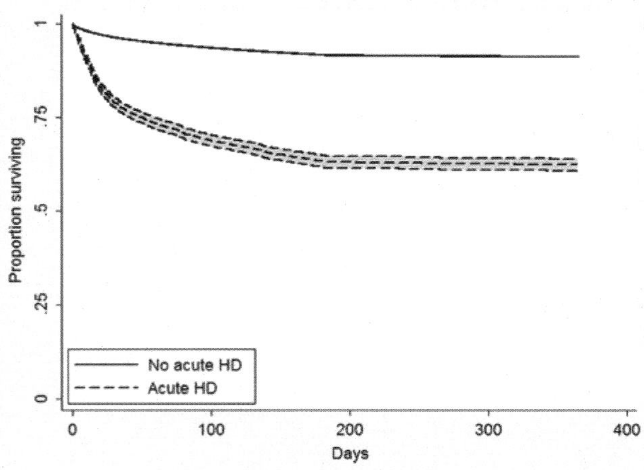

Figure 2. Unadjusted survival among patients with and without acute hemodialysis, Pennsylvania 2005–2007. Kaplan-Meier survival curves for patients who did and did not receive acute hemodialysis, with 95% confidence intervals.

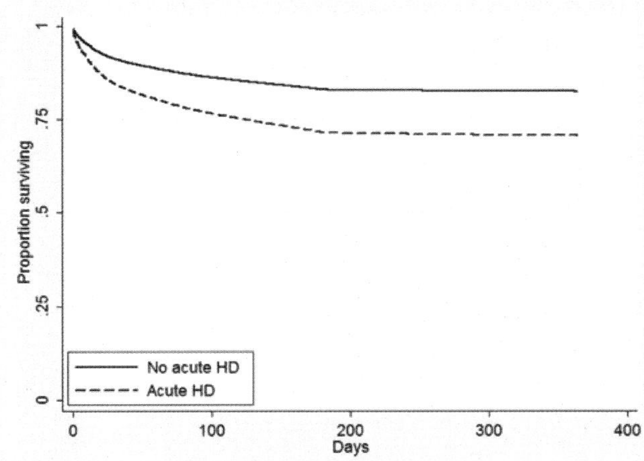

Figure 3. Adjusted survival among propensity-score matched patients with and without acute hemodialysis, Pennsylvania 2005–2007. Cox-adjusted survival curves with covariate adjustment for patients who did and did not receive acute hemodialysis after matching on propensity to receive acute hemodialysis. Variables included in covariate risk adjustment included age; female sex; black race; insurance with Medicare or private insurance vs. no insurance; insurance with Medicaid and/or Medicare vs. no insurance; MediQual predicted probability of death; and the top 25 Clinical Classification Software admission diagnoses for people who received acute hemodialysis, with the exception of hypertension with complications and secondary hypertension (#6) and peripheral and visceral atherosclerosis (#25), which were dropped in the model selection phase.

result more from choices by the uninsured patients and their surrogates than from healthcare providers' decisions—unconscious or otherwise—to forego these interventions in the uninsured. The reasons underlying the observed disparity merit further investigation, perhaps using survey-based or qualitative methods.

Perhaps the most striking finding from our study is the increased mortality risk for patients who received acute HD, even after robust risk-adjustment, including propensity score matching. Even after we limited the sample to the sickest patients, those admitted to the ICU, this increased mortality risk persisted. This finding runs counter to the commonly accepted notion that acute HD decreases mortality for those in whom it is initiated. Certainly, despite our best efforts to match by propensity to receive acute HD patients who did and did not receive it, the possibility of unmeasured confounding by illness severity remains. Though a principal diagnosis of AKI was a covariate in our propensity scoring and survival models, we could not match patients on severity of AKI (e.g., by serum BUN or creatinine or urine output), as our dataset did not include that information.

However, we also cannot rule out the possibility that acute HD is deleterious to patient survival. Elseviers and colleagues reported similar results from a nonrandomized prospective study of 1,303 patients in 9 ICUs [25]. They found that differences in illness severity did not account for the higher in-hospital mortality observed in patients who received acute HD. Intriguingly, they also noted wide variations between ICUs in initiation of acute HD, underscoring the general lack of consensus in nephrology and critical care about the relative indications for this therapy. In our study, we attempted to account for between-institution variations by including each hospital's standardized rate of HD among patients at a high probability of dying in our propensity score calculation and appropriately adjusting Cox model standard errors for clustering of patients within hospitals.

Two even more recent studies, though they did not find higher mortality with acute HD, did find lack of survival benefit. For Clec'h and colleagues, this lack of benefit was in patients who received acute HD versus those who did not after matching on propensity to receive acute HD using detailed clinical information [26]. For Wilson and colleagues, this lack of benefit was in patients who developed severe AKI on days other than Sundays compared to patients who developed severe AKI on Sundays, despite lower frequency of acute HD initiation on Sundays [27]. Moreover, Wilson and colleagues, in their most recent study, observed an association between dialysis for AKI and increased survival when dialysis was initiated in patients with higher serum creatinine but not when it was initiated in patients with lower serum creatinine. In fact, in patients with lower serum creatinine, initiation of dialysis for AKI was associated with increased mortality [28]. Though the reasons that acute HD might exert either no effect or a negative effect on patient survival are far from clear and merit further research, the known risks of HD—episodic hypotension, an indwelling catheter, immune and coagulation disturbances, changes in medication clearance, to name a few—all might play a role.

Our study has several strengths that should be noted. Our sample includes over 2 million observations from a dataset that captured admissions of all adults in almost every hospital in a populous US state, not just Medicare beneficiaries or hospitals within a particular commercial or government healthcare system. Our analyses benefitted from the precise risk adjustment of the MediQual model for predicted probability of death. Furthermore, by restricting our sample to admissions from the last quarter of 2005 onwards, we were able to take advantage of updated ICD-9-CM codes that allow for separation of CKD and ESRD. As such, we can have reasonable confidence in our ability to differentiate between acute and chronic HD using administrative data.

This study is not without weaknesses, however. Though we carefully crafted our strategy to exclude ESRD patients from the sample and backed it up with a sensitivity analysis, without medical records we are unable to fully validate the strategy. Despite adjusting for a wide variety of covariates in our models and propensity-score matching patients who received acute HD with patients who did not, as well as replicating our main results with a sensitivity analysis limited to patients sick enough to be admitted to the ICU, there is still likely to be some degree of unmeasured confounding contributing to the survival difference between the groups. In the most extreme case, if the only patients dialyzed were those who would have definitely died from their illness, then acute HD had to confer a survival benefit, as some patients did survive. While we cannot exclude this possibility using our dataset, we mitigated it to the fullest extent that our dataset would allow. Finally, in order to use the precise risk adjustment of the MediQual model, we excluded all those admissions for which PHC4 did not require calculation of predicted probability of death. Our sample must therefore be considered nonrandom. In fact one of our sensitivity analyses did demonstrate that the inclusion of all admissions in our sample would have altered the results. But the most important finding, the hazard ratio for death in patients who received acute HD versus those who did not, actually became larger in this case.

Taken in the context of previous research, our findings regarding predictors of acute HD suggest factors other than clinical indication at play in determining who receives this therapy; our findings regarding survival after acute HD raise questions about its presumed benefits. Given the extraordinary costs of intensive interventions such as acute HD in the US, and the ever-expanding population of patients who might become ill enough to be viewed as candidates for it, healthcare providers and policy-makers alike must carefully consider why exactly patients receive the therapies they do and whether those reasons impact eventual outcomes.

Supporting Information

Figure S1 Standardized (observed-to-expected) hemodialysis use for patients at high probability of dying upon admission, by hospital, Pennsylvania 2001–2007. Each dot represents 1 hospital.

Figure S2 Covariate balance before and after inverse probability treatment weighting by propensity score. Movement of the open dots towards a Z-value of 0 represents better covariate balance after weighting, with a value of 0 reflecting perfect balance.

Text S1 Diagnosis-related groups or International Classification of Diseases, 9th Revision, Clinical Modification principal diagnoses for which the Pennsylvania Health Care Cost Containment Council required predicted probability of inpatient death to be calculated, by year.

Acknowledgments

The authors wish to thank Khaled Abdel-Kader, MD, MS for his suggestion of the method for one of the sensitivity analyses and his helpful input regarding propensity score matching.

Disclaimer: The Pennsylvania Health Care Cost Containment Council (PHC4) is an independent state agency responsible for addressing the problem of escalating health costs, ensuring the quality of health care, and increasing access to healthcare for all citizens regardless of ability to pay. PHC4 has provided data to this entity in an effort to further PHC4's mission of educating the public and containing health care costs in Pennsylvania. PHC4, its agents, and staff, have made no representation, guarantee, or warranty, express or implied, that the data — financial, patient, payor, and physician specific information — provided to this entity, are error free, or that the use of the data will avoid differences of opinion or interpretation. This analysis was not prepared by PHC4. This analysis was done by the University of Pittsburgh. PHC4, its agents and staff, bear no responsibility or liability for the results of the analysis, which are solely the responsibility of the University of Pittsburgh.

Author Contributions

Conceived and designed the experiments: SR EC CC MU AB. Performed the experiments: SR EC CC AB. Analyzed the data: SR EC CC AB. Contributed reagents/materials/analysis tools: EC CC AB. Contributed to the writing of the manuscript: SR EC MU AB.

References

1. Xue JL, Daniels F, Star RA, Kimmel PL, Eggers PW, et al. (2006) Incidence and mortality of acute renal failure in Medicare beneficiaries, 1992 to 2001. J Am Soc Nephrol 17: 1135–1142.
2. Mehta RL, Pascual MT, Gruta CG, Zhuang S, Chertow GM (2002) Refining predictive models in critically ill patients with acute renal failure. J Am Soc Nephrol 13: 1350–1357.
3. Palevsky PM, Zhang JH, O'Connor TZ, Chertow GM, Crowley ST, et al. (2008) Intensity of renal support in critically ill patients with acute kidney injury. N Engl J Med 359: 7–20.
4. Bellomo R, Cass A, Cole L, Finfer S, Gallagher M, et al. (2009) Intensity of continuous renal-replacement therapy in critically ill patients. N Engl J Med 361: 1627–1638.
5. Mehta RL, Pascual MT, Soroko S, Chertow GM (2002) Diuretics, mortality, and nonrecovery of renal function in acute renal failure. JAMA 288: 2547–2553.
6. Mehta RL, Pascual MT, Soroko S, Savage BR, Himmelfarb J, et al. (2004) Spectrum of acute renal failure in the intensive care unit: the PICARD experience. Kidney Int 66: 1613–1621.
7. Bagshaw SM, Laupland KB, Doig CJ, Mortis G, Fick GH, et al. (2005) Prognosis for long-term survival and renal recovery in critically ill patients with severe acute renal failure: a population-based study. Crit Care 9: R700–709.
8. Hsu CY, Chertow GM, McCulloch CE, Fan D, Ordonez JD, et al. (2009) Nonrecovery of kidney function and death after acute on chronic renal failure. Clin J Am Soc Nephrol 4: 891–898.
9. Wald R, Quinn RR, Luo J, Li P, Scales DC, et al. (2009) Chronic dialysis and death among survivors of acute kidney injury requiring dialysis. JAMA 302: 1179–1185.
10. Gopal I, Bhonagiri S, Ronco C, Bellomo R (1997) Out of hospital outcome and quality of life in survivors of combined acute multiple organ and renal failure treated with continuous venovenous hemofiltration/hemodiafiltration. Intensive Care Med 23: 766–772.
11. Ahlstrom A, Tallgren M, Peltonen S, Rasanen P, Pettila V (2005) Survival and quality of life of patients requiring acute renal replacement therapy. Intensive Care Med 31: 1222–1228.
12. Johansen KL, Smith MW, Unruh ML, Siroka AM, O'Connor TZ, et al. (2010) Predictors of health utility among 60-day survivors of acute kidney injury in the Veterans Affairs/National Institutes of Health Acute Renal Failure Trial Network Study. Clin J Am Soc Nephrol 5: 1366–1372.
13. Hamel MB, Phillips RS, Davis RB, Desbiens N, Connors AF, et al. (1997) Outcomes and cost-effectiveness of initiating dialysis and continuing aggressive care in seriously ill hospitalized adults. SUPPORT Investigators. Study to Understand Prognoses and Preferences for Outcomes and Risks of Treatments. Ann Intern Med 127: 195–202.
14. Rauf AA, Long KH, Gajic O, Anderson SS, Swaminathan L, et al. (2008) Intermittent hemodialysis versus continuous renal replacement therapy for acute renal failure in the intensive care unit: an observational outcomes analysis. J Intensive Care Med 23: 195–203.
15. Pine M, Jordan HS, Elixhauser A, Fry DE, Hoaglin DC, et al. (2007) Enhancement of claims data to improve risk adjustment of hospital mortality. JAMA 297: 71–76.
16. Barnato AE, Farrell MH, Chang CC, Lave JR, Roberts MS, et al. (2009) Development and validation of hospital "end-of-life" treatment intensity measures. Med Care 47: 1098–1105.
17. Charlson ME, Pompei P, Ales KL, MacKenzie CR (1987) A new method of classifying prognostic comorbidity in longitudinal studies: development and validation. J Chronic Dis 40: 373–383.
18. Deyo RA, Cherkin DC, Ciol MA (1992) Adapting a clinical comorbidity index for use with ICD-9-CM administrative databases. J Clin Epidemiol 45: 613–619.
19. Valentin A, Jordan B, Lang T, Hiesmayr M, Metnitz PG (2003) Gender-related differences in intensive care: a multiple-center cohort study of therapeutic interventions and outcome in critically ill patients. Crit Care Med 31: 1901–1907.
20. Fowler RA, Sabur N, Li P, Juurlink DN, Pinto R, et al. (2007) Sex-and age-based differences in the delivery and outcomes of critical care. CMAJ 177: 1513–1519.
21. Pietropaoli AP, Glance LG, Oakes D, Fisher SG (2010) Gender differences in mortality in patients with severe sepsis or septic shock. Gend Med 7: 422–437.
22. Ehlenbach WJ, Barnato AE, Curtis JR, Kreuter W, Koepsell TD, et al. (2009) Epidemiologic study of in-hospital cardiopulmonary resuscitation in the elderly. N Engl J Med 361: 22–31.
23. Lyon SM, Benson NM, Cooke CR, Iwashyna TJ, Ratcliffe SJ, et al. (2011) The effect of insurance status on mortality and procedural use in critically ill patients. Am J Respir Crit Care Med 184: 809–815.
24. Elixhauser A, Steiner C, Harris DR, Coffey RM (1998) Comorbidity measures for use with administrative data. Med Care 36: 8–27.
25. Elseviers MM, Lins RL, Van der Niepen P, Hoste E, Malbrain ML, et al. (2010) Renal replacement therapy is an independent risk factor for mortality in critically ill patients with acute kidney injury. Crit Care 14: R221.
26. Clec'h C, Darmon M, Lautrette A, Chemouni F, Azoulay E, et al. (2012) Efficacy of renal replacement therapy in critically ill patients: a propensity analysis. Crit Care 16: R236.
27. Wilson FP, Yang W, Schrauben S, Machado C, Lin JJ, et al. (2013) Sundays and mortality in patients with AKI. Clin J Am Soc Nephrol 8: 1863–1869.
28. Wilson FP, Yang W, Machado CA, Mariani LH, Borovskiy Y, et al. (2014) Dialysis versus Nondialysis in Patients with AKI: A Propensity-Matched Cohort Study. Clin J Am Soc Nephrol 9: 673–681.

Low-Dose Aspirin for Prevention of Cardiovascular Disease in Patients with Chronic Kidney Disease

Ae Jin Kim[1], Hye Jin Lim[1], Han Ro[1,2], Kwang-Pil Ko[3], Song Yi Han[1], Jae Hyun Chang[1,2], Hyun Hee Lee[1,2], Wookyung Chung[1,2], Ji Yong Jung[1,2]*

1 Division of Nephrology, Department of Internal Medicine, Gachon University Gil Medical Center, Incheon, Korea, **2** Gachon University School of Medicine, Incheon, Korea, **3** Department of Preventive Medicine, Gachon University School of Medicine, Incheon, Korea

Abstract

Background: Chronic kidney disease (CKD) is a major risk factor for the development of cardiovascular disease (CVD). Previous trials have investigated the effects of low-dose aspirin on CVD prevention in patients with diabetes; however, patients with CKD were not examined. The role of aspirin in diabetics is controversial, and the available literature is contradictory. Therefore, we studied whether low-dose aspirin would be beneficial for patients with CKD, a group that is at high risk for CVD.

Method: From a total of 25340 patients with CKD, 1884 recipients of low-dose aspirin (100 mg/day) were paired 1:1 with non-recipients for analysis using propensity score matching. The primary endpoint was the development of atherosclerotic CVD, including coronary arterial disease, stroke, and peripheral arterial disease. Secondary endpoints included death from any cause, bleeding events, doubling of serum creatinine, and renal death.

Results: The incidence of a primary endpoint of any atherosclerotic CVD was significantly higher in the aspirin users than in the non-users ($P<0.001$). Secondary endpoints, including all-cause mortality and composite bleeding events, were not significantly different between the aspirin users and the non-users. However, the doubling of serum creatinine levels ($P=0.001$) and renal death ($P=0.042$) were significantly associated with the use of aspirin.

Conclusion: These results suggest that the use of low-dose aspirin in patients with CKD may have harmful consequences related to the development of CVD and renal progression.

Editor: Valquiria Bueno, UNIFESP Federal University of São Paulo, Brazil

Funding: This study was supported by Chong Kun Dang Pharmaceutical Corp. in Korea. The funders had no role in the study design, data collection and analysis, decision to publish, or preparation of the manuscript.

Competing Interests: The authors have read the journal's policy and the authors of this manuscript have the following competing interests: this study was supported by Chong Kun Dang Pharmaceutical Corp. in Korea.

* Email: jyjung@gachon.ac.kr

Introduction

Compared with the general population, individuals with chronic kidney disease (CKD) are at an increased risk for cardiovascular disease (CVD) and death from cardiovascular events [1]. CVD is the leading cause of mortality in individuals with varying degrees of CKD. Therefore, preventive measures for CVD are of great importance in patients with CKD. Previous studies have demonstrated that efforts to lower blood pressure [2,3] and lipid levels [4] are effective for reducing the risk of CVD in patients with CKD. However, the importance of other potential preventive therapies, such as antiplatelet agents, remains controversial.

Aspirin has been shown to be effective in reducing cardiovascular morbidity and mortality in high-risk patients who have experienced myocardial infarction (MI) or stroke [5] and is recommended as a secondary prevention strategy for individuals with multiple risk factors such as hypertension, dyslipidemia, obesity, diabetes, and a family history of ischemic heart disease [6,7]. The American Diabetes Association and the American Heart Association recommend low-dose aspirin (75–162 mg) for adults with diabetes who have no previous history of vascular disease, a 10-year risk of CVD events that is greater than 10%, and no increased risk of bleeding [6].

Several potential mechanisms have been proposed for the increased risk of CVD in patients with CKD, including increased oxidative stress [8], inflammation [8], platelet dysfunction [9], accelerated atherosclerosis [10], and attenuated response to antiplatelet agents [11]. Similar to diabetes, CKD has recently been considered to be equivalent to coronary artery disease [12,13]. Although antiplatelet agents have been shown to reduce the risk for major CVD events in patients with coronary artery disease and in those with an equivalent disease such as diabetes, limited data exist regarding the use of antiplatelet agents in patients with CKD. This is largely because these patients were systematically excluded from large randomized trials [14]. Additionally, there is concern over whether chronic aspirin use can potentially lead to an increased risk of hemorrhage after

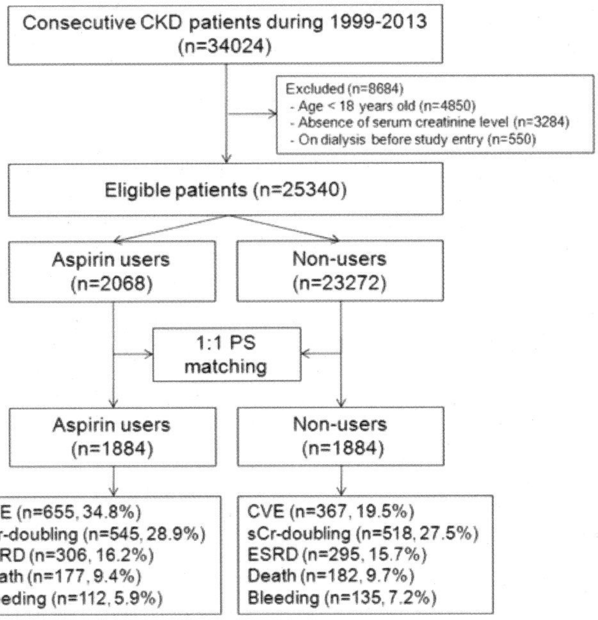

Figure 1. Cohort formation.

treatment with an antiplatelet agent, as patients with CKD have abnormal platelet function [15]. There is substantial uncertainty regarding the risk/benefit balance associated with the use of antiplatelet agents by CKD patients. Accordingly, the purpose of this study was to evaluate the effects and safety of low-dose aspirin used for the prevention of CVD in patients with CKD, a group that is at high risk for CVD.

Materials and Methods

Ethics statement

This investigation was approved by the institutional review board (IRB) in Gachon University Gil Medical Center and was in accordance with the principle of the Helsinki Declaration II (GCIRB2938-2012). This study was a retrospective observational design and did not include any interventions, therefore written informed consent was waived after confirmation of IRB.

Study design and setting

This study was a retrospective Propensity score (PS)-matched analysis of the effect of low-dose aspirin therapy on the development of CVD.

Participants

Patients who presented to Gachon University Gil Medical Center, which is a tertiary teaching hospital, with renal problems between November 1, 1999 and June 30, 2013 were screened for inclusion in this study. A total of 34024 patients with CKD were identified. The following groups of patients were excluded: (i) patients who were under 18 years of age (n = 4850); (ii) patients whose medical records were lacking information on serum creatinine levels (n = 3284); and (iii) patients who received dialysis prior to entry in the study (n = 550). Therefore, 25340 patients were included in the final analysis (Figure 1). The Institutional Review Board of our hospital approved the research protocol and methods.

Variables

The patients' demographic and clinical and laboratory data were obtained from electronic medical records. We obtained the following demographic data: age, gender, Body mass index (BMI), comorbidities (diabetes, hypertension, history of CVD, and history of peptic ulcer disease). Other comorbid conditions, such as angina pectoris, myocardial infarction, other ischemic heart disease, atrial fibrillation, heart failure, hypertension, and cerebrovascular disease, were identified using the validated *ICD-10* codes. Cardiovascular disease (CVD) was defined as angina pectoris, myocardial infarction, other ischemic heart disease, atrial fibrillation, heart failure, or cerebrovascular disease. Medications included renin-angiotensin-aldosterone system (RAAS) blockers (angiotensin-converting enzyme inhibitors and angiotensin receptor blockers), statins, beta-blockers, calcium channel blockers (CCBs), diuretics, warfarin, clopidogrel and cilostazol. The laboratory data included levels of proteinuria as measured by a dipstick test, serum creatinine levels, and the levels of hemoglobin, albumin, cholesterol, triglycerides, high-density lipoprotein (HDL)-cholesterol, calcium, phosphorus, and uric acid at the time of the initial hospital visit. We estimated the glomerular filtration rate (eGFR) using the following 4-variable Modification of Diet in Renal Disease (MDRD) Study equation. CKD was defined by a specific value of the eGFR (<60 ml/min/1.73 m^2), the presence of proteinuria (defined as trace or greater by dipstick), or both on at least 2 occasions ≥ 3 months apart [16].

Outcome end points

The primary end point was the development of any atherosclerotic event, which was a composite of significant coronary artery disease that required angioplasty (including ballooning and stenting), ischemic stroke, and peripheral vascular disease. Adverse events that were defined as composite bleeding included gastrointestinal bleeding, hemorrhagic stroke, and hemoptysis. Other secondary endpoints included death from any cause, time to doubling of serum creatinine, and renal failure that was defined by the occurrence of end-stage renal disease (ESRD) that required renal replacement therapy. Comparisons of outcome end points were performed on the basis of time until the first event according to the intention-to-treat principle, and they included all patients in the groups to which they were assigned (follow-up was censored on the day of the last visit).

Statistical analysis

Because the patients in this study were not randomly assigned to an aspirin treatment group, we used the PS to reduce any potential confounding and selection biases. Two different types of analyses in assessing the association of aspirin with outcomes were used; intention to treat (ITT) for the unmatched cohort and PS for the matched cohort. In addition, to reduce potential confounding and treatment selection bias, we performed rigorous adjustment for significant differences in baseline covariates with the use of PS matching. We calculated the PS for each patient by modeling the probability of receiving aspirin. A multivariable logistic regression analysis model was generated to predict the probability of receiving aspirin, given the following set of covariates: age, gender, BMI, diabetes, hypertension, history of CVD and peptic ulcer disease, proteinuria, baseline eGFR, baseline levels of hemoglobin, white blood cells, platelets, albumin, cholesterol, triglycerides, HDL-cholesterol, calcium, phosphorus, and uric acid in addition to the use of RAAS blockers, statins, beta-blockers, CCBs, diuretics, warfarin, clopidogrel and cilostazol. Using these covariates, a PS was calculated for each patient. We subsequently used the derived PS values to match 2068 aspirin users with non-

Table 1. Baseline characteristics of study participants (before after propensity score 1:1 matching).

Variable	Before matching				After propensity matching			
	Aspirin users, (N = 2068)	Non-users, (N = 23272)	*p*-value	Standardized differences	Aspirin users, (N = 1884)	Non-users, (N = 1884)	*p*-value	Standardized differences
Age, year	61.7±13.0	48.5±15.7	**<0.001**	1.269	61.0±13.0	61.5±13.6	0.180	0.046
Male gender, n (%)	1213 (58.7)	11207 (48.2)	**<0.001**	0.212	1091 (57.9)	1048 (55.6)	0.164	0.046
Diabetes, n (%)	895 (43.3)	3606 (15.5)	**<0.001**	0.641	769 (40.8)	784 (41.6)	0.630	0.016
Hypertension, n (%)	1369 (66.2)	6285 (27.0)	**<0.001**	0.855	1203 (63.9)	1244 (66.0)	0.137	0.044
BMI, kg/m^2	25.3±5.6	25.3±6.1	0.881	0.006	25.4±5.6	25.4±5.8	0.116	0.001
Previous CVD, n (%)	718 (34.7)	1082 (4.6)	**<0.001**	0.818	621 (33.0)	579 (30.7)	0.068	0.049
Previous PUD, n (%)	54 (2.6)	1089 (4.7)	**<0.001**	0.112	53 (2.8)	56 (3.0)	0.847	0.012
eGFR, ml/min/1.73 m^2	42.3±28.1	69.8±29.3	**<0.001**	1.283	43.2±28.7	43.7±26.4	0.544	0.025
Proteinuria, n (%)	1268 (61.3)	10955 (47.1)	**<0.001**	0.288	1143 (60.7)	1185 (62.9)	0.261	0.045
Laboratory								
Hemoglobin, g/dl	12.3±2.6	13.2±2.2	**<0.001**	0.282	12.3±2.6	12.2±2.7	0.640	0.015
White blood cells, ×10^3/μl	8.9±3.9	8.0±4.5	**<0.001**	0.267	8.8±3.8	8.8±4.1	0.891	0.008
Platelet, ×10^3/μl	246.1±84.8	256.1±80.0	**<0.001**	0.164	246.6±85.0	252.5±102.4	0.052	0.080
Albumin, g/dl	3.8±0.7	4.2±0.6	**<0.001**	0.250	3.8±0.7	3.8±0.7	0.981	0.005
Cholesterol, mg/dl	193.2±60.3	188.3±47.3	**0.004**	0.112	193.1±60.3	192.4±59.1	0.854	0.017
Triglycerides, mg/dl	169.6±126.1	146.1±117.6	**<0.001**	0.263	168.9±127.5	173.9±142.4	0.347	0.049
HDL-cholesterol, mg/dl	44.6±13.7	50.9±14.7	**<0.001**	0.573	44.9±13.9	45.0±14.8	0.573	0.009
Calcium, mg/dl	8.9±0.8	9.1±0.7	**<0.001**	0.106	8.9±0.9	8.9±0.8	0.615	0.014
Phosphorus, mg/dl	3.9±1.2	3.7±1.6	**<0.001**	0.120	3.9±1.2	4.0±4.5	0.199	0.036
Uric acid, mg/dl	6.6±2.3	5.5±2.0	**<0.001**	0.478	6.6±2.3	6.5±2.4	0.638	0.037
Medications								
RAAS blockers, n (%)	1443 (69.8)	4973 (21.4)	**<0.001**	1.112	54 (2.9)	64 (3.4)	0.399	0.029
Statin, n (%)	813 (39.3)	2563 (11.0)	**<0.001**	0.690	10 (0.5)	21 (1.1)	0.072	0.067
Beta-blockers, n (%)	1205 (58.3)	3561 (15.3)	**<0.001**	0.996	37 (2.0)	39 (2.1)	0.907	0.020
CCB, n (%)	1275 (61.7)	4385 (18.8)	**<0.001**	0.973	44 (2.3)	55 (2.9)	0.315	0.038
Diuretics, n (%)	1250 (60.4)	4243 (18.2)	**<0.001**	0.958	65 (3.5)	74 (3.9)	0.488	0.021
Warfarin, n (%)	160 (7.7)	370 (1.6)	**<0.001**	0.293	2 (0.1)	0 (0)	0.500	0.045
Clopidogrel, n (%)	287 (13.9)	1084 (4.7)	**<0.001**	0.321	1 (0.1)	6 (0.3)	0.125	0.045
Cilostazol, n (%)	626 (30.3)	662 (2.8)	**<0.001**	0.797	3 (0.2)	2 (0.1)	>0.999	0.026

BMI: body mass index;
CVD: cardiovascular disease;
PUD: peptic ulcer disease;
eGFR: estimated glomerular filtration rate;
HDL: high-density lipoprotein;
RAAS: renin-angiotensin-aldosterone system;
CCB: calcium channel blocker.
Note: Conversion factors for units were as follows: hemoglobin in g/dl to g/l, ×10; white blood cell in ×10^3/μl to ×10^9/l, equal; platelets in ×10^3/μl to ×10^9/l, equal; albumin in mg/dl to g/l,×10; cholesterol in mg/dl to mmol/l,×0.02586; triglycerides in mg/dl to mmol/l,×0.01129; HDL-cholesterol in mg/dl to mmol/l,×0.02586; calcium in mg/dl to mmol/l, ×0.2495; phosphorus in mg/dl to mmol/l, ×0.3229; uric acid in mg/dl to μmol/l, ×59.48.

users at a ratio of 1:1 using the Greedy matching algorithm (8 to 1 digit match). After all PS matches were performed, we assessed the balance in baseline covariates using the standardized mean difference, paired t-test, and McNemar's tests, as appropriate, for continuous and categorical variables (Table 1). We analyzed all available data without the imputation of missing values. PS matching was performed with the Statistical Analysis Systems software package (SAS Institute, Cary, NC).

The continuous variable data are reported as the mean ± SD unless otherwise specified. The categorical data are expressed as the absolute values and percentages. Continuous variables were compared by Student's t-tests, and categorical variables were compared by χ^2 or Fisher's exact tests, as appropriate before PS matching. Following the descriptive statistics, cumulative incidences of primary and secondary end points were estimated by the Kaplan-Meier method, and differences between groups were assessed with the log-rank test. A Cox proportional hazard model was used to determine the independent risk factors for incidence of atherosclerotic CVD and to estimate hazard ratio (HR) of aspirin use along with 95% confidence intervals (CIs) for incidence of doubling of serum creatinine and ESRD. The adjustment variables included age (10-year increase), diabetic status, hypertension, history of CVD, proteinuria, baseline eGFR, hemoglobin level (<10 g/dl), albumin level (<3.5 g/dl), and cholesterol as well as the use of RAAS blockers, statins, beta-blockers, CCBs, diuretics, warfarin, clopidogrel and cilostazol. A Cox proportional hazard model stratified by matched pairs was also used for the matched cohort. All analyses except PS matching were performed with SPSS version 15.0 software (SPSS, Inc., Chicago, IL). Statistical significance was defined as $P<0.05$.

Results

Study population and baseline characteristics

A total of 34024 patients who presented with renal complications were screened for inclusion in this study, and a total of 25340 patients fulfilled the inclusion criteria. The cohort with aspirin use included patients who were already taking aspirin at the time they enrolled in the study. Aspirin was prescribed for 8.2% (2068 of 25340) of the total number of patients. The characteristics of the study population are summarized in Table 1. Patients who were prescribed aspirin were more likely than non-users to be older and male. These patients were also more likely to have diabetes; hypertension; previous CVD; proteinuria; low baseline kidney function; low levels of hemoglobin, platelets, albumin, HDL cholesterol, and calcium; and high levels of total cholesterol, triglycerides, phosphorus, uric acid, and white blood cells. In addition, these patients were less likely to have peptic ulcer disease.

BMI and medication status (e.g., RAAS blockers, statins, beta-blockers, CCB, diuretics, warfarin, clopidogrel, and cilostazol) did not vary significantly between aspirin users and non-users. Using PS matching, 1884 aspirin users were successfully matched to non-users (Figure 1). After PS matching, there were no statistically significant clinical differences between the aspirin users and the non-users (Table 1).

Risk factors for atherosclerotic CVD

Atherosclerotic CVD occurred significantly more often in aspirin users before and after PS matching ($P<0.001$; Figure 2). We used Cox proportional hazard analyses to evaluate the possible risk factors for the development of atherosclerotic CVD. In a multivariate Cox proportional analysis adjusted for aspirin use, age (10-year increase), baseline eGFR, presence of proteinuria, previous CVD, diabetes, hypertension, hemoglobin level <10 g/dl, albumin level <3.5 g/dl, cholesterol level, and use of medications (RAAS blockers, statins, beta-blockers, CCBs, diuretics, warfarin, clopidogrel, and cilostazol), the risk of atherosclerotic CVD was significantly higher in aspirin users than in non-users in the unmatched cohort (HR, 2.577; 95% CI, 2.238–2.967; $P<0.001$; Table 2). In the matched cohort, the use of aspirin was also associated with a higher incidence of atherosclerotic CVD (HR, 2.259; 95% CI, 1.880–2.714; $P<0.001$; Table 2).

Association between aspirin use and diabetes and between aspirin use and beta-blockers for cardiovascular events

Of the 3768 patients included in the study, 1553 (41.2%) were diagnosed with diabetes. A total of 319 of 769 (41.5%) PS-matched diabetic patients used aspirin, while 336 of 1115 (30.1%) PS-matched non-diabetic patients used aspirin. The HRs (95% CIs) for CVD among those with and without diabetes were 1.826 (1.538–2.168, $P<0.001$) and 2.646 (2.171–3.225, $P<0.001$), respectively (P for interaction, 0.002; Figure 3). A total of 646 of 1847 (35.0%) matched patients treated with beta-blockers used aspirin, while 9 of 37 (24.3%) matched patients treated without beta-blockers used aspirin. The HRs (95% CIs) for CVD among those treated with and without beta-blockers were 2.179 (1.912–2.482, $P<0.001$) and 0.642 (0.280–1.470, $P=0.294$), respectively (P for interaction, 0.004; Figure 3). The associations between aspirin use and CVD were generally homogeneous across the other patient subgroups (Figure 3).

Risk of bleeding associated with aspirin use

The composite of gastrointestinal bleeding, hemorrhagic stroke, and hemoptysis was not significantly different between the aspirin users and non-users in the matched cohort ($P=0.763$; Figure 4A).

Other secondary endpoints: survival and renal outcome

We also analyzed the cumulative survival rate between patients who were prescribed aspirin and those who were not. There were no significant differences in the cumulative overall survival rate between aspirin users and non-users in the matched cohort ($P=0.157$; Figure 4(B)). The event-free survival, the doubling of serum creatinine ($P=0.001$; Figure 4C), and renal death ($P=0.042$; Figure 4D) were significantly lower in the aspirin users than in the non-users. We performed a multivariate Cox proportional analysis that was adjusted for aspirin use, age (10–year increase), baseline eGFR, presence of proteinuria, previous CVD, diabetes, hypertension, hemoglobin level (<10 g/dl), albumin level (<3.5 g/dl), and the use of medications (e.g., RAAS blockers, statins, beta-blockers, CCBs, diuretics, warfarin, clopidogrel, and cilostazol). Even after adjustment, the risks of serum creatinine doubling and renal death were significantly higher in aspirin users than in non-users in the unmatched cohort (HR, 1.390; 95% CI, 1.255–1.540; $P<0.001$ for doubling of serum creatinine and HR, 1.467; CI, 1.279–1.683; $P<0.001$ for renal death; Table 3) and matched cohort (HR, 1.325; 95% CI, 1.160–1.513; $P<0.001$ for doubling of serum creatinine and HR, 1.310; CI, 1.096–1.566; $P=0.003$ for renal death; Table 3).

Discussion

In the present study, we evaluated the role of low-dose aspirin in the prevention of atherosclerotic CVD in patients with CKD. Using PS matching, we found that patients with CKD who were on a regimen of low-dose aspirin were significantly more likely to develop atherosclerotic CVD than those who did not use aspirin. Even after the adjustment for underlying CVD, the use of aspirin

Table 2. Multivariate Cox proportional analyses for atherosclerotic cardiovascular disease.

	Unmatched cohort		Matched cohort	
	HR (95% CI)	*p*-value	HR (95% CI)	*p*-value
Aspirin	2.577 (2.238–2.967)	**<0.001**	2.259 (1.880–2.714)	**<0.001**
Age, 10-year increase	1.383 (1.314–1.456)	**<0.001**	1.171 (1.085–1.264)	**<0.001**
Baseline eGFR	0.995 (0.993–0.998)	**0.001**	0.995 (0.991–0.999)	**0.013**
Proteinuria	1.032 (0.903–1.178)	0.645	0.929 (0.763–1.131)	0.463
Previous CVD	3.282 (2.870–3.754)	**<0.001**	2.866 (2.393–3.431)	**<0.001**
Diabetes	1.731 (1.525–1.964)	**<0.001**	1.592 (1.334–1.899)	**<0.001**
Hypertension	2.291 (1.968–2.666)	**<0.001**	1.493 (1.203–1.851)	**<0.001**
Hemoglobin<10 g/dl	0.728 (0.569–0.932)	**0.012**	0.657 (0.481–0.897)	**0.008**
Albumin <3.5 g/dl	1.026 (0.845–1.247)	0.794	0.935 (0.722–1.210)	0.608
Cholesterol	1.002 (1.001–1.003)	**<0.001**	1.001 (1.000–1.003)	0.068
'RAAS blockers	0.685 (0.495–0.947)	**0.022**	0.802 (0.466–1.380)	0.426
Statin	1.021 (0.613–1.702)	0.935	0.320 (0.045–2.298)	0.257
Beta-blockers	0.954 (0.695–1.310)	0.772	0.998 (0.582–1.710)	0.994
CCB	1.146 (0.883–1.488)	0.306	0.837 (0.482–1.454)	0.528
Diuretics	0.676 (0.488–0.936)	**0.018**	0.649 (0.351–1.198)	0.167
Warfarin	1.079 (0.473–2.458)	0.857	3.820 (0.495–29.509)	0.199
Clopidogrel	3.049 (1.438–6.465)	**0.004**	3.384 (0.826–13.863)	0.090
Cilostazol	2.159 (1.237–3.767)	**0.007**	1.294 (0.178–9.405)	0.799

Abbreviations: HR: hazards ratio;
eGFR: estimated glomerular filtration rate;
CVD: cardiovascular disease;
RAAS: renin-angiotensin-aldosterone system;
CCB: calcium channel blocker.

remained an independent and significant predictor of CVD. In the subgroup analyses, almost all subgroups were consistently associated with an increased risk of CVD. Although there were no significant differences in all-cause mortality or composite bleeding events between the aspirin users and non-users, doubling of serum creatinine and renal death occurred more frequently in the aspirin users. These findings are interesting in light of the use of low-dose aspirin for protection against CVD in this population.

The burden of CVD among patients with CKD is substantial. The increased risk of CVD and mortality in patients with CKD

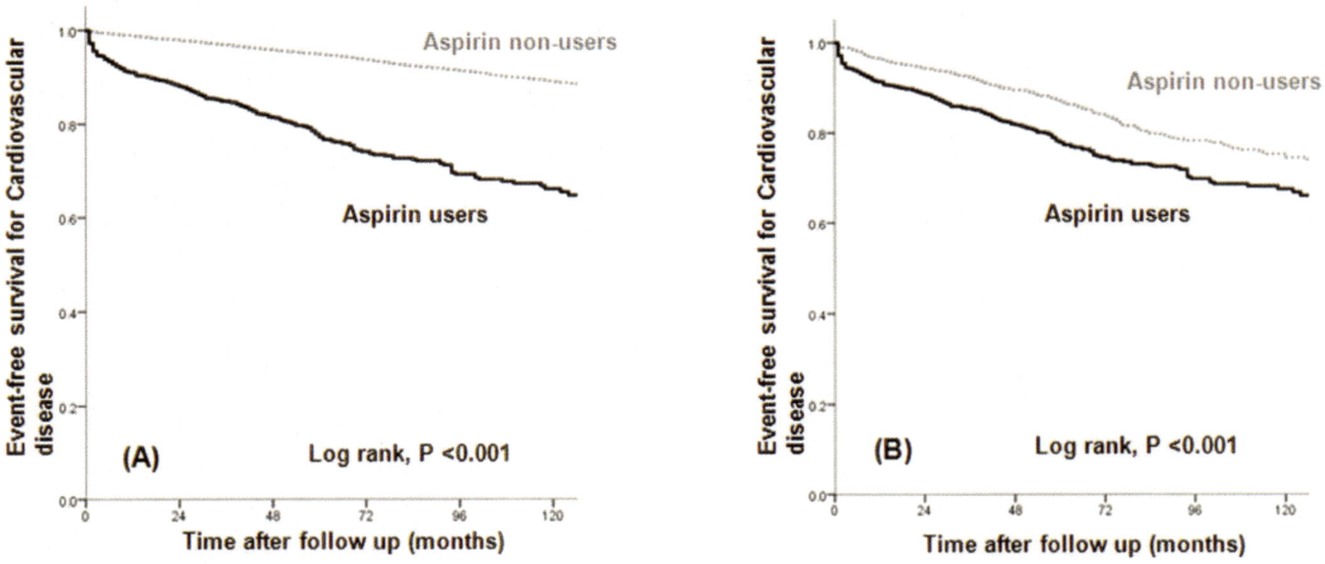

Figure 2. The event-free survival of patients with atherosclerotic cardiovascular disease according to treatment group (A) before and (B) after PS matching. Atherosclerotic cardiovascular disease occurred more frequently in aspirin users versus non-users.

Total patients (n=3768)	Aspirin user (n=1884) No. of events/ No. of at risk (%)	Aspirin non-user (n=1884) No. of events/ No. of at risk (%)	HR (95% CI)	p-value Effect	p-value Interaction
Age (years)					
< 70 (n=2688)	479 / 1384 (34.6)	266 / 1304 (20.4)	2.066 (1.777-2.402)	<0.001	0.492
≥ 70 (n=1080)	176 / 500 (35.2)	101 / 580 (17.4)	2.296 (1.796-2.936)	<0.001	
Gender					
Male (n=2139)	411 / 1091 (37.7)	222 / 1048 (21.2)	2.086 (1.771-2.458)	<0.001	0.999
Female (n=1629)	244 / 793 (30.8)	145 / 836 (17.3)	2.141 (1.741-2.633)	<0.001	
DM					
No (n=2215)	336 / 1115 (30.1)	140 / 1100 (12.7)	2.646 (2.171-3.225)	<0.001	**0.002**
Yes (n=1553)	319 / 769 (41.5)	227 / 784 (29.0)	1.826 (1.538-2.168)	<0.001	
HTN					
No (n=1321)	148 / 681 (21.7)	68 / 640 (10.6)	2.176 (1.632-2.900)	<0.001	0.936
Yes (n=2447)	507 / 1203 (42.1)	299 /1244 (24.0)	2.164 (1.874-2.498)	<0.001	
Previous CVD					
No (n=2568)	304 / 1263 (24.1)	150 / 1305 (11.5)	2.552 (2.097-3.106)	<0.001	0.074
Yes (n=1200)	351 / 621 (56.5)	217 / 579 (37.5)	1.771 (1.494-2.100)	<0.001	
eGFR<60					
No (n=1017)	165 / 504 (32.7)	88 / 513 (17.2)	2.185 (1.685-2.833)	<0.001	0.644
Yes (n = 2751)	490 / 1380 (35.5)	279 / 1371 (20.4)	2.106 (1.817-2.442)	<0.001	
Hb <10					
No (n=2714)	533 / 1366 (39.0)	283 / 1348 (21.0)	2.212 (1.914-2.558)	<0.001	0.156
Yes (n=702)	73 / 342 (21.3)	51 / 360 (14.2)	1.874 (1.306-2.687)	0.001	
RAAS blockers					
No (n=3650)	640 / 1830 (35.0)	353 / 1820 (19.4)	2.149 (1.886-2.450)	<0.001	0.188
Yes (n=118)	15 / 54 (27.8)	14 / 64 (21.9)	1.307 (0.631-2.709)	0.471	
Beta-blockers					
No (n=3692)	646 / 1847 (35.0)	352 / 1845 (19.1)	2.179 (1.912-2.482)	<0.001	**0.004**
Yes (n=76)	9 / 37 (24.3)	15 / 39 (38.5)	0.642 (0.280-1.470)	0.294	

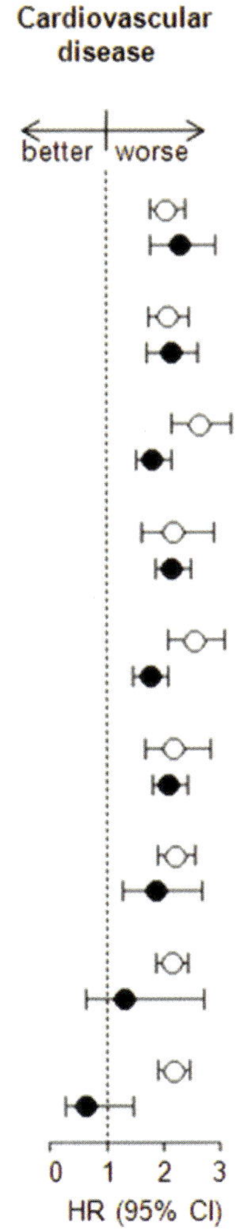

Figure 3. Association of aspirin use and cardiovascular disease in subgroups of the matched cohort.

has stimulated interest in identifying effective methods for reducing the risk of CVD. Although the effects of aspirin in individuals with CKD are uncertain, several studies support the beneficial effect of aspirin in this population. Sciahbasi et al [17] and McCullough et al [18] reported that aspirin use was associated with reduced odds of admission with ST elevation MI and reduced in-hospital mortality after MI. In a post hoc subgroup analysis of a randomized controlled trial, Jardine et al [19] also reported that aspirin therapy led to greater absolute reduction in major CVD and greater mortality in hypertensive patients with CKD than in patients with normal kidney function. These authors explain that the increased benefit lies partially in the high baseline risk of these patients, which translates a similar proportional benefit into a greater absolute benefit.

A recent meta-analysis by Palmer et al [20] evaluated the effects of aspirin and clopidogrel in 9 trials (all post hoc subgroup analyses for CKD) involving 9969 patients who had acute ACS or who were undergoing percutaneous coronary intervention (PCI) and in 31 trials involving 11,701 patients with stable or no CVD. These authors concluded that the use of antiplatelet agents in patients with CKD had little or no effect on all-cause or cardiovascular mortality or on myocardial infarction. However, these authors acknowledged the limitations of low-quality or very low-quality evidence (i.e., significant heterogeneity in the study populations, considerable variation among the studies, and variations in the post hoc subgroup analyses of the trials).There are several potential mechanisms that may explain the poor response to treatment with antiplatelet agents in patients with CKD, including increased platelet activation [11], high residual platelet reactivity [11,21], altered pharmacokinetic effects of uremia on drug transport and non-renal metabolism [22,23], and elevated Von Willebrand antigen levels [24,25] in these patients. In addition, patients with CKD not only have thrombotic predisposition [26] but also, paradoxically, have bleeding diathesis [27] due to the underlying complex hemostatic disorder found in individuals with progressive kidney failure. Uremia is associated with prolongation of bleeding time as well as abnormal platelet aggregation and adhesion due to intrinsic and extrinsic factors [28].

In the subgroup analysis, all subgroups were associated with an increased risk for CVD, except the subjects who were being treated with RAAS blockers and beta-blockers. We evaluated the association between aspirin use (in addition to diabetes and beta-blockers) and other factors for CVD. Aspirin use is associated with a lower HR for CVD in diabetic patients compared to non-diabetic patients. This finding may support the recommendation of low-dose aspirin for secondary prevention of CVD in diabetic patients. In addition, aspirin use is also associated with a lower HR for CVD in individuals who use beta-blockers compared to those

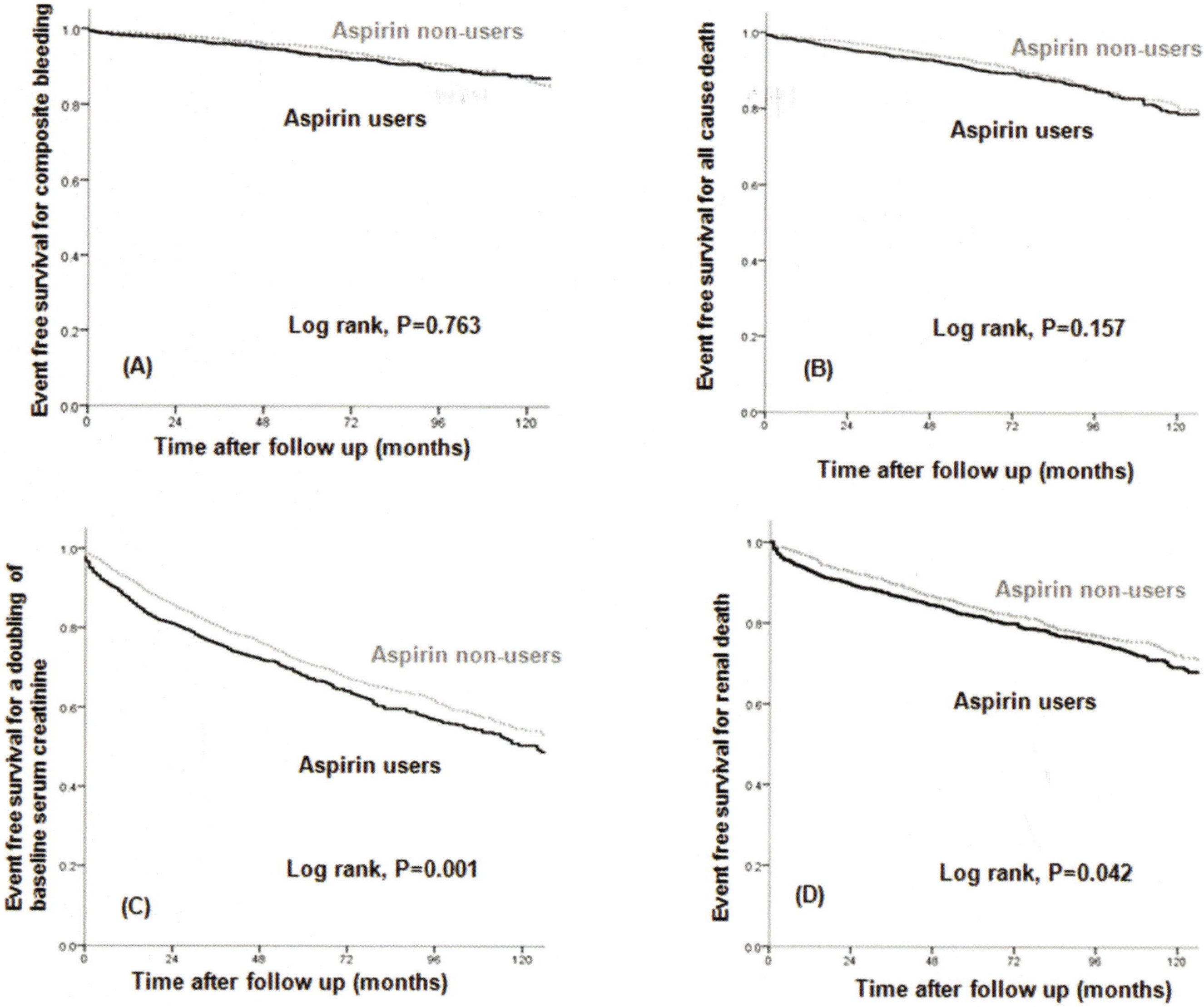

Figure 4. The event-free survival for (A) composite bleeding, (B) all-cause death, (C) a doubling of baseline serum creatinine, and (D) renal death according to treatment group in the matched cohort. There were no significant differences in the incidence of composite bleeding and the cumulative overall survival rate between aspirin users and non-users. Aspirin users showed a higher incidence of doubling of baseline serum creatinine and an increased renal death rate compared with non-users.

Table 3. Multivariate Cox proportional analyses for a doubling of serum creatinine and ESRD[a].

	Unmatched cohort		Matched cohort	
	HR (95% CI)	**p-value**	**HR (95% CI)**	**p-value**
SCr x 2b	1.390 (1.255–1.540)	**<0.001**	1.325 (1.160–1.513)	**<0.001**
ESRD	1.467 (1.279–1.683)	**<0.001**	1.310 (1.096–1.566)	**0.003**

Abbreviations: HR: hazards ratio;
CI: confidence interval;
SCr: serum creatinine;
ESRD: end-stage renal disease.
[a]adjusted for aspirin treatment, age (10 year increase), baseline eGFR, proteinuria, previous CVD, diabetes, hypertension, hemoglobin (<10 g/dl), and albumin (<3.5 g/dl) levels and use of medications (RAAS blockers, statin, beta-blockers, CCB, diuretics, warfarin, clopidogrel, cilostazol).
[b]SCr x 2: a doubling of the baseline serum creatinine concentration.

who do not. This effect may also be due to the protective role of beta-blockers against CVD.

The question of whether the use of aspirin by patients with CKD increases the risk for bleeding is controversial. The first United Kingdom Heart and Renal Protection (UK-HARP) trial [29] and the Dialysis Outcomes and Practice Patterns Study (DOPPS) [30] showed no increased risk of major bleeding, gastrointestinal bleeding in those who were taking an aspirin dose of 100 mg/day, respectively. However, in the meta-analysis by Palmer et al [20], there was an increase in major and minor bleeding events with the use of antiplatelet agents in patients with CKD and ACS who required PCI. These findings were generated using low-quality evidence, with considerable variation in trial duration, heterogeneity in the definitions and assessment of bleeding outcomes, and reliance on subgroup data from major trials. The incidence of a bleeding event in our study may be lower than the incidence in these other studies because we defined the bleeding risk as a composite bleeding event that includes hemorrhagic stroke, gastrointestinal bleeding, and hemoptysis and does not include minor bleeding such as epistaxis, ecchymosis, or bruising. However, we believe that our criteria are also suitable for defining a clinically significant bleeding event. Additional well-designed and controlled studies are needed to confirm the association between the use of antiplatelet agents and the risk of bleeding in patients with CKD.

We assessed the effect of low-dose aspirin on renal outcome in patients with CKD. The doubling of serum creatinine and the occurrence of ESRD that requires renal replacement therapy were significantly associated with low-dose aspirin use in patients with CKD. Unlike our study, The UK-HARP-1 trial [29] showed that low-dose aspirin use in patients with CKD was not associated with progression of CKD (as measured by a decrease in renal function, >20% increase in creatinine, and the initiation of dialysis). Subsequently, in the subgroup analysis of a randomized controlled trial, Jardine et al [19] reported that aspirin use did not affect renal function in the overall study population, but data were scarce regarding the effects of low-dose aspirin on the renal outcome in patients within any eGFR category. However, because the study of Jardine et al is a post hoc subgroup analysis of hypertension optimal treatment (HOT), which mainly included diastolic hypertensive patients, only 2.9% of the study population had an eGFR<45 ml/min/1.73 m^2, in contrast to 53.1% in our study.

Although our study showed that the use of aspirin was associated with a higher risk for CVD even after the adjustment for any underlying CVD, there were some limitations. First, the participants in this study were from a single center and single ethnic groups. There need to be a further investigation about the effect of low-dose aspirin on atherosclerotic cardiovascular disease among patients with chronic kidney disease in multi-center, other ethnic and racial groups. Second, this study was an observational study rather than a controlled interventional trial. Thus, some important baseline covariates were not distributed equally. To address this issue, we used PS matching to minimize the differences in baseline characteristics. Despite these efforts, differences in unmeasured characteristics could have led to biased results. Third, we could not evaluate whether non-use of aspirin could lead to beneficial effects on CVD development in these patients because our study was not an interventional trial.

Despite these limitations, our study is the only large observational cohort study with PS matching that provides evidence that the use of low-dose aspirin is associated with a higher risk for atherosclerotic CVD in patients with CKD.

In conclusion, although the role of low-dose aspirin in the development of atherosclerotic CVD in patients with CKD is debatable, our results show that the use of low-dose aspirin in patients with CKD has potentially harmful effects, as it increases the risk for CVD and renal progression. Further randomized clinical trials are warranted to confirm the effect of low-dose aspirin therapy on the development of CVD in these patients.

Author Contributions

Conceived and designed the experiments: JYJ. Performed the experiments: AJK JYJ. Analyzed the data: AJK KPK JYJ. Contributed to the writing of the manuscript: AJK JYJ. Reviewed the manuscript and approved the final version: AJK HJL SYH HR KPK JHC HHL WC JYJ.

References

1. Coresh J, Selvin E, Stevens LA, Manzi J, Kusek JW, et al. (2007) Prevalence of chronic kidney disease in the United States. JAMA 298: 2038–2047.
2. Ninomiya T, Perkovic V, Turnbull F, Neal B, Barzi F, et al. (2013) Blood pressure lowering and major cardiovascular events in people with and without chronic kidney disease: meta-analysis of randomised controlled trials. BMJ 347: f5680.
3. Mann JF, Gerstein HC, Pogue J, Bosch J, Yusuf S (2001) Renal insufficiency as a predictor of cardiovascular outcomes and the impact of ramipril: the HOPE randomized trial. Ann Intern Med 134: 629–636.
4. Palmer SC, Craig JC, Navaneethan SD, Tonelli M, Pellegrini F, et al. (2012) Benefits and harms of statin therapy for persons with chronic kidney disease: a systematic review and meta-analysis. Ann Intern Med 157: 263–275.
5. Baigent C, Blackwell L, Collins R, Emberson J, Godwin J, et al. (2009) Aspirin in the primary and secondary prevention of vascular disease: collaborative meta-analysis of individual participant data from randomised trials. Lancet 373: 1849–1860.
6. Pignone M, Alberts MJ, Colwell JA, Cushman M, Inzucchi SE, et al. (2010) Aspirin for primary prevention of cardiovascular events in people with diabetes: a position statement of the American Diabetes Association, a scientific statement of the American Heart Association, and an expert consensus document of the American College of Cardiology Foundation. Circulation 121: 2694–2701.
7. U.S. Preventive Services Task Force (2009) Aspirin for the prevention of cardiovascular disease: U.S. Preventive Services Task Force recommendation statement. Ann Intern Med 150: 396–404.
8. Oberg BP, McMenamin E, Lucas FL, McMonagle E, Morrow J, et al. (2004) Increased prevalence of oxidant stress and inflammation in patients with moderate to severe chronic kidney disease. Kidney Int 65: 1009–1016.
9. Boccardo P, Remuzzi G, Galbusera M (2004) Platelet dysfunction in renal failure. Semin Thromb Hemost 30: 579–589.
10. Adeseun GA, Xie D, Wang X, Joffe MM, Mohler ER 3rd, et al. (2012) Carotid plaque, carotid intima-media thickness, and coronary calcification equally discriminate prevalent cardiovascular disease in kidney disease. Am J Nephrol 36: 342–347.
11. Gremmel T, Muller M, Steiner S, Seidinger D, Koppensteiner R, et al. (2013) Chronic kidney disease is associated with increased platelet activation and poor response to antiplatelet therapy. Nephrol Dial Transplant 28: 2116–2122.
12. Debella YT, Giduma HD, Light RP, Agarwal R (2011) Chronic kidney disease as a coronary disease equivalent–a comparison with diabetes over a decade. Clin J Am Soc Nephrol 6: 1385–1392.
13. Briasoulis A, Bakris GL (2013) Chronic kidney disease as a coronary artery disease risk equivalent. Curr Cardiol Rep 15: 340.
14. Charytan D, Kuntz RE (2006) The exclusion of patients with chronic kidney disease from clinical trials in coronary artery disease. Kidney Int 70: 2021–2030.
15. Weigert AL, Schafer AI (1998) Uremic bleeding: pathogenesis and therapy. Am J Med Sci 316: 94–104.
16. National Kidney Foundation (2002) K/DOQI clinical practice guidelines for chronic kidney disease: evaluation, classification, and stratification. Am J Kidney Dis 39: S1–266.
17. Sciahbasi A, Arcieri R, Quarto M, Pendenza G, Lanzillo C, et al. (2010) Impact of chronic aspirin and statin therapy on presentation of patients with acute myocardial infarction and impaired renal function. Prev Cardiol 13: 18–22.
18. McCullough PA, Sandberg KR, Borzak S, Hudson MP, Garg M, et al. (2002) Benefits of aspirin and beta-blockade after myocardial infarction in patients with chronic kidney disease. Am Heart J 144: 226–232.
19. Jardine MJ, Ninomiya T, Perkovic V, Cass A, Turnbull F, et al. (2010) Aspirin is beneficial in hypertensive patients with chronic kidney disease: a post-hoc subgroup analysis of a randomized controlled trial. J Am Coll Cardiol 56: 956–965.
20. Palmer SC, Di Micco L, Razavian M, Craig JC, Perkovic V, et al. (2012) Effects of antiplatelet therapy on mortality and cardiovascular and bleeding outcomes in persons with chronic kidney disease: a systematic review and meta-analysis. Ann Intern Med 156: 445–459.

21. Angiolillo DJ, Bernardo E, Capodanno D, Vivas D, Sabate M, et al. (2010) Impact of chronic kidney disease on platelet function profiles in diabetes mellitus patients with coronary artery disease taking dual antiplatelet therapy. J Am Coll Cardiol 55: 1139–1146.
22. Dreisbach AW (2009) The influence of chronic renal failure on drug metabolism and transport. Clin Pharmacol Ther 86: 553–556.
23. Nolin TD, Frye RF, Le P, Sadr H, Naud J, et al. (2009) ESRD impairs nonrenal clearance of fexofenadine but not midazolam. J Am Soc Nephrol 20: 2269–2276.
24. Shen L, Lu G, Dong N, Jiang L, Ma Z, et al. (2012) Von Willebrand factor, ADAMTS13 activity, TNF-alpha and their relationships in patients with chronic kidney disease. Exp Ther Med 3: 530–534.
25. Spiel AO, Gilbert JC, Jilma B (2008) von Willebrand factor in cardiovascular disease: focus on acute coronary syndromes. Circulation 117: 1449–1459.
26. Wattanakit K, Cushman M, Stehman-Breen C, Heckbert SR, Folsom AR (2008) Chronic kidney disease increases risk for venous thromboembolism. J Am Soc Nephrol 19: 135–140.
27. Mezzano D, Tagle R, Panes O, Perez M, Downey P, et al. (1996) Hemostatic disorder of uremia: the platelet defect, main determinant of the prolonged bleeding time, is correlated with indices of activation of coagulation and fibrinolysis. Thromb Haemost 76: 312–321.
28. Washam JB, Adams GL (2008) Risks and benefits of antiplatelet therapy in uremic patients. Adv Chronic Kidney Dis 15: 370–377.
29. Baigent C, Landray M, Leaper C, Altmann P, Armitage J, et al. (2005) First United Kingdom Heart and Renal Protection (UK-HARP-I) study: biochemical efficacy and safety of simvastatin and safety of low-dose aspirin in chronic kidney disease. Am J Kidney Dis 45: 473–484.
30. Ethier J, Bragg-Gresham JL, Piera L, Akizawa T, Asano Y, et al. (2007) Aspirin prescription and outcomes in hemodialysis patients: the Dialysis Outcomes and Practice Patterns Study (DOPPS). Am J Kidney Dis 50: 602–611.

Effect of Information and Telephone-Guided Access to Community Support for People with Chronic Kidney Disease: Randomised Controlled Trial

Tom Blakeman[1¶], Christian Blickem[1*¶], Anne Kennedy[2], David Reeves[1], Peter Bower[3], Hannah Gaffney[1], Caroline Gardner[3], Victoria Lee[3], Praksha Jariwala[1], Shoba Dawson[1], Rahena Mossabir[1], Helen Brooks[1], Gerry Richardson[4], Eldon Spackman[4], Ivaylo Vassilev[2], Carolyn Chew-Graham[5], Anne Rogers[2]

1 NIHR Collaboration for Leadership in Applied Health Research (CLAHRC) Greater Manchester, Centre for Primary Care, Institute of Population Health, University of Manchester, Manchester, United Kingdom, **2** NIHR CLAHRC Wessex, Health Sciences, University of Southampton, Highfield Campus, Southampton, United Kingdom, **3** NIHR School for Primary Care Research, Centre for Primary Care, Institute of Population Health, University of Manchester, Manchester, United Kingdom, **4** Centre for Health Economics, University of York, Heslington, York, United Kingdom, **5** Primary Care & Health Services, University of Keele, Staffordshire, United Kingdom

Abstract

Background: Implementation of self-management support in traditional primary care settings has proved difficult, encouraging the development of alternative models which actively link to community resources. Chronic kidney disease (CKD) is a common condition usually diagnosed in the presence of other co-morbidities. This trial aimed to determine the effectiveness of an intervention to provide information and telephone-guided access to community support versus usual care for patients with stage 3 CKD.

Methods and Findings: In a pragmatic, two-arm, patient level randomised controlled trial 436 patients with a diagnosis of stage 3 CKD were recruited from 24 general practices in Greater Manchester. Patients were randomised to intervention (215) or usual care (221). Primary outcome measures were health related quality of life (EQ-5D health questionnaire), blood pressure control, and positive and active engagement in life (heiQ) at 6 months. At 6 months, mean health related quality of life was significantly higher for the intervention group (adjusted mean difference = 0.05; 95% CI = 0.01, 0.08) and blood pressure was controlled for a significantly greater proportion of patients in the intervention group (adjusted odds-ratio = 1.85; 95% CI = 1.25, 2.72). Patients did not differ significantly in positive and active engagement in life. The intervention group reported a reduction in costs compared with control.

Conclusions: An intervention to provide tailored information and telephone-guided access to community resources was associated with modest but significant improvements in health related quality of life and better maintenance of blood pressure control for patients with stage 3 CKD compared with usual care. However, further research is required to identify the mechanisms of action of the intervention.

Editor: Gozde Ozakinci, University of St Andrews, United Kingdom

Funding: The study was conducted as part of the NIHR Collaboration for Leadership in Applied Health Research and Care (CLAHRC) Greater Manchester. The views expressed in this article are those of the authors and not necessarily those of the NHS, NIHR or the Department of Health. No funding bodies had any role in study design, data collection and analysis, decision to publish, or preparation of the manuscript.

Competing Interests: The authors have declared that no competing interests exist.

* Email: christian.blickem@manchester.ac.uk

¶ TB and CB are joint first authors on this work.

Introduction

Self-management support is seen as a priority for people with long-term health problems and primary care has been identified as an important site of delivery [1] [2]. However implementation in traditional primary care settings has proved difficult, encouraging the development of alternative models [3] [4] [5] [6] [7] [8]. This, together with evidence that health-related phenomena (such as smoking cessation and weight loss) spread across social networks [9], suggests the need for a paradigm shift in how to support people with long-term health problems [1] [10].

Rather than focussing exclusively on individual factors such as self-efficacy and behaviour, self-management support might better utilize personal networks and resources within the community [11]. Self-management support undertaken within and utilising the social networks of people living with long-term conditions draws on a broader set of resources including practical and emotional support ('illness work') [11] [12] [13] [14]. This approach which focuses on personal communities and resources highlights the centrality of relationships in self-management, such as friends and family, and the importance of encouraging links within local communities which lie outside formal healthcare. This has the advantage of potentially building sustainable strategies for self-management over the long term, which may be of particular benefit to socially disadvantaged communities who have struggled to engage with traditional models of self-management support [15]. These populations are likely to be more amenable to self-management support options, which are more closely aligned to their everyday lives and personal preferences [11] [12] [14].

Effective management of CKD may prevent progression of the disease, and reduce the risk of cardiovascular disease [16] [17]. As emphasised by NICE guidance in the management of CKD, a key element of recommended practice is to offer high quality education at appropriate stages of the person's condition to enable understanding and informed choices about treatment [17]. It is recommended that information should be tailored to their stage and cause of CKD, any complications and the risk of progression.

However, whilst discussions around CKD may be viewed as a platform to address vascular risk and support lifestyle change, concerns have also been raised over unnecessary disease labelling, with both general practitioners and practice nurses having expressed a reticence to disclose a diagnosis of stage 3 CKD [18] [19] [20] [21] [22]. This includes a need to underplay CKD, with efforts focused on reassuring patients, particularly in older people and patients with CKD stage 3A [22]. This tension is reflected in inconsistent use of disease registers for patients who fulfil the criteria for CKD, evidence of infrequent clinical discussions about CKD, as well as low patient awareness of early stage CKD [23] [24] [25] [26]. Chronic kidney disease is also patterned by socio-economic deprivation, is usually diagnosed in the presence of other co-morbidities. CKD is therefore a good exemplar to explore the possibilities of innovative community and network focused models of self-management [27] [28] [29] [30].

This trial was conducted as part of a wider programme of work that aimed to improve health care and reduce inequalities in health for people living with chronic vascular conditions (http://clahrc-gm.nihr.ac.uk/). A key element of the programme was to improve links between different providers of support for health, including professionals, voluntary, and community resources in order to widen the options of self-management support [31]. This approach emphasises the support for people with long-term conditions outside conventional services, and the distinction between professionally-defined and patient-defined priorities in the management of long-term conditions. With a particular focus on the interface between primary care and resources in the community, the BRinging Information and Guided Help Together (BRIGHT) intervention aimed to explore the potential of network focused self-management support in the context of CKD. The BRIGHT intervention was delivered to patients with stage 3 CKD and aimed to: 1) provide patient information that incorporated both clinical and lay knowledge; 2) provide telephone-guided help by lay health workers to support patient access to community support; and 3) broaden the scope of self-management support by tailoring access to local community resources [14].

The primary aim of the trial was to test whether an intervention which provides information about self-management, tailored access to local community resources and telephone-guidance can improve health outcomes for patients with stage 3 CKD.

Methods

The protocol for this trial and supporting CONSORT checklist are available as supporting information; see Checklist S1 and Protocol S1.

Ethics Statement

The trial was approved by NRES Committee NorthWest Greater Manchester Central reference: 11/NW/0855. Participants provided their written consent to participate in this study.

We conducted a pragmatic, two-arm, patient level randomised controlled trial to test whether this model of self-management support is effective and cost-effective compared to usual primary care for patients with a diagnosis of stage 3 CKD. Intervention and trial design were informed by the principles of minimally disruptive medicine [32] and sought to ensure that: CKD was understood and prioritised from a patient perspective; it built on rather than disrupted existing clinical dialogue; it prioritised linkage with community resources; and recognised that CKD is a condition that is rarely diagnosed in isolation but rather needs to be discussed in the context of managing other risk factors and co-morbidities [27]. Full details of the protocol have been published elsewhere (see protocol S1) [14].

The trial was registered 5 months after recruitment of patients started, due to an error in the application of our procedures. Registration was completed during the recruitment period, and prior to follow up, analysis of the data and interpretation. Patient recruitment and follow-up took place between April 2012 and November 2012. Patients were recruited from practice CKD registers. Patients provided their written consent to participate in this study. The authors confirm that all ongoing and related trials for this intervention are registered.

Population and setting

Eligible patients were registered with 24 general practices in Greater Manchester. This included 13 practices that participated in a renal collaborative project established by CLAHRC for Greater Manchester designed to improve identification and management of patients with CKD [33]. Patients coded with an existing clinical diagnosis of stage 3 CKD (both stages 3a and 3b, with and without proteinuria) were eligible and invited through the practice registers at GP practices. Participating general practices provided data on stage of CKD including evidence of proteinuria according to the disease classification system for CKD outlined in 2008 NICE guidance. Patients were excluded if they were unable to communicate in English, had reduced capacity to provide informed consent or were in receipt of palliative care. Only one person per household was eligible to take part to avoid potential contamination. Areas for practice recruitment were chosen because they served some of the most deprived populations of the UK: 20.4% of participants lived in the 20% most deprived local areas in England [34].

Telephone contact was made by a member of the practice team to patients due to be seen for a vascular disease review and/or if the GP or nurse prefered, through raising the study at the end of the consultation. These patients were informed about the BRIGHT trial and asked if their contact details could be forwarded to the BRIGHT team for them to be contacted for further information. If patients agreed to participate a meeting with a researcher was arranged and the first part of the questionnaire was sent.

The BRIGHT intervention was designed to align with patients' routine disease review appointments conducted by participating general practices. Informed consent and baseline data collection was carried out by a member of the research team, where possible subsequent to a patient's disease review appointment at their general practice so that we could ensure blood pressure readings were collected at or as near to baseline as possible and to ensure practices had the opportunity to discuss CKD diagnosis with patients prior to the trial. Recruitment took place between April and November 2012 and 637 eligible patients identified by practices agreed to be contacted by a researcher. The number of patients approached to be involved with the study were frequently requested by the trial team but unfortunately this information was very patchy and so it is not possible to report accurately.

Intervention

The intervention entailed provision of a kidney information guidebook; a booklet and interactive website that tailored access to community resources; and telephone-guided help from a lay health worker. Details of the BRIGHT intervention are detailed in the published study protocol [14].

The kidney information guidebook. The 'Keeping Your Kidneys Healthy' guidebook was developed in response to findings that emerged during an initial study, which identified a need for an information resource to support patients diagnosed with stage 3 CKD [22]. This was developed with patients with stage 3 CKD and provided information based on the experiences of patients, their expressed information needs and medical evidence about treatment options. The process of development followed established principles [35] [36] [37]. The guidebook was intended to encourage patients to consider changes they could make to maintain general vascular health in the context of having a diagnosis of early stage CKD.

PLANS: Tailored access to community resources. The PLANS (Patient-Led Assessment for Networks Support) booklet and website have been designed to address the range of health and social problems related to living with a long-term health problem [38]. PLANS is a needs-led self-assessment tool for users to assess and prioritise their health and social needs, with links to relevant community resources and local support (collated in a database and aligned via the website to the PLANS questions). As well as offering lifestyle options (weight management classes, exercise groups, etc.), PLANS has been designed to increase social contact and promote community support awareness and engagement to sustain independent living. Patients who received the intervention were given access to the PLANS website and also given a PLANS booklet. The telephone support guided participants through the PLANS questions and options on the database.

Telephone facilitation from a lay health worker. The telephone facilitation model was informed by a systematic review of telephone-based self-management interventions to prevent and manage vascular disease conducted by members of the BRIGHT team [39]. Two telephone calls from a lay health worker were delivered to patients in the intervention arm; one call at one-week post-administration of the kidney information guidebook and the PLANS booklet, followed by another call four-weeks later. For the first call, a lay health worker guided patients through the PLANS booklet and website and discussed the PLANS results (e.g. local groups and resources). PLANS and the telephone support were designed to focus on patients' needs, everyday living arrangements, and personal preferences. For example, patients were asked to provide background information about themselves including how they felt they were coping with their health; living circumstances (e.g. married, family, etc); personal and social interests and current social activity. Patients were then taken through the online PLANS questionnaire by a telephone support worker to identify needs and preferences related to wellbeing, health education, adult learning, support, independent living and volunteering opportunities. Following this they were offered a set of results of local activities and services. Brief descriptions of these results were given to patients who were then asked if they were interested in any further information about any of the groups, activities or services. Hence, the intervention was tailored to meet the expressed needs of patients based on their personal preferences and the background information provided. After the first telephone call, information about the groups, activities or services were sent to the patient. For the second call, patients were asked if they had tried any of the recommended activities and were offered another opportunity to complete the PLANS questionnaire. Telephone support was available (Monday to Friday) throughout the course of the trial for unscheduled enquiries from patients.

Lay health workers participated in a three-hour training session facilitated by CB (who led the development of PLANS) about how to facilitate appropriate referrals to local resources. For the training, lay health workers received a detailed workbook and guidance on how to deliver the intervention by telephone. There were 8 telephone support workers: 3 members of staff, 4 postgraduate students, and one undergraduate student at the University of Manchester. One support worker (PJ) was employed specifically to oversee the delivery of the telephone support. Most of the support workers had a limited background in health and social care and all but one were psychology graduates.

Participants in the control arm were sent the kidney information guidebook and the PLANS booklet with links to the website at the end of the trial period. Both arms had usual access to primary care.

Sample size

We powered the study to have 80% power to detect a standardised effect size of 0.25 between the control and intervention arms on any continuous outcome measure. This also provided 80% power to detect a change of at least 10% in the percentage of patients achieving blood pressure control. These are relatively small effects, but in line with most sizes of effect observed in our previous trials of self-management interventions [40] [41]. Basing power on an alpha level of 0.05 and a regression analysis treating outcome measures at baseline as a covariate correlated at 0.5 with follow-up (a conservative estimate), and 25% attrition of participants, we aimed to recruit between 16 and 18 general practices and a total of 500 patients across these. In the event, we recruited a higher number of practices, 24, but a slightly lower number of patients, 436, though due to a lower than anticipated attrition rate, without any loss of power.

Randomisation

Immediately after consent and baseline data collection, an independent clinical trials unit was contacted by telephone and the participant was allocated to receive either the intervention or usual care (1:1) via a minimisation algorithm. The minimisation procedure ensured that within each practice, as each subsequent patient was recruited the two trial arms remained well-balanced on three key prognostic factors (age, smoking status and evidence of other vascular disease). The method also includes a degree of random allocation to avoid complete determination.

Outcomes

We collected patient level outcomes at baseline and at six months. We had three primary outcomes: positive and active and engagement in life, blood pressure control; and health related quality of life. Engagement was measured using the 'The Positive and Active Engagement in Life' domain of the validated Health

Education Impact Questionnaire (heiQ) [42] because the item content fitted with the goal of the intervention which was to provide access to meaningful support and rewarding activities. The items are:

- I am doing interesting things in my life
- Most days I am doing some of the things I really enjoy
- I try to make the most of my life
- I have plans to do enjoyable things for myself.
- I feel like I am actively involved in life

As stated by Osborne et al. 'this scale assesses motivation to be active and embodies the notion of participants in self-management/patient education programs engaging or re-engaging in life-fulfilling activities as a result of program involvement. Items in this construct aim to measure the individuals' activities to convert intention into positive outcomes, and implies a change of lifestyle and life activities.' [42]

Blood pressure was dichotomised as 'controlled' versus poorly controlled in accordance with 2008 NICE guidance [17] on the management of CKD for patients with stage 3 CKD with and without proteinuria (i.e. <140/90 for patients without proteinuria and <130/80 for patients with proteinuria). Blood pressure recordings were collected from general practice records; we used the readings taken closest to date of randomisation and 6 month follow up. Generic health related quality of life was measured using the EuroQoL EQ-5D index of health-related quality of life (three-level version) [43].

Secondary outcomes included: an additional five domains of the heiQ (social integration and support, skill and technique acquisition, emotional wellbeing, self-monitoring and insight, and health service navigation); the Summary of Diabetes SelfCare Activities Measure (SDSCA) [44]; the anxiety sub-scale from the Hospital Anxiety and Depression Scale (HADS-A) [45], and as a measure of CKD-specific anxiety the Emotional Response item from the Brief Illness Perception Questionnaire (BIPQ) in relation to the patient's CKD [46]; four physical and psychological well-being health education outcome measures taken from the Medical Outcomes Study (general health, social role/limitation, energy/vitality and psychological wellbeing) [47]; the UCLA Loneliness Scale [48]; the Medication Knowledge and Medication Motivation subscales from the Modified Morisky Medication Adherence Scale (MMMAS) [49]; Social capital [50] service use (frequency of contact with primary care services and hospital outpatient services); and levels of Illness, practical everyday and emotional work done by social network members (see Protocol S1). [14]

With the exception of blood pressure which was measured by a health care professional at a clinic, all outcomes were administered by post and collected by a researcher. Neither the researchers nor health care practitioners were blinded to allocation.

Service utilisation measured primary health care (GP home and practice visits, pharmacy), community health and social care, secondary health care services, out of pocket costs and costs of lost productivity. Unit cost estimates were then applied to these resource use data to generate patient level cost estimates. The cost of developing and delivering the intervention were also estimated.

Statistical analysis

Analysis followed intention to treat principles and a pre-specified plan (see analysis plan S1). Binary outcomes (i.e. blood pressure control) were analysed using logistic regression and continuous outcomes using linear regression, using robust standard errors adjusted for the clustering of patients within practices. We controlled for baseline values of each outcome, design (i.e. minimisation) factors (age-group, smoking status, additional vascular disease) and self-report of CKD as an additional pre-specified covariate. We applied multiple imputation (MI) to baseline and 6 month variables with missing values by the chained equations approach using scores on all primary and secondary outcomes (at baseline and follow-up), CKD stage, patient demographics (age, gender, education, area deprivation, smoking status) and comorbidities. We used 20 MI sets, as examination of Monte Carlo errors indicated that this provided stability of results [51].

MI was adopted for the main analysis because this provides less biased estimates of effect than those from complete cases analysis [51] but a sensitivity analysis was conducted based on complete cases. We also conducted a further post-hoc sensitivity analysis to examine stability against two blood pressure related factors. First, the NICE criteria for blood pressure control differs between patients with and without diabetes or proteinuria; second, we found wide variation in the dates of patient routine blood pressure readings relative to dates of randomisation and 6 month follow-up [17]. To test the stability of our results to these factors we repeated the primary analysis including covariates for presence of diabetes/proteinuria and for length of time between baseline and follow-up blood pressure readings. Where either sensitivity analysis produced a result differing in significance from the primary analysis, this is indicated in the text and tables.

Analyses were conducted using STATA IC (version 12.1) with an alpha significance value of 5%. For outcomes with skewness or kurtosis ≥1.5, we used standard errors based on 1000 bootstrapped samples to derive confidence intervals and p values. We report effect sizes standardised on baseline standard deviations across all participants.

Cost effectiveness analysis

Utilisation and Resource use. Resource use data and EQ5D data were collected using patient questionnaires at baseline and 6 month follow up. Missing data was imputed using multiple imputation methods. Unit cost estimates were applied to relevant resource use data to generate a total cost per patient (post-randomisation). Quality Adjusted Life Years (QALYs) were generated by applying the UK "tariff" [52] to EQ5D responses and used the Area under the Curve method with adjustment for baseline scores on the EQ5D [53]. Cost and QALY data were then synthesised to calculate an Incremental Cost Effectiveness Ratio (ICER).

Results

Figure 1 presents the trial CONSORT diagram. 34 practices were initially approached and 10 practices declined to participate in the trial prior to data collection. 440 patients were recruited from 24 GP practices (mean list size; 5815 patients) with an average of 18 patients per practice. Subsequently, 4 patients were excluded post-randomisation because they were identified as not meeting the criteria of having stage 3 CKD. Their registered GPs and the patients were informed. In total, 436 patients completed baseline data and 374 (85.7%) patients returned 6 month follow up data. We excluded two baseline blood pressure readings taken more than 15 months prior to randomisation; all other blood pressure readings were within 6 months of the target dates, with an average deviation of minus 27 days at baseline and minus 17 days at 6 month follow up.

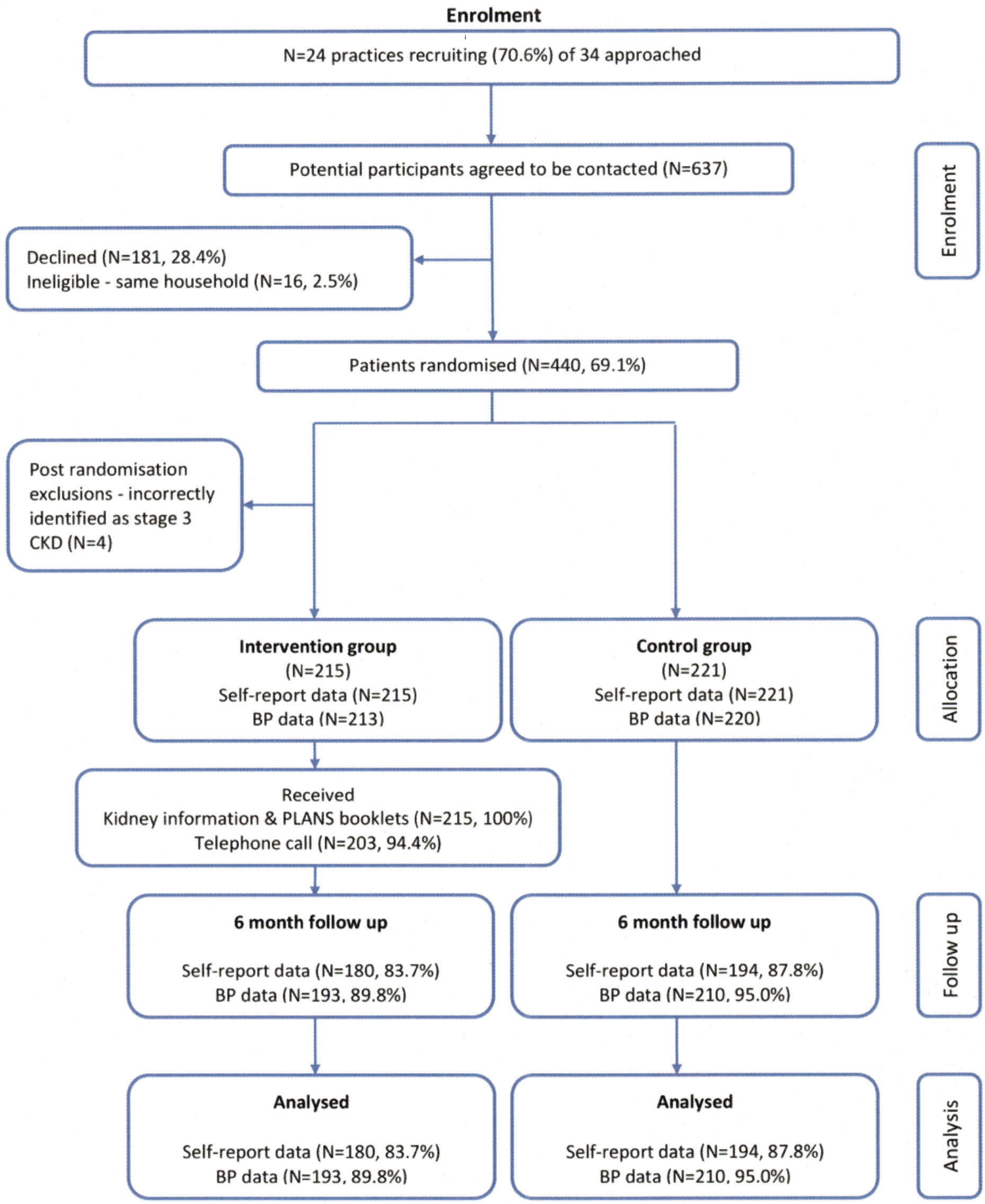

Figure 1. Trial CONSORT Diagram.

Baseline characteristics of study participants

58.5% (n = 255) of patients were female and few patients were non-white (1.4%). The mean age of patients was 72.1 years and 41.7% (n = 182) of patients had co-morbid established cardiovascular disease. Just over half of patients did not self-report CKD (52.1%, n = 227) (table 1).

Engagement with intervention

The intervention comprised of the kidney information guidebook, the telephone service and the PLANS booklet and/or interactive website aimed at encouraging patients to contact and participate in local community activities or services. In summary, 82.2% (n = 147) of the 179 intervention patients who returned 6-month follow-up data reported using the 'Keeping Your Kidneys Healthy' guidebook at least once and 91.9% (n = 135) of these

Table 1. Baseline characteristics of participants.

Characteristics	BRIGHT intervention (n = 215)	Usual care (n = 221)	Total (n = 436)
Gender:			
Male	90 (41.9)	91 (41.2)	181 (41.5)
Female	125 (58.1)	130 (58.8)	255 (58.5)
Mean age in years (SD):	72.4 (9.2)	71.8 (9.0)	72.1 (9.1)
Age group:			
<75 years	118 (54.9)	132 (59.7)	250 (57.3)
75 years or older	97 (45.1)	89 (40.3)	186 (42.7)
CKD Stage:			
3a−proteinuria	156 (72.6)	156 (70.6)	312 (71.6)
3a+proteinuria	8 (3.7)	10 (4.5)	18 (4.1)
3b−proteinuria	37 (17.2)	39 (17.7)	76 (17.4)
3b+proteinuria	14 (6.5)	16 (7.2)	30 (6.9)
Education:			
No qualifications	104 (49.5)	84 (39.3)	188 (44.3)
1 or more O levels	18 (8.6)	19 (8.9)	37 (8.7)
1 or more A levels	3 (1.4)	10 (4.7)	13 (3.1)
NVQ/other trade/professional	64 (30.5)	90 (42.1)	154 (36.3)
Degree	21 (10.0)	11 (5.1)	32 (7.6)
Ethnicity:			
White	202 (98.1)	213 (99.1)	415 (98.6)
Non-white	4 (1.9)	2 (0.9)	6 (1.4)
Mean Index of multiple deprivation (SD) (Higher score = greater deprivation):	21.9 (15.2)	23.4 (17.5)	22.7 (16.4)
Co-morbid established cardiovascular disease (Angina, Irregular heartbeat, Stroke, PVD, heart failure):			
No	126 (58.6)	128 (57.9)	254 (58.3)
Yes	89 (41.4)	93 (42.1)	182 (41.7)
Diabetes:			
No	166 (77.2)	169 (76.5)	335 (76.8)
Yes	49 (22.8)	52 (23.5)	101 (23.2)
No of co morbid long-term conditions (excluding kidney problems):			
0	3 (1.4)	2 (0.9)	5 (1.2)
1–2	63 (29.3)	68 (30.8)	131 (30.1)
3–4	102 (47.4)	90 (40.7)	192 (44.0)
5–6	30 (14.0)	49 (22.2)	79 (18.1)
7+	17 (7.9)	12 (5.4)	29 (6.7)
Smoker:			
No	198 (92.1)	201 (91.0)	399 (91.5)
Yes	17 (7.9)	20 (9.1)	37 (8.5)
Recruited from collaborative practice:			
No	87 (40.5)	87 (39.4)	174 (39.9)
Yes	128 (59.5)	134 (60.6)	262 (60.1)
Mean General Health score (SD):	2.8 (0.9)	2.7 (1.0)	2.8 (0.9)
Self-report CKD:			
No	111 (51.6)	116 (52.5)	227 (52.1)
Yes	104 (48.4)	105 (47.5)	209 (47.9)
Blood pressure control:			
Uncontrolled	66 (31.0)	57 (25.9)	123 (28.4)
Controlled	147 (69.0)	163 (74.1)	310 (71.6)
Mean heiQ, positive and active engagement in life (SD):	64.6 (19.7)	65.6 (18.5)	65.1 (19.1)
Mean EQ-5D (SD):	0.67 (0.30)	0.67 (0.30)	0.67 (0.30)

Table 1. Cont.

Characteristics	BRIGHT intervention (n = 215)	Usual care (n = 221)	Total (n = 436)
Mean service use in previous 6 months (SD):	7.4 (7.1)	8.1 (14.1)	7.8 (11.2)

Values are number (percentage) unless stated otherwise.

patients reported that they found it 'useful' or 'very useful'. Furthermore, 87.2% (n = 156) of patients reported that the kidney information guidebook was 'easy to read' and 48% (n = 86) reported that the guidebook made them 'feel less anxious' (table 2).

Overall, 94.4% (n = 203) of patients in the intervention arm received an initial telephone support call and 97.5% (n = 198) of these received a follow up support call 4 weeks later. 62% (n = 111) of patients reported that they found the telephone support call 'useful' or 'very useful' and 40.2% (n = 72) stated that the call encouraged them to 'think about trying local activities'.

Around a quarter of patients reported accessing the website (26.3%, n = 47) and 66.5% (n = 119) reported that the PLANS booklet was 'useful' or 'very useful'. Forty (22.3%) patients contacted at least one PLANS group, 28 (15.6%) attended at least one PLANS group and 14 (7.8%) reported that they were currently attending at least one PLANS group at 6-month follow-up.

Analysis of outcomes

In analyses of primary outcomes, blood pressure was within NICE guidance for a significantly greater proportion of patients in the intervention group at 6 months, relative to baseline (adjusted odds-ratio = 1.85; 95% CI = 1.25, 2.72) (table 3). Mean health related quality of life was also significantly higher for the intervention group (adjusted mean difference = 0.05; 95% CI = 0.01, 0.08). However, patients in the intervention group did not differ significantly on positive and active engagement in life [42]. These results were confirmed by a sensitivity analysis using complete cases and a further post-hoc analysis adjusted for differing sub-group criteria for blood pressure control and differing times of measurement.

Figure 2 depicts the unadjusted rates of blood pressure control for the two groups, across time. The rate of control remained stable in the intervention group over the 6 months, but dropped very considerably in control patients, suggesting that the effect of the intervention was to help patients maintain, but not increase, blood pressure control. Mean systolic and diastolic blood pressure in intervention patients changed very little over the 6 months (from 131.6 to 131.5 and 73.6 to 73.4 respectively), but increased in control patients (129.0 to 135.2 and 73.4 to 74.5 respectively). For health related quality of life however, there was an increase in mean score for intervention patients, compared to no change in the control group mean (Figure 3).

Analysis of secondary outcomes (table 3) indicated that patients in the intervention group reported significantly higher levels of self-care activity at 6 months compared to control patients (adjusted mean difference = 0.23; 95% CI = 0.04, 0.41). In contrast to our hypothesis, patients in the intervention group experienced a significant reduction in practical work undertaken by their social network at 6 months (adjusted mean difference = −2.02; 95% CI = −3.68, −0.36). All results remained unchanged under both sensitivity analyses, with the exception of a significant ($p<0.05$) increase in energy/vitality scores for intervention patients under complete cases analysis.

Cost effectiveness. Based on a multiple imputation analysis, there were statistically significant differences between the groups in terms of Quality Adjusted Life Years generated over the 6 month time horizon of the trial. The absolute difference, in favour of the BRIGHT intervention, of 0.012 QALYs (95%CI 0.002 to 0.022) after adjustment including baseline EQ5D scores would be considered statistically significant at conventional levels. Again based on multiple imputation data, the intervention group was associated with a reduction in costs compared with control due to lower secondary care attendance. The mean difference in total cost was £175 (95%CI −£284 to £635). Control groups costs were inflated by two individuals spending 60+ days as inpatients. However, even when these are removed, the intervention is associated with reduced costs (mean difference £123, 95% CI −£103 to £349). Results from the multiple imputation were consistent with the complete case analysis, where again QALYs were significantly higher in BRIGHT group and costs were reduced.

Discussion

Principal findings of the study

The BRIGHT intervention used tailored information and telephone-facilitated help to enhance self-management by sign-posting patients to community resources. The intervention was associated with modest but significant improvements in health related quality of life and better blood pressure control, which was maintained in the intervention arm but not in the control arm. However, with the exception of a small increase in self-care activities, these effects were not matched by improvements in patient-reported positive and active engagement in life.

These modest but significant benefits occurred in the context of relatively limited engagement with some aspects of the interventions. Relatively few patients in the intervention arm of the trial reported engagement with a PLANS group, with only 7.8% reporting attending at least one PLANS group at 6-months. This data might suggest that the PLANS component was ineffective and could be omitted from the intervention. We argue that would be premature. It is difficult to remove individual components from a complex intervention without potentially threatening the effectiveness of the whole. Qualitative work conducted as part of the BRIGHT trial [54] shows that the PLANS and telephone-guided help components of the intervention were more challenging for patients, and also provided some evidence that the process encouraged positive action by giving patients the opportunity to reflect on their current circumstances. A better focus may be on enhancing the intervention, by increasing the number of follow up consultations, or providing supported access to groups (such as transport). However, lack of clarity about the causal mechanisms suggests that further work is needed to explore these issues before more widespread commissioning can be recommended.

Strengths and limitations of this study

The intervention is a generic model that could be adapted for any chronic condition, but CKD was selected because of its

Table 2. Intervention uptake and evaluation.

Outcome	Total intervention group 6mfu data (n = 179)
Kidney booklet uptake	
How useful did you find the 'Keeping your kidneys healthy booklet':	
Very useful or useful	150 (83.8)
Not very useful or useful at all	8 (4.5)
Didn't use	17 (9.5)
Missing	4 (2.2)
How often did you refer to the 'Keeping your kidneys healthy booklet':	
Used occasionally or now and then	81 (45.3)
Used only once	66 (36.9)
Haven't used	27 (15.1)
Missing	5 (2.8)
Kidney booklet evaluation	
The 'Keeping your kidneys healthy booklet' was easy to read:	
Strongly agree or agree	156 (87.2)
Neither agree nor disagree	11 (6.2)
Disagree or strongly disagree	1 (0.6)
Missing	11 (6.2)
The 'Keeping your kidneys healthy booklet' made me feel less anxious:	
Strongly agree or agree	86 (48.0)
Neither agree nor disagree	65 (36.3)
Disagree or strongly disagree	15 (8.4)
Missing	13 (7.3)
The 'Keeping your kidneys healthy booklet' helped me discuss care with my doctor:	
Strongly agree or agree	101 (56.4)
Neither agree nor disagree	53 (29.6)
Disagree or strongly disagree	12 (6.7)
Missing	13 (7.3)
The 'Keeping your kidneys healthy booklet' helped me understand how the NHS will support my care:	
Strongly agree or agree	117 (65.4)
Neither agree nor disagree	44 (24.6)
Disagree or strongly disagree	3 (1.7)
Missing	15 (8.4)
The 'Keeping your kidneys healthy booklet' enabled you to cope with life:	
Much better or better	70 (39.1)
Same or less	74 (41.3)
Missing/not applicable	35 (19.6)
The 'Keeping your kidneys healthy booklet' enabled you to understand your condition:	
Much better or better	93 (52.0)
Same or less	56 (31.3)
Missing/not applicable	30 (16.8)
The 'Keeping your kidneys healthy booklet' enabled you to cope with your condition:	
Much better or better	80 (44.7)
Same or less	63 (35.2)
Missing/not applicable	36 (20.1)
The 'Keeping your kidneys healthy booklet' enabled you to keep yourself healthy:	
Much better or better	93 (52.0)
Same or less	57 (31.8)
Missing/NA	29 (16.2)
The 'Keeping your kidneys healthy booklet' enabled you to feel confident about your health:	
Much more or more	69 (38.6)

Table 2. Cont.

Outcome	Total intervention group 6mfu data (n = 179)
Same or less	79 (44.1)
Missing/NA	31 (17.3)
The 'Keeping your kidneys healthy booklet' enabled you to help yourself:	
Much more or more	74 (41.3)
Same or less	72 (40.2)
Missing/NA	33 (18.4)
Telephone support call uptake:	
How useful did you find the telephone support call:	
Very useful or useful	111 (62.0)
Not very useful or useful at all	14 (7.8)
Didn't use	47 (26.3)
Missing	7 (3.9)
Telephone support call evaluation:	
I would like to use this type of service again:	
Strongly agree or agree	47 (26.3)
Neither agree nor disagree	86 (48.0)
Disagree or strongly disagree	29 (16.2)
Missing	17 (9.5)
I felt the conversation with the telephone support worker was relevant to me:	
Strongly agree or agree	91 (50.8)
Neither agree nor disagree	59 (33.0)
Disagree or strongly disagree	15 (8.4)
Missing	14 (7.8)
I felt the conversation with the telephone support worker understood my needs and concerns:	
Strongly agree or agree	99 (55.3)
Neither agree nor disagree	58 (32.4)
Disagree or strongly disagree	7 (3.9)
Missing	15 (8.4)
The conversation encouraged me to think about trying local activities:	
Strongly agree or agree	72 (40.2)
Neither agree nor disagree	64 (35.8)
Disagree or strongly disagree	28 (15.7)
Missing	15 (8.4)
The conversation was easy to follow:	
Strongly agree or agree	131 (73.2)
Neither agree nor disagree	28 (15.6)
Disagree or strongly disagree	4 (2.2)
Missing	16 (8.9)
Website uptake:	
How useful did you find the website:	
Very useful or useful	41 (22.9)
Not very useful or useful at all	14 (7.8)
Didn't use	108 (60.3)
Missing/not applicable	16 (8.9)
How many times did you visit the website?:	
Used occasionally or now and then	18 (10.1)
Used only once	29 (16.2)
Haven't used	90 (50.3)
Missing/not applicable	42 (23.5)

Table 2. Cont.

Outcome	Total intervention group 6mfu data (n = 179)
Website evaluation:	
I found the website easy to use:	
Strongly agree or agree	26 (14.5)
Neither agree nor disagree	52 (29.1)
Disagree or strongly disagree	12 (6.7)
Missing/not applicable	89 (49.7)
I found the website relevant to me:	
Strongly agree or agree	14 (7.8)
Neither agree nor disagree	62 (34.6)
Disagree or strongly disagree	13 (7.3)
Missing/not applicable	90 (50.3)
PLANS booklet uptake:	
How useful did you find the PLANS booklet:	
Very useful or useful	119 (66.5)
Not very useful or useful at all	29 (16.2)
Didn't use	26 (14.5)
Missing	5 (2.8)
PLANS groups uptake:	
Total number of PLANS groups patient's contacted:	
0	101 (56.1)
1–2	34 (18.9)
3+	6 (3.4)
Missing	6 (3.3)
Not applicable - No group information requested	33 (18.3)
Total number of PLANS groups patient's attended:	
0	108 (60.0)
1	19 (10.6)
2	6 (3.3)
3	3 (1.7)
Missing	11 (6.1)
Not applicable - No group information requested	33 (18.3)
Total number of PLANS groups patient's currently attending:	
0	122 (67.8)
1	10 (5.6)
2	2 (1.1)
3	2 (1.1)
Missing	11 (6.1)
Not applicable - No group information requested	33 (18.3)

Values are number (percentage).

association with socioeconomic deprivation as well as controversies over the relevance of the condition to patients and practitioners. The majority of patients with stage 3 CKD are managed in primary care and though effective self-management support is highlighted as a key aspect of care for this practice population [17], thus far there has been limited research and evidence on how to achieve this [55]. Intervention and study design was informed by the principles of minimally disruptive medicine [32] in order to support the embedding and integration of recruitment for the BRIGHT intervention with primary care procedures. We achieved high levels of participation by general practices. Respecting GP judgement on eligibility, 440 out of 637 (69%) potential participants agreed to take part in the trial. In addition, participant self-report indicated that the components of the intervention were both acceptable and useful.

We recognise that the provision of information may also be relevant to patients with CKD stages 1 or 2 with proteinuria, who are also at increased cardiovascular risk [16]. However, for trial purposes, in order to be confident of recruiting patients with a recorded diagnosis, we limited recruitment to patients with stage 3 CKD - a stage incentivised by the Quality and Outcomes Framework of the new General Medical Services contract [56].

Table 3. Results of regression analyses of primary and secondary outcomes at 6 months.

	Unadjusted mean (SD); N					
Outcome	**BRIGHT intervention[1]**	**Usual care[1]**	**Adjusted mean difference[2] (95% CI)**	**P Value[2]**	**Effect size[2]**	**Effect size from complete cases analysis[1]**
Primary Outcomes						
Blood pressure control	67.3%[3]; 193	55.3%[3]; 210	1.85[4] (1.25, 2.72)	0.002*	1.85[4] (1.25, 2.72)	1.90[4] (1.28, 2.83)
Positive and active engagement with life (heiQ) positive and active engagement in life *Higher score = higher engagement with life*	66.4 (19.7); 180	66.5 (17.6); 194	0.00 (−3.20, 3.21)	0.999	0.00 (−0.16, 0.16)	−0.01 (−0.17, 0.16)
Health-related Quality of Life (EQ-5D)	0.71 (0.28); 179	0.67 (0.29); 193	0.05 (0.01, 0.08)	0.027*	0.16 (0.03, 0.29)	0.18 (0.06, 0.30)
Secondary Outcomes						
heiQ, social integration and support *Higher score = Higher social integration*	69.6 (20.3); 178	69.4 (15.6); 193	0.78 (−1.70, 3.26)	0.537¶	0.05 (−0.10, 0.20)	0.01 (−0.16, 0.19)
heiQ, skills and technique acquisition *Higher score = Higher skills and technique acquisition*	65.4 (14.6); 177	65.0(13.1); 192	1.49 (−0.88, 3.85)	0.218¶	0.10 (−0.06, 0.27)	0.13 (−0.05, 0.31)
heiQ, emotional wellbeing *Higher score = Higher negative affect*	31.4 (22.2); 180	34.0 (22.2); 194	−1.85 (−5.75, 2.05)	0.329	−0.09 (−0.25, 0.07)	−0.09 (−0.25, 0.07)
heiQ, self-monitoring and insight *Higher score = Higher self monitoring and insight*	70.7 (12.2); 180	70.7 (11.5); 194	0.47 (−1.65, 2.58)	0.644	0.04 (−0.11, 0.20)	0.03 (−0.13, 0.18)
heiQ, health services navigation *Higher score = higher health service navigation*	70.5 (16.2); 179	69.4 (15.9); 193	1.88 (−1.28, 5.04)	0.226	0.14 (−0.06, 0.34)	0.12 (−0.08, 0.32)
SelfCare Activities (SDSCA) *Higher score = higher self-care*	4.5 (1.2); 172	4.2 (1.2); 191	0.23 (0.04, 0.41)	0.019*	0.20 (0.06, 0.34)	0.17 (0.05, 0.29)
Anxiety (HADS-A) *Higher score = greater anxiety*	4.6 (3.7); 179	5.2 (4.1); 194	−0.51 (−1.05, 0.02)	0.060	−0.14 (−0.28, 0.01)	−0.14 (−0.27, 0.00)
CKD-specific anxiety (BIPQ Emotional Response item asked in relation to CKD) (6 months only) *Higher score = greater anxiety*	1.2 (2.0); 179	1.6 (2.2); 190	−0.46 (−0.97, 0.05)	0.073	−0.21 (−0.42, 0.00)	−0.18 (−0.39, 0.02)
MOS, General Health *Higher score = Better general health*	2.8 (1.0); 179	2.8 (0.9); 193	0.01 (−0.12, 0.14)	0.832	0.01 (−0.12, 0.14)	−0.02 (−0.14, 0.10)
MOS, Social/Role Activities Limitations *Higher score = LOWER social limitations*	73.2 (28.2); 177	68.7 (30.5); 194	1.85 (−3.68, 7.37)	0.492	0.06 (−0.10, 0.22)	0.05 (−0.13, 0.22)
MOS, Energy/Vitality *Higher score = higher energy and vitality*	52.4 (22.0); 179	50.8 (21.8); 194	2.77 (−0.39, 5.93)	0.082	0.13 (0.00, 0.26)	0.16 (0.04, 0.28)
MOS, Psychological Wellbeing *Higher score = higher psychological wellbeing*	74.7 (18.8); 179	74.0 (19.9); 193	1.28 (−1.18, 3.73)	0.286	0.06 (−0.06, 0.18)	0.08 (−0.04, 0.19)
Loneliness (UCLA Loneliness Scale) *Higher score = LOWER loneliness.*	30.3 (5.3); 177	31.0 (4.4); 192	−0.06 (−0.82, 0.69)	0.861	−0.01 (−0.15, 0.14)	−0.01 (−0.15, 0.14)

Table 3. Cont.

Outcome	Unadjusted mean (SD); N — BRIGHT intervention[1]	Usual care[1]	Adjusted mean difference[2] (95% CI)	P Value[2]	Effect size[2]	Effect size from complete cases analysis[1]
MMMAS, Medication knowledge (6 months only) *Higher score = higher medication knowledge*	2.6 (0.6); 175	2.6 (0.6); 191	−0.05 (−0.16, 0.05)	0.331¶	−0.09 (−0.26, 0.09)	−0.07 (−0.26, 0.12)
MMMAS, Medication motivation (6 months only) *Higher score = higher medication motivation*	2.7 (0.6); 177	2.7 (0.5); 192	−0.03 (−0.13, 0.07)	0.568¶	−0.06 (−0.25, 0.14)	−0.05 (−0.25, 0.16)
Social capital: Health Survey for England *Higher score = greater satisfaction with opportunities to participate in the community*	3.7 (0.8); 178	3.6 (0.8); 188	0.08 (−0.08, 0.23)	0.325	0.09 (−0.08, 0.26)	0.09 (−0.08, 0.25)
Service use	6.1 (5.5); 180	6.5 (4.7); 194	−0.30 (−1.10, 0.49)	0.455¶	−0.03 (−0.10, 0.04)	−0.03 (−0.1, 0.04)
Social network - Illness work *Higher score = greater help with illness work from social network*	10.3 (8.4); 160	11.5 (9.0); 182	−1.18 (−3.02, 0.66)	0.208¶	−0.21 (−0.54, 0.12)	−0.24 (−0.61, 0.13)
Social network - Practical work *Higher score = greater help with practical work from social network*	6.2 (6.2); 159	8.1 (7.1); 176	−2.02 (−3.68, −0.36)	0.017*¶	−0.46 (−0.83, −0.08)	−0.53 (−0.93, −0.12)
Social network - Emotional work *Higher score = greater help with emotional work from social network*	13.4 (10.4); 163	14.9 (11.4); 182	−0.67 (−2.47, 1.12)	0.463¶	−0.09 (−0.31, 0.14)	−0.13 (−0.35, 0.09)

[1]Values from complete cases.
[2]Values from multiple imputation analysis.
[3]Percentage of patients with controlled blood pressure.
[4]Adjusted odds ratio.
¶P value based on boot strapped estimate of variance.
*Significant at $p<0.05$.

Participation was restricted to patients able to read and understand English so we cannot assume that the findings of this study would be similar for patients in whom English is not their first language. None of the staff who delivered the intervention had clinical training (though one was a member of the research team and all but one were psychology graduates), and the BRIGHT training was brief. If the intervention was to be rolled out, it is likely that it could be delivered by a range of staff, including staff in voluntary groups, more established lay health workers such as health trainers, or telecare staff.

Limitations of the study are that a longer follow-up would have been preferable to show if the improvements could be sustained. The trial used validated instruments to measure health related quality of life and positive and active engagement in life [42] [52], though we recognise there is potential for bias in patient self-report outcomes in an unblinded trial. Resource use was also collected using patient questionnaires at baseline and follow up, which is a potential limitation as self-report may not always agree with sources such as service records. Blood pressure measurement was based on routine data collection rather than formal research assessments, and there was also a small difference in retention rates between arms. However, we used robust allocation concealment, achieved high levels of retention overall, and used appropriate imputation to account for missing data, and have no reason to doubt that the blood pressure outcomes are valid. Nevertheless, caution is required with interpretation of the blood pressure outcome, since the mechanism of action remains unclear. There were no significant differences between the two arms of the study in terms of positive and active engagement in life (primary outcome), GP and nurse visits, or medication adherence (secondary outcomes). We did not collect data on prescribing of antihypertensive medication, which is a potential limitation in understanding mechanisms of action though an effect was observed on self-management activities (secondary outcomes) using a validated measure that assesses diet, exercise and smoking behaviour. The intervention was intended to facilitate greater engagement with community groups and resources, but contrary to our original hypothesis, in addition to no significant effect in positive and active engagement in life, levels of support from personal social networks (for practical work) were significantly reduced in the intervention arm. One plausible explanation is that intervention patients felt enabled to do more for themselves, thus reducing dependence on others: high dependency has negative emotional effects and greater autonomy is a desired objective of many people with limiting health problems [57]. A better understanding of the mechanisms by which these innovative network interventions achieve their effects is a key research question for the future.

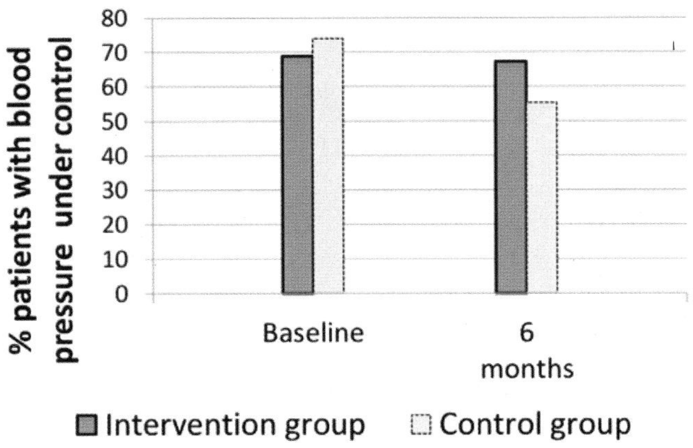

Figure 2. Percentages of intervention and control patients with controlled blood pressure.

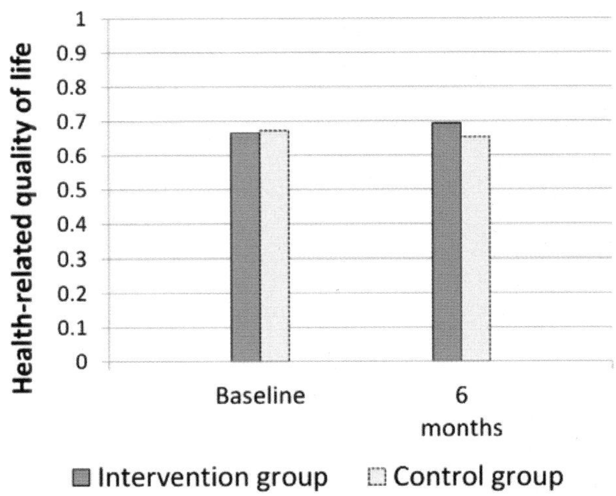

Figure 3. Health related quality of life for intervention and control patients.

Comparison with other studies and key implications of the research

The BRIGHT trial aimed to connect people to resources in order to support vascular health and broader wellbeing, and builds on growing evidence that diverse and supportive networks can improve health [9]. This approach values support provided outside healthcare settings, though it may be important that such support is legitimised by a GP or nurse [58]. Our intervention may have created a critical moment or tipping point for patients. Perhaps this method of increasing awareness of CKD gave control to the patient enabling them to initiate responses or actions.

A recent meta-analysis highlighted the importance of blood pressure lowering as an effective strategy for reducing cardiovascular events in people with CKD [59]. Our results demonstrated deterioration in blood pressure control in usual care patients and maintenance of control in those receiving the intervention, but the comparative benefits were similar in magnitude to structured care in general practice for patients with poorly controlled hypertension [60].

There have been concerns among GPs and nurses that raising awareness of CKD could have detrimental effects on patients because of raised anxiety [22], but the current study provides a model for informing patients about the diagnosis in the context of the maintenance of general vascular health, with good evidence for benefits in both clinical and quality of life outcomes and no noticeable increase in anxiety. Broadening and personalising discussions around kidney health may address fears over disease labelling and support the practise of effective minimally disruptive medicine [21] [32]. In light of recent clinical guidance, in addition to the BRIGHT trial's focus on placing CKD in the context of general vascular health, patient and carer involvement in the development of information resources to support the prevention and management of acute kidney injury (AKI) may also be warranted [61]. Elderly housebound patients living with complex co-morbidities are particularly at risk of AKI - a syndrome that is common, harmful, costly and potentially avoidable [62].

These findings provide support for an effective and cost-effective strategy to improve outcomes for people with CKD and other vascular diseases, which takes health management into everyday contexts. Moving away from traditional individually-focused models of self-management allows for appreciation of the everyday challenges faced by people with long-term conditions and draws attention towards potentially valuable forms of non-clinical support [12].

Conclusions

Findings that an intervention delivered outside the health encounter can have a significant (albeit modest) impact on health outcomes and can be cost effective demonstrate the merit of a community focussed approach to self-management support. The BRIGHT trial highlights the potential importance of widening the types of support offered to people with long-term conditions, in particular by shifting the emphasis of self-management support towards community resources and personal networks of support. Although further work on mechanisms of effect is clearly warranted, these findings, alongside evidence that interventions to change professional behaviour to support self-management are of limited benefit, suggest that better outcomes may be achieved by placing more effort and resources in communities and that more research should be directed towards determining ways and means of embedding health management activities into everyday life.

Acknowledgments

The authors would like to thank the participating practices, staff and patients for their contribution. The authors would also like to thank Yvonne Rossi, Angela Swallow, Kerin Hannon, Brook Butler, Abigail Methley, Amy Degnan, Anna Chisholm, Christina Pearce, Susan Moschogianis, Emily Haythornthwaite, Nicola Small and John Humphries for their contributions to the design and conduct of this study.

Author Contributions

Conceived and designed the experiments: CB TB AK AR IV PB DR CCG GR ES HB. Performed the experiments: TB CB AK AR PB DR HG HB SD CG RM VL PJ. Analyzed the data: CB TB AK AR PB DR GR HG ES HB SD CG RM VL PJ. Wrote the paper: CB TB AK AR PB DR GR HG ES HB SD CG RM VL PJ IV CCG. Designed the intervention: CB TB AK AR IV PJ HB.

References

1. Wagner EH (1998) Chronic disease management: what will it take to improve care for chronic illness? Eff Clin Pract 1: 2–4.
2. Dennis SM, Zwar N, Griffiths R, Roland M, Hasan I, et al. (2008) Chronic disease management in primary care: from evidence to policy. Medical Journal of Australia 188: S53.
3. Kennedy A, Bower P, Reeves D, Blakeman T, Bowen R, et al. (2013) Implementation of self management support for long term conditions in routine primary care settings: cluster randomised controlled trial. BMJ: British Medical Journal 346.
4. Warsi A, Wang PS, LaValley MP, Avorn J, Solomon DH (2004) Self-management education programs in chronic disease: a systematic review and methodological critique of the literature. Archives of Internal Medicine 164: 1641.
5. McCall N, Cromwell J (2011) Results of the Medicare Health Support disease-management pilot program. New England Journal of Medicine 365: 1704–1712.
6. Powell LH, Calvin Jr JE, Richardson D, Janssen I, de Leon CFM, et al. (2010) Self-management counseling in patients with heart failure. JAMA: the Journal of the American Medical Association 304: 1331–1338.
7. Egginton JS, Ridgeway JL, Shah ND, Balasubramaniam S, Emmanuel JR, et al. (2012) Care management for Type 2 diabetes in the United States: a systematic review and meta-analysis. BMC Health Services Research 12: 72.
8. Motheral BR (2011) Telephone-Based Disease Management: Why It Does Not Save Money-Page 2. Am J Manag Care 17: e10-e16.
9. Christakis NA, Fowler JH (2008) The collective dynamics of smoking in a large social network. N Engl J Med 358: 2249–2258.
10. Marmot M (2010) Fair Society, Healthy Lives: Strategic Review of Health Inequalities in England post 2010
11. Bower P, Kennedy A, Reeves D, Rogers A, Blakeman T, et al. (2012) A cluster randomised controlled trial of the clinical and cost-effectiveness of a 'whole systems' model of self-management support for the management of long- term conditions in primary care: trial protocol. Implementation Science 7.
12. Vassilev I, Rogers A, Blickem C, Brooks H, Kapadia D, et al. (2013) Social Networks, the 'Work' and Work Force of Chronic Illness Self-Management: A Survey Analysis of Personal Communities. PloS one 8: e59723.
13. Furler J (2008) Changing paradigms in chronic condition care. Chronic Illness 4: 157–159.
14. Blickem C, Blakeman T, Kennedy A, Bower P, Reeves D, et al. (2013) The clinical and cost-effectiveness of the BRinging Information and Guided Help Together (BRIGHT) intervention for the self-management support of people with stage 3 chronic kidney disease in primary care: study protocol for a randomized controlled trial. Trials 14: 28.
15. Wanless D (2003) Securing good health for the whole population: population health trends. London: HM Treasury. 51 p. p.
16. Matsushita K, van der Velde M, Astor BC, Woodward M, Levey AS, et al. (2010) Association of estimated glomerular filtration rate and albuminuria with all-cause and cardiovascular mortality in general population cohorts: a collaborative meta-analysis. Lancet 375: 2073.
17. NICE (2008) Chronic kidney disease Early identification and management of chronic kidney disease in adults in primary and secondary care. London: National Institute for Health and Clinical Excellence. Clinical guidelines CG73 Clinical guidelines CG73.
18. Abdi Z, Gallagher H, O'Donoghue D (2012) Telling the truth: why disclosure matters in chronic kidney disease. The British Journal of General Practice 62: 172.
19. Crinson I, Gallagher H, Thomas N, de Lusignan S (2010) How ready is general practice to improve quality in chronic kidney disease? A diagnostic analysis. The British Journal of General Practice 60: 403.
20. Remuzzi G, Benigni A, Finkelstein FO, Grunfeld JP, Joly D, et al. (2013) Kidney failure: aims for the next 10 years and barriers to success. Lancet 382: 353–362.
21. Moynihan R, Glassock R, Doust J (2013) Chronic kidney disease controversy: how expanding definitions are unnecessarily labelling many people as diseased. BMJ: British Medical Journal 347.
22. Blakeman T, Protheroe J, Chew-Graham C, Rogers A, Kennedy A (2012) Understanding the management of early-stage chronic kidney disease in primary care: a qualitative study. British Journal of General Practice 62: e233–e242.
23. Fraser SD, Roderick P, Bailey L, Sanderson H (2012) Novel use of a combined primary and secondary care data resource: investigation of inequalities in chronic kidney disease identification in the UK Hampshire Health Record. The Lancet 380: S40.
24. Greer RC, Cooper LA, Crews DC, Powe NR, Boulware L (2011) Quality of patient-physician discussions about CKD in primary care: a cross-sectional study. American Journal of Kidney Diseases 57: 583–591.
25. Plantinga LC, Tuot DS, Powe NR (2010) Awareness of chronic kidney disease among patients and providers. Advances in chronic kidney disease 17: 225–236.
26. McIntyre NJ, Fluck R, McIntyre C, Taal M (2012) Treatment needs and diagnosis awareness in primary care patients with chronic kidney disease. British Journal of General Practice 62: e227–e232.
27. De Lusignan S, Gallagher H, Stevens P, Harris K, Dmitrieva O, et al. (2011) Chronic kidney disease frequently asked questions. London: NHS Employers and BMA.
28. Jha V, Garcia-Garcia G, Iseki K, Li Z, Naicker S, et al. (2013) Chronic kidney disease: global dimension and perspectives. The Lancet.
29. Coresh J, Selvin E, Stevens LA, Manzi J, Kusek JW, et al. (2007) Prevalence of chronic kidney disease in the United States. JAMA: the journal of the American Medical Association 298: 2038–2047.
30. Hossain M, Palmer D, Goyder E, El Nahas A (2012) Social deprivation and prevalence of chronic kidney disease in the UK: workload implications for primary care. QJM 105: 167–175.
31. Rogers A, Vassilev I, Sanders C, Kirk S, Chew-Graham C, et al. (2011) Social networks, work and network-based resources for the management of long-term conditions: a framework and study protocol for developing self-management support. Implementation Science 6.
32. May C, Montori VM, Mair FS (2009) We need minimally disruptive medicine. BMJ 339.
33. Humphreys J, Harvey G, Coleiro M, Butler B, Barclay A, et al. (2012) A collaborative project to improve identification and management of patients with chronic kidney disease in a primary care setting in Greater Manchester. BMJ Quality & Safety 21: 700–708.
34. Statistics OfN (2007) Index of Multiple Deprivation (IMD).
35. Kennedy A, Robinson A, Thompson D, Wilkin D (1999) Development of a guidebook to promote patient participation in the management of ulcerative colitis. Health Soc Care Community 7: 177–186.
36. Kennedy A, Rogers A (2002) Improving patient involvement in chronic disease management: the views of patients, GPs and specialists on a guidebook for ulcerative colitis Pat Educ Couns 47: 257–263.
37. Kennedy A, Robinson A, Rogers A (2003) Incorporating patients' views and experiences of life with IBS in the development of an evidence based self-help guidebook. Pat Educ Couns 50: 303–310.
38. Blickem C, Kennedy A, Vassilev I, Morris R, Brooks H, et al. (2013) Linking people with long-term health conditions to healthy community activities: development of Patient-Led Assessment for Network Support (PLANS). Health Expect 16: e48–59.
39. Small N, Blickem C, Blakeman T, Panagioti M, Chew-Graham CA, et al. (2013) Telephone based self-management support by 'lay health workers' and 'peer support workers' to prevent and manage vascular diseases: a systematic review and meta-analysis. BMC Health Serv Res 13: 533.
40. Kennedy A, Nelson E, Reeves D, Richardson G, Roberts C, et al. (2003) A randomised controlled trial to assess the impact of a package comprising a patient-orientated, evidence-based self-help guidebook and patient-centred consultations on disease management and satisfaction in inflammatory bowel disease. Health Technol Assess 7: iii, 1–113.
41. Kennedy A, Reeves D, Bower P, Lee V, Middleton E, et al. (2007) The effectiveness and cost effectiveness of a national lay-led self care support programme for patients with long-term conditions: a pragmatic randomised controlled trial. Journal of Epidemiology and Community Health 61: 254–261.
42. Osborne RH, Elsworth GR, Whitfield K (2007) The Health Education Impact Questionnaire (heiQ): An outcomes and evaluation measure for patient education and self-management interventions for people with chronic conditions. Patient Education and Counseling 66: 192–201.
43. Kind P (1996) The EuroQoL instrument: an index of health-related quality of life. Quality of Life and Pharmacoeconomics in Clinical Trials. Philadelphia: LippincottRaven.
44. Toobert D, Hanson S, Glasgow R (2000) The summary of Diabetes SelfCare Activities Measure. Diabetes Care 23: 943–950.
45. Zigmond A, Snaith R (1983) The hospital anxiety and depression scale. Acta Psychiatric Scandinavica 67: 361–370.
46. Broadbent E, Petrie KJ, Main J, Weinman J (2006) The Brief Illness Perception Questionnaire. Journal of Psychosomatic Research: 60.
47. Lorig K, Stewart A, Ritter P, Gonzalez V, Laurent D, et al. (1996) Outcome measures for health education and other health care interventions Thousand Oaks: Sage.
48. Russell DW (1996) UCLA Loneliness Scale (Version 3): Reliability, Validity, and Factor Structure. Journal of Personality Assessment 66: 20–40.
49. Morisky DE, Green LW, Levine DM (1986) Concurrent and Predictive Validity of a Self-Reported Measure of Medication Adherence. Medical Care 24: 67–74.
50. Bajekal M, Purdon S (2011) Social capital and social exclusion: development of a condensed module for the Health Survey for England. Available: http://wwwdhgovuk/prod_consum_dh/groups/dh_digitalassets/@dh/@en/documents/digitalasset/dh_4058955pdf.

51. White IR, Royston P, Wood AM (2011) Multiple imputation using chained equations: Issues and guidance for practice. Statistics in medicine 30: 377–399.
52. Dolan P, Gudex C, Kind P, Williams A (1995) A social tariff for EuroQol: results from a UK general population survey: Centre for Health Economics.
53. Manca A, Hawkins N, Sculpher MJ (2005) Estimating mean QALYs in trial-based cost-effectiveness analysis: the importance of controlling for baseline utility. Health economics 14: 487–496.
54. Blickem C, Kennedy A, Jariwala P, Morris R, Bowen R, et al. (2014) Aligning everyday life priorities with people's self-management support networks: an exploration of the work and implementation of a needs-led telephone support system. BMC health services research 14: 262.
55. Li T, Wu HM, Wang F, Huang CQ, Yang M, et al. (2011) Education programmes for people with diabetic kidney disease. Cochrane Database of Systematic Reviews 15.
56. Prescribing and Primary Care team HaSCIC Quality and Outcomes Framework, Achievement, Prevalence and exceptions data 2011/2012. Health and Social Care Information Centre, 2012.
57. Cornwell B (2009) Network Bridging Potential in Later Life Life-Course Experiences and Social Network Position. Journal of aging and health 21: 129–154.
58. Rogers A, Lee V, Kennedy A (2007) Continuity and change?: Exploring reactions to a guided self-management intervention in a randomised controlled trial for IBS with reference to prior experience of managing a long term condition. Trials 8: 6.
59. Trialists'Collaboration BPLT (2013) Blood pressure lowering and major cardiovascular events in people with and without chronic kidney disease: meta-analysis of randomised controlled trials. BMJ: British Medical Journal 347.
60. Stewart S, Carrington MJ, Swemmer CH, Anderson C, Kurstjens NP, et al. (2012) Effect of intensive structured care on individual blood pressure targets in primary care: multicentre randomised controlled trial. BMJ: British Medical Journal 345.
61. Excellence NIfHaC (2013) Acute Kidney Injury. Prevention, detection and management of acute kidney injury up to the point of renal replacement therapy. London: National Institute for Health and Care Excellence.
62. Khwaja A (2012) KDIGO clinical practice guidelines for acute kidney injury. Nephron Clinical Practice 120: c179–c184.

Soluble α-Klotho as a Novel Biomarker in the Early Stage of Nephropathy in Patients with Type 2 Diabetes

Eun Young Lee[1*¶], Sang Soo Kim[2¶], Ji-Sung Lee[3], In Joo Kim[2], Sang Heon Song[2], Seung-Kuy Cha[4], Kyu-Sang Park[4], Jeong Suk Kang[1], Choon Hee Chung[5]

1 Department of Internal Medicine, Soonchunhyang University Cheonan Hospital, Cheonan, Korea, 2 Department of Internal Medicine, Pusan National University Hospital, Busan, Korea, 3 Biostatistical Consulting Unit, Soonchunhyang University Medical Center, Seoul, Korea, 4 Department of Physiology, Yonsei University Wonju College of Medicine, Wonju, Korea, 5 Department of Internal Medicine, Yonsei University Wonju College of Medicine, Wonju, Korea

Abstract

Objective: Although α-klotho is known as an anti-aging, antioxidant, and cardio-renal protective protein, the clinical implications of soluble α-klotho levels in patients with diabetes have not been evaluated. Therefore, this study evaluated whether plasma and urinary α-klotho levels are associated with albuminuria in kidney disease in diabetes.

Research Design and Methods: A total of 147 patients with type 2 diabetes and 25 healthy control subjects were enrolled. The plasma and urine concentrations of α-klotho were analyzed by enzyme-linked immunosorbent assay.

Results: Plasma α-klotho (572.4 pg/mL [95% CI, 541.9–604.6 pg/mL] *vs.* 476.9 pg/mL [95% CI, 416.9–545.5 pg/mL]) and urinary α-klotho levels (59.8 pg/mg creatinine [95% CI, 43.6–82.0 pg/mg creatinine] *vs.* 21.0 pg/mg creatinine [95% CI, 9.7–45.6 pg/mg creatinine]) were significantly higher in diabetic patients than non-diabetic controls. Among diabetic patients, plasma α-klotho concentration was inversely associated with albuminuria stages (normoalbuminuria, 612.6 pg/mL [95% CI, 568.9–659.6 pg/mL], microalbuminuria, 551.8 pg/mL [95% CI, 500.5–608.3 pg/mL], and macroalbuminuria, 505.7 pg/mL [95% CI, 439.7–581.7 pg/mL] (p for trend $=0.0081$), while urinary α-klotho levels were remained constantly high with increasing urinary albumin excretion.

Conclusions: Soluble α-klotho levels in plasma and urine may be novel and useful early markers of diabetic renal injury.

Editor: Leighton R James, University of Florida, United States of America

Funding: This research was supported by Basic Science Research Program through the National Research Foundation of Korea (NRF) funded by the Ministry of Education, Science, and Technology (2012R1A1A2044121) and the Soonchunhyang University Research Fund (No. 20130626). The funders had no role in study design, data collection and analysis, decision to publish, or preparation of the manuscript.

Competing Interests: The authors have declared that no competing interests exist.

* Email: eylee@sch.ac.kr

¶ These authors contributed equally to this work.

Introduction

Although α-klotho was first described as an anti-aging factor, recent experimental and clinical studies suggest α-klotho also has important pleotroic effects on the kidneys [1]. Soluble α-klotho is derived from the proteolytic cleavage of the extracellular portion of the membrane-bound α-klotho; alternatively, it can be generated directly by the alterative splicing of the α-klotho transcript [2]. It can be measured in blood, urine, and cerebrospinal fluid [1]. Animals with chronic kidney disease have very low renal, plasma, and urinary α-klotho levels [3]. Furthermore, humans with chronic kidney disease exhibit markedly reduced α-klotho in serum [4] and urine [3,5] in the early stages of kidney disease, progressively decreasing in more advanced stages.

However, with regard to diabetic nephropathy, the role of α-klotho in the pathogenesis of kidney injury has not been fully studied. Renal α-klotho expression is markedly decreased in diabetic nephropathy in humans and mice [6–8]. A similar decline is observed in kidney cells treated with methylglyoxal-modified albumin [8]. These findings collectively suggest renal α-klotho deficiency is part of an underlying mechanism involved in diabetic kidney injury. However, the actual role of soluble α-klotho in diabetic kidney disease has not been evaluated.

This study determined whether diabetes influences soluble circulating or urinary α-klotho level and investigated the relationship between these soluble α-klotho levels and albuminuria in patients with type 2 diabetes.

Research Design And Methods

Ethics statement

This study was carried out in accordance with the Declaration of Helsinki and study protocol was approved by the Institutional Review Board of Pusan National University Hospital (Busan, Korea). All patients provided their written informed consent before entering the study. Data are available to all interested researchers on request to the Institutional Review Board of Pusan National University Hospital.

Subjects

A total of 147 consecutive patients with type 2 diabetes were enrolled at outpatient clinics between February 2010 and February 2012. All patients met the following inclusion criteria: age ≥18 years and estimated GFR (eGFR) ≥60 mL min^{-1} 1.73 m^{-2}, serum creatinine <1.2 mg/dL, stable renal function status without 2-fold elevation of serum creatinine for at least 5 months, and no history of administration of RAS inhibitors. If patients took RAS inhibitors, these medications were withdrawn and replaced with other antihypertensive agents for at least 2 months before enrollment in this study. A random spot urine sample and a blood sample were obtained from each patient at the clinic visit. Medical histories and anthropometric measurements were also recorded on the same day. The eGFR was calculated using the Modification of Diet in Renal Disease (MDRD) Study formula as follows: MDRD = 186× (serum creatinine [mg/dL]$)^{-1.154}$ × age [years]$^{-0.203}$ [9]; a correction factor of 0.742 was used for women.

Patients with active urinary tract infection; renal disease other than diabetic nephropathy; neoplastic disorders; severe liver dysfunction; active or chronic infection or inflammatory disorders; pregnancy; or a recent (i.e., within 6 months) history of acute myocardial infarction, stroke, or occlusive peripheral vascular disease were excluded. Nondiabetic control subjects were randomly selected from the Center for Health Promotion at Pusan National University Hospital for a comprehensive medical check-up. They were enrolled in this study if they had fasting plasma glucose levels of <100 mg/dL after an overnight fasting, eGFR of ≥60 mL min^{-1} 1.73 m^{-2} and had no prior history of diabetes, renal disease or cardiovascular diseases including hypertension and dyslipidemia.

Soluble α-klotho enzyme-linked immunosorbent assays

Plasma samples were centrifuged for 15 minutes at 3,000 rpm within 30 minutes of collection; plasma was removed and stored at −70°C until analysis. Urine samples were centrifuged for 10 minutes at 3,000 rpm to remove particulate matter and stored at −70°C until analysis. The plasma and urine concentrations of α-klotho were analyzed by human soluble α-klotho immunoassay kits (Immuno-Biological Laboratories, Gunma, Japan) according to the manufacturer's protocol. All samples were run in duplicate and were within the range of the standard curve (93.75–6,000 pg/mL). Values below the detection limit (6.15 pg/mL) were approximated using the mean value between zero and the lower limit of detection. The intra- and inter-assay coefficients of variation were less than 10%. The levels of urinary α-klotho were expressed as the ratio of urinary α-klotho to urinary creatinine in order to assess the hydration states and renal functions of the patients.

Statistical analysis

Categorical variables, continuous variables with a normal distribution, and non-normally distributed variables are presented as number (percentage), mean ± SD, and median (interquartile range), respectively. Statistical analyses were performed after log-transforming the data of all skewed variables. Geometric means (i.e., antilogarithms of the transformed means) are presented with 95% CIs. The significance of differences between continuous variables was tested by ANOVA or the Kruskal–Wallis test, with polynomial contrasts for linear trends or Tukey's multiple comparison test where appropriate. Categorical variables were analyzed using the Pearson χ^2 test. Pearson correlation analysis was used to determine the correlations between individual variables. Multivariate regression analyses were used to determine the associations of plasma α-klotho with several parameters. All statistical analyses were performed using SPSS version 15.0 (SPSS Inc., Chicago, IL). The level of significance was set at $p<0.05$. All hypothesis tests were 2-sided.

Results

Elevated plasma and urinary α-klotho levels in patients with type 2 diabetes

A total of 172 subjects were enrolled in this study; their mean age was 55.8±10.4 years (range, 24–82 years), and there were 77 men and 95 women. Age, systolic, diastolic blood pressure, alanine aminotransferase, insulin, and eGFR were significantly higher in diabetic patients than non-diabetic control. Meanwhile, hemoglobin, total bilirubin, and direct bilirubin were significantly lower in diabetic patients than in non-diabetic controls. Other parameters did not differ significantly between the diabetes group and non-diabetic controls (Table 1). Plasma α-klotho was significantly higher in diabetic patients (Fig. 1*A*, 572.4 pg/mL [95% CI, 541.9–604.6 pg/mL] *vs.* 476.9 pg/mL [95% CI, 416.9–545.5 pg/mL], $p=0.016$). Urinary α-klotho levels were also significantly higher in diabetic patients than in non-diabetic controls (Fig. 1*C*, 59.8 pg/mg creatinine [95% CI, 43.6–82.0 pg/mg creatinine] *vs.* 21.0 pg/mg creatinine [95% CI, 9.7–45.6 pg/mg creatinine], $p=0.006$).

Inverse correlation between plasma α-klotho levels and albuminuria in patients with type 2 diabetes

Categories of progressively worse albuminuria were linearly associated with lower plasma α-klotho levels. The diabetic patients were categorized into 3 groups according to urine albumin creatinine ratio (ACR): ACR <30 mg/g creatinine (normoalbuminuria group, $n=75$), ACR 30–299 mg/g creatinine (microalbuminuria group, $n=42$), and ACR ≥300 mg/g creatinine (macroalbuminuria group, $n=30$) (Table 2). Age, sex, BMI, diastolic blood pressure, aspartate aminotransferase, alanine aminotransferase, HDL cholesterol, uric acid, phosphorous, serum creatinine, eGFR, C-reactive protein, and insulin did not differ significantly among the 3 groups.

The mean plasma α-klotho concentration in the normoalbuminuria group was 612.58 pg/mL compared to 505.70 pg/mL in the macroalbuminuria group (average difference, 106.88 pg/mL). Fig. 1 shows a clear inverse association between plasma α-klotho level and albuminuria level. Plasma α-klotho concentrations were the highest in the normoalbuminuria group and tended to decrease with increasing degrees of albuminuria (Fig. 1*B*, p for linear trend $=0.008$). In contrast to plasma α-klotho levels, no albuminuria level was significantly associated with urinary α-klotho creatinine ratio (Fig. 1*D*).

Correlations between plasma α-klotho levels and other parameters in patients with type 2 diabetes

As shown in Table 3, plasma α-klotho was significantly correlated with hemoglobin, aspartate aminotransferase, alanine aminotransferase, and insulin. Meanwhile, plasma α-klotho was negatively correlated with phosphorus, urine protein creatinine ratio, and urine ACR ($P<0.05$). However, there were no significant correlations between plasma α-klotho and HbA_{1C}, eGFR, or urine α-klotho. We performed multivariate regression analyses for the associations of plasma α-klotho with several parameters. In a multiple linear regression analysis, plasma α-klotho was significantly associated with hemoglobin ($r=0.01344$, $P=0.0095$) and urine ACR ($r=0.00154$, $P<0.0001$, Table 4).

Table 1. Clinical characteristics and laboratory findings of non-diabetic control subjects and type 2 diabetic patients.

	Normal (n=25)	DM (n=147)	P-value[†]
Age, years	50.9±7.6	56.6±10.6	0.0101
Sex, male	14(56.0)	63(42.9)	0.2218
BMI, kg/m^2	23.4±2.9	23.5±3.4	0.8408
SBP, mmHg	119.4±14.3	126.3±14.8	0.0333
DBP, mmHg	74.4±7.9	79.0±10.3	0.0335
Hemoglobin, g/dL	14.7±1.6	13.3±1.6	0.0002
Albumin, g/dL	4.5±0.3	4.4±0.5	0.2321
AST, IU/L	22.2±6.1	23.1±11.5	0.5364
ALT, IU/L	18.4±6.0	24.7±16.9	0.0009
Total cholesterol, mg/dL	193.68±33.60	180.03±40.64	0.1141
HDL cholesterol, mg/dL	55.32±13.42	50.04±16.87	0.1392
Triglycerides, mg/dL*	110.35(87.61 138.99)	140.78(126.98 156.09)	0.0726
Total bilirubin, mg/dL	1.07±0.36	0.64±0.21	<.0001
Direct bilirubin, mg/dL	0.21±0.07	0.14±0.05	0.0002
Uric acid, mg/dL	5.10±0.91	4.75±1.31	0.1027
Calcium, mg/dL	9.44±0.45	9.36±0.49	0.4258
Phosphorus, mg/dL	3.50±0.63	3.65±0.60	0.2621
Serum creatinine, mg/dL	0.85±0.14	0.80±0.17	0.1885
eGFR, mL/min/1.73 m^2*	85.49(81.70 89.45)	90.62(87.4293.94)	0.0449
C-reactive protein, mg/L*	0.05 (0.04 0.08)	0.08 (0.06 0.09)	0.1924
Insulin, μIU/mL	1.24(0.63 2.23)	5.83(3.35 11.62)	<.0001

Values are mean ± SD, number of patients (%), median (interquartile range), and geometric means (95% CI) unless otherwise indicated. DM, diabetes mellitus; SBP, systolic blood pressure; DBP, diastolic blood pressure; AST, aspartate aminotransferase; ALT, alanine aminotransferase; eGFR, estimated glomerular filtration rate. *P-values were calculated using log-transformed values. †P-values were calculated by Student's t-test, Mann-Whitney u-test or Pearson χ^2 test where appropriate.

Conclusions

This study is the first to demonstrate the plasma and urine levels of soluble α-klotho are significantly elevated in the diabetic patients with relatively preserved renal function compared to control subjects. The results also show plasma α-klotho levels decreased in proportion to urinary albumin excretion, although urinary α-klotho levels were stable with increasing urinary albumin excretion.

α-Klotho is a single-pass transmembrane protein that is highly expressed in the kidneys and is known to act as a co-receptor for fibroblast growth factor-23 [1]. Circulating soluble α-klotho can be generated directly by the alterative splicing of the α-klotho transcript or the extracellular domain of membrane α-klotho can be released from membrane-anchored α-klotho on the cell surface [2]. Unlike membrane α-klotho, which functions as a co-receptor for fibroblast growth factor-23, soluble α-klotho acts as a hormonal factor and plays important roles in anti-aging, anti-oxidation, ion transport modulation, and Wnt signaling. Previous studies aiming to clarify the role of α-klotho as a potential biomarker of kidney injury show the blood and urinary concentrations of α-klotho decrease early in the course of chronic kidney disease in mice with experimentally induced chronic kidney disease [3] as well as humans [4]. Although blood α-klotho concentration was found to be linearly associated with eGFR in previous studies [3,4], plasma α-klotho was not associated with the eGFR in the present study. The reason for this discrepancy is that only patients with an eGFR >60 mL min^{-1} 1.73 m^{-2} were enrolled; the geometric mean of eGFR was 90.6 mL min^{-1} 1.73 m^{-2} in the present study. The concentration of α-klotho in human urine is estimated to be 20–200 pM [10]. Urinary α-klotho is known to be correlated with eGFR and is reported to be a surrogate marker of functioning nephrons in the patients with chronic kidney disease [3,5]. The present finding that urinary α-klotho was higher in the diabetic patients whose eGFR is also higher than that of normal people, further corroborates this.

Meanwhile, little is known about circulating α-klotho levels in diabetes-related nephropathy. Recent studies in patients with diabetes report conflicting data. One study found serum α-klotho level was not significantly different between patients with diabetes without nephropathy and non-diabetic controls [11,12]. In contrast, another study reports a significant reduction in serum klotho levels in patients with glycated hemoglobin (HbA1c) levels ≥6.5% compared to control samples (HbA1c <6.5%) [13].

Kacso *et al.* [12] report α-klotho decreases in early chronic kidney disease and increases thereafter in the diabetic patient. However, they did not evaluate the association between soluble α-klotho levels and the extent of albuminuria in the early stage of diabetic nephropathy, specifically in patients with normal renal function. Asai *et al.* previously showed that renal α-klotho levels were significantly decreased in early diabetic nephropathy patients [7], however, they've never compared renal α-klotho levels between diabetic patients and normal control. They've just showed reduction in renal α-klotho levels in diabetic nephropathy patients than patients with minimal change disease or IgA nephropathy. Furthermore, the mean age of diabetic nephropathy patients was significantly older than patients with minimal change disease and IgA nephropathy. They also showed that renal α-klotho levels were significantly decreased in diabetic mice at 8

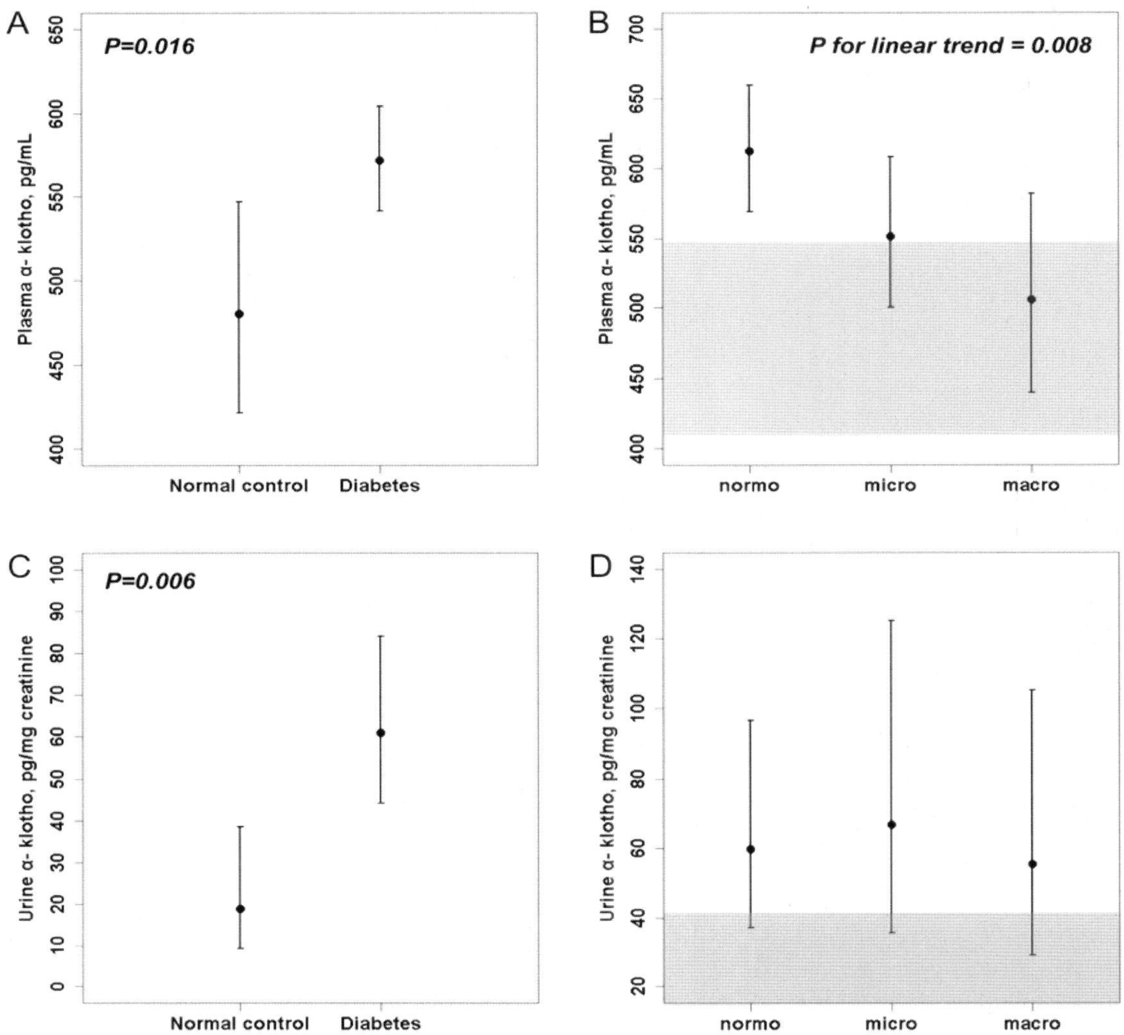

Figure 1. Plasma (A,B) and urine (C,D) levels of soluble α-klotho in normal participants (n=25) and patients with type 2 diabetes (n=147). Plasma and urine α-klotho levels were higher in diabetes patients with relatively preserved renal function than the non-diabetic controls (A,C). The diabetes patients were categorized into 3 groups according to urine ACR: ACR <30 mg/g creatinine (normoalbuminuria group, n = 75), ACR 30–299 mg/g creatinine (microalbuminuria group, n = 42), and ACR ≥300 mg/g creatinine (macroalbuminuria group, n = 30). Plasma α-klotho levels decreased in proportion to urinary albumin excretion, although urinary α-klotho levels were stable with increasing urinary albumin excretion (B,D). Data of non-diabetic control are expressed as a shaded area for the reference (B, D). Data are presented as geometric means and 95% CIs as an error bar plot. *P*-values calculated using the log-transformed values are shown in the graph. normo; normoalbuminuria, micro; microalbuminuria, macro; macroalbuminuria.

weeks after development of diabetes mellitus. They showed that albuminuria was increased at 2, 4, 6, and 8 weeks after onset of diabetes, however, renal α-klotho levels were not decreased until 4 weeks after development of diabetes. And they've not reported the renal α-klotho levels in early stage of albuminuric diabetic mice before 4 weeks of diabetes.

Zhao *et al.* showed decreased renal klotho expression in *db/db* mouse [8]. Although they did not indicate the levels of albuminuria or renal function data, they used *db/db* mouse at 20 weeks of age, which is regarded as relatively late stage of diabetic nephropathy. Deveraj *et al.* reported that soluble fraction of klotho was decreased in diabetic patients than non-diabetic controls, however they never mentioned the albuminuria status of their diabetic patients [13]. According to our data, there was a clear inverse association between plasma α-klotho level and albuminuria level in diabetic patients with relatively preserved renal function. van Ark J *et al.* measured circulating α-klotho levels in diabetes patients. Although they reported that circulating α-klotho levels were not changed in diabetic patients compared to control, their sample size was very small (n = 35) and they never mentioned the albuminuria status of their diabetic patients [11]. In the present study, plasma α-klotho levels in patients with type 2 diabetes were highest in the normoalbuminuria stage and decreased with increasing urinary albumin excretion. It is surprising that the plasma α-klotho levels in the macroalbuminuria group were still comparable with those in the non-diabetic controls.

Both acute kidney injury and chronic kidney disease exhibit renal and systemic α-klotho deficiency. Levels of α-klotho plummet very early and severely in acute kidney injury, representing a pathogenic factor that exacerbates acute kidney damage [14]. In chronic kidney disease, α-klotho deficiency significantly impacts the progression of renal disease as well as extrarenal complications [3,4]. Meanwhile, soluble α-klotho levels

Table 2. Baseline clinical and laboratory parameters in patients with type 2 diabetes according to albuminuria status.

	Normoalbuminuria (n=75)	Microalbuminuria (n=42)	Macroalbuminuria (n=30)	P-value[†]
Age, years	56.8±10.5	56.9±11.9	55.8±9.1	0.8995
Sex, male	31(41.3)	15(35.7)	17 (56.7)	0.1938
Duration of diabetes, years	4^{ab}(2–6)	8^{a}(5–14)	9^{b}(6–15)	0.0007
Diabetic retinopathy, %	17(22.7)	19(45.2)	17(56.7)	0.0016
Diabetic neuropathy, %	8(10.7)	20(47.6)	13(43.3)	<.0001
BMI, kg/m^2	23.4±3.0	23.7±4.2	23.4±3.4	0.8957
SBP, mmHg	123.5^{a}±12.0	126.1±12.3	133.4^{a}±21.2	0.0077
DBP, mmHg	78.0±8.8	78.3±10.5	82.5±12.6	0.1073
HbA$_{1c}$, %	7.8^{ab}±1.4	8.4^{a}±1.6	8.6^{b}±2.0	<.0001
Glycated albumin, %*	18.40^{ab}(17.24 19.64)	24.32^{a}(22.15 26.70)	21.87^{b}(18.68 25.61)	<.0001
Hemoglobin, g/dL	13.6^{a}±1.3	13.3±1.6	12.7^{a}±2.2	0.0297
Albumin, g/dL	4.5^{a}±0.3	4.4^{b}±0.4	4.1^{ab}±0.7	<.0001
AST, IU/L	23.3±8.7	23.0±14.3	22.9±13.2	0.9882
ALT, IU/L	24.7±13.6	25.2±21.2	23.8±18.5	0.9417
Total cholesterol, mg/dL	170.44^{a}±37.18	181.57±37.83	201.87^{a}±45.03	0.0013
LDL cholesterol, mg/dL	98.6^{a}±30.6	111.2±34.4	123.8^{a}±57.7	0.0090
HDL cholesterol, mg/dL	49.0±15.7	49.9±12.9	52.8±23.7	0.5944
Triglycerides, mg/dL*	128.11^{a}(110.14 149.01)	139.63(117.92 165.33)	180.31^{a}(141.72 229.41)	0.0428
Total bilirubin, mg/dL	0.66^{a}±0.21	0.67^{b}±0.19	0.53^{ab}±0.23	0.0067
Direct bilirubin, mg/dL	0.15^{a}±0.05	0.15^{b}±0.05	0.12^{ab}±0.06	0.0076
Uric acid, mg/dL	4.6±1.2	4.7±1.4	5.2±1.3	0.1393
Calcium, mg/dL	9.39±0.37	9.44^{a}±0.46	9.15^{a}±0.72	0.0362
Phosphorus, mg/dL	3.56±0.57	3.73±0.60	3.74±0.67	0.2406
Serum creatinine, mg/dL	0.79±0.15	0.77±0.16	0.85±0.20	0.1387
eGFR, mL/min/1.73 m^2*	90.3(86.5 94.2)	92.3(85.7 99.5)	89.2(80.4 98.8)	0.7856
C-reactive protein, mg/L*	0.07(0.05 0.09)	0.09(0.06 0.13)	0.07(0.04 0.12)	0.5280
Insulin, μIU/mL	5.87(3.35 11.62)	5.19(1.49 13.05)	7.54(4.26 11.70)	0.5165
Urine ACR, mg/g*	9.85^{ab}(6.74 9.85)	103.04^{ac} (68.11 103.04)	1131.12^{bc}(609.53 1131.12)	<.0001
Urine PCR, mg/g*	100.67^{ab}(83.22 100.67)	356.16^{ac}(222.33 356.16)	2261.86^{bc}(1146.68 2261.86)	<.0001

Values are mean ± SD, number of patients (%), median (interquartile range), and geometric means (95% CI) unless otherwise indicated. DR, diabetic retinopathy; DN, diabetic neuropathy; SBP, systolic blood pressure; DBP, diastolic blood pressure; TC, total cholesterol; TG, triglycerides; TB, total bilirubin; DB, direct bilirubin; UA, uric acid; Ca, calcium; P, phosphorous; Scr, serum creatinine; eGFR, estimated glomerular filtration rate; CRP, C-reactive protein; ACR, Urine albumin creatinine ratio; PCR, Urine protein creatinine ratio. *P-values were calculated using log-transformed values. [†]P-values were calculated by ANOVA or Pearson χ^2 test where appropriate. The same superscripted letters indicate statistical significance according to Tukey's multiple comparison test.

in plasma and/or urine may serve as early biomarkers of kidney parenchymal injury [15].

Recent studies indicate the potential contribution of absolute α-klotho deficiency to acute and chronic kidney injury [14,15]. Emerging evidence suggests α-klotho deficiency is an early biomarker of kidney disease as well as a pathogenic factor. α-Klotho deficiency is associated with progression and chronic complications in chronic kidney disease, including vascular calcification, cardiac hypertrophy, and secondary hyperparathyroidism; in particular, α-klotho deficiency induces resistance to fibroblast growth factor-23 and predisposition to hyperphosphatemia, which represents a critical feature of chronic kidney disease [1]. In the present study, plasma α-klotho concentrations tended to decrease with increasing degrees of albuminuria. Surprisingly, plasma α-klotho levels in diabetes-related nephropathy were still not lower than those in the normal controls, whereas they were lower in chronic kidney disease patients than normal controls in previous studies. Although absolute plasma α-klotho levels were not lower than normal, it is possible these levels are insufficient to prevent albuminuria in the microalbuminuria and macroalbuminuria stages of diabetes-related kidney disease. The results of the present study may help further elucidate the role of α-klotho in the development and progression of albuminuria in type 2 diabetes.

It is worth noting that the significance of urine α-klotho concentration as an early biomarker has not been evaluated in chronic kidney disease. The most important finding of the present study is that for the first time, high urine α-klotho levels were found to be associated with diabetes in humans even in the normoalbuminuria stage.

Nevertheless, the underlying mechanisms explaining the present results require further investigation. The present results may be explained by increased α-klotho synthesis or its cleavage process, although requires further study. The extracellular domain of α-klotho protein is subject to ectodomain shedding and is released into the blood and urine [1]; therefore, it may function as a hormone [16]. Hyperglycemia does not affect renal α-klotho

Table 3. Correlations between plasma α-klotho levels and other parameters in patients with diabetes (n = 147).

	Plasma klotho*	
	r	*P*-value
BMI, kg/m^2	0.098	0.2398
SBP, mmHg	−0.013	0.8740
DBP, mmHg	0.046	0.5820
HbA_{1c}, %	0.046	0.5773
Glycated albumin, %*	0.069	0.4076
Hemoglobin, g/dL	0.287	0.0005
Albumin, g/dL	0.050	0.5511
AST, IU/L	0.243	0.0030
ALT, IU/L	0.194	0.0188
Total cholesterol, mg/dL	0.005	0.9547
LDL cholesterol, mg/dL	0.040	0.6308
HDL cholesterol, mg/dL	−0.013	0.8763
Triglycerides, mg/dL*	−0.116	0.1622
Total bilirubin, mg/dL	0.137	0.0978
Direct bilirubin, mg/dL	0.155	0.0626
Uric acid, mg/dL	−0.117	0.1604
Calcium, mg/dL	0.060	0.4671
Phosphorus, mg/dL	−0.240	0.0037
Serum creatinine, mg/dL	0.059	0.4749
eGFR, mL/min/1.73 m^2*	−0.018	0.8265
C-reactive protein, mg/L*	−0.080	0.3335
Insulin, μIU/mL	0.183	0.0273
Urine ACR, mg/g*	−0.214	0.0093
Urine PCR, mg/g*	−0.237	0.0040
Urine klotho, pg/mg*	−0.011	0.8967

SBP, systolic blood pressure; DBP, diastolic blood pressure; AST, aspartate aminotransferase; ALT, alanine aminotransferase; eGFR, estimated glomerular filtration rate; ACR, albumin creatinine ratio; PCR, protein creatinine ratio. *Log transformed data before analysis, *r:* Pearson correlation coefficient.

production per se, because high glucose does not alter α-klotho expression in kidney cells and diabetes does not affect renal α-klotho mRNA expression in mice [11]. The lack of an association between HbA_{1c} or glycated albumin with soluble α-klotho concentrations in the present study also corroborates previous observations. Insulin can increase soluble α-klotho concentration through the cleavage and release of the extracellular domain of α-klotho [17]. In type 2 diabetes at early stage, soluble α-klotho level

Table 4. Multiple linear regression analysis between plasma α-klotho levels and other parameters in patients with diabetes (*n* = 147).

	Plasma Klotho*		
	β	SE	P-value
Age, years	0.00038	0.00066	0.5690
Hemoglobin, g/dL	0.01344	0.00511	0.0095
ALT, IU/L	−0.00035	0.00042	0.4047
Phosphorus, mg/dL	0.02243	0.01211	0.0661
Total bilirubin, mg/dL	−0.02343	0.03553	0.5108
Insulin, μIU/mL	−0.00009	0.00014	0.5321
Urine ACR, mg/g	0.00154	0.00003	<.0001
Urine PCR, mg/g	0.00000	0.00001	0.9961

ALT, alanine aminotransferase; ACR, albumin creatinine ratio; PCR, protein creatinine ratio. *Log transformed data before analysis.

is increased in plasma that may result in increased amount of α-klotho protein in urine. α-Klotho protein is expressed in both apical and basolateral membrane of kidney tubule [18]. Soluble α-klotho level may be determined by two possible mechanisms; 1) cleavage of α-klotho protein by proteases such as ADAM10 or 17 [17] and 2) secretion of splice variant form of α-klotho into blood or urine. Extracellular domain of α-klotho can be released into urine and blood from apical and basolateral membranes, respectively. Insulin receptor is also expressed in both apical and basolateral membrane of kidney tubular cells. At early stagy of type 2 diabetes, blood insulin level is increased that can stimulate the cleavage and release of the extracellular domain of α-klotho [17] into blood and/or urine. In this study, blood insulin level was also increased in diabetic patients than non-diabetic controls as expected. Increased level of soluble α-klotho may be filtered in glomeruli and present in urine. Cha *et al.* [10] reported that intraperitoneal administration of soluble klotho increased urinary K^+ excretion in rat by ROMK channel activation which is expressed in apical membrane. Interestingly, epitope-tagged klotho was appeared in urine at 2 hr after intravenous administration [19] indicating that klotho protein may be filtered in glomeruli and regulates ROMK channel from luminal side.

We found an interesting decrease in hemoglobin concentration from 13.6 g/dL in patients with normoalbuminuria to 13.3 g/dL in patients with microalbuminuria and then low to 12.7 g/dL in macroalbuminuria (Table 2). The decrease of hemoglobin concentration in the absence of significant excretory dysfunction has also been demonstrated in other study [20]. The decrease in hemoglobin in macroalbuminuria as compared to normoalbuminuria cannot be explained by reduced renal function as there was no significant difference in eGFR between the groups (Table 2). Our and the previous findings may suggest that erythropoietin deficiency, which has a major etiological role in the anemia associated with renal failure, begins even before there is evidence of deterioration in renal function. Other possibility includes eryptosis. Enhanced eryptosis, suicidal erythrocyte death, is observed in diabetes [21] and eryptosis is further enhanced in klotho-deficient mice [22].

Plasma and urinary α-klotho were not correlated in a previous study [5] or the present study.

Exogenous supplementation or stimulation of endogenous α-klotho may prevent and/or ameliorate kidney injury and mitigate chronic kidney disease development. The correction of α-klotho deficiency may delay the progression and forestall the development of extrarenal complications in chronic kidney disease. Angiotensin II receptor blocker treatment was recently shown to increase blood α-klotho levels while reducing albuminuria in type 2 diabetes with nephropathy [23,24]. The findings that both exogenous soluble α-klotho administration and overexpression of membranous α-klotho in kidney cell culture suppress NF-κB activation and subsequent inflammatory cytokine production in the response to TNF-α stimulation suggest α-klotho serves as an anti-inflammatory modulator [8]. Therefore, preventing deceases in α-klotho and α-klotho supplementation are potential novel therapeutic strategies for early diabetic nephropathy. In multiple experimental models of chronic kidney disease, the replacement or endogenous upregulation of α-klotho protects the kidneys from renal insults, preserves kidney function, and suppresses renal fibrosis. Thus, α-klotho is a highly promising candidate early biomarker as well as a novel therapeutic agent for chronic kidney disease [2].

The results of this study are subject to some limitations. First, the sample size was relatively small. We measured the urinary levels of α-klotho with single random spot urine samples, although urine samples were collected at the outpatient clinic from patients without illness or renal diseases besides diabetic nephropathy; moreover, a moderate linear association was observed between the amount of urine α-klotho in 24 hours and urinary α-klotho/creatinine ratio in random urine specimens ($r = 0.726$, $p < 0.01$) [5]. Despite these limitations, it is noteworthy that blood and urine α-klotho concentrations can easily be checked and used to assess the development of diabetic nephropathy prior to the onset of microalbuminuria, which is the earliest sign of diabetic nephropathy in clinical settings. Second, In addition, we measured and evaluated plasma and urinary α-klotho concentrations at a single time point in this cross-sectional study. Therefore, it is unclear whether plasma and/or urine α-klotho causes albuminuria in diabetes. Furthermore, all enrolled patients on medication with RAS inhibitors had a sufficient washout period for these drugs in order to role out the effect of RAS inhibitors on plasma and/or urinary klotho levels and albuminuria.

In conclusion, the results of the present study suggest plasma and urinary α-klotho may be the early markers for predicting renal injury in patients with type 2 diabetes and we need to do long-term prospective study in order to elucidate the role of α-klotho in the pathophysiological mechanisms of the development and progression of albuminuria in type 2 diabetes.

Author Contributions

Performed the experiments: SSK. Analyzed the data: EYL JSL. Contributed reagents/materials/analysis tools: SSK IJK SHS. Wrote the paper: EYL. Contributed to the discussion, and reviewed and edited the manuscript: SKC KSP JSK CHC.

References

1. Kuro-o M (2012) Klotho in health and disease. Curr Opin Nephrol Hypertens 21: 362–368.
2. Hu MC, Kuro-o M, Moe OW (2012) Secreted klotho and chronic kidney disease. Adv Exp Med Biol 728: 126–157.
3. Hu MC, Shi M, Zhang J, Quiñones H, Griffith C, et al. (2011) Klotho deficiency causes vascular calcification in chronic kidney disease. J Am Soc Nephrol 22: 124–136.
4. Kim HR, Nam BY, Kim DW, Kang MW, Han JH, et al. (2013) Circulating α-klotho levels in CKD and relationship to progression. Am J Kidney Dis 61: 899–909.
5. Akimoto T, Yoshizawa H, Watanabe Y, Numata A, Yamazaki T, et al. (2012) Characteristics of urinary and serum soluble Klotho protein in patients with different degrees of chronic kidney disease. BMC Nephrol 13:155.
6. Lin Y, Kuro-O M, Sun Z (2013) Genetic deficiency of anti-aging gene Klotho exacerbates early nephropathy in STZ-induced diabetes in male mice. Endocrinology 154: 3855–3863.
7. Asai O, Nakatani K, Tanaka T, Sakan H, Imura A, et al. (2012) Decreased renal α-Klotho expression in early diabetic nephropathy in humans and mice and its possible role in urinary calcium excretion. Kidney Int 81: 539–547.
8. Zhao Y, Banerjee S, Dey N, LeJeune WS, Sarkar PS, et al. (2011) Klotho depletion contributes to increased inflammation in kidney of the db/db mouse model of diabetes via RelA (serine)536 phosphorylation. Diabetes 60: 1907–1916.
9. Myers GL, Miller WG, Coresh J, Fleming J, Greenberg N, et al. (2006) Recommendations for improving serum creatinine measurement: a report from the Laboratory Working Group of the National Kidney Disease Education Program. Clin Chem 52: 5–18.
10. Cha SK, Ortega B, Kurosu H, Rosenblatt KP, Kuro-O M, et al. (2008) Removal of sialic acid involving Klotho causes cell-surface retention of TRPV5 channel via binding to galectin-1. Proc Natl Acad Sci U S A 105: 9805–9810.
11. Van Ark J, Hammes HP, Van Dijk MC, Vervloet MG, Wolffenbuttel BH, et al. (2013) Circulating alpha-klotho levels are not disturbed in patients with type 2 diabetes with and without macrovascular disease in the absence of nephropathy. Cardiovasc Diabetol 12: 116.
12. Kacso IM, Bondor CI, Kacso G (2012) Soluble serum Klotho in diabetic nephropathy: relationship to VEGF-A. Clin Biochem 45: 1415–1420.

13. Devaraj S, Syed B, Chien A, Jialal I (2012) Validation of an immunoassay for soluble Klotho protein: decreased levels in diabetes and increased levels in chronic kidney disease. Am J Clin Pathol 137: 479–485.
14. Hu MC, Moe OW (2012) Klotho as a potential biomarker and therapy for acute kidney injury. Nat Rev Nephrol 8: 423–429.
15. Hu MC, Kuro-o M, Moe OW (2012) The emerging role of Klotho in clinical nephrology. Nephrol Dial Transplant 27: 2650–2657.
16. Kurosu H, Yamamoto M, Clark JD, Pastor JV, Nandi A, et al. (2005) Suppression of aging in mice by the hormone Klotho. Science 309: 1829–1833.
17. Chen CD, Podvin S, Gillespie E, Leeman SE, Abraham CR (2007) Insulin stimulates the cleavage and release of the extracellular domain of Klotho by ADAM10 and ADAM17. Proc Natl Acad Sci USA 104: 19796–19801.
18. Chang Q, Hoefs S, van der Kemp AW, Topala CN, Bindels RJ, et al. (2005) The beta-glucuronidase klotho hydrolyzes and activates the TRPV5 channel. Science 21;310: 490–493.
19. Cha SK, Hu MC, Kurosu H, Kuro-o M, Moe O, et al. (2009) Regulation of renal outer medullary potassium channel and renal K(+) excretion by Klotho. Mol Pharmacol 76: 38–46.
20. Adetunji OR, Mani H, Olujohungbe A, Abraham KA, Gill GV (2009) 'Microalbuminuric anaemia'—the relationship between haemoglobin levels and albuminuria in diabetes. Diabetes Res Clin Pract 85: 179–182.
21. Lang F, Lang E, Föller M (2012) Physiology and pathophysiology of eryptosis. Transfus Med Hemother 39: 308–314.
22. Kempe DS, Ackermann TF, Fischer SS, Koka S, Boini KM, et al. (2009) Accelerated suicidal erythrocyte death in Klotho-deficient mice. Pflugers Arch 458: 503–512.
23. Lim SC, Liu JJ, Subramaniam T, Sum CF (2013) Elevated circulating alpha-klotho by angiotensin II receptor blocker losartan is associated with reduction of albuminuria in type 2 diabetes patients. J Renin Angiotensin Aldosterone Syst [Epub ahead of print].
24. Karalliedde J, Maltese G, Hill B, Viberti G, Gnudi L (2013) Effect of renin-angiotensin system blockade on soluble Klotho in patients with type 2 diabetes, systolic hypertension, and albuminuria. Clin J Am Soc Nephrol 8: 1899–1905.

Permissions

All chapters in this book were first published in PLOS ONE, by The Public Library of Science; hereby published with permission under the Creative Commons Attribution License or equivalent. Every chapter published in this book has been scrutinized by our experts. Their significance has been extensively debated. The topics covered herein carry significant findings which will fuel the growth of the discipline. They may even be implemented as practical applications or may be referred to as a beginning point for another development.

The contributors of this book come from diverse backgrounds, making this book a truly international effort. This book will bring forth new frontiers with its revolutionizing research information and detailed analysis of the nascent developments around the world.

We would like to thank all the contributing authors for lending their expertise to make the book truly unique. They have played a crucial role in the development of this book. Without their invaluable contributions this book wouldn't have been possible. They have made vital efforts to compile up to date information on the varied aspects of this subject to make this book a valuable addition to the collection of many professionals and students.

This book was conceptualized with the vision of imparting up-to-date information and advanced data in this field. To ensure the same, a matchless editorial board was set up. Every individual on the board went through rigorous rounds of assessment to prove their worth. After which they invested a large part of their time researching and compiling the most relevant data for our readers.

The editorial board has been involved in producing this book since its inception. They have spent rigorous hours researching and exploring the diverse topics which have resulted in the successful publishing of this book. They have passed on their knowledge of decades through this book. To expedite this challenging task, the publisher supported the team at every step. A small team of assistant editors was also appointed to further simplify the editing procedure and attain best results for the readers.

Apart from the editorial board, the designing team has also invested a significant amount of their time in understanding the subject and creating the most relevant covers. They scrutinized every image to scout for the most suitable representation of the subject and create an appropriate cover for the book.

The publishing team has been an ardent support to the editorial, designing and production team. Their endless efforts to recruit the best for this project, has resulted in the accomplishment of this book. They are a veteran in the field of academics and their pool of knowledge is as vast as their experience in printing. Their expertise and guidance has proved useful at every step. Their uncompromising quality standards have made this book an exceptional effort. Their encouragement from time to time has been an inspiration for everyone.

The publisher and the editorial board hope that this book will prove to be a valuable piece of knowledge for researchers, students, practitioners and scholars across the globe.

Contributors

Jeonghwan Lee
Department of Internal Medicine, Hallym University Hangang Sacred Heart Hospital, Seoul, Korea
Clinical Research Center for End Stage Renal Disease (CRC for ESRD), Daegu, Korea

Jung Pyo Lee
Clinical Research Center for End Stage Renal Disease (CRC for ESRD), Daegu, Korea
Department of Internal Medicine, Seoul National University Boramae Medical Center, Seoul, Korea

Ji In Park and Yon Su Kim
Clinical Research Center for End Stage Renal Disease (CRC for ESRD), Daegu, Korea
Department of Internal Medicine, Seoul National University College of Medicine, Seoul, Korea

Jin Ho Hwang
Clinical Research Center for End Stage Renal Disease (CRC for ESRD), Daegu, Korea
Department of Internal Medicine, Chung-Ang University Hospital, Seoul, Korea

Hye Min Jang
Clinical Research Center for End Stage Renal Disease (CRC for ESRD), Daegu, Korea
Department of Statistics, Kyungpook National University, Daegu, Korea

Ji-Young Choi and Yong-Lim Kim
Clinical Research Center for End Stage Renal Disease (CRC for ESRD), Daegu, Korea
Department of Internal Medicine, Kyungpook National University School of Medicine, Daegu, Korea

Chul Woo Yang
Clinical Research Center for End Stage Renal Disease (CRC for ESRD), Daegu, Korea
Department of Internal Medicine, The Catholic University of Korea College of Medicine, Seoul, Korea

Shin-Wook Kang
Clinical Research Center for End Stage Renal Disease (CRC for ESRD), Daegu, Korea
Department of Internal Medicine, Yonsei University College of Medicine, Seoul, Korea

Nam-Ho Kim
Clinical Research Center for End Stage Renal Disease (CRC for ESRD), Daegu, Korea
Department of Internal Medicine, Chonnam National University Medical School, Gwangju, Korea

Chun Soo Lim
Clinical Research Center for End Stage Renal Disease (CRC for ESRD), Daegu, Korea
Department of Internal Medicine, Seoul National University Boramae Medical Center, Seoul, Korea
Department of Internal Medicine, Seoul National University College of Medicine, Seoul, Korea

CRC for ESRD investigators
Clinical Research Center for End Stage Renal Disease (CRC for ESRD), Daegu, Korea

Chuan Wang, Jun Song, Xinguo Hou, Yu Sun, Peng Lin, Kai Liang, Lei Gong, Meijian Wang, Fuqiang Liu, Wenjuan Li, Fei Yan, Junpeng Yang, Lingshu Wang, Meng Tian, Jidong Liu, Ruxing Zhao and Li Chen
Department of Endocrinology, Qilu Hospital of Shandong University, Jinan, Shandong, China

Zeqiang Ma
China National Heavy Duty Truck Group Corporation Hospital, Jinan, Shandong, China

Weifang Yang
Lukang Hospital of Jining, Jining, Shandong, China

Chengqiao Li
Department of Endocrinology, Second People's Hospital of Jining, Jining, Shandong, China

Xiuping Zhang
Shantui Community Health Center, Jining, Shandong, China

Samantha J. Borland
Institute of Cardiovascular Sciences, Faculty of Medical and Human Sciences, University of Manchester, Manchester, United Kingdom

Gareth D. Hyde, Rebecca F. Taylor and Ann E. Canfield
Institute of Cardiovascular Sciences, Faculty of Medical and Human Sciences, University of Manchester, Manchester, United Kingdom
Wellcome Trust Centre for Cell-Matrix Research, University of Manchester, Manchester, United Kingdom

Andrew P. Gilmore
Wellcome Trust Centre for Cell-Matrix Research, University of Manchester, Manchester, United Kingdom
Faculty of Life Sciences, University of Manchester, Manchester, United Kingdom

Nick Ashton and Hon Sing Geoffrey Wu
Faculty of Life Sciences, University of Manchester, Manchester, United Kingdom

Poorva Jain and Melanie Calvert
Primary Care Clinical Sciences, NIHR School of Primary Care Research, University of Birmingham, Birmingham, United Kingdom

Paul Cockwell
Department of Renal Medicine, Queen Elizabeth Hospital Birmingham, University Hospital Birmingham, Birmingham, United Kingdom
Division of Immunity and Infection, Medical School, University of Birmingham, Birmingham, United Kingdom

Richard J. McManus
Department of Primary Care Health Sciences, NIHR School of Primary Care Research, University of Oxford, Oxford, United Kingdom

Paul R. Kalra
Portsmouth Hospitals NHS Trust, Portsmouth, United Kingdom
NHLI Imperial College, ICMS, London, United Kingdom

Xavier García-Moll
Unitat Hospitalització, Servei de Cardiologia, Hospital de la Santa Creu i Sant Pau, Barcelona, Spain

José Zamorano
University Hospital Ramón y Cajal, Madrid, Spain,

Philip A. Kalra
Salford Royal NHS Foundation Trust, Salford, United Kingdom

Kim M. Fox
NHLI Imperial College, ICMS, London, United Kingdom
Royal Brompton Hospital, London, United Kingdom

Ian Ford
University of Glasgow, Glasgow, United Kingdom

Roberto Ferrari
Department of Cardiology, Azienda Ospedaliero-Universitaria di Ferrara, Ospedale di Cona, Cona, Italy

Jean-Claude Tardif
Montreal Heart Institute, Université de Montreal, Montreal, Canada

Michal Tendera
Medical University of Silesia, Katowice, Poland

Nicola Greenlaw
University of Glasgow, Glasgow, United Kingdom

Ph. Gabriel Steg for the CLARIFY Investigators
Royal Brompton Hospital, London, United Kingdom
Université Paris-Diderot, Sorbonne-Paris Cité, Paris, France
INSERM U-1148, Paris, France
Département Hospitalo-Universitaire FIRE, Hôpital Bichat, Assistance Publique – Hôpitaux de Paris, Paris, France

Makoto Yamaguchi, Shinichi Akiyama, Sawako Kato, Takayuki Katsuno, Tomoki Kosugi, Waichi Sato, Naotake Tsuboi, Yoshinari Yasuda, Masashi Mizuno, Yasuhiko Ito, Seiichi Matsuo and Shoichi Maruyama
Department of Nephrology, Nagoya University Graduate School of Medicine, Nagoya, Japan,

Masahiko Ando
Center for Advanced Medicine and Clinical Research, Nagoya University Hospital, Nagoya, Japan

Ryohei Yamamoto
Department of Geriatric Medicine and Nephrology, Osaka University Graduate School of Medicine, Suita, Japan

Eun Young Lee and Jeong Suk Kang
Department of Internal Medicine, Soonchunhyang University Cheonan Hospital, Cheonan, Korea

Sang Soo Kim, In Joo Kim and Sang Heon Song
Department of Internal Medicine, Pusan National University Hospital, Busan, Korea

Ji-Sung Lee
Biostatistical Consulting Unit, Soonchunhyang University Medical Center, Seoul, Korea

Seung-Kuy Cha and Kyu- Sang Park
Department of Physiology, Yonsei University Wonju College of Medicine, Wonju, Korea

Choon Hee Chung
Department of Internal Medicine, Yonsei University Wonju College of Medicine, Wonju, Korea

Xian-Hui Gao and Guo-Yi Zhang
Laboratory of Preventive Medicine, School of Public Health, Liaoning Medical University, Jinzhou, China

Ying Wang
Department of Toxicology, School of Public Health, Liaoning Medical University, Jinzhou, China

Hui-Ying Zhang
Sleep Monitoring Center, First Affiliated Hospital of Liaoning Medical University, Jinzhou, China

Noriaki Kitamura, Takahiro Yamaguchi and Yoshiko Iwai
Department of Molecular Biology, School of Medicine, University of Occupational and Environmental Health, Kitakyushu, Japan

Masahito Tamura and Yutaka Otsuji
Second Department of Internal Medicine, Cardiology and Nephrology, School of Medicine, University of Occupational and Environmental Health, Kitakyushu, Japan

Akihiro Kuma
Department of Molecular Biology, School of Medicine, University of Occupational and Environmental Health, Kitakyushu, Japan
Second Department of Internal Medicine, Cardiology and Nephrology, School of Medicine, University of Occupational and Environmental Health, Kitakyushu, Japan

Sohsuke Yamada
Department of Pathology and Cell Biology, School of Medicine, University of Occupational and Environmental Health, Kitakyushu, Japan

Ke-Yong Wang
Bio-information Research Center, University of Occupational and Environmental Health, Kitakyushu, Japan

Hiroto Izumi
Department of Occupational Pneumology, Institute of Industrial Ecological Science, University of Occupational and Environmental Health, Kitakyushu, Japan

Kimitoshi Kohno
The President Laboratory, University of Occupational and Environmental Health, Kitakyushu, Japan

Yasuaki Nakagawa, Toshio Nishikimi, Koichiro Kuwahara, Hideyuki Kinoshita, Yoshihiro Kuwabara, Kazuhiro Nakao, Takeya Minami, Chinatsu Yamada and Kazuwa Nakao
Department of Medicine and Clinical Science, Kyoto University Graduate School of Medicine, Kyoto, Japan

Shinji Yasuno and Kenji Ueshima
Department of EBM Research, Kyoto University Hospital, Institute for Advancement of Clinical and Translational Science, Kyoto, Japan

Yoshihiro Ikeda
Medical corporation, Ikeda Clinic, Kyoto, Japan

Hiroyuki Okamoto, Kazukiyo Horii and Kiyoshi Nagata
Diagnostics Division, Shionogi and Co., Ltd, Oska, Japan

Kenji Kangawa
Department of Biochemistry, National Cerebral and Cardiovascular Center Research Institute, Fujishirodai, Suita, Osaka, Japan

Naoto Minamino
Department of Molecular Pharmacology, National Cerebral and Cardiovascular Center Research Institute, Fujishirodai, Suita, Osaka, Japan

Hayato Sasaki, Tomohiro Nishino, Daisuke Torigoe and Takashi Agui
Laboratory of Laboratory Animal Science and Medicine, Department of Disease Control, Graduate School of Veterinary Medicine, Hokkaido University, Sapporo, Japan

Nobuya Sasaki
Laboratory of Laboratory Animal Science and Medicine, Faculty of Veterinary Medicine, Kitasato University, Towada, Japan

Ken-ichi Nagasaki
Section of Biological Safety Research, Chitose Laboratory, Japan Food Research Laboratories, Chitose, Japan,

Hiroshi Kitamura
Department of Veterinary Physiology, School of Veterinary Medicine, Rakuno Gakuen University, Ebetsu, Japan

Marine L. Croze and Christophe O. Soulage
Université de Lyon, F-69600, Oullins, France
INSERM, U1060, CarMeN, INSA-Lyon, Univ. Lyon-1, Villeurbanne, France

Caroline C. Pelletier, Laetitia Koppe, Pascaline M. Alix, Emilie Kalbacher and Fitsum Guebre-Egziabher
Université de Lyon, F-69600, Oullins, France
INSERM, U1060, CarMeN, INSA-Lyon, Univ. Lyon-1, Villeurbanne, France
Hospices Civils de Lyon, Service de Néphrologie Hôpital E Herriot, Lyon, France

Aoumeur Hadj-Aissa
Université de Lyon, F-69600, Oullins, France
Hospices Civils de Lyon, Exploration Fonctionnelle Rénale et Métabolique, Hôpital E Herriot, Lyon, France

Denis Fouque
Université de Lyon, F-69600, Oullins, France
INSERM, U1060, CarMeN, INSA-Lyon, Univ. Lyon-1, Villeurbanne, France
Hospices Civils de Lyon, Service de Néphrologie, Centre Hospitalier Lyon-SUD, Pierre-Bénite, France

Hung-Ta Wo, Po-Cheng Chang, Chun-Chieh Wang, Ming-Shien Wen and Chung-Chuan Chou
Department of Cardiology, Chang-Gung Memorial Hospital, Linko, Taiwan

Tien-Hsing Chen
Department of Cardiology, Chang-Gung Memorial Hospital, Linko, Taiwan
Department of Cardiology, Chang-Gung Memorial Hospital, Xiamen, China, Chang Gung
University College of Medicine, Kaohsiung, Taiwan

Jiun-Chi Huang
Division of Nephrology, Department of Internal Medicine, Kaohsiung Medical University Hospital, Kaohsiung Medical University, Kaohsiung, Taiwan
Department of Internal Medicine, Kaohsiung Municipal Hsiao-Kang Hospital, Kaohsiung Medical University, Kaohsiung, Taiwan

Szu-Chia Chen and Jer-Ming Chang
Division of Nephrology, Department of Internal Medicine, Kaohsiung Medical University Hospital, Kaohsiung Medical University, Kaohsiung, Taiwan
Department of Internal Medicine, Kaohsiung Municipal Hsiao-Kang Hospital, Kaohsiung Medical University, Kaohsiung, Taiwan
Faculty of Medicine, College of Medicine, Kaohsiung Medical University, Kaohsiung, Taiwan

Chi-Chih Hung
Division of Nephrology, Department of Internal Medicine, Kaohsiung Medical University Hospital, Kaohsiung Medical University, Kaohsiung, Taiwan
Faculty of Medicine, College of Medicine, Kaohsiung Medical University, Kaohsiung, Taiwan

Ho-Ming Su
Division of Cardiology, Department of Internal Medicine, Kaohsiung Medical University Hospital, Kaohsiung Medical University, Kaohsiung, Taiwan

Department of Internal Medicine, Kaohsiung Municipal Hsiao-Kang Hospital, Kaohsiung Medical University, Kaohsiung, Taiwan
Faculty of Medicine, College of Medicine, Kaohsiung Medical University, Kaohsiung, Taiwan

Shang-Jyh Hwang and Hung-Chun Chen
Division of Nephrology, Department of Internal Medicine, Kaohsiung Medical University Hospital, Kaohsiung Medical University, Kaohsiung, Taiwan
Faculty of Renal Care, College of Medicine, Kaohsiung Medical University, Kaohsiung, Taiwan

Shu-Yi Wei
Department of Internal Medicine, Kaohsiung Municipal United Hospital, Kaohsiung, Taiwan
Yuh-Ing Junior College of Health Care and Management, Kaohsiung, Taiwan

Badreldin H. Ali, Mohammed Al Za'abi, Khalid A. Al Balushi and Aishwarya Ramkumar
Department of Pharmacology and Clinical Pharmacy, College of Medicine and Health Sciences, Sultan Qaboos University, Alkhod, Muscat, Oman

Suhail Al-Salam
Department of Pathology, College of Medicine and Health Sciences, United Arab Emirates, Alin, United Arab Emirates

Mostafa I. Waly
Department of Food Sciences and Nutrition, College of Agricultural and Marine Sciences, Sultan Qaboos University, Alkhod, Muscat, Oman

Javid Yasin
Department of Medicine, College of Medicine and Health Sciences, United Arab
Emirates, Alin, United Arab Emirates

Sirin A. Adham
Department of Biology, College of Science, Sultan Qaboos University, Sultan Qaboos University, Alkhod, Muscat, Oman

Abderrahim Nemmar
Department of Physiology, College of Medicine and Health Sciences, United Arab Emirates, Alin, United Arab Emirates

Julia M. Hofstra, Jo H. M. Berden, Johan van der Vlag, Jack F. M. Wetzels and Tom Nijenhuis
Department of Nephrology, Radboud university medical center, Nijmegen, the Netherlands

Marieke J. H. Coenen, Mascha M. V. A. P. Schijvenaars, Lies H. Hoefsloot and Nine V. A. M. Knoers
Department of Human Genetics, Radboud university medical center, Nijmegen, the Netherlands

Michael E. Matheny
Geriatrics Research Education and Clinical Center (GRECC), Tennessee Valley Healthcare System (TVHS), Veteran's Health Administration, Nashville, TN, United States of America
Department of Biomedical Informatics, Vanderbilt University School of Medicine, Nashville, TN, United States of America
Division of General Internal Medicine, Department of Medicine, Vanderbilt University School of Medicine, Nashville, TN, United States of America
Department of Biostatistics, Vanderbilt University School of Medicine, Nashville, TN, United States of America

Josh F. Peterson
Department of Biomedical Informatics, Vanderbilt University School of Medicine, Nashville, TN, United States of America
Division of General Internal Medicine, Department of Medicine, Vanderbilt University School of Medicine, Nashville, TN, United States of America

Svetlana K. Eden
Department of Biostatistics, Vanderbilt University School of Medicine, Nashville, TN, United States of America

Adriana M. Hung
Geriatrics Research Education and Clinical Center (GRECC), Tennessee Valley Healthcare System (TVHS), Veteran's Health Administration, Nashville, TN, United States of America
Division of Nephrology, Department of Medicine, Vanderbilt University School of Medicine, Nashville, TN, United States of America

Theodore Speroff
Geriatrics Research Education and Clinical Center (GRECC), Tennessee Valley Healthcare System (TVHS), Veteran's Health Administration, Nashville, TN, United States of America
Division of General Internal Medicine, Department of Medicine, Vanderbilt University School of Medicine, Nashville, TN, United States of America
Department of Biostatistics, Vanderbilt University School of Medicine, Nashville, TN, United States of America

Khaled Abdel-Kader, Sharidan K. Parr, T. Alp Ikizler and Edward D. Siew
Division of Nephrology, Department of Medicine, Vanderbilt University School of Medicine, Nashville, TN, United States of America

Milan Gautam, Atsushi Izawa, Yuji Shiba, Hirohiko Motoki, Takahiro Takeuchi, Ayako Okada, Takeshi Tomita, Yusuke Miyashita, Jun Koyama and Uichi Ikeda
Department of Cardiovascular Medicine, Shinshu University School of Medicine, Matsumoto, Nagano, Japan

Khalid Bashar, Donagh Healy, Elrasheid A. H. Kheirelseid, Mary Clarke – Moloney, Paul E. Burke and Eamon G. Kavanagh
Department of vascular surgery, University Hospital Limerick, Limerick, Ireland

Leonard D. Browne and Michael T. Walsh
Centre for Applied Biomedical Engineering Research (CABER), Department of Mechanical, Aeronautical and Biomedical Engineering, Materials and Surface Science Institute, University of Limerick, Limerick, Ireland

Stewart Redmond Walsh
Department of surgery, National University of Ireland, Galway, Ireland

Marine Baron, Renata Belo, Lucia Moreira-Teixeira and Maria Leite-de-Moraes
INEM (Institut Necker Enfants Malades), CNRS UMR 8253, INSERM UMR 1151, Université Paris Descartes, Sorbonne Paris Cité, France, Hôpital Necker Enfants Malades, Paris, France

Dominique Cathelin, Eric Rondeau and Laurent Mesnard
INSERM UMR S 702, Université Pierre et Marie Curie, Assistance Publique-Hôpitaux de Paris, Hôpital Tenon, Paris, France
AP-HP, Hôpital Tenon, Urgences Néphrologiques and Transplantation Rénale, Universite Pierre et Marie Curie, Paris, France

Claire Cartery
Nephrology and Dialysis, Tenon Hospital, Assistance Publique-Hôpitaux de Paris, Hôpital Tenon, Paris, France

Carlos Martínez-Salgado and Francisco J. López-Hernández
Instituto de Estudios de Ciencias de la Salud de Castilla y León-Instituto de Investigación Biomédica de Salamanca (IECSCYL-IBSAL), Unidad de Investigación, Hospital Universitario de Salamanca, Salamanca, Spain
Departamento de Fisiología y Farmacología, Universidad de Salamanca, Salamanca, Spain
Instituto Reina Sofía de Investigación Nefrológica, Fundación Iñigo Álvarez de Toledo, Madrid, Spain

Ana M. Blázquez-Medela, Omar García-Sánchez and José M. López-Novoa
Departamento de Fisiología y Farmacología, Universidad de Salamanca, Salamanca, Spain
Instituto Reina Sofía de Investigación Nefrológica, Fundación Iñigo Álvarez de Toledo, Madrid, Spain

María J. Montero
Departamento de Fisiología y Farmacología, Universidad de Salamanca, Salamanca, Spain

Víctor Blanco-Gozalo
Instituto de Estudios de Ciencias de la Salud de Castilla y León-Instituto de Investigación Biomédica de Salamanca (IECSCYL-IBSAL), Unidad de Investigación, Hospital Universitario de Salamanca, Salamanca, Spain
Departamento de Fisiología y Farmacología, Universidad de Salamanca, Salamanca, Spain
Bio-inRen, S.L., Salamanca, Spain

Yaremi Quiros
Departamento de Fisiología y Farmacología, Universidad de Salamanca, Salamanca, Spain
Bio-inRen, S.L., Salamanca, Spain

Veronica Dimuccio and Benedetta Bussolati
Department of Molecular Biotechnology and Health Sciences, University of Torino, Torino, Italy

Andrea Ranghino, Biancone and Giovanni Camussi
Department of Medical Sciences, University of Torino, Torino, Italy,

Loredana Praticò Barbato
Immunogenetics and Transplant Biology Service, Città della Salute e della Scienza Hospital, Torino, Italy

Fabrizio Fop
Division of Nephrology, Dialysis and Transplantation, Città della Salute e della Scienza Hospital, Torino, Italy

Der-Sheng Han
Department of Physical Medicine and Rehabilitation, National Taiwan University Hospital BeiHu Branch, Taipei, Taiwan
Department of Physical Medicine and Rehabilitation, National Taiwan University Hospital, Taipei, Taiwan

Yu Chu-Su
Department of Laboratory Medicine, National Taiwan University Hospital, Taipei, Taiwan
Institute of Biomedical Engineering, National Taiwan University, Taipei, Taiwan

Chih-Kang Chiang, Fen-Yu Tseng and Kwan-Dun Wu
Department of Internal Medicine, National Taiwan University Hospital, Taipei, Taiwan

Ping-Huei Tseng
Department of Internal Medicine, National Taiwan University Hospital, Taipei, Taiwan
Graduate Institute of Clinical Medicine, College of Medicine, National Taiwan University, Taipei, Taiwan

Chi-Ling Chen
Graduate Institute of Clinical Medicine, College of Medicine, National Taiwan University, Taipei, Taiwan
Graduate Institute of Epidemiology and Preventive Medicine, College of Public Health, National Taiwan University, Taipei, Taiwan

Wei-Shiung Yang
Department of Internal Medicine, National Taiwan University Hospital, Taipei, Taiwan
Graduate Institute of Clinical Medicine, College of Medicine, National Taiwan University, Taipei, Taiwan
Research Center for Developmental Biology and Regenerative Medicine, National Taiwan University, Taipei, Taiwan

Shia T. Kent and Lei Huang
Department of Epidemiology, University of Alabama at Birmingham, Birmingham, Alabama, United States of America

Daichi Shimbo and Keith M. Diaz
Center for Behavioral Cardiovascular Health, Department of Medicine, Columbia University Medical Center, New York, New York, United States of America

Meredith L. Kilgore
Department of Health Care Organization and Policy, University of Alabama at Birmingham, Birmingham, Alabama, United States of America

Suzanne Oparil
Department of Medicine, Division of Cardiovascular Disease, University of Alabama at Birmingham, Birmingham, Alabama, United States of America

Paul Muntner
Department of Epidemiology, University of Alabama at Birmingham, Birmingham, Alabama, United States of America
Department of Medicine, Division of Cardiovascular Disease, University of Alabama at Birmingham, Birmingham, Alabama, United States of America

Ping-Fang Chiu
Institute of Medicine, Chung Shan Medical University, Taichung, Taiwan
School of Medicine, Chung Shan Medical University, Taichung, Taiwan
Nephrology Division, Department of Internal Medicine, Changhua Christian Hospital, Changhua, Taiwan

Chia-Lin Wu, Hung-Hsiang Liou and Chirn-Bin Chang
Nephrology Division, Department of Internal Medicine, Changhua Christian Hospital, Changhua, Taiwan

Ching-Hui Huang
Division of Cardiology, Department of Internal Medicine, Changhua Christian Hospital, Changhua, Taiwan

Horng-Rong Chang
Institute of Medicine, Chung Shan Medical University, Taichung, Taiwan
School of Medicine, Chung Shan Medical University, Taichung, Taiwan
Division of Nephrology, Department of Internal Medicine, Chung Shan Medical University Hospital, Taichung, Taiwan

Chia-Chu Chang
School of Medicine, Chung Shan Medical University, Taichung, Taiwan
Nephrology Division, Department of Internal Medicine, Changhua Christian Hospital, Changhua, Taiwan
Ph.D. Program for Aging, College of Medicine, China Medical University, Taichung, Taiwan

Sarah J. Ramer
Rutgers New Jersey Medical School, Newark, New Jersey, United States of America

Elan D. Cohen
Division of General Internal Medicine, Department of Medicine, University of Pittsburgh School of Medicine, Pittsburgh, Pennsylvania, United States of America

Chung-Chou H. Chang
Division of General Internal Medicine, Department of Medicine, University of Pittsburgh School of Medicine, Pittsburgh, Pennsylvania, United States of America
Department of Biostatistics, University of Pittsburgh Graduate School of Public
Health, Pittsburgh, Pennsylvania, United States of America

Mark L. Unruh
Division of Nephrology, Department of Internal Medicine, University of New Mexico School of Medicine, Albuquerque, New Mexico, United States of America

Amber E. Barnato
Division of General Internal Medicine, Department of Medicine, University of Pittsburgh School of Medicine, Pittsburgh, Pennsylvania, United States of America
Department of Clinical and Translational Science, University of Pittsburgh School of Medicine, Pittsburgh, Pennsylvania, United States of America
Department of Health Policy and Management, University of Pittsburgh Graduate School of Public Health, Pittsburgh, Pennsylvania, United States of America
The CRISMA Laboratory (Clinical Research, Investigation, and Systems Modeling of Acute Illness), Department of Critical Care Medicine, University of Pittsburgh, Pittsburgh, Pennsylvania, United States of America

Song Yi Han, Ae Jin Kim and Hye Jin Lim
Division of Nephrology, Department of Internal Medicine, Gachon University Gil Medical Center, Incheon, Korea

Han Ro, Jae Hyun Chang, Hyun Hee Lee, Wookyung Chung and Ji Yong Jung
Division of Nephrology, Department of Internal Medicine, Gachon University Gil Medical Center, Incheon, Korea
Gachon University School of Medicine, Incheon, Korea

Kwang-Pil Ko
Department of Preventive Medicine, Gachon University School of Medicine, Incheon, Korea

Tom Blakeman, Christian Blickem, David Reeves, Hannah Gaffney, Praksha Jariwala, Shoba Dawson, Rahena Mossabir and Helen Brooks
NIHR Collaboration for Leadership in Applied Health Research (CLAHRC) Greater Manchester, Centre for Primary Care, Institute of Population Health, University of Manchester, Manchester, United Kingdom

Anne Kennedy, Ivaylo Vassilev and Anne Rogers
NIHR CLAHRC Wessex, Health Sciences, University of Southampton, Highfield Campus, Southampton, United Kingdom

Peter Bower, Caroline Gardner and Victoria Lee
NIHR School for Primary Care Research, Centre for Primary Care, Institute of Population Health, University of Manchester, Manchester, United Kingdom

Gerry Richardson and Eldon Spackman
Centre for Health Economics, University of York, Heslington, York, United Kingdom

Carolyn Chew-Graham
Primary Care and Health Services, University of Keele, Staffordshire, United Kingdom

Charles Hobson
Department of Surgery, Malcom Randall VA Medical Center, Gainesville, Florida, United States of America
Department of Health Services Research, Management and Policy, University of Florida, Gainesville, Florida, United States of America

John Dortch, Tezcan Ozrazgat Baslanti, Daniel R. Layon, Alina Roche, Alison Rioux, Brenda Fahy and Azra Bihorac
Department of Anesthesiology, University of Florida, Gainesville, Florida, United States of America

Jeffrey S. Harman
Department of Health Services Research, Management and Policy, University of Florida, Gainesville, Florida, United States of America

Chao-Ju Chen and Po-Liang Lu
Department of Internal Medicine, Kaohsiung Medical University Hospital, Kaohsiung, Taiwan College of Medicine, Kaohsiung Medical University, Kaohsiung, Taiwan

Tsu-Lan Wu
Department of Clinical Pathology, Linkou Chang Gung Memorial Hospital, Taoyuan, Taiwan

Ying-Tsong Chen
Institute of Genomics and Bioinformatics, National Chung Hsing University, Taichung, Taiwan
Biotechnology Center, National Chung Hsing University, Taichung, Taiwan
Institute of Molecular and Genomic Medicine, National Health Research Institutes, Miaoli, Taiwan

Chang-Phone Fung
Section of Infectious Diseases, Department of Medicine, Taipei Veterans General Hospital, Taipei, Taiwan

Yin-Ching Chuang
Department of Internal Medicine and Medical Research, Chi Mei Medical Center, Tainan, Taiwan
Department of Internal Medicine, Chi Mei Medical Center, Liouying, Tainan, Taiwan

Jung-Chung Lin
Division of Infectious Diseases and Tropical Medicine, Department of Internal Medicine, Tri-Service General Hospital, National Defense Medical Center, Taipei, Taiwan
Institute of Microbiology and Immunology, National Defense Medical Center, Taipei, Taiwan,

L. Kristopher Siu
Division of Infectious Diseases and Tropical Medicine, Department of Internal Medicine, Tri-Service General Hospital, National Defense Medical Center, Taipei, Taiwan
Graduate Institute of Basic Medical Science, China Medical University, Taichung, Taiwan
National Institute of Infectious Diseases and Vaccinology, National Health Research Institutes, Miaoli, Taiwan

Index